RNA INTERFERENCE

Edited by **Ibrokhim Y. Abdurakhmonov**

RNA Interference

http://dx.doi.org/10.5772/60631
Edited by Ibrokhim Y. Abdurakhmonov

Contributors

Gyung Whan Kim, Kyoungjoo Cho, Utpal Bhadra, Debabani Roy Chowdhury, Manika Pal Bhadra, Constanca Figueiredo, Rainer Blasczyk, Qiuju Han, Zhaohua Hou, Cai Zhang, Jian Zhang, Devi Singh, Preeti Sirohi, Rajendra Kumar, Sarika Chaudhary, Kamiya Mehla, Pankaj Kumar Singh, Shashi Kumar, Pooran Chand, Tetsuya Tanaka, Remil Galay, Rika Umemiya-Shirafuji, Kozo Fujisaki, Masami Mochizuki, Emine Salva, Ceyda Ekentok, Suna Özbaş Turan, Jülide Akbuğa, Omar Bagasra, Zhabiz Golkar, Donald Gene Pace, Elena Chernolovskaya, Olga Gvozdeva, Yuxia Yang, Mengyu Hu, Qiankun Ni, Bin Yang, Cheng Yang, Santosh Kumar Upadhyay, Nidhi Thakur, Jaspreet Kaur Mundey, Thais B. Rodrigues, Antonio Figueira, Anne Meinhardt, Barbara Seliger, Doerte Falke, Thomas Boldicke, Oliver Backhaus, Covadonga Paneda, Wenyi Gu, Taisen Iguchi, Kenji Toyota, Wayne Hunter, Eduardo Andrade, Ibrokhim Abdurakhmonov

Published by InTech

Janeza Trdine 9, 51000 Rijeka, Croatia

Publishing Process Manager Iva Simcic

Technical Editor InTech DTP team

Cover InTech Design team

First published April, 2016

Printed in Croatia

Additional hard copies can be obtained from orders@intechopen.com

RNA Interference, Edited by Ibrokhim Y. Abdurakhmonov

p. cm.

ISBN 978-953-51-2272-2

For EU product safety concerns:
IN TECH d.o.o., Prolaz Marije Krucifikse Kozulić 3, 51000 Rijeka, Croatia,
info@intechopen.com or visit our website at intechopen.com.

Meet the editor

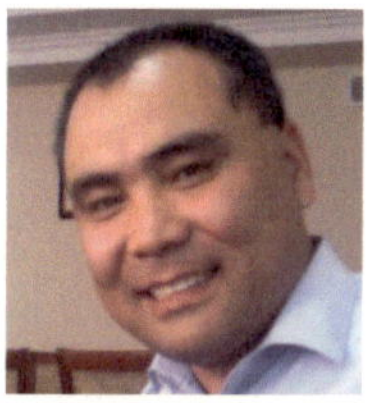

Ibrokhim Y. Abdurakhmonov received his B.S. Degree (1997) *in biotechnology* from the National University of Uzbekistan, M.S. degree *in plant breeding* (2001) from Texas A&M University of USA, Ph.D. degree (2002) *in molecular genetics*, Doctor of Science degree (2009) *in genetics*, and full professorship (2011) *in molecular genetics and molecular biotechnology* from the Institute of Genetics and Plant Experimental Biology, Academy of Sciences of Uzbekistan. He founded (2012) and is currently leading the Center of Genomics and Bioinformatics of Uzbekistan. He serves as an associate editor/editorial board member of several international and national journals on plant sciences. He received Government award, 2010 chest badge "Sign of Uzbekistan," 2010 TWAS prize, and "ICAC Cotton Researcher of the Year 2013" for his outstanding contribution to cotton genomics and biotechnology. He was elected as the World Academy of Sciences (TWAS) Fellow (2014) on *Agricultural Science* and as a co-chair/chair of "Comparative Genomics and Bioinformatics" workgroup (2015) of International Cotton Genome Initiative (ICGI).

Contents

Preface

RNA interference (RNAi), being a revolutionary discovery of all biological sciences of twenty-first century and historically known as *co-suppression, quelling,* and/or *post-transcriptional gene silencing* (PTGS), is an evolutionarily conserved, double-stranded RNA-dependent, universal eukaryotic process to clean "foreign-like" mRNA transcripts in a sequence-specific manner before they generate harmful proteins or invade the genome. Opportunity to induce and trigger RNAi for any desired sequence signature and its systematic spreading property from cell-to cell, tissue to tissue, or in whole body system made it an efficient approach to study the function of any genes and/or sequence signatures of an organism.

Increasing body of our knowledge on a sequence/gene of interest, improved design of RNAi inducers with its various modifications, development of efficient and specific delivery systems, and optimized targeting strategies as well as the use of organism's own gene or gene fragment further made RNAi advantageous over existing gene manipulation "transgenic" technologies. Hence, RNAi holds a great potential for agricultural biotechnology and crop improvement, food security, industrial biotechnology and biofuel production, molecular pharmacology, and treatment of various inflammatory, infectious, and hereditary diseases such as complex immune and cancer therapy. Addressing all of these, RNAi research and application significantly advanced in past decade period.

The book *RNA interference,* a collection of 19 chapters from distinguished laboratories and eminent scientists of the world conducting state-of-the-art RNAi research, aims to provide readers "up-to-date" knowledge and progress on basics; types of inducers, triggers, and delivery systems; design and optimization requirements; and performance of RNAi in various cell models and organisms. Further, chapters of this book discuss a wide variety of potential "bench-to-clinic" applications of RNAi and lessons learned in crop improvement and protection, veterinary and animal protection, molecular pharmacology, and medicine, including its current and future therapeutic potential on inflammatory, blood, central nervous system, eye, liver, immune and cancer disease therapies with some aspects of limitations, alternative tools, safety, and risk assessment.

Although we missed the latest developments on RNAi repositories, screens, and databases as well as in-depth coverage of crop RNAi applications and commercialization efforts, I trust that various topics on advancements of RNAi research and its application, compiled in this single book, should add information to currently available literature sources and be useful for university students as well as private and public life science researchers, enhancing the reader's knowledge.

I would like to express my sincere appreciation to all eminent authors of the book chapters for their contributions, hard work, and full cooperation with my editorial requests. I thank the InTech book department, for giving me an editorship opportunity of this book, and Ms. Sandra Bakic and Ms. Iva Simcic, InTech's Publishing Process Managers, for their initiation of this book project, coordination of entire book processing, correspondence with authors, and support and help with this book publication.

Ibrokhim Y. Abdurakhmonov
Center of Genomics and Bioinformatics,
Academy of Sciences of Uzbekistan,
Ministry of Agriculture and Water Resource,
"Uzcottonindustry" association,
Tashkent, Uzbekistan

Section 1

Introductory

Chapter 1

RNA Interference – A Hallmark of Cellular Function and Gene Manipulation

Ibrokhim Y. Abdurakhmonov

Additional information is available at the end of the chapter

http://dx.doi.org/10.5772/62038

Abstract

The discovery of RNA interference (RNAi) and its utilization in downregulation of specific target transcripts have revolutionized gene function analysis and elucidation of many key biochemical/genetic pathways. The insights into gene function, combined with a technology that made silencing of gene function possible using the potent, highly specific and selective RNAi approaches, provided the solution to longstanding complex obstacles in targeted crop improvementsfor agriculture, and disease therapies for medicine. In this introductory chapter, I aim briefly to cover the basics and peculiarities of RNAi and the advances made in understanding the mechanisms, components, function, evolution, application, safety and risk assessment of RNAi, while at the same time highlighting the related chapters of this book.

Keywords: Gene silencing, RNA interference, RNAi inducers and delivery, RNAi-based disease therapy, biosafety

1. Introduction

The "central dogma" of genetics as first presented by Francis Crick is that genes, packed inside the cell as the deoxyribonucleic acid (DNA) molecule, are transcribed into messenger ribonucleic acids (mRNA), which are subsequently translated into proteins (or enzymes). These final protein products provide all life functions, and together with DNA and RNA, constitute the molecules of life. Therefore, if there is a disruption (interference) of a gene function, messenger RNA synthesis, or protein translation, normal life processes get altered or even stopped. "No gene-no messenger", or "no messenger-no protein", has been the basis of understanding biological processes. One of the easy-to-access points in cellular processes is messenger RNA due to its cytoplasmic location, "naked" structure, comparatively short half-life, and temporal existence between transcription and translation. Further, mRNA is in between the chain of events from DNA to protein; it has the universal chemical structure, consisting of only four nucleotides, regardless of the encoded message. In contrast, proteins are chemically much more variable, consisting of combinations of 21 different amino acids, with side chains that vary from very hydrophilic to highly hydrophobic. If mRNA is altered or eliminated before translation, there is no functional gene product, which results in changing the cellular process from the native state. This is the entire rationale of RNA interference (RNAi).

RNA interference is a process in eukaryotic cells in which double stranded endogenous or exogenous RNA molecules trigger a cytoplasmic response, which involves sequence specific target identification and destruction. This may include native messenger RNAs (mRNAs) that code vitally important proteins [1]. Any type of double-stranded RNA (dsRNA) molecules can activate RNAi where long dsRNAs, microRNAs (miRNAs) and small interfering RNAs (siRNAs) and their various forms and modifications are considered the main players/inducers [1]. Let us take a look at RNAi discovery history.

Plant scientists in the 1990s first used targeted gene silencing by introducing an antisense gene into plants. The first example was silencing of a nopaline synthase (NOS) gene, for which the silencing was only visible by loss of a band on a Norther blot and loss of NOS activity [2]. The second antisense gene used in plants targeted the petunia chalcone synthase (CHS) gene, encoding the first step in floral pigment production, and the result was visible in the loss of petal pigmentation [3]. Curiously, attempts to create dark pigmented petunia flowers by overexpression of the same CHS gene resulted in similar colorless petunia petals [4, 5]. It was thought that such a phenotype was "*due to post-transcriptional inhibition of gene expression via an increased rate of mRNA degradation*" [6]. The observed phenomenon was named as "*co-suppression*" of gene expression and the molecular mechanism behind "*co-suppression*" remained unknown for many years [7]. Later, a transient gene inactivation of the carotenogenic *albino-3* (*AL-3*) and *albino-1* (*AL-1*) genes was reported after transformation with homologous sequences in *Neurospora crassa* [8]. This phenomenon, named as gene "*quelling*", was observed to be severely destructive but spontaneously and progressively reversible and monodirectional, resulting in mutant, intermediate, and wild-type phenotypes [8]. In the years to follow, the co-suppression phenomenon were attributed to inverted repeat T-DNA insertions, which result in RNA transcripts with internal complementary sequences that can fold back on themselves, generating double-stranded RNA and can seed the now well-known Argonaute/dicer silencing system.

Following these seminal discoveries, similar phenomena were discovered in other organisms including the nematode (*Caenorhabditis elegans*) and insects (*Drosophila melanogaster*) from studying the function of a *PAR-1* gene (required for establishing embryo polarity) in the former and alcohol dehydrogenase in the latter (*ADH*) [9, 10]. These studies not only demonstrated a wide range of functionality of "*co-suppression*" phenomenon but also prompted an intense effort to understand the exact mechanism causing this process. In one experiment, injection of dsRNAs associated with muscle protein production into nematodes successfully silenced the targeted gene. The effect on muscle production was not observed using either mRNA or antisense RNA [11]. With this work, for the first time, the agent directly responsible for "*co-suppression*" was identified and formally named as "*RNA interference*" or RNAi. This work was later recognized with the 2006 Nobel Prize.

http://dx.doi.org/10.5772/62038

In plants, the suppression of targeted genes during viral infections was discovered [12] and subsequently developed into a system by which plant gene function may be studied through inhibition by infection with viruses bearing a short sequence targeted against plant mRNAs [13]. This phenomenon was termed as "*virus-induced gene silencing*" (VIGS) and is often used to study gene function in plant species that are recalcitrant to transformation or just take a very long time to regenerate.

Over the past decade, RNAi has been demonstrated in many eukaryotes including humans as well as some prokaryotic life forms [14] and has been recognized to form an integral part of many gene regulatory networks during development. This revolutionary breakthrough in biological science has become a valuable *in vitro, in vivo,* and *ex vivo* manipulation of gene expression, allowing for large-scale studies of gene function. It is now a routine laboratory practice to introduce the desired gene-specific dsRNA inducers into cells and selectively, robustly, and systematically silence the targeted sequence signature revealing its cellular function. In addition, RNAi has become an efficient tool for agricultural biotechnology to improve production [15] and combat disease pests as well as for medicine and molecular pharmacology to cure complex infectious, inflammatory, and hereditary diseases [16].

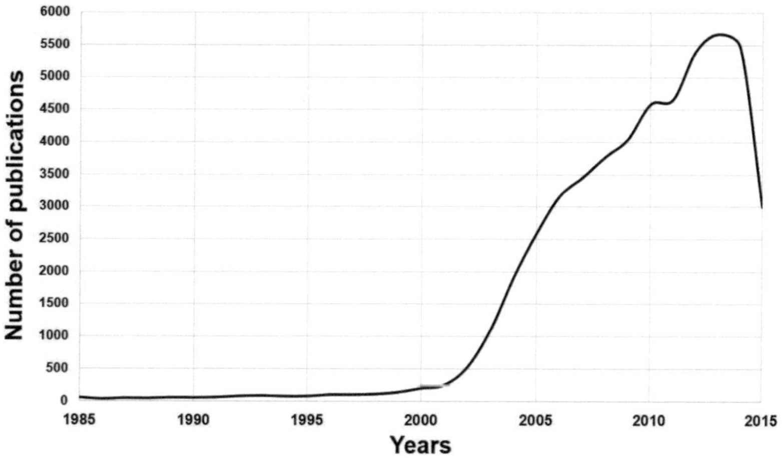

Figure 1. Dynamics of scientific publications devoted to the RNA interference for the past three decades. Source: PubMed [18] data sorted by the year of publications, which were retrieved by the search with the unquoted keyword "*RNA interference*"]

RNAi research has rapidly advanced and expanded over the past decade, evidenced by increasing numbers of publications, research projects, and practical applications in both agriculture and medicine. For example, searching *Google Scholar* [17] with the unquoted keyword "*RNA interference*" retrieved over 1 million (1,110,000) documents. Repeating the same search with "organism-specified RNA interference" in *PubMed* database [18] on the same date returned a total of 50,824 indexed scientific documents with a major pick after 2002 reaching to over 1,000 scientific publications per year (Figure 1). The distribution of specified search results revealed a number of PubMed-indexed, RNAi-related publications for human (32,007), plant (3,701), animal (27,751), insect (4,145), fungal (690), and prokaryotic (119) organisms. Moreover, the therapeutic application of RNAi is also expanding rapidly with 9,953 articles related to this topic and found in *PubMed* searching with "RNA interference therapy" keyword. In this brief introductory chapter, I aim to cover the basic understanding behind RNAi and an update knowledge on its applications, limitations, safety, and risks, highlighting and discussing some of the key points presented in this book.

2. Components, mechanism, and function

The principle mechanism of RNAi is complex, but very straightforward and easy to understand. RNAi is induced by the introduction of specific exogenous dsRNA either by virus genome RNAs, injection of synthetic dsRNAs or, in plants, is mediated by Agrobacterium. RNAi is also part of the normal development and dsRNAs are produced by endogenous genes encoding miRNA precursors or other long dsRNA molecules. In either case, the dsRNAs are recognized by the enzyme dicer and cleaved into short, double-stranded fragments of ~19-25 base pair long siRNAs [1]. These siRNAs are separated into two single-stranded RNAs (ssRNAs), which are referred to as the "*passenger*" and the "*guide*" strands. The passenger strand is degraded, while the guide strand is picked up by the RNA-induced silencing complex (RISC) that has enzymatic digestion activity and contains the key components of Argonaute (AGO) and P-element induced wimpy testis (PIWI) proteins [1]. The RISC proteins perform the unwinding of the *guide* and *passenger* strands in ATP-independent manner [19, 20]; however, ATP is required to unwind and remove the cleaved mRNA strand from the RISC complex after catalysis [21]. There are effector proteins such as RDE-4 (nematodes) and R2D2 (insects) that recognize exogenous dsRNAs and stimulate dicer activity. R2D2 also has a differentiating function for siRNA strands by stably binding to 5' end of the *passenger* strand, thus directing the *guide* strand to the RISC [22]. Here, it should be noted that the 5′ end of the *guide* strand is involved in matching and binding the target mRNA while the 3′ end physically arranges target mRNAs into the cleavage-favorable site of the RISC complex [21]. AGO/PIWI proteins localize within the specific P-body regions in the cytoplasm, considered to be a critical site for RNAi [23–25].

It is not clear as yet how the *guide* strand-bound active RISC complex finds mRNA targets within the cell, but it is known that this process is sequence-specific. Once the target mRNA is identified and captured though RNAi machinery, RISC cleaves the target mRNA rendering it untranslatable [1]. In most cases, the entire process is triggered by amplification of the cleavage process through synthesis of additional dsRNAs from primarily digested fragments of mRNA. Upon annealing to the mRNA target, the guide RNA may also be extended by RNA-dependent RNA polymerase (RdRP), resulting in extended "secondary" dsRNAs which in turn may lead to the formation of new siRNAs that enhance and further systematically spread the degradation of the target mRNA in cytoplasm [26, 27].

Although the pathways toward RNAi from exogenous and endogenous dsRNA converge at the RISC and use the same downstream RNAi machinery, there are also some clear differences in their processing and handling [1]. Endogenous dsRNAs cleaved by dicer (**1**) produce 20–25 bp fragments with a two-nucleotide overhang at the 3′end of siRNA duplex [1], while the length of exogenous dsRNAs-derived siRNAs, required for specificity, is unknown. Exogenous dsRNAs are distinctly (**2**) handled by the above-mentioned effector proteins, RDE-4 or R2D2 [26, 27], whereas siRNA derived from endogenous dsRNAs (i.e., miRNA precursors) are handled by double-stranded miRNA precursor-binding DGCR8 and Drosha proteins with RNAse III enzyme activity. Plants do not have Drosha homologs, instead, processing of miRNA to siRNAs is carried out by one of four dicer-like proteins. Endogenous miRNAs (**3**), except some plant miRNAs, typically have several mismatches to the target sequence, while siRNAs derived from exogenous dsRNAs usually are designed to have a perfect match to the target. Most importantly, (**4**) endogenous dsRNA-derived miRNAs are capable of mildly inhibiting the translation of hundreds of mRNAs [28–30], while exogenous dsRNA-derived ones usually silence only single specific target [31]. Depending on organisms, for instance in *C. elegans* and *D. melanogaster*, (**5**) distinct Argonaute proteins and dicer enzymes [32, 33] process miRNAs and exogenous siRNAs. Furthermore, endogenously processed miRNAs prevalently (**6**) interact with miRNA response elements (MREs) located within the 3'-UTRs region of target mRNAs. Upon binding to MREs, miRNAs can decrease the gene expression of various mRNAs by either inhibiting translation (in animals) or directly causing degradation of the transcript (in plants). In contrast, exogenous dsRNA-derived siRNAs may interact with any complementary sequence region of the target mRNA, causing direct cleavage of the transcript [1]. miRNAs may actually regulate translation of target mRNAs in dual ways, as translation regulation by miRNAs oscillates between repression and activation during the cell cycle through a yet unknown mechanism [34].

The main biological function of RNAi is regulation of gene activity of cells at the post-transcriptional level (PTGS) either by the inhibition of translation of mRNA or by direct degradation of the mRNA. In addition to PTGS, RNAi pathway components may contribute to maintenance of genome organization and structure, mediated by RNA-induced histone modification. Histone modification in turn affects heterochromatin formation and may silence gene activity at the pre-transcriptional level [35]. This process is referred to as "RNA-induced gene silencing (RITS) and requires dicer, siRNA and RISC component proteins such as AGO and R2D2 [36]. In addition, RNAi components and inducers (siRNA/dicer/AGO) may also possibly upregulate expression of genes in binding into a promoter region and through histone demethylation, a process dubbed RNA activation [37, 38].

Because of sequence-specific recognition, regulatory properties, and the possibility of systemic spreading of dsRNAs, RNAi is the key "sterilizing agent" of cells and tissues, and it functions as potent immune response against foreign nucleic acids from viruses, transposons, or transformation events which can invade and harm the genome and its stability [39]. The chapters presented in Section 2 of this book have a more detailed coverage of the history of the RNAi discovery, mechanism, and functional components and on the biological role of RNAi including natural small RNAs/microRNAs as well as long noncoding RNAs in gene regulations.

3. Differences among organisms

Although the RNAi pathway is a universal process in eukaryotic cells, and it consists of similar component(s), mechanisms, and functions as described above, there are some variations among organisms in both up-take of exogenous dsRNAs and induction of RNAi. First, RNAi is systemic and heritable in plants and *C. elegans*. The systemic spreading of RNAi in plants occurs because of transfer of siRNAs between cells through plasmodesmata and the phloem [40]. Second, in plants, RNAi induces epigenetic silencing of genes through methylation of promoters of targeted genes which may be passed to the next generation [41], while in Drosophila and mammals this is not the case. Third, plant miRNAs have perfect or nearly perfect complementary to their target genes and directly cleave and degrade targeted mRNA. In contrast, animal miRNAs have one or more mismatches to target sequence and halt the translation process [42].

RNAi is not found in some eukaryotic protozoa (e.g., *Leishmania major* and *Trypanosoma cruzi*) [43, 44]. Some fungi (e.g., *Saccharomyces cerevisiae*) lack specific RNAi component(s) and the reintroduction of these missing components can recover RNAi [45, 46]. Further, prokaryotic organisms have distinctive RNA-dependent gene regulation system controlled by RNA products of translation-inhibiting genes. These regulatory RNAs are not processed by dicer enzymes, differentiating them from eukaryotic RNAi [47]. However, recently, the clustered regularly interspaced short palindromic repeats (CRISPR/Cas9) interference system has been characterized in prokaryotes, which is a gene silencing pathway analogous to eukaryotic RNAi systems [14]. The CRISPR interference system has its specific components, advantages, and limitations that are well described in the literature [48, 49], but will not be presented here. The chapter by Dr. Devi Singh and his colleagues in Section 2 of this book has a detailed coverage of RNAi in various organisms. RNAi in various organisms is also discussed in the chapter by Galay et al. presented in Section 6 of this book, highlighting the specifics of RNAi in ticks while Dr. Tayota and his colleagues present an interesting methodological paper on RNAi in the water flea in Section 3.

4. Evolution

Studies on components, mechanisms, and functions of RNAi have demonstrated variations among organisms, differences in eukaryotes and prokaryotes, and indicate that RNAi is derived from an ancestral immune defense function against transcripts of transposons and viruses [50, 51]. Although some eukaryotes might have lost RNAi components or, even, the entire pathway following the emergence of the Eukaryota, parsimony-based phylogenetic analyses suggest that an ancestral lineage of all eukaryotes possibly had a primitive RNAi capability including relevant components for some key functions such as histone modification [50]. Phylogenetic studies also indicate that miRNAs of plants and animals may have evolved independently, but the conservation of some key proteins involved in RNAi also indicate that the last common ancestor of modern eukaryotes already possessed an siRNA-based gene silencing system. The RNAi-like defense system of prokaryotes is functionally similar, but structurally distinct from the eukaryotic RNAi system [52]. It seems likely that a proto-RNAi system possessed at least some form of dicer-like, AGO, PIWI, and RdRP proteins. These basic components were shared by major eukaryotic lineages and functioned within an RNA degradation exosome complex [53].

Being an important component of an antiviral innate immune defense system in eukaryotes, RNAi components and various interaction/regulatory mechanisms, including the miRNA pathway, evolved later but at faster rates under strong directional selection [54]. This could have been a means of generating an improved response to the evolutionary arms race with viral genes. Correspondingly, some plant viruses have evolved the means to suppress the RNAi response in their host cells [55]. Extensive studies reported that an ancient duplication of RNAi components followed by species-specific gene duplications and losses provided evolutionary diversification, specificity and adaptation of the RNAi system in many organisms [56]. Chapter(s) presented in Section 2 has covered some evolutionary aspects of RNAi.

5. Applications

Since its first discovery as anti-sense gene suppression, *co-suppression* or *quelling* phenomenon, the sequence specificity, efficiency, and systemic spreading (in some organisms) characteristics of RNAi to suppress target gene expression have caught researchers' attention and soon became an attractive and powerful tool for gene function discovery in life sciences [1]. By full or partial suppression of target gene expression using RNAi, the change in cell physiology and/or developmental phenotype helps to reveal the function of the target gene. Therefore, a utilization of RNAi has revolutionized the annotation of cellular functions of many unknown and unique genes, adding to our understanding the complex genetic/biochemical pathways and their interactions. Thanks to its partial silencing effect, RNAi also helped to discover the function of genes when complete knockout would cause lethality [57]. Moreover, by targeting homologous sequences within a gene family, a single RNAi construct can suppress the expression of multiple members of a gene family, and thus reveal phenotypes that would have been missed in a single mutant due to redundancy in gene function.

The results of the functional genomics studies, advances in the understanding of the RNAi mechanism, improved design of trait-specific RNAi inducers (such as miRNAs), selection of target gene sequences combined with the development of proper delivery systems, as well as screens for "off-target" and cross reactivity have brought the practical applications of RNAi far beyond its initial experimental reach.

Agricultural application of RNAi through tissue culture-derived genetic modifications and transgenic research in a wide range of technical, food, and horticulture crops have been particularly successful and have solved many problems. Examples include, but are not limited to, crop yield and quality improvements [15, 58], food/nutrient quality improvements and fortification [59–62], decreasing the harmful precursors and carcinogens [63, 64], and improvement of plant pest and disease resistance [65–66]. Many of these applications are now evaluated for commercialization or are already in commercial production [67]. In this context, targeting far red (FR) photoreceptor gene (*PHYA1*) using RNAi approach [15], our team succeed to develop the world's first RNAi cotton cultivars with improved fiber quality and other key agronomic traits without adversely affecting the yield, which successfully passed multi-environmental large field trials and have been approved for cotton farming in Uzbekistan.

Therapeutic application of RNAi has also been successful in medicine and molecular pharmacology with examples in inflammatory and infectious disease [68-71], cancer [72-75], as well as hereditary and neurodegenerative diseases [76]. Indeed, for many other disorders RNAi may have great potential. To highlight advances made on this field, in Section 4 of this book, we present several relevant chapters on advances of RNAi application in key human diseases of blood, ocular, nervous, kidney, and oncogenic origin. In addition, Section 5 chapters discuss RNAi utilization in various immune and infectious diseases. Section 6 chapters present the latest advances of RNAi application in studies of insects and parasitic pests such as ticks. All of these chapters highlight various aspects of RNAi and add interesting insights to the present RNAi discussions.

6. Safety and risk assessment

Manipulation of the organisms' own genetic sequence signature(s) (cis-genesis) is usually considered safer compared to "trans-genesis" that utilizes "foreign" genetic material to create genetically modified (GM) crops and its products [77]. However, for RNAi, when broken down to ~21 nucleotides this quickly may lose its meaning, as a trans-RNAi will only work if it has sufficient homology to an endogenous target transcript. Chemically, RNA is "*generally recognized as safe (GRAS)*" or it is "*rarely formally considered in risk assessment*" [67]. Despite this and many other examples of successful application of RNAi technology in agriculture and medicine, there may be risks associated with high or repeated dosages of dsRNA, which inadvertently may interfere with unintended target sequences. A growing body of evidences suggests that testing for the safety and assessing possible risks associated with the use of RNAi-derived products sound practical, in particular, evidence of the remarkable stability of dsRNAs in the environment, their survival and resistance in the acidic conditions of the digestive tracts of higher organisms, and consequent transmissibility of dsRNA from foods to humans/animals. Further, production of possibly harmful "secondary" dsRNAs [67] by primary RNAi inducers raised an early warning signal regarding the GRAS signature of any RNA molecule and the possibility of risks for human health and environment.

Safety concerns about RNAi-based drugs are exemplified by the lethality of 23 out of 49 distinct RNAi therapy experiments in mice because of potential "off-target" effects that could shut down non-targeted gene(s) with sequence similarity to therapeutic RNAi inducer [78]. This observed lethality, however, could be due to "oversaturation" of the dsRNA pathway and delivery issues of short hairpin RNAs [79] that needs to be optimized for harmless therapeutic applications. There are several suggested approaches to minimize or eliminate such "off-target", "oversaturation" or delivery issues, in particular through the use of (1) comprehensive *in silico* target and off-target analyses [80], (2) modified designing of RNAi inducers with improved target selectivity, and (3) efficient delivery systems.

There may also be concerns about the uptake of intact plant miRNA by consumers through plant diet. Plant microRNAs and some long dsRNA molecules, with sequence complimentary and perfect matches to endogenous human genes, were demonstrated to survive the digestive tract of humans and can freely and routinely enter the blood system [67, 81]. *In vitro* human cell culture experiments further showed that such plant siRNA entered into human blood system could silence endogenous human genes due to sequence complementarity. While this may require attention of regulatory systems on one hand, on the other hand, human consumption of food crops with natural occurring siRNAs is considered safe and so far has not caused any dramatic biohazards or risk [81]. The chapters in Section 3 of this book also present updated information on RNAi delivery methods (e.g. Tayota et al.); synthesis, chemical and structural modifications, and designing for high specificity and selectivity of RNAi inducers (see Gvozdeva and Chernolovskaya), and limitations of RNAi and possible alternative technology such as ER-targeted intrabodies for gene silencing (see chapter by Backhaus and Böldicke).

Risk assessment and available protocols/guidelines are in the early stages of development. Some suggest that dsRNA-derived products must be subject to risk assessment studies [67]. Other findings indirectly support the safety of RNAi [81, 82], provided its use is within specific dosage ranges, the correct delivery system is in place and RNAi inducers without possible off-target effects, unintended gene silencing and secondary dsRNA production can be designed. However, it is always advisable to admit to possible risks of any novel genomic technology, including RNAi, and consider potential biohazards and evaluate risks for environmental health, before release of a new product [58, 81–85]. To accomplish this, Heinemann et al. [67] proposed the following five-step guidance: (1) to perform detailed *in silico* comparative bioinformatics analyses for targets of designed dsRNA and identify possible "off-targets" in key consumers; (2) to experimentally quantify designed dsRNAs, and the processing of any other unknown sequence signatures or secondary dsRNA as a result of introducing intended RNAi inducer into recipient or its product; (3) to test possible biohazards and risks due to exposure of RNAi product in animal and human cell/tissue culture; (4) to conduct animal feeding experiments for the long-term physiological and toxicological patterns and possible chronic effects; and (5) to perform clinical trials of RNAi-derived products in humans.

7. Conclusions and future perspectives

Thus, being a revolutionizing discovery in genome biology to characterize functions of any desired unknown genetic sequences, the discovery of RNAi has significantly widened our knowledge on core cellular processes. This knowledge has created opportunities and solutions to longstanding obstacles in conventional agriculture and medicine, offering a bright future to curing complex human and animal diseases, improve crop production and protection, and a sustained global food security through proper manipulation of key genes with agricultural or medicinal importance. Although key issues on specificity, selectivity, and delivery of RNAi inducing structures still exist, and some safety risks associated with the use of RNAi products have been recognized, the general believe is that RNAi is a safer technology than transgenomics utilizing "foreign" genetic information. Safe applications, however, require proper designing, dosage and delivery of RNAi inducers, and before its delivery for wide consumer market, the safety risks should be assessed. Addressing the advances made over the past three decades in RNAi research and commercialization, in this book, we have compiled and presented a diverse collection of chapters contributed by the science research communities. We all believe that RNAi, in combination with the rapidly expanding genomic information in key organisms and novel genome editing tools, will become even more powerful and efficient, and that we will all enjoy its benefits far into the future.

Acknowledgements

I thank the Academy of Sciences of Uzbekistan and Committee for Coordination Science and Technology Development of Uzbekistan for basic science FA-F5-T030; and several applied (FA-A6-T081 and FA-A6-T085) and innovation (I-2015-6-15/2 and I5-FQ-0-89-870) research grants. I am particularly grateful and thank the Office of International Research Programs (OIRP) of the United States Department of Agriculture (USDA) – Agricultural Research Service (ARS) and U.S. Civilian Research & Development Foundation (CRDF) for international cooperative grants P121, P121B, and UZB-TA-2292, which are devoted to study, development, application, risk assessment, and commercialization of RNAi cotton cultivars and their products. I sincerely thank Dr. Alexander R. van der Krol, Waginengen University, Netherlands, and Dr. Eric J. Devor, Iowa State University, the USA, for their critical reading and suggestions to this chapter manuscript.

Author details

Ibrokhim Y. Abdurakhmonov*

Address all correspondence to: genomics@uzsci.net

Center of Genomics and Bioinformatics, Academy of Science, Ministry of Agriculture and Water Resources, and "UzCottonIndustry" Association of the Republic of Uzbekistan, Tashkent, Uzbekistan

References

[1] Hannon GJ. RNA interference. Nature. 2002;418:244–51. DOI: 10.1038/418244a

[2] Rothstein SJ, Dimaio J, Strand M, Rice D. Stable and heritable inhibition of the expression of nopaline synthase in tobacco expressing antisense RNA. Proc Natl Acad Sci U S A. 1987;84:8439–8443. DOI:10.1073/pnas.84.23.8439

[3] van der Krol AR, Lenting PE, Veenstra J, van der Meer IM, Koes RE, Gerats AGM, Joseph N. M. Mol JNM, Stuitje AR. An anti-sense chalcone synthase gene in transgenic plants inhibits flower pigmentation. Nature 1988;333:866–869.DOI: 10.1038/333866a0

[4] van der Krol AR, Mur LA, Beld M, Mol JN, Stuitje AR. Flavonoid genes in petunia: addition of a limited number of gene copies may lead to a suppression of gene expression. Plant Cell. 1990;2:291–-99. DOI:10.1105/tpc.2.4.291

[5] Napoli C, Lemieux C, Jorgensen R. Introduction of a chimeric chalcone synthase gene into petunia results in reversible co-suppression of homologous genes in trans". Plant Cell. 1990; 2:279–289. DOI:10.1105/tpc.2.4.279

[6] van Blokland R, van der Geest N, Mol JNM, Kooter JM. Transgene-mediated suppression of chalcone synthase expression in Petunia hybrida results from an increase in RNA turnover. Plant J. 1994;6:861–877. DOI:10.1046/j.1365-313X.1994.6060861.x.

[7] Mol JNM, van der Krol AR. Antisense nucleic acids and proteins: fundamentals and applications. New York: Marcel Dekker; 1991. 231 p. ISBN 0-8247-8516-9.

[8] Romano N, Macino G (1992). Quelling: transient inactivation of gene expression in *Neurospora crassa* by transformation with homologous sequences. Mol Microbiol. 1992;6:3343–3353. DOI:10.1111/j.1365-2958.1992.tb02202.x

[9] Guo S, Kemphues K. par-1, a gene required for establishing polarity in *C. elegans* embryos, encodes a putative Ser/Thr kinase that is asymmetrically distributed. Cell. 1995;81:611–620. DOI:10.1016/0092-8674(95)90082-9

[10] Pal-Bhadra M, Bhadra U, Birchler J. Cosuppression in Drosophila: gene silencing of alcohol dehydrogenase by white-Adh transgenes is polycomb dependent. Cell. 1997;90: 479–490. DOI:10.1016/S0092-8674(00)80508-5

[11] Fire A, Xu S, Montgomery M, Kostas S, Driver S, Mello C. Potent and specific genetic interference by double-stranded RNA in *Caenorhabditis elegans*. Nature. 1998;391: 806–811. DOI:10.1038/35888. PMID 9486653

[12] Ratcliff F, Harrison B, Baulcombe D. A similarity between viral defense and gene silencing in plants. Science. 1997;276:1558. DOI:10.1126/science.276.5318.1558.

[13] Godge MR, Purkayastha A, Dasgupta I, Kumar PP.Virus-induced gene silencing for functional analysis of selected genes. Plant Cell Rep. 2008;27: 209-219. DOI:

[14] Hale C, Kleppe K, Terns RM, Terns MP. Prokaryotic silencing (psi)RNAs in Pyrococcus furiosus. RNA. 2008;14:2572–2579. DOI: 10.1261/rna.1246808

[15] Abdurakhmonov IY, Buriev ZT, Saha S, Jenkins JN, Abdukarimov A, Pepper AE. Cotton *PHYA1* RNAi enhances major fiber quality and agronomic traits of cotton (Gossypium hirsutum L). Nature Communications.2014;4:3062; DOI:10. 1038/ncomms4062

[16] Kupferschmidt K. A Lethal Dose of RNA. Science. 2013;341:732–733. DOI:10.1126/science.341.6147.732

[17] Google Scholar. 2015. Available from: http://scholar.google.com [Accessed 2015-09-06]

[18] PubMed database. 2015. Available from: http://www.ncbi.nlm.nih.gov/pubmed [Accessed from 2015-09-06]

[19] Matranga C, Tomari Y, Shin C, Bartel D, Zamore P. Passenger-strand cleavage facilitates assembly of siRNA into Ago2-containing RNAi enzyme complexes. Cell. 2005;123: 607–620. DOI:10.1016/j.cell.2005.08.044

[20] Leuschner P, Ameres S, Kueng S, Martinez J. Cleavage of the siRNA passenger strand during RISC assembly in human cells. EMBO Rep. 2006;7:314–320. DOI: 10.1038/sj.embor.7400637

[21] Haley B, Zamore B. Kinetic analysis of the RNAi enzyme complex. Nature Structural & Molecular Biology. 2004;11:599–606. DOI:10.1038/nsmb780

[22] Tomari Y, Matranga C, Haley B, Martinez N, Zamore P; Matranga; Haley; Martinez; Zamore. A protein sensor for siRNA asymmetry. Science. 2004;306:1377–1380. DOI: 10.1126/science.1102755

[23] Sen G, Blau H. Argonaute 2/RISC resides in sites of mammalian mRNA decay known as cytoplasmic bodies. Nat Cell Biol. 2005;7: 633–636. DOI:10.1038/ncb1265. PMID 15908945

[24] Lian S, Jakymiw A, Eystathioy T, Hamel J, Fritzler M, Chan E. GW bodies, microRNAs and the cell cycle. Cell Cycle. 2006;5:242–245. DOI:10.4161/cc.5.3.2410

[25] Jakymiw A, Lian S, Eystathioy T, Li S, Satoh M, Hamel J, Fritzler M, Chan E. Disruption of P bodies impairs mammalian RNA interference. Nat Cell Biol.2005;7:1267–1274. DOI:10.1038/ncb1334

[26] Parker G, Eckert D, Bass B. RDE-4 preferentially binds long dsRNA and its dimerization is necessary for cleavage of dsRNA to siRNA. RNA. 2006;12:807–818. DOI: 10.1261/rna.2338706

[27] Liu Q, Rand T, Kalidas S, Du F, Kim H, Smith D, Wang X. R2D2, a bridge between the initiation and effector steps of the Drosophila RNAi pathway. Science. 2003;301: 1921–1925. DOI:10.1126/science.1088710

[28] Lim LP, Lau NC, Garrett-Engele P, Grimson A, Schelter JM, Castle J, Bartel DP, Linsley PS, Johnson JM. Microarray analysis shows that some microRNAs downregulate large numbers of target mRNAs. Nature. 2005;433:769–773. DOI:10.1038/nature03315. PMID 15685193

[29] Selbach M, Schwanhäusser B, Thierfelder N, Fang Z, Khanin R, Rajewsky N. Widespread changes in protein synthesis induced by microRNAs. Nature. 2008:455: 58–63. DOI:10.1038/nature07228

[30] Baek D, Villén J, Shin C, Camargo FD, Gygi SP, Bartel DP.The impact of microRNAs on protein output. Nature.2008;455: 64–71. DOI:10.1038/nature07242

[31] Pillai RS, Bhattacharyya SN, Filipowicz W. Repression of protein synthesis by miRNAs: how many mechanisms? Trends Cell Biol 2007;17:118–126. DOI:10.1016/j.tcb.2006.12.007

[32] Okamura K, Ishizuka A, Siomi H, Siomi M (2004). "Distinct roles for Argonaute proteins in small RNA-directed RNA cleavage pathways". Genes Dev. 2004;18:1655–1666. DOI:10.1101/gad.1210204

[33] Lee Y, Nakahara K, Pham J, Kim K, He Z, Sontheimer E, Carthew R. Distinct roles for Drosophila Dicer-1 and Dicer-2 in the siRNA/miRNA silencing pathways. Cell. 2004;117:69–81. DOI:10.1016/S0092-8674(04)00261-2

[34] Vasudevan S, Tong Y, Steitz JA. Switching from Repression to Activation: MicroRNAs Can Up-Regulate Translation. Science. 2007;318:1931–1934. DOI:10.1126/science

[35] Holmquist G, Ashley T. Chromosome organization and chromatin modification: influence on genome function and evolution. Cytogenet Genome Res.2006;114:96–125. DOI:10.1159/000093326

[36] Verdel A, Jia S, Gerber S, Sugiyama T, Gygi S, Grewal S, Moazed D. RNAi-mediated targeting of heterochromatin by the RITS complex. Science. 2004;303:672–676. DOI:10.1126/science.1093686

[37] Li LC, Okino ST, Zhao H, Pookot D, Place RF, Urakami S, Enokida H, Dahiya R. Small dsRNAs induce transcriptional activation in human cells. Proc Natl Acad Sci USA.2006;103:17337–17342. DOI:10.1073/pnas.0607015103

[38] Check E. RNA interference: hitting the on switch. Nature. 2007;448: 855–858.DOI:10.1038/448855a

[39] Stram Y, Kuzntzova L. Inhibition of viruses by RNA interference. Virus Genes. 2006;32:299–306. DOI:10.1007/s11262-005-6914-0

[40] Lodish H, Berk A, Matsudaira P, Kaiser CA, Krieger M, Scott MP, Zipurksy SL, Darnell J. Molecular Cell Biology. 5th ed. New York; W.H; 2004.963 p. ISBN 978-0-7167-4366-8.

[41] Jones L, Ratcliff F, Baulcombe DC. RNA-directed transcriptional gene silencing in plants can be inherited independently of the RNA trigger and requires Met1 for maintenance. Curr Biol. 2001;11:747–757. DOI:10.1016/S0960-9822(01)00226-3

[42] Saumet A, Lecellier CH. Anti-viral RNA silencing: do we look like plants ?. Retrovirology. 2006;3:3. DOI:10.1186/1742-4690-3-3

[43] DaRocha W, Otsu K, Teixeira S, Donelson J. Tests of cytoplasmic RNA interference (RNAi) and construction of a tetracycline-inducible T7 promoter system in Trypanosoma cruzi. Mol Biochem Parasitol. 2004;133:175–86. DOI:10.1016/j.molbiopara.2003.10.005

[44] Robinson K, Beverley S. Improvements in transfection efficiency and tests of RNA interference (RNAi) approaches in the protozoan parasite Leishmania. Mol Biochem Parasitol. 2003;28:217–228. DOI:10.1016/S0166-6851(03)00079-3

[45] Aravind L, Watanabe H, Lipman DJ, Koonin EJ. Lineage-specific loss and divergence of functionally linked genes in eukaryotes. Proc Natl Acad Sci USA. 2000;97:11319–11324. DOI:10.1073/pnas.200346997

[46] Drinnenberg IA, Weinberg DE, Xie KT, Nower JP, Wolfe KH, Fink GR, Bartel DP. RNAi in budding yeast. Science 2009;326:544–550. DOI:10.1126/science.

[47] Morita T, Mochizuki Y, Aiba H. Translational repression is sufficient for gene silencing by bacterial small noncoding RNAs in the absence of mRNA destruction". Proc Natl Acad Sci USA. 2006;103:4858–486. DOI:10.1073/pnas.0509638103

[48] Larson MH, Gilbert LA, Wang X, Lim WA, Weissman JS, Qi LS. CRISPR interference (CRISPRi) for sequence-specific control of gene expression. Nature Protocols 2013;8:2180–2196. DOI:10.1038/nprot.2013.132

[49] Gilbert LA, Larson MH, Morsut L, Liu Z, Brar GA, Torres SE, Stern-Ginossar N, Brandman O, Whitehead EH, Doudna JA, Lim WA, Weissman JS, Qi LS. CRISPR-mediated modular RNA-guided regulation of transcription in eukaryotes. Cell. 2013;154:442–451. DOI:10.1016/j.cell.2013.06.044

[50] Cerutti H, Casas-Mollano J. On the origin and functions of RNA-mediated silencing: from protists to man". Curr Genet. 2006;50:81–99. DOI:10.1007/s00294-006-0078-x

[51] Buchon N, Vaury C. RNAi: a defensive RNA-silencing against viruses and transposable elements. Heredity. 2006;96:195–202. DOI:10.1038/sj.hdy.6800789.

[52] Shabalina S, Koonin EV. Origins and evolution of eukaryotic RNA interference Ecol Evol. 2008;23:578–587. DOI: 10.1016/j.tree.2008.06.005

[53] Anantharaman V, Koonin E, Aravind L. Comparative genomics and evolution of proteins involved in RNA metabolism. Nucleic Acids Res. 2002;30:1427–64. DOI: 10.1093/nar/30.7.1427

[54] Obbard DJ; Jiggins FM; Halligan DL; Little TJ. Natural selection drives extremely rapid evolution in antiviral RNAi genes. Curr Biol. 2006;16:580–585. DOI:10.1016/j.cub.2006.01.065

[55] Lucy A, Guo H, Li W, Ding S. Suppression of post-transcriptional gene silencing by a plant viral protein localized in the nucleus. EMBO J. 2000;19:1672–1680. DOI:10.1093/emboj/19.7.1672

[56] Hu Y, Stenlid J, Elfstrand M, Olson A. Evolution of RNA interference proteins dicer and argonaute in Basidiomycota. Mycologia. 2013;105:1489–1498.DOI: 10.3852/13-171

[57] Voorhoeve PM, Agami R. Knockdown stands up. Trends Biotechnol. 2003;21:2–4. DOI:10.1016/S0167-7799(02)00002-1

[58] Saurabh Satyajit, Vidyarthi AS, Prasad D. RNA interference: concept to reality in crop improvement. Planta. 2014;239:543–564. DOI:10.1007/s00425-013-2019-5

[59] Sunilkumar G, Campbell L, Puckhaber L; Stipanovic R, Rathore K. Engineering cottonseed for use in human nutrition by tissue-specific reduction of toxic gossypol. Proc Natl Acad Sci USA.2006:103:18054–18059. DOI:10.1073/pnas.0605389103

[60] Siritunga D, Sayre R. Generation of cyanogen-free transgenic cassava. Planta. 2003;217:367–373. DOI:10.1007/s00425-003-1005-8

[61] Le L, Lorenz Y, Scheurer, S, Fötisch K, Enrique E, Bartra J, Biemelt S, Vieths S, Sonnewald U. Design of tomato fruits with reduced allergenicity by dsRNAi-mediated inhibition of ns-LTP (Lyc e 3) expression. Plant Biotechnol J. 2006;4:231–242. DOI: 10.1111/j.1467-7652.2005.00175.x

[62] Niggeweg R, Michael A, Martin C.Engineering plants with increased levels of the antioxidant chlorogenic acid. Nat Biotechnol.2004;22:746–54. DOI:10.1038/nbt966

[63] Gavilano L, Coleman N, Burnley L, Bowman M, Kalengamaliro, Hayes A, Bush L, Siminszky B. Genetic engineering of Nicotiana tabacum for reduced nornicotine content". J Agric Food Chem. 2006;54:9071–9078. DOI:10.1021/jf0610458

[64] Allen R, Millgate A, Chitty J, Thisleton J, Miller J, Fist A, Gerlach W, Larkin P. RNAi-mediated replacement of morphine with the nonnarcotic alkaloid reticuline in opium poppy". Nat Biotechnol.2004;22:1559–1566. DOI:10.1038/nbt1033

[65] Zadeh A, Foster G. Transgenic resistance to tobacco ringspot virus. Acta Virol. 2004;48:145–152

[66] Mao YB, Cai WJ, Wang JW, Hong GJ, Tao XY, Wang LJ, Huang YP, Chen XY. Silencing a cotton bollworm P450 monooxygenase gene by plant-mediated RNAi impairs larval tolerance of gossypol. Nat Biotechnol. 2007;25:1307–1313. DOI: 10.1038/nbt1352

[67] Heinemann JA, Agapito-Tenfen SZ, Carman JA. A comparative evaluation of the regulation of GM crops or products containing dsRNA and suggested improvements to risk assessments. Environ Int. 2013;55:43–55. DOI: 10.1016/j.envint.2013.02.010

[68] Crowe S. Suppression of chemokine receptor expression by RNA interference allows for inhibition of HIV-1 replication. AIDS. 2003;17 Suppl 4:S103–S105. DOI: 10.1097/00002030-200317004-00014

[69] Kusov Y, Kanda T, Palmenberg A, Sgro J, Gauss-Müller V. Silencing of Hepatitis A Virus Infection by Small Interfering RNAs. J Virol. 2006;80:5599–610. DOI:10.1128/JVI.01773-05

[70] Jia F, Zhang Y, Liu C.A retrovirus-based system to stably silence hepatitis B virus genes by RNA interference. Biotechnol Lett. 2006;8:1679–1685. DOI:10.1007/s10529-006-9138-z

[71] Hu L, Wang Z, Hu C, Liu X, Yao L, Li W, Qi Y. Inhibition of Measles virus multiplication in cell culture by RNA interference. Acta Virol. 2005;49:227–234. DOI: Not availble

[72] Putral L, Gu W, McMillan N. RNA interference for the treatment of cancer". Drug News Perspect. 2006;19:317–324. DOI:10.1358/dnp.2006.19.6.985937

[73] Izquierdo M. Short interfering RNAs as a tool for cancer gene therapy". Cancer Gene Ther. 2005;12:217–227. DOI:10.1038/sj.cgt.7700791

[74] Li C, Parker A, Menocal E, Xiang S, Borodyansky L, Fruehauf J. Delivery of RNA interference. Cell Cycle. 2006;5:2103–2109. DOI:10.4161/cc.5.18.3192

[75] Takeshita F, Ochiya T. Therapeutic potential of RNA interference against cancer. Cancer Sci. 2006;97:689–696. DOI:10.1111/j.1349-7006.2006.00234.x

[76] Raoul C, Barker S, Aebischer P. Viral-based modelling and correction of neurodegenerative diseases by RNA interference. Gene Ther. 2006;3:487–495. DOI:10.1038/sj.gt.3302690

[77] Hou H, Atlihan N, Lu ZX. New biotechnology enhances the application of cisgenesis in plant breeding. Front Plant Sci. 2014;5:389. DOI: 10.3389/fpls.2014.00389.

[78] Check E. RNA treatment kills mice. Nature. 2006; DOI:10.1038/news060522-10

[79] Grimm D, Streetz K, Jopling C, Storm T; Pandey K, Davis C, Marion P, Salazar Kay F, Kay M. Fatality in mice due to oversaturation of cellular microRNA/short hairpin RNA pathways. Nature. 2006;441:537–541. DOI:10.1038/nature04791

[80] Qiu S, Adema C, Lane T. A computational study of off-target effects of RNA interference. Nucleic Acids Res. 2005;33:1834–1847. DOI:10.1093/nar/gki324

[81] Petrick JS, Brower-Toland B, Jackson AL, Kier LD. Safety assessment of food and feed from biotechnology-derived crops employing RNA-mediated gene regulation to achieve desired traits: a scientific review. Regul Toxicol Pharmacol. 2013;66:167–176. DOI: 10.1016/j.yrtph.2013.03.008

[82] Kamthan A, Chaudhuri A, Kamthan M, Datta A. Small RNAs in plants: recent development and application for crop improvement. Front Plant Sci. 2015;6:208. DOI: 10.3389/fpls.2015.00208

[83] Lemgo GN, Sabbadini S, Pandolfini T, Mezzetti B. Biosafety considerations of RNAi-mediated virus resistance in fruit-tree cultivars and in rootstock. Transgenic Res. 2013;22:1073–1088. DOI: 10.1007/s11248-013-9728-1.

[84] Ramesh SV. Non-coding RNAs in crop genetic modification: considerations and predictable environmental risk assessments (ERA). Mol Biotechnol. 2013;55:87–100. DOI: 10.1007/s12033-013-9648-6

[85] Auer C, Frederick R. Crop improvement using small RNAs: applications and predictive ecological risk assessments. Trends Biotechnol. 2009;27:644–651. DOI: 10.1016/j.tibtech.2009.08.005

Section 2

Gene Regulation by Small RNA Molecules

Chapter 2

RNA Interference Technology — Applications and Limitations

Devi Singh, Sarika Chaudhary, Rajendra Kumar, Preeti Sirohi, Kamiya Mehla, Anil Sirohi, Shashi Kumar, Pooran Chand and Pankaj Kumar Singh

Additional information is available at the end of the chapter

http://dx.doi.org/10.5772/61760

Abstract

RNA interference (RNAi), an evolutionarily conserved mechanism triggered by double-stranded RNA (dsRNA), causes gene silencing in a sequence-specific manner. RNAi evolved naturally to mediate protection from both endogenous and exogenous pathogenic nucleic acids and to modulate gene expression. Multiple technological advancements and precision in gene targeting have allowed a plethora of potential applications, ranging from targeting infections in crop plants to improving health in human patients, which have been reviewed in this chapter.

Keywords: RNA interference, miRNA, RNAi mediated gene silencing, RNA-induced silencing complex

1. Introduction

Ascribing the structure and function relationship to a gene and modulating its expression to manifest the desired phenotype have been major challenges for scientists. [1] In order to elucidate the phenotype(s) associated with a given gene, various gene-targeting techniques have been tried with mixed success. Gene silencing can be executed at transcriptional gene silencing (TGS) and posttranscriptional gene silencing (PTGS) levels. [2] The TGS involves targeting genes at DNA level by altering promoter and enhancer efficiencies, methylation status of genes, and deleting parts of genes by homologous recombination, transcription activator-like effector nucleases (TALENs), and clustered regularly interspaced short palindromic repeats (CRISPR)/Cas9 systems. [3] The PTGS techniques rely upon the breakdown of mRNA by various technologies, including antisense RNA, ribozymes, DNAzymes, micro-

RNAs, and RNA interference (RNAi). [4] Among all these techniques, RNAi is the most efficient tool for targeted gene silencing. RNAi is now routinely utilized across multiple biological disciplines to determine gene function. RNAi is also being utilized for therapeutic interventions to downregulate the expression of genes involved in disease pathogenesis. The current review is focused on recent advancements in the biology and applications of RNAi.

2. RNAi-mediated gene silencing: A historical perspective across multiple species

2.1. Discovery of RNAi in plants and fungi

R. Jorgensen and his colleagues identified a novel mechanism of post-transcriptional gene silencing in *Petunia*. [5] They were attempting to introduce a chalcone synthase gene under a strong promoter to deepen the purple color of *Petunia* flowers; however, instead of getting a stronger purple color flower they observed that most flowers lost their color. Thus, they observed diminished expression of both the homologous endogenous gene and the exogenously introduced transgenic copy of the gene and termed the phenomenon as co-suppression. [5] Although the exact mechanism of this phenomenon remained undeciphered at that time, the posttranscriptional nature of gene silencing was still appreciated. [5-7]The suppression of endogenous gene expression by transformation of exogenous homologous sequences was later termed as quelling in *Neurospora crassa*. [8, 9]

2.2. RNAi in Ceanorhabdites elegans

In 1995, Guo and Kempheus attempted to knock down the expression of PAR-1 gene by antisense RNA in *C. elegans*; they observed a similar loss of gene expression with sense RNA controls as well [10]. At that time, they could not explain the mechanistic basis of such an observation. In 1998, Andrew Fire, Craig C. Mello, and their colleagues demonstrated efficient and specific interference of gene expression by introducing double-stranded RNA in the nematode *C. elegans* [11]. The genetic interference was genetically heritable and was stronger than the antisense strategy. This novel phenomenon was termed as RNA interference or RNAi by Fire and colleagues [11].

Subsequently, Lisa Timmons and Andrew Fire demonstrated that *C. elegans*, when fed on bacteria genetically engineered to express dsRNA for unc-22 and fem-1 genes, showed specific and reversible silencing of unc-22 and fem-1 genes in the worm [12, 13]. High-throughput genetic screens have been developed by either feeding the worms on genetically engineered bacteria expressing dsRNA or soaking or injecting the nematode with dsRNA. Functional genomic analysis of chromosomes I and III in *C. elegans* have been performed by Fraser and Gonczy, respectively, utilizing the RNA interference strategy [14, 15].

2.3. RNAi technology in *Drosophila*

Specific gene silencing has been achieved in the embryo extracts and cultured cells of *Drosophila* flies by utilizing the RNAi tool [16]. Zamore and colleagues utilized *Drosophila melanogaster* embryo lysates to demonstrate the cleavage of long dsRNA strands into short interfering dsRNA fragments (siRNA) of ~22 nucleotides (nt) [16]. Later Elbashir and colleagues demonstrated that chemically synthesized 21- or 22-nt-long dsRNA carrying 3′ overhangs could induce efficient RNA cleavage in embryo extracts from *Drosophila* [17].

2.4. RNAi in mammalian systems

A global nonspecific inhibition of protein synthesis was observed in mammalian cells by exposing them to dsRNAs that were greater than 30 base pairs (bp) in length [18]. RNA-dependent protein kinase (PKR), and 2′, 5′ oligoadenylate synthetase (2′, 5′-OAS) were responsible for the nonspecific silencing. PKR phosphorylates eIF-2α, a translation initiation factor, to shut down global protein synthesis. A synthesis product of enzyme 2′,5′-OAS activates RNase L, which induces nonspecific degradation of all mRNAs in a mammalian cell [18]. Long dsRNAs induce interferon response that activates both of these enzymes in mammalian cells [19]. The nonspecific interference pathways represent the mammalian cell response to viral infection or other stress [20]. Tuschl and colleagues demonstrated that RNA interference could be directly mediated by small interference RNA (siRNA) in cultured mammalian cells [21]. However, because siRNA does not integrate into the genome, the RNAi response from siRNA is only transient. In order to induce stable gene suppression in mammalian cells, Hannon and his colleagues utilized RNA Pol III promoter-driven (e.g., U6 or H1) expression of short hairpin RNAs (shRNAs) [22]. Various approaches have since been developed for mammalian cells to obtain successful gene silencing. Some of the successful gene silencing approaches are listed in Table 1.

Kingdom	Species	Silencing process	Induction stimulus
Fungi	*Neurospora*	Quelling	Transgene(s)
	Saccharomyces pombe	RNAi	dsRNA
Plants	*Arabidopsis, Coffea canéfora, Nicotiana, Petunia*	Transcriptional or Post-transcriptional gene silencing, co-suppression	Transgene(s) and viruses
Invertebrates	*Paramecium*	Homology-dependent gene silencing	Transgene(s)
	Amblyomma americanum, Anopheles, Brugia malayi, Dugesia japonica, Hydra, Leishmania donovani, Schistosoma mansoni, Tribolium castaneum, Trypanosoma brucei, etc.	RNAi	dsRNA
	Ceanorhabditis elegans	RNAi, TGS	dsRNA, Transgene(s)
	Drosophila melanogaster	Co-suppression, RNAi, Transcriptional gene silencing	dsRNA Transgene(s)
Vertebrates	Human, Mouse, Zebrafish,	RNAi	dsRNA

Table 1. Gene silencing approaches

3. The mechanism of silencing

RNAi-mediated gene silencing is executed by siRNAs. The process of silencing begins with the cleavage of long dsRNAs into 21–25 -nt fragments of siRNAs in cytoplasm [16, 17]. The process is catalyzed by Dicer enzyme [23]. These siRNAs are inserted into multiprotein silencing complex, which is known as RNA-induced silencing complex (RISC). Subsequent unwinding of siRNA duplex, in turn, leads to active confirmation of RISC complex (RISC*). Next, target mRNA (mRNA to be degraded) is recognized by antisense RNA, which signals RISC complex for the endonucleolytic degradation of the homologous mRNA. Tuschl and his colleagues have defined the directionality of dsRNA processing and the target RNA cleavage sites [17]. According to their results, target mRNA is cleaved in the centre of the region that is recognized by complimentary guide siRNA, which is 10–12 -nt away from the 5′ terminus of siRNA [17]. The RNAi process is completed by the last step of siRNA molecule amplification. It is well established that the next generation of siRNAs is derived from the priming on the target mRNA by RNA-dependent RNA polymerase (RdRp) enzyme by existing siRNAs. The second generation of siRNAs is effective in inducing a secondary RNA interference that is defined as transitive RNAi. The transitive RNAi causes a systemic genetic interference in plants and *C. elegans*. Interestingly, transitive and systemic RNAi is absent in *Drosophila* and mammals owing to the lack of RdRp in both organisms [24]. An illustration of the function of RNAi is demonstrated in Figure 1.

A multitude of studies suggests a possible link between RNAi and chromatin remodeling [24]. The dsRNA works at TGS and PTGS in plants, where both pathways related and assist in gene silencing. Only TGS is heritable and drives methylation of endogenous sequences. Multiple proteins, including Polycomb in *Drosophila* and *C. elegans* [22], and Piwi in *Drosophila* [25], execute silencing at both TGS and PTGS levels. Volpe and his colleagues documented that RNAi complex proteins, including Dicer, Agronaute, and RdRp, assist in centromeric silencing in *Schizosaccharomyces pombe* [26]. This suggests that RNAi contributes to the maintenance of genomic stability [26].

4. Enzymes involved in RNAi

4.1. Dicer

Dicer was first characterized and defined in *Drosophila* by Bernstein et al. [27]. Dicer belongs to the RNase III-class and assists in ATP-dependent siRNA generation from long dsRNAs. Importantly, human Dicer does not require ATP for the cleavage of long dsRNAs [28]. Structurally, Dicer is a large (~220-kDa) multi-modular protein that acts as an antiparallel dimer. Dicer has multiple domains, including an N-terminal putative DExH/DEAH box RNA helicase/ATPase domain, an evolutionarily conserved PAZ domain, two neighboring domains that resemble RNase III, and a dsRNA-binding domain. PAZ domain in dicer helps in recognizing the end of dsRNA, whereas RNase III domain helps in the cleavage of dsRNA. Function of other domains is not fully known. Dicer orthologs has been defined in many

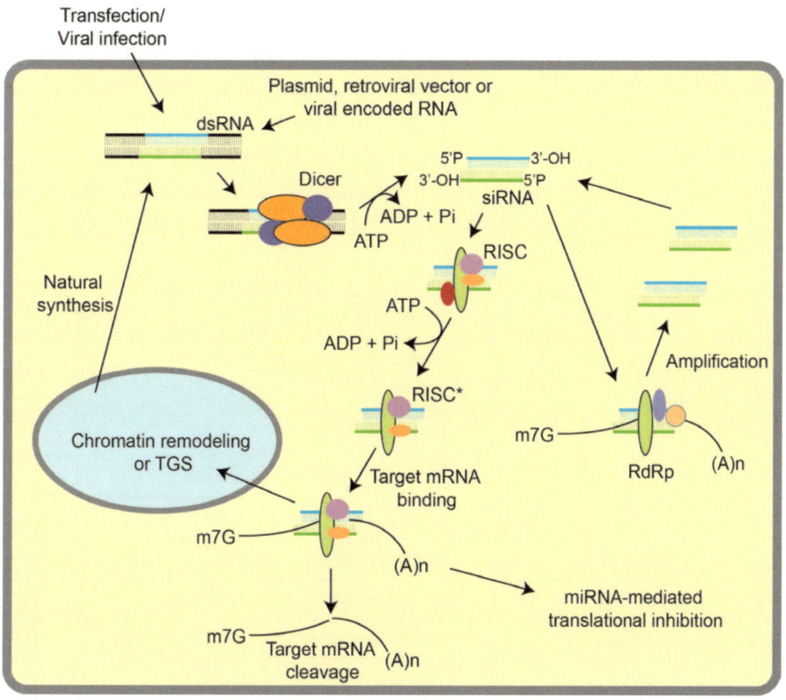

Figure 1. Mechanism of RNAi-mediated silencing. The model demonstrates double-stranded RNA (dsRNA) can generate either from exogenous natural sources, such as a viral infection, exogenous artificial sources such as transfection, or natural synthesis. The dsRNA is then processed by a multimeric Dicer enzyme to generate siRNA that can be further amplified by RNA-dependent RNA polymerase (RdRp). The siRNA subsequently interacts with an array of proteins to form RNA-induced silencing complex (RISC) that is activated in an ATP-dependent manner. The activated RISC (RISC*) can then induce chromatin remodeling or TGS, or induce target RNA cleavage, or cause miRNA-mediated translational inhibition.

organisms, including *S. pombe*, *Arabidopsis thaliana* (CARPEL FACTORY [CAF]), *Drosophila* (DCR-1 and DCR-2), *C. elegans* (DCR-1), mouse, and humans. In addition to RNAi, Dicer also assists in the generation of microRNAs in multiple organisms [29].

4.2. RNA-Induced Silencing Complex (RISC)

RISC is a ribonucleoprotein complex that fragments mRNAs through the production of a sequence-specific nuclease. At first, while working on *Drosophila* embryo extracts, Zamore and his colleagues identified ~250 kDa precursor complex, which turns into an activated complex of 100 kDa upon addition of ATP. However, Hannon and his colleagues found a 500-kDa complex from *Drosophila* S2 cells [30, 31]. The siRNA is an important part of RISC and was the first to be identified. It acts as a template and guides RISC to the target mRNA molecule. To date, a number of RISC protein components are known in *Drosophila* and mammalian species. Interestingly, these components are not completely overlapping, which suggests the developmental stage-specific or evolutionarily non-conserved nature of the components of RISC complex [24].

The first RISC protein component identified was Agronaute-2, a *C. elegans* RDE-1 homologue [32]. Argonaute (AGO) proteins are part of an evolutionarily conserved protein family and they play a central role in RNAi, determination of stem cell developmental regulation, and tumorigenesis. AGOs are ~100 kDa highly basic proteins that contain N-terminal PAZ and mid- and C-terminal PIWI domains [33]. The PAZ domain is an RNA-binding module, which is involved in protein–protein interactions, whereas PIWI is essentially required for target cleavage. Some AGO proteins that are involved in RNAi are listed in the Table 2.

Species	Argonaute homolog	Essentiality for RNAi	Citations
Arabidopsis	AGO1	Essential for co-suppression and PTGS	
	ZWILE	Non-essential	
Tetrahymena	TWI1	Essential for DNA elimination	
Neurospora	QDE2	Required component of RISC	
C. elegans	RDE-1	Forms complex with Dicer	
	ALG-1	Nonessential	
	ALG-2	Nonessential	
	PPW-1	Essential for germline RNAi	
Drosophila	Aubergine	Localizes with dsRBP Staufen and RNA helicase Vasa. Essential for maturation-dependent RNAi generation.	
	dAgro1	Essential in embryos, acts downstream of RNAi generation	
	dAgo2	Required component of RISC	
	dAgo3	Prediction based on DNA sequence	
	PIWI	Essential for PTGS and TGS	
Mammals (human)	EIF2C2/hAgo2	Part of RISC complex and catalyzes the miRNA –directed cleavage	

Table 2. Argonaute homolog proteins in RNAi

Some RISC components are non-AGO proteins, including dFXR and VIG in *Drosophila,* the fragile X mental retardation 1 (FMR1) homolog in *Drosophila*, and germin3/4 in mammals [34].

4.3. RNA helicase

RNA helicases cause unwinding of dsRNA. However, Dicer contains its own helicase activity in the N-terminal helicase domain. Hence, the helicase proteins putatively function downstream of the RISC complex. Two major RNA helicase families are involved in RNAi [35]. SDE3 from *A. thaliana* and its homologous proteins in mouse, human, and *Drosophila* constitute the first such helicase family. The second family contains Upf1p from yeast and an Upf1 homologue (SMG-2) in *C. elegans*. The Upf1/SMG-2 is characterized by cysteine-rich motif conserved across species and multiple C-terminal Ser-Gln (SQ) doublets. MUT-6, a DEAH-box helicase in *C. elegans* is also putatively involved in transposon suppression. Another RNA helicase Germin3 resides in complex with human AGO protein EIF2C2/hAgo2 [36].

4.4. RNA-dependent RNA polymerase (RdRp)

RdRp catalyzes the amplification and triggering of RNAi, which is usually in small amounts. RdRp catalyzes the siRNA-primed amplification by polymerase chain reaction to convert mRNA into dsRNAs, a long form that is cleaved to produce new siRNAs [37]. Lipardi and his colleagues demonstrated RdRp-like activity in *Drosophila* embryo extracts, but the enzyme responsible for the RdRp activity in the *Drosophila* or human is not known. Some of the RdRps involved in RNAi have been summarized in Table 3.

Species	RdRp homolog	Essentiality for RNAi	Citations
Arabidopsis	SDE1	Essential for PTGS by transgenes but not by viruses	
Neurospora	QDE1	Essential for co-suppression	
C. elegans	EGO1	Essential for germline RNAi	
	RRF1	Essential for RNAi in soma	
	RDE9	Forms complexes with Dicer	

Table 3. RdRps involved in RNAi

5. Various small RNA isoforms related to RNAi

5.1. Small interfering RNAs (siRNAs)

Small interfering RNAs are 21–23-nt-long double-stranded RNA molecules with 2–3-nt overhangs at the 3′ termini. siRNAs are normally generated, as mentioned in the above sections, by the cleavage of long double-stranded RNAs by RNase III (Dicer) [16]. siRNAs must be phosphorylated at the 5′ termini by endogenous kinases to enter into the RISC complex [31]. It is thought that the hydroxylated 3′ termini are essential for the siRNA-primed amplification step catalyzed by RdRps. However, Zamore et al. showed that non-priming alterations in the 3′ hydroxyl group did not adversely affect RNAi-mediated silencing [38]. They went on to explain that siRNAs operate as guide RNAs for gene repression but not as primers in the human and *Drosophila* RNAi pathways [38]. Conversely, Hamada et al. showed in mammalian cells that modifying the 3′ end of the antisense strand of siRNA abolished the RNAi effect, while modifying the 3′ end of the sense strand did not affect the RNAi silencing [39]. These findings support the model that each strand of siRNA has different functions in the RNAi process, and the 3′ hydroxylated end of the antisense strand may prime the amplification. Ambros et al. discovered endogenous siRNA in more than 500 genes in wild-type *C. elegans* [39]. This suggests that siRNA may be a globally conserved and common molecule among species.

5.2. Micro RNAs (miRNAs)

miRNAs are 19–25-nt small RNA species produced by Dicer-mediated cleavage of endogenous ~70-nt noncoding stem-loop precursors. The miRNAs, while allowing mismatches, can either repress the target mRNA translation (mostly in mammals) or facilitate mRNA destruction (mostly in plants) [40]. miRNAs *lin*-4 and *let*-7 were the first ones to be identified in *C. elegans* [40]. So far, about 2000 different miRNAs have been identified in plants, animals, and lower species. While some miRNAs are evolutionarily conserved, others are specific for some developmental stages or are species-specific. Different terminologies are referred to in literature. According to one terminology, the miRNAs with well-characterized functions (e.g., *lin-4 and let-7*) are referred to as small temporal RNAs (stRNAs), while other similar small RNAs of unknown functions are called miRNAs [40]. Multiple miRNAs have been characterized for their physiological roles in cancer and other diseases [41, 42]. Comparisons between siRNA and miRNA have been listed in the Table 4.

Resemblences	
siRNA	**miRNA**
1. The siRNAs require processing from long dsRNAs.	1. The miRNAs require processing from stem-loop precursors that are ~70 nt long.
2. An RNase III enzyme Dicer is required for processing.	2. Dicer is required.
3. The siRNAs are usually ~22 nt long.	3. The miRNAs are also ~22 nt long.
Disparities	
siRNA	**miRNA**
1. The siRNAs are double-stranded structures with 2-nt 3′ overhangs that are formed during cleavage by Dicer.	1. The miRNAs are single-stranded structures.
2. The siRNA require high homology with the mRNA to bind and cleave.	2. The miRNAs can function even with a few mismatched nucleotides.
3. The siRNAs mediate target mRNA cleavage by RISC.	3. The miRNAs can either block target mRNA translation by binding to it or mediate target mRNA cleavage by RISC.
4. The siRNAs are usually triggered by transgene incorporation, viral infection, or active transposons.	4. The miRNAs are constitutively expressed cellular RNA moieties with potential roles in development, and cell proliferation and death.

Table 4. Comparative characteristics of siRNA and miRNA

5.3. Tiny noncoding RNAs (tncRNAs)

Ambros and his colleagues discovered the first tncRNAs in *C. elegans*. They identified and characterized 33 new tncRNAs in *C. elegans* by performing cDNA sequencing and comparative genetics [40]. The tncRNAs are very similar to miRNAs with regard to their size, single-stranded structure, and lack of a precise complementarity to a given mRNA. However, they are distinct with regard to their lack of processing from a "miRNA-like hairpin precursor", and phylogenetic nonconservation. Similarly to miRNA, tncRNAs are transcribed from noncoding sequences. However, their developmental role is not fully understood. According to Ambros and his colleagues, it is plausible that some of the miRNAs might be processed from noncoding mRNAs in the course of RNAi [40].

6. Evolutionary relevance of RNAi in the immunological responses

RNAi may provide a systemic way to immunize an organism against the invasive nucleic acids from viruses and transposons via inducing the RNAi responses. Virus-induced gene silencing (VIGS) in plants is accomplished by RNAi. Multiple genetic links between RNAi and virulence are known. Many plant viruses code for viral suppressors of gene silencing (VSGS). VSGS acts as a virulence determinant, and hence, is required for developing anti-virulence response in the host. In response to the virulence, the host can also modify its PTGS/RNAi mechanisms to prevent future infections. RNAi can even target DNA virus amplification in plants [43]. VIGS mechanisms exist not only in plants and nematodes but also in other species; for example, flock house virus (FHV), a virus that infects *Drosophila*, also codes for a potential silencing suppressor (b2) [24]. Nonetheless, the precise function of RNAi in mammalian antiviral defense is not clear.

RNAi also plays a crucial role in the development process of multicellular organisms. When mutated, *CARPEL FACTORY*, a Dicer homologue in *Arabidopsis*, can cause developmentally defective leaves and induce overproliferation of floral meristems. Inactivation of Dicer by mutations causes developmental problems and sterility in *C. elegans*. Mutations in AGO protein influence normal development in *Drosophila* as well. Hence, components of RNAi pathway play a significant role in normal development, but such components and the affiliated gene products play crucial roles in related but distinct gene regulation pathways [23].

A potential role of RNAi and human disease pathogenesis has been proposed due to association of RNA binding proteins with RISC complex, such as Vasa intronic gene (VIG) and the fragile X mental retardation protein (FMRP) *Drosophila* homologue [36].

7. RNAi as a functional genomics tool and its applications for therapy

RNAi technology is applicable for gene silencing in many species. RNAi has been used extensively in *C. elegans* for functional genomics. High-throughput investigation of most of the

~19,000 genes has been accomplished. Ahringer and his colleagues produced an RNAi library, representing ~86% of the genes of *C. elegans* [15]. This strategy has been successfully attempted in multiple other model organisms, including human [44].

RNAi has also been utilized successfully in mammalian cells [44]. Various methods have been employed for siRNA knockdown of specific genes in mammalian cells. DNA-vector-mediated RNAi silences genes transiently in mammalian cells, while other expression systems are used for stable silencing. The promoters of RNA polymerase (pol) II and III (U6 and H1, alone or together) have been used for stable silencing. Furthermore, tRNA promoter-based systems have been used for this purpose. However, pol III-based short hairpin RNA (shRNA) expression systems (e.g., H1 RNA pol-based pSuper vector) are suitable choices. Retroviral-vector-based delivery of siRNAs has also been utilized for more efficient silencing. Two classes of retrovirus vectors have been employed: (1) HIV-1-derived lentivirus vectors and (2) Oncoretrovirus-based vectors, such as Moloney murine leukemia virus (MoMuLV) and Murine stem cell virus (MSCV). Transgenic mice have been established with germline transmission of a shRNA expression cassette for silencing of genes not targeted by homologous recombination-based approaches [45]. Desirable applications of this technique include inducible and cell type-specific expression patterns.

The use of RNAi is not limited to the determination of mammalian gene function, and also could be used for treating viral infections and cancer [46, 47]. Viral and human genes that are needed for viral replication can be attacked to generate viral-resistant host cells or to treat viral infections [47]. Oncogenes, which accelerate cancer growth, can be targeted by RNAi [48, 49]. Targeting of molecules important for neovascularization could prevent tumor growth [50]. This book presented several chapters with detailed discussions of therapeutic aspects of the RNAi in immune, blood, cancer, and brain diseases. We refer readers to those chapters (by Hu et al.; Gu; and Cho and Kim) rather to continue repeated information here.

8. Conclusions

Fast progress in RNAi technology has shown promise for use in reverse genetics and therapy. However, mechanistic complexities of this technology still need to be determined. RNAi has now been established as a revolutionary tool for functional genomics in organisms. Multiple studies have defined the role of RNAi in mammalian and plant defense systems. A plethora of studies have utilized RNAi technology to modulate gene expression. RNAi-based full genomic screens have allowed identification of specific genes, controlling a given trait with high accuracy. Further studies will continue to unravel the unlimited potential of RNAi to serve humankind.

http://dx.doi.org/10.5772/61760

Author details

Devi Singh[1*], Sarika Chaudhary[2], Rajendra Kumar[3], Preeti Sirohi[1], Kamiya Mehla[4], Anil Sirohi[1], Shashi Kumar[5], Pooran Chand[1] and Pankaj Kumar Singh[4]

*Address all correspondence to: devisingh11@gmail.com

1 Molecular Biology laboratory, Department of Genetics and Plant Breeding, Sardar Vallabhbhai Patel University of Agriculture and Technology, Meerut, India

2 Institute of Genomics and Integrative Biology, New Delhi, India

3 Department of Agri-Biotechnology, SardarVallabhbhai Patel University of Agricultureand Technology, Meerut, India

4 Eppley Institute for Research in Cancer and Allied Diseases, UNMC, Omaha, Nebraska, USA

5 International Centre for Genetic Engineering and Biotechnology, New Delhi, India

References

[1] Yanai I, DeLisi C. The society of genes: Networks of functional links between genes from comparative genomics. Genome Biol. 2002;3:research0064. DOI: 10.1186/gb-2002-3-11-research0064

[2] Gura T. A silence that speaks volumes. Nature. 2000;404:804–808. DOI: 10.1038/35009245

[3] Kim H, Kim JS. A guide to genome engineering with programmable nucleases. Nat Rev Genet. 2014;15:321–334. DOI: 10.1038/nrg3686

[4] Scherer LJ, Rossi JJ. Approaches for the sequence-specific knockdown of mRNA. Nat Biotechnol. 2003;21:1457–1465. DOI: 10.1038/nbt915

[5] Jorgensen RA, Cluster PD, English J, Que Q, Napoli CA. Chalcone synthase cosuppression phenotypes in petunia flowers: Comparison of sense vs. antisense constructs and single-copy vs. complex T-DNA sequences. Plant Mol Biol. 1996;31:957–973. DOI: 10.1007/BF00040715

[6] Cogoni C, Macino G. Post-transcriptional gene silencing across kingdoms. Curr Opin Genet Dev. 2000;10:638–643. DOI: 10.1016/S0959-437X(00)00134-9

[7] Napoli C, Lemieux C, Jorgensen R. Introduction of a chimeric chalcone synthase gene into petunia results in reversible co-suppression of homologous genes in trans. Plant Cell. 1990;2:279–289. DOI: 10.1105/tpc.2.4.279

[8] Romano N, Macino G. Quelling: Transient inactivation of gene expression in Neurospora crassa by transformation with homologous sequences. Mol Microbiol. 1992;6:3343–3353. DOI: 10.1111/j.1365-2958.1992.tb02202.x

[9] Hammond SM, Caudy AA, Hannon GJ. Post-transcriptional gene silencing by double-stranded RNA. Nat Rev Genet. 2001;2:110–119. DOI: 10.1038/35052556

[10] Guo S, Kemphues KJ. par-1, a gene required for establishing polarity in C. elegans embryos, encodes a putative Ser/Thr kinase that is asymmetrically distributed. Cell. 1995;81:611–620. DOI: 10.1016/0092-8674(95)90082-9

[11] Fire A, Xu S, Montgomery MK, Kostas SA, Driver SE, Mello CC. Potent and specific genetic interference by double-stranded RNA in Caenorhabditis elegans. Nature. 1998;391:806–811. DOI: 10.1038/35888

[12] Timmons L, Fire A. Specific interference by ingested dsRNA. Nature. 1998;395:854. DOI: 10.1038/27579

[13] Timmons L, Court DL, Fire A. Ingestion of bacterially expressed dsRNAs can produce specific and potent genetic interference in Caenorhabditis elegans. Gene. 2001;263:103–112. DOI: 10.1016/S0378-1119(00)00579-5

[14] Dykxhoorn DM, Novina CD, Sharp PA. Killing the messenger: Short RNAs that silence gene expression. Nat Rev Mol Cell Biol. 2003;4:457–467. DOI: 10.1038/nrm1129

[15] Fraser AG, Kamath RS, Zipperlen P, Martinez-Campos M, Sohrmann M, Ahringer J. Functional genomic analysis of C. elegans chromosome I by systematic RNA interference. Nature. 2000;408:325–330. DOI: 10.1038/35042517

[16] Zamore PD, Tuschl T, Sharp PA, Bartel DP. RNAi: Double-stranded RNA directs the ATP-dependent cleavage of mRNA at 21 to 23 nucleotide intervals. Cell. 2000;101:25–33. DOI: 10.1016/S0092-8674(00)80620-0

[17] Elbashir SM, Lendeckel W, Tuschl T. RNA interference is mediated by 21- and 22-nucleotide RNAs. Genes Dev. 2001;15:188–200. DOI: 10.1101/gad.862301

[18] Tran N, Raponi M, Dawes IW, Arndt GM. Control of specific gene expression in mammalian cells by co-expression of long complementary RNAs. FEBS Lett. 2004;573:127–134. DOI: 10.1016/j.febslet.2004.07.075

[19] Gantier MP, Williams BR. The response of mammalian cells to double-stranded RNA. Cytokine Growth Factor Rev. 2007;18:363–371. DOI: 10.1016/j.cytogfr.2007.06.016

[20] Bass BL. RNA interference. The short answer. Nature. 2001;411:428–429. DOI: 10.1038/35078175

[21] Elbashir SM, Harborth J, Lendeckel W, Yalcin A, Weber K, Tuschl T. Duplexes of 21-nucleotide RNAs mediate RNA interference in cultured mammalian cells. Nature. 2001;411:494–498. DOI: 10.1038/35078107

[22] Hannon GJ. RNA interference. Nature. 2002;418:244–251. DOI: 10.1038/418244a

[23] Zeng Y, Cullen BR. RNA interference in human cells is restricted to the cytoplasm. RNA. 2002;8:855–860. DOI: 10.1017.S1355838202020071

[24] Denli AM, Hannon GJ. RNAi: An ever-growing puzzle. Trends Biochem Sci. 2003;28:196–201. DOI: 10.1016/S0968-0004(03)00058-6

[25] Pal-Bhadra M, Bhadra U, Birchler JA. RNAi related mechanisms affect both transcriptional and posttranscriptional transgene silencing in Drosophila. Mol Cell. 2002;9:315–327. DOI: 10.1016/S1097-2765(02)00440-9

[26] Volpe TA, Kidner C, Hall IM, Teng G, Grewal SI, Martienssen RA. Regulation of heterochromatic silencing and histone H3 lysine-9 methylation by RNAi. Science. 2002;297:1833–1837. DOI: 10.1126/science.1074973

[27] Bernstein E, Caudy AA, Hammond SM, Hannon GJ. Role for a bidentate ribonuclease in the initiation step of RNA interference. Nature. 2001;409:363–366. DOI: 10.1038/35053110

[28] Zhang H, Kolb FA, Brondani V, Billy E, Filipowicz W. Human Dicer preferentially cleaves dsRNAs at their termini without a requirement for ATP. EMBO J. 2002;21:5875–5885. DOI: 10.1093/emboj/cdf582

[29] Hutvagner G, McLachlan J, Pasquinelli AE, Balint E, Tuschl T, Zamore PD. A cellular function for the RNA-interference enzyme Dicer in the maturation of the let-7 small temporal RNA. Science. 2001;293:834–838. DOI: 10.1126/science.1062961

[30] Nykanen A, Haley B, Zamore PD. ATP requirements and small interfering RNA structure in the RNA interference pathway. Cell. 2001;107:309–321. DOI: 10.1016/S0092-8674(01)00547-5

[31] Denli AM, Tops BB, Plasterk RH, Ketting RF, Hannon GJ. Processing of primary microRNAs by the Microprocessor complex. Nature. 2004;432:231–235. DOI: 10.1038/nature03049

[32] Tabara H, Sarkissian M, Kelly WG, Fleenor J, Grishok A, Timmons L, Fire A, Mello CC. The rde-1 gene, RNA interference, and transposon silencing in C. elegans. Cell. 1999;99:123–132. DOI: 10.1016/S0092-8674(00)81644-X

[33] Szweykowska-Kulinska Z, Jarmolowski A, Figlerowicz M. RNA interference and its role in the regulation of eucaryotic gene expression. Acta Biochim Pol. 2003;50:217–229. DOI: 035001217

[34] Caudy AA, Myers M, Hannon GJ, Hammond SM. Fragile X-related protein and VIG associate with the RNA interference machinery. Genes Dev. 2002;16:2491–2496. DOI: 10.1101/gad.1025202

[35] Carmell MA, Xuan Z, Zhang MQ, Hannon GJ. The Argonaute family: Tentacles that reach into RNAi, developmental control, stem cell maintenance, and tumorigenesis. Genes Dev. 2002;16:2733–2742. DOI: 10.1101/gad.1026102

[36] Martinez J, Patkaniowska A, Urlaub H, Luhrmann R, Tuschl T. Single-stranded antisense siRNAs guide target RNA cleavage in RNAi. Cell. 2002;110:563–574. DOI: 10.1016/S0092-8674(02)00908-X

[37] Lipardi C, Wei Q, Paterson BM. RNAi as random degradative PCR: siRNA primers convert mRNA into dsRNAs that are degraded to generate new siRNAs. Cell. 2001;107:297–307. DOI: 10.1016/S0092-8674(01)00537-2

[38] Schwarz DS, Hutvagner G, Haley B, Zamore PD. Evidence that siRNAs function as guides, not primers, in the Drosophila and human RNAi pathways. Mol Cell. 2002;10:537–548. DOI: 10.1016/S1097-2765(02)00651-2

[39] Hamada M, Ohtsuka T, Kawaida R, Koizumi M, Morita K, Furukawa H, Imanishi T, Miyagishi M, Taira K. Effects on RNA interference in gene expression (RNAi) in cultured mammalian cells of mismatches and the introduction of chemical modifications at the 3'-ends of siRNAs. Antisense Nucleic Acid Drug Dev. 2002;12:301–309. DOI: 10.1089/108729002761381285

[40] Ambros V, Lee RC, Lavanway A, Williams PT, Jewell D. MicroRNAs and other tiny endogenous RNAs in C. elegans. Curr Biol. 2003;13:807–818. DOI: 10.1016/S0960-9822(03)00287-2

[41] Singh PK, Brand RE, Mehla K. MicroRNAs in pancreatic cancer metabolism. Nat Rev Gastroenterol Hepatol. 2012;9:334–344. DOI: 10.1038/nrgastro.2012.63

[42] Singh PK, Mehla K, Hollingsworth MA, Johnson KR. Regulation of aerobic glycolysis by microRNAs in Cancer. Mol Cell Pharmacol. 2011;3:125–134. DOI: 10.4255/mcpharmacol.11.17

[43] Pooggin M, Shivaprasad PV, Veluthambi K, Hohn T. RNAi targeting of DNA virus in plants. Nat Biotechnol. 2003;21:131–132. DOI: 10.1038/nbt0203-131b

[44] Hu G, Kim J, Xu Q, Leng Y, Orkin SH, Elledge SJ. A genome-wide RNAi screen identifies a new transcriptional module required for self-renewal. Genes Dev. 2009;23:837–848. DOI: 10.1101/gad.1769609

[45] Tiscornia G, Singer O, Ikawa M, Verma IM. A general method for gene knockdown in mice by using lentiviral vectors expressing small interfering RNA. Proc Natl Acad Sci U S A. 2003;100:1844–1848. DOI: 10.1073/pnas.0437912100

[46] Whitehurst AW, Bodemann BO, Cardenas J, Ferguson D, Girard L, Peyton M, Minna JD, Michnoff C, Hao W, Roth MG, Xie XJ, White MA. Synthetic lethal screen identification of chemosensitizer loci in cancer cells. Nature. 2007;446:815–819. DOI: 10.1038/nature05697

[47] Smith JA, White EA, Sowa ME, Powell ML, Ottinger M, Harper JW, Howley PM. Genome-wide siRNA screen identifies SMCX, EP400, and Brd4 as E2-dependent regulators of human papillomavirus oncogene expression. Proc Natl Acad Sci U S A. 2010;107:3752–3757. DOI: 10.1073/pnas.0914818107

[48] Shukla SK, Gunda V, Abrego J, Haridas D, Mishra A, Souchek J, Chaika NV, Yu F, Sasson AR, Lazenby AJ, Batra SK, Singh PK. MUC16-mediated activation of mTOR and c-Myc reprograms pancreatic cancer metabolism. Oncotarget. 2015;6:19118–19131. DOI: NA

[49] Chaika NV, Gebregiworgis T, Lewallen ME, Purohit V, Radhakrishnan P, Liu X, Zhang B, Mehla K, Brown RB, Caffrey T, Yu F, Johnson KR, Powers R, Hollingsworth MA, Singh PK. MUC1 mucin stabilizes and activates hypoxia-inducible factor 1 alpha to regulate metabolism in pancreatic cancer. Proc Natl Acad Sci U S A. 2012;109:13787–13792. DOI: 10.1073/pnas.1203339109

[50] Swanton C, Marani M, Pardo O, Warne PH, Kelly G, Sahai E, Elustondo F, Chang J, Temple J, Ahmed AA, Brenton JD, Downward J, Nicke B. Regulators of mitotic arrest and ceramide metabolism are determinants of sensitivity to paclitaxel and other chemotherapeutic drugs. Cancer Cell. 2007;11:498–512. DOI: 10.1016/j.ccr.2007.04.011

[51] Fagard M, Boutet S, Morel JB, Bellini C, Vaucheret H. AGO1, QDE-2, and RDE-1 are related proteins required for post-transcriptional gene silencing in plants, quelling in fungi, and RNA interference in animals. Proc Natl Acad Sci U S A. 2000;97:11650–11654. DOI: 10.1073/pnas.200217597

[52] Morel JB, Godon C, Mourrain P, Beclin C, Boutet S, Feuerbach F, Proux F, Vaucheret H. Fertile hypomorphic ARGONAUTE (ago1) mutants impaired in post-transcriptional gene silencing and virus resistance. Plant Cell. 2002;14:629–639. DOI: 10.1105/tpc.010358

[53] Mochizuki K, Fine NA, Fujisawa T, Gorovsky MA. Analysis of a piwi-related gene implicates small RNAs in genome rearrangement in tetrahymena. Cell. 2002;110:689–699. DOI: 10.1016/S0092-8674(02)00909-1

[54] Catalanotto C, Azzalin G, Macino G, Cogoni C. Involvement of small RNAs and role of the qde genes in the gene silencing pathway in Neurospora. Genes Dev. 2002;16:790–795. DOI: 10.1101/gad.222402

[55] Tabara H, Yigit E, Siomi H, Mello CC. The dsRNA binding protein RDE-4 interacts with RDE-1, DCR-1, and a DExH-box helicase to direct RNAi in C. elegans. Cell. 2002;109:861–871. DOI: 10.1016/S0092-8674(02)00793-6

[56] Grishok A, Pasquinelli AE, Conte D, Li N, Parrish S, Ha I, Baillie DL, Fire A, Ruvkun G, Mello CC. Genes and mechanisms related to RNA interference regulate expression of the small temporal RNAs that control C. elegans developmental timing. Cell. 2001;106:23–34. DOI: 10.1016/S0092-8674(01)00431-7

[57] Tijsterman M, Ketting RF, Plasterk RH. The genetics of RNA silencing. Annu Rev Genet. 2002;36:489–519. DOI: 10.1146/annurev.genet.36.043002.091619

[58] Kennerdell JR, Yamaguchi S, Carthew RW. RNAi is activated during Drosophila oocyte maturation in a manner dependent on aubergine and spindle-E. Genes Dev. 2002;16:1884–1889. DOI: 10.1101/gad.990802

[59] Williams RW, Rubin GM. ARGONAUTE1 is required for efficient RNA interference in Drosophila embryos. Proc Natl Acad Sci U S A. 2002;99:6889–6894. DOI: 10.1073/pnas.072190799

[60] Hammond SM, Boettcher S, Caudy AA, Kobayashi R, Hannon GJ. Argonaute2, a link between genetic and biochemical analyses of RNAi. Science. 2001;293:1146–1150. DOI: 10.1126/science.1064023

[61] Hutvagner G, Zamore PD. A microRNA in a multiple-turnover RNAi enzyme complex. Science. 2002;297:2056–2060. DOI: 10.1126/science.1073827

[62] Dalmay T, Hamilton A, Rudd S, Angell S, Baulcombe DC. An RNA-dependent RNA polymerase gene in Arabidopsis is required for posttranscriptional gene silencing mediated by a transgene but not by a virus. Cell. 2000;101:543–553. DOI: 10.1016/S0092-8674(00)80864-8

[63] Cogoni C, Macino G. Homology-dependent gene silencing in plants and fungi: a number of variations on the same theme. Curr Opin Microbiol. 1999;2:657–662. DOI: 10.1016/S1369-5274(99)00041-7

[64] Smardon A, Spoerke JM, Stacey SC, Klein ME, Mackin N, Maine EM. EGO-1 is related to RNA-directed RNA polymerase and functions in germ-line development and RNA interference in C. elegans. Curr Biol. 2000;10:169–178. DOI: 10.1016/S0960-9822(00)00323-7

[65] Sijen T, Fleenor J, Simmer F, Thijssen KL, Parrish S, Timmons L, Plasterk RH, Fire A. On the role of RNA amplification in dsRNA-triggered gene silencing. Cell. 2001;107:465–476. DOI: 10.1016/S0092-8674(01)00576-1

Chapter 3

The Role of Immune Modulatory MicroRNAs in Tumors

Barbara Seliger, Anne Meinhardt and Doerte Falke

Additional information is available at the end of the chapter

http://dx.doi.org/10.5772/61805

Abstract

Tumors could evade the control of $CD8^+$ T and/or NK cell-mediated surveillance by distinct immune escape strategies. These include the aberrant expression of HLA class I antigens, coinhibitory or costimulatory molecules, and components of the interferon (IFN) signal transduction pathway. In addition, alterations of the tumor microenvironment could interfere with a proper antitumoral immune response by downregulating or inhibiting the frequency and/or activity of immune effector cells and professional antigen presenting cells. Based on the identification as major mediators of the posttranscriptional silencing of gene expression, microRNAs (miRNAs) have been suggested to play a key role in many biological processes known to be involved in neoplastic transformation. Indeed, miRNA expression is frequently deregulated in many cancer types and could have tumor-suppressive as well as oncogenic potential. This review focused on the characterization of miRNAs, which are involved in the control of the immune surveillance or immune escape of tumors and their use as potential diagnostic and prognostic biomarkers as well as therapeutic targets. Moreover, miRNAs can have dual activities by affecting the neoplastic and immunogenic phenotype of tumors.

Keywords: APM, IFN, immune escape, microRNA, tumor microenvironment

1. Introduction

Tumors have developed different strategies to evade immune recognition by cytotoxic T lymphocytes (CTLs) as well as natural killer (NK) cells. This is caused by alterations of the tumor itself, changes of the tumor microenvironment (TME), reduced frequency, and impaired function of diverse immune subpopulations. The processes leading to immune evasion of tumors are diverse and could be associated with structural alterations and/or deregulation of genes/proteins from tumor cells, but also from different immune cells important for recognition and killing of tumor cells or in the induction of immune suppression. The identification of microRNAs (miRNAs), involved in the RNA interference (RNAi)-based control of these immune modulatory molecules, clarified the complexity of the mechanisms conditioning tumor immune escape. This review is focused on the identification and characterization of immune modulatory miRNAs (im-miRNAs) in tumors, thereby altering the antitumoral immune response by miRNAi-mediated RNAi.

2. The MHC class I antigen processing and presentation machinery (APM)

The major histocompatibility complex class I (MHC) molecules present an array of peptide epitopes for surveillance by $CD8^+$ T cells. These peptides are classically derived from proteins synthesized in the cytosol. Upon proteasomal degradation of ubiquitinated proteins, the yielded peptides are then transported into the endoplasmic reticulum (ER) via the heterodimeric peptide transporter associated with antigen processing (TAP). The peptide transport into the ER is ATP dependent and sequence specific. The TAP heterodimer associates in ER with a number of other proteins to form the peptide loading complex (PLC). These include the chaperone tapasin, which recruits MHC class I heavy chain (HC)/β_2-microglobulin (β_2-m) dimers and calreticulin. The peptides are either trimmed by ER-resident aminopeptidases or directly loaded onto MHC class I molecules [1]. Upon peptide loading, the PLC dissociates from the trimer consisting of the MHC class I HC, β_2-m, and peptide is then transported via the trans Golgi to the cell surface and exposed to $CD8^+$ CTLs [1].

3. Immune stimulatory and immune inhibitory molecules and immune response

An effective T-cell response requires two signals. The first is mediated by the interaction with MHC class I antigens on the antigen-presenting cells (APC), and the second is mediated by the interaction of B7 family members on APC with CD28 or CTLA4 on T cells. The prototypes of B7 family members are B7-1 (CD80) and B7-2 (CD86). During the last years, the B7 family was growing consisting of B7-H1 (PDL-1), B7-H2, B7-H3, B7-H4, and B7-H6 molecules [2, 3]. While B7-H1 and B7-H4 represent coinhibitory molecules, B7-H2 was identified as costimulatory molecule, which is mainly expressed on B cells, monocytes and dendritic cells (DC): B7-H2 binds to the receptor ICOS, which results in activation of T cells through phosphatidylinositol-3-kinase-dependent signal transduction pathways and in the induction of Th2 cell-mediated immune response, proliferation, and cytokine production [4]. The role of B7-H3 is currently controversially discussed and depends on the cell types analyzed, demonstrating either costimulatory or coinhibitory activity. Regarding B7-H4, its expression is primarily restricted to activated T cells, B cells, monocytes, and DCs [5, 6]. B7-H4 is not detected in the majority of normal tissues and cells but is overexpressed in a variety of tumor tissues. B7-H6 has been identified as ligand for the NK cell receptor NKp30 and is detectable on surface or in the cytosol of tumor cells and as soluble factor in the peritoneal fluid [7], while it is not expressed on healthy cells. The interaction of B7-H6 with NKp30 is involved in NK cell

http://dx.doi.org/10.5772/61805

responses [8]. It is noteworthy that many other coinhibitory molecules have also been identified and their role on immune responses is currently under investigation [2, 3].

4. Features of the interferon-γ-mediated signal transduction

Interferons (IFN) are a group of pleiotropic cytokines that play a key role in the intercellular communication during innate and adaptive immune responses, in particular in the host defense against viral and bacterial infections and neoplastic transformation [9]. The IFN family could be classified into type I and type II IFNs, which differ in their activity regarding immune modulation [10].

IFN-γ belongs to the type II IFN and is a central regulator of immune responses by controlling and modulating the expression of targets essential for cell-cell communication and cellular interactions. It is secreted by activated T cells, NK cells, and macrophages and induced by DC and monocytes stimulated with bacterial cell wall components [11]. IFN-γ exerts its activity by binding to its heterodimeric receptor consisting of IFN-γ-R1 and IFN-γ-R2 subunits [12, 13]. This results in the dimerization of the receptor subunits followed by activation (transphosphorylation) of the receptor-associated tyrosine kinases JAK1 and JAK2 belonging to the Janus kinase (JAK) family and phosphorylation and dimerization of the JAK-associated STAT1 transcription factor. The activated STAT1 is translocated into the nucleus and recruited to the IFN-γ-activated sequence (GAS) element of the promoters of the STAT1 target genes leading to their transcriptional activation.

IFN-γ-regulated genes can be classified into primary and secondary responsive genes. Primary responsive genes are induced early due to the binding of STAT dimers to the GAS element in the promoter region of target genes, like IRF1, CXCL9, and CXCL10 [14]. IRF1 binds to IFN-stimulated response elements (ISRE) and modulates gene induction of the secondary responsive genes. IFN-γ induced the transcription of MHC class I and class II antigens and of many APM components and at high concentrations could lead to a caspase-dependent apoptosis. In addition, IFN-γ is involved in amplifying toll-like receptor (TLR) signaling by increasing or inhibiting the transcription of TLRs, chemokines, and cytokines [15, 16]. Furthermore, IFN-γ promotes the induction of SOCs proteins (suppressor of cytokine signaling), which inhibit IFN-γ signaling by a negative feedback loop, resulting in the inactivation of JAK1 and JAK2 [17]. Moreover, IFN-γ signaling is controlled by inhibiting JAK1, JAK2, and IFN-γ-R1 via dephosphorylation mediated by SH2-domain-containing protein tyrosine phosphatase 2 [18], by proteasomal degradation of JAK1 and JAK2 [18] and by inhibition of STAT1, which is mediated by the protein inhibitor of activated STAT1 [19].

5. Distinct levels of tumor immune escape

Tumors have developed different strategies to escape immune surveillance, which could occur at the level of immune cells, tumor micromilieu, and the tumor itself (Figure 1). The frequency, activity, and function of CD8+ and CD4+ T lymphocytes, DC, NK cells, and B cells are often downregulated in peripheral blood of tumor patients, while the number of immune-suppressive myeloid-derived suppressor cells (MDSC), NKT cells, and regulatory T cells (Treg) is upregulated [20-23].

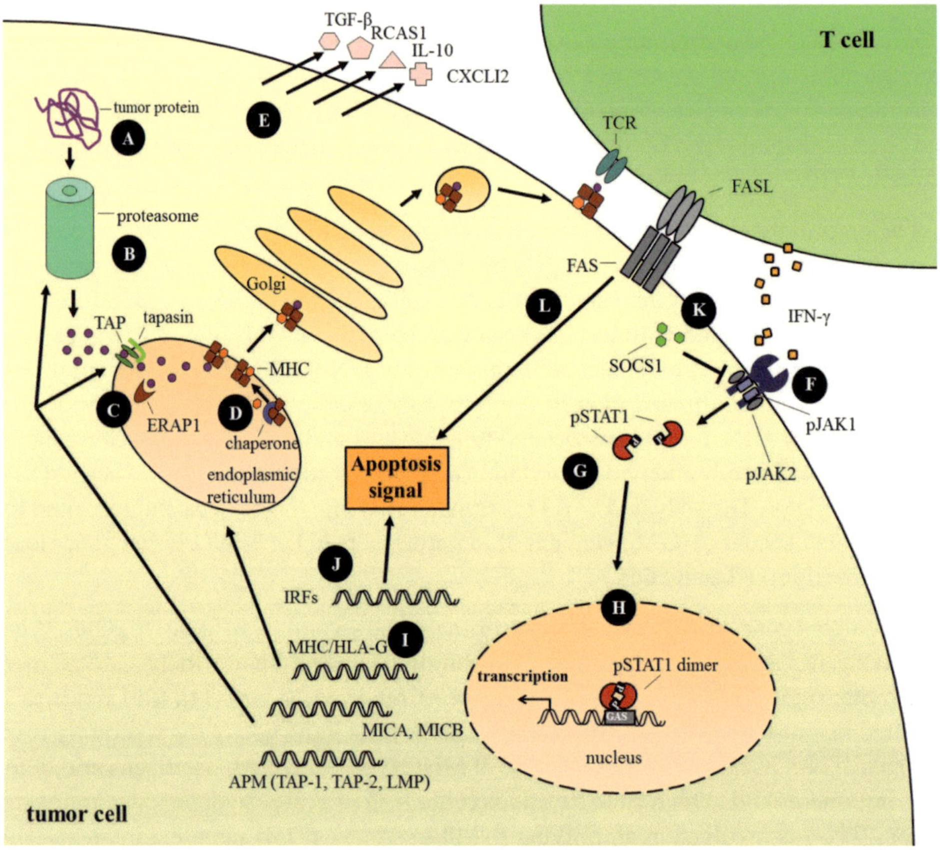

Figure 1. Tumor immune escape mechanisms containing (A) loss of tumor antigen expression; (B) variations in tumor antigen processing; (C) defects in the peptide transporter TAP, chaperone tapasin, and protease ERAP1; (D) defects in expression of MHC class I heavy chain and β_2-microglobulin; (E) release of anti-inflammatory cytokines; (F) downregulation of IFN-γ-R1, JAK1, JAK2, STAT1, and STAT2; (G) altered phosphorylation states of STAT1; (H) impaired upregulation of IFN-γ regulated genes (MHC class I, APM); (I) upregulated expression of HLA-G; (J) altered methylation pattern of IRF; (K) overexpression of SOCS1; and (L) protection from T-cell-mediated apoptosis.

The tumor microenvironment (TME) consists of various cellular and soluble factors and is of clinical relevance since its composition significantly correlates with the tumor patients' outcome. These include different cellular components, such as fibroblasts, blood vessels, immune cells, stroma cells, extracellular matrix, and soluble factors such as immune-suppressive cytokines, like interleukin (IL)-10, transforming growth factor (TGF)-β, metabolites, arginase and prostaglandin, hypoxia, and pH, which negatively interfere with the antitumoral immune responses.

In tumors, an aggressive and deregulated growth of neoplastic transformed cells, which overexpress proangiogenic factors, such as the vascular endothelial growth factor (VEGF), leads to the development of organized blood vessels. These blood vessels are fundamentally different from the normal vasculature. Tumor-associated fibroblasts (TAF) represent the major constituents of the tumor stroma and produce growth factors, including the VEGF and inhibitory cytokines that activate extracellular matrix thereby contributing to the tumor growth.

Furthermore, cancer is often driven by inflammation mediated by monocytes and tumor-associated macrophages (TAM), which belong to the innate immune cells. Macrophages could be classified in type 1 and 2 macrophages. While M1 macrophages express a series of proinflammatory cytokines, chemokines and effector molecules, the M2 macrophages express a wide array of anti-inflammatory molecules, including IL-10, IL-35, TGF-β, and adenosine. TAMs are mainly of the M2 phenotype and secrete different cytokines, chemokines and proteases, which promote tumor angiogenesis, growth, metastasis as well as immune suppression.

In addition to TAM and TAF, MDSC represent a heterogeneous population derived from myeloid progenitors [20]. They can promote tumor growth by enhancing angiogenesis or suppression of innate and adaptive immune responses. Regarding the innate immune cells, MDSCs suppress NK cell cytotoxicity, promote M2 macrophage differentiation, and modulate the priming activity of mature DC [24]. Moreover, MDSCs suppress T-cell responses by induction of apoptosis, secretion of immune modulatory factors, modulation of amino acid metabolism, restriction of T-cell homing, and induction of Treg [25-28]. Tregs suppress the activity of immune cells and maintain immune tolerance to self-antigens. They express CD4, CD25 and FoxP3 [22]. The elevated numbers of Tregs in cancer is due to their efficient migration into the tumor sites [29], local expansion in the tumor environment[29], and *de novo* generation within the tumor [30].

5.1. Alterations of the tumors

Immune escape mechanisms include loss or downregulation of HLA class I antigens and/or components of the antigen processing machinery (APM), upregulation of nonclassical HLA-G and HLA-E antigens, and coinhibitory molecules, including PDL-1, as well as alterations of signaling transduction cascades, including in particular the IFN signaling pathway [31]. The frequency of these different mechanisms highly varied between tumor (sub)types and is often correlated with a worse prognosis and reduced survival of tumor patients.

5.1.1. MHC class I abnormalities

The classical MHC class I pathway and the APM components are involved in eradication of developing tumors [32]. Since $CD8^+$ CTLs recognize and eliminate cells presenting tumor antigens via HLA class I molecules, loss of HLA class I expression results in evasion of CTL-mediated cell death [33]. Abnormalities of HLA class I antigens are often due to downregulation of various components of the MHC class I APM, in particular of TAP, tapasin, β_2-m, and MHC class I HC. Structural alterations of these components are rare, while MHC class I defects are mainly due to deregulation of the different components, which could be controlled at the transcriptional, epigenetic (methylation, acetylation), posttranscriptional (e.g., microRNAs, protein degradation), or posttranslational (phosphorylation) level.

HLA-G has been demonstrated as a nonclassical HLA class I antigen, which is in general only expressed on immune privileged organs, but also on many tumors of distinct origin [34]. The overexpression of HLA-G or secretion of soluble HLA-G are directly associated with tumor progression and reduced patients' survival. It suppresses antitumoral immune responses by binding to receptors of various immune populations, thereby inhibiting the sensitivity to CTL- and NK cell-mediated lysis in particular [34]. In contrast, tumor cells with deficient expression of classical HLA class I molecules are eradicated by NK cells.

5.1.2. Check points as important regulators of immune response

During carcinogenesis, members of the B7-family play a key regulatory role of both stimulatory and inhibitory T-cell responses, which depends on the available B7 ligand and receptor on the respective target and immune cells [35, 36]. Interestingly, B7-H1 and B7-H4 were often overexpressed on tumors leading to impaired immune recognition. By interaction with these coinhibitory molecules, the intensity of the T-cell responses is reduced by raising the threshold of activation, halting proliferation, enhancing apoptosis, and inhibiting the differentiation of effector cells [37].

5.1.3. Role of IFN-γ in cancer immunogenicity

Abnormalities of MHC class I expression on tumor cells due to the downregulation or loss of APM component expression are common mechanisms, by which tumor cells can escape from anti-tumor-specific immunity [38, 39]. In addition, tumor cells are often not susceptible to treatment with IFN-γ, which could be due to structural alterations or deregulation of constituents of the IFN signal pathway. Several studies confirmed that defects in the IFN-γ receptor signaling cascade could be occur at multiple steps of this pathway, including lack of the expression of the IFN-γ-R1, abnormal forms of JAK2, lack of expression of JAK1 [40], altered phosphorylation, repressed STAT1 expression, and overexpression of SOCS1. The latter results in an increased negative feedback regulation of the IFN-γ signal cascade. The defects in the IFN-γ receptor signaling cascade caused impaired expression of IFN-γ regulated genes.

Previous studies demonstrated that IFN-γ responsive genes are frequently downregulated in tumor cells due to impaired IRF1 expression as well as defective transcriptional and posttranscriptional regulation of components involved in the IFN-γ signal transduction pathway. The loss of the IFN-γ-mediated upregulation of TAP in a renal cell carcinoma is associated with the lack of IRF1 and STAT1 binding activities as well as JAK1, JAK2, and STAT1 phosphorylation [41]. This impaired IFN-γ-mediated phosphorylation could not be restored by JAK1 and/or JAK2 gene transfer. Furthermore, an impaired STAT1-phosphorylation associated with the loss of IFN-γ-mediated MHC class I upregulation was also reported in melanoma and colorectal carcinoma cells [42].

IFN-γ treatment is able to restore the expression of many genes belonging to the MHC class I APM [43, 44]. As a consequence, anti-tumor-specific immune responses can be induced, suggesting that IFN-γ acts as key regulator of immunogenicity [45]. Its antitumoral activity includes also the induction of apoptosis and inhibition of cell proliferation by STAT1 activation, which induces expression of cell cycle inhibitor, CDKN1A [46]. In addition, the IFN-γ-mediated upregulation of MHC class I antigens could be due to DNA demethylation of MHC class I APM genes, suggesting that IFN-γ acts as an epigenetic modifier of APM components [47]. Therefore, IFN-γ is a major player in the regulatory network combating tumor cell proliferation and tumor survival.

6. Features of miRNAs

miRNAs are small noncoding ~22 nucleotide long regulatory RNAs encoded in the human genome, which control the posttranscriptional gene expression by binding to the 3′-untranslated region (UTR) of mRNA of target genes, thereby affecting their stability and/or their translation [48]. An individual miRNA could target numerous cellular mRNAs, while single miRNA can be regulated by several proteins [49, 50]. miRNAs have emerged as key players in the posttranscriptional control of gene expression and based on their prediction appear to be directly involved in the expression of at least 50% of all protein-coding genes in mammals [51].

A strong relationship between miRNAs and human cancer has been developed during the past years. High throughput analysis allows the comparison of miRNA expression pattern in normal and tumor tissues demonstrating global changes within the miRNA expression in different malignancies. Interestingly, the miRNA genes were frequently located at fragile sites and cancer-associated chromosomal regions. The deregulation of the biogenesis and expression of miRNAs is involved in the initiation as well as progression of tumors, metastasis formation, and therapy resistance [52]. Furthermore, miRNAs can participate in reprogramming components of the tissue tumor microenvironment (TME) in order to promote tumorgenicity [53]. In the following sections, miRNAs are described as powerful RNAi inducing regulators of immune modulatory genes involved in escape from immune surveillance. Moreover, this review highlights some miRNAs and their roles in immune escape and discusses these miRNAs as putative targets for (immune) therapy (Figure 2).

6.1. Antigen processing and presentation machinery and miRNAs

Recent studies showed identified miRNAs able to affect the expression of APM components. Microarray analysis of miRNA-9 overexpressing nasopharyngeal carcinoma cells demonstrated that miRNA-9 controls the expression of components of the classical MHC class I pathway. miRNA-9 targets many IFN-induced genes and MHC class I APM molecules, such as the proteasome subunits PSMB8 and PSMB10, TAP1, β_2-m, HLA-B, HLA-C, and the nonclassical HLA-F and HLA-H antigens [54]. However, the binding of miRNA-9 to the 3′-UTR of these molecules has not yet been shown. miRNA-9 is involved in the cellular differentiation [55] and

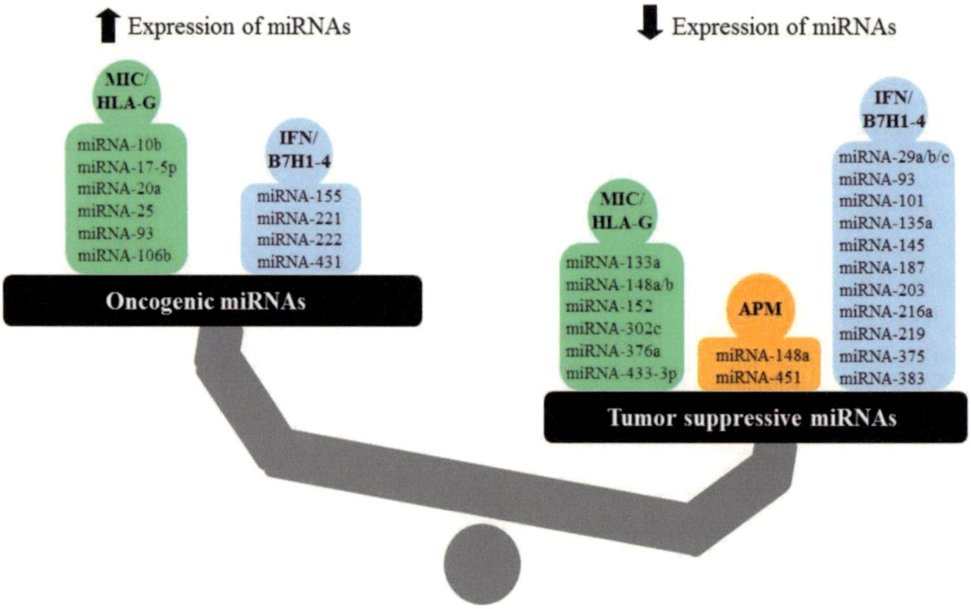

Figure 2. Scale of miRNAs targeting immune pathways in cancer exhibit an imbalance of tumor-suppressive miRNAs, which occur more frequent than oncogenic miRNAs as per knowledge from today. Oncogenic miRNA are highly expressed in cancer, while tumor-suppressive miRNAs possess a reduced expression.

aberrantly expressed in many cancer types breast cancer[56], colon cancer [57], nasopharyngeal carcinoma [58], and melanoma [59], suggesting that the decreased miRNA-9 expression is associated with tumor suppressor activity. In contrast, miRNA-9 expression is increased in brain cancer [60] and in Hodgkin's lymphoma [61], implying an oncomir potential. Furthermore, miRNA-9 has been shown to regulate the proliferation [56, 60-62] epithelial-mesenchymal transition (EMT), invasion and metastasis [62-64], apoptosis [56], tumor angiogenesis [63-64], and evasion of immune surveillance in many cancer types [54]. Although the function of miRNA-9 in the classical MHC class I pathway has still to be characterized in extent, miRNA-9-mediated regulation of APM deficiencies might be at least partially responsible for the T cell-mediated immune escape.

Besides miRNA-9, the ER stress-induced miRNA-346 modulates the expression of APM components and IFN-induced genes as shown by miRNA arrays. Functional studies revealed that TAP1 is a direct target of miRNA-346 using overexpression and RNAi knockdown experiments with miRNA mimic and miRNA inhibitors. The ER stress-mediated MHC class I-associated antigen presentation decrease might be explained by increased miRNA-346 expression [65], although the function of miRNA-346 in cancer has not yet been fully analyzed.

The inflammation and overexpression of miRNA-451 are associated with the carcinogenesis of lung cancer. A decrease in the proliferation, invasion, and metastatic potential of lung cancer cells was detected after the overexpression of miRNA-451. In addition, the proteasome subunit

PSMB8 has been identified as a direct target of miRNA-451 using both bioinformatics and dual luciferase reporter assays. This was confirmed by miRNA-451-overexpressing lung cancer cells, demonstrating a reduced PSMB8 protein expression. These data suggest that miRNA-451 inhibits the development and metastasis of lung cancer [66].

There are variations that exist in the 3′-UTR of HLA-C, which modulate the miRNA-binding capacity and consequently the HLA-C surface expression. miR-148a has been shown to bind to the HLA-C 3′-UTR. Next to cancer, the miRNA-148a expression is associated with the control of HIV [67-70]. Furthermore, miRNA-181a is upregulated in Hepatitis B virus infected cells and has a binding site in the 3′-UTR of the HLA-A gene, which might be a target of miRNA-181a [71]. Moreover, viral DNA or RNA can encode miRNAs, e.g., miRNA-US4-1 from the human cytomegalovirus, which targets the amino-peptidase ERAP1, thereby blocking CTL response [72].

6.2. Control of HLA-G and MHC-related proteins by miRNAs

Recently, a number of HLA-G-specific miRNAs have been identified, which belong to the miRNA-148 family consisting of three members, miRNA-148a, miRNA-148b, and miRNA-152. These miRNAs have been shown to act as tumor suppressors in many tumors, including prostate, ovarian, endometrial, and colorectal cancer [69, 73, 74]. In addition, other miRNAs such as miRNA-133, miRNA-548, and miRNA-628 have been identified to inhibit HLA-G expression. The HLA-C-regulating miRNAs are involved in inducing T and/or NK cell responses and have a tumor-suppressive capacity. Moreover, some of the HLA-G-regulated miRNAs are inversely expressed when compared to HLA-G in tumor lesions and are associated with disease progression [74].

The cytotoxicity of NK cells is determined by activating and inactivating signals. The ligands of the activating NK cell receptor NKG2D are the major histocompatibility complex class I-related molecules (MIC) A and B and the human cytomegalovirus UL16-binding proteins (ULBP) [73]. The expression of MICA and MICB is controlled by several oncogenic miRNAs, like miRNA-10b, miRNA-17-5p, miRNA-20a, miRNA-25, miRNA-93, and miRNA-106b, which increase the proliferative, invasive, and angiogenic potential of tumors [73, 75-83] and affect the NK cell cytotoxicity. The tumor-suppressive miRNA-302c, miRNA-376a, and miRNA-433-3p showed a reduced expression in cancer and target the 3′-UTR of MIC [73, 84-87]. Furthermore, the expression of ULBP is regulated by many tumor-suppressive miRNAs, e.g., miRNA-34a/c, miRNA-140-5p, miRNA-302c, miRNA-409-3p, and miRNA-433-p, and by the oncogenic miRNA-650 [73, 83, 85, 87].

6.3. Control of B7 family members by miRNA

The expression of B7 family members is subject to the regulatory control of miRNAs: B7-H1 could act as a costimulatory molecule, which is expressed on B cells, T cells, macrophages, and DCs [88], and acts as a ligand for PDL-1. miRNA-513 targets B7-H1 and inhibits its expression by translational repression [89]. In this context, Tamura and coworkers identified an association between low expression of B7-H2 and the escape from immune surveillance indicating that B7-H2 has a potential role in tumorigenesis. B7-H2 [90] is a direct target of miRNA-24, which inhibits B7-H3 expression and therefore is involved in cancer immune evasion. B7-H3 is an immune regulatory molecule, which is often overexpressed in different cancers and associated with metastasis and poor prognosis [91, 92]. Its expression could be posttranscriptionally regulated by miRNA-29c. The miRNA-29c-mediated downregulation of B7-H3 expression was found in breast cancer and acts therefore as tumor-suppressive miRNA [93]. Furthermore, another B7-H3-regulating miRNA, miRNA-187, has been identified in clear renal cell carcinoma, and its expression is downregulated in this disease [94]. The coinhibitor B7-H4 functions as a negative mediator of immune responses. So far, no information exists about the role of miRNAs in the regulation of B7-H4 expression. In addition, miRNAs binding to the 3′-UTR of B7-H6 have not yet been identified.

6.4. Control of the IFN-γ pathway by miRNAs

The regulation of IFN-γ signaling includes negative as well as positive regulators, such as kinases and phosphatases as well as transcription factors. A main regulatory role of IFN-γ signaling is attributed to miRNAs, affecting genes involved in proliferation, differentiation, signal transduction, immune response, and carcinogenesis [50, 95].

IFN-γ can modulate the expression levels of miRNAs and to regulate miRNAs at the level of miRNA biogenesis [96], whereas miRNAs can inhibit IFN expression directly or indirectly. In addition, studies have confirmed that miRNAs are able to target components of the IFN-γ signaling pathway and components of the JAK/STAT-pathway can regulate miRNAs simultaneously. The latter has been described by controlling miRNA expression via transcription factors, such as c-myc, the hypoxia-induced factor (HIF), and STATs [97]. The contribution and regulatory role of miRNAs in IFN-γ signaling is still under investigation and an emerging research area. Here, to highlight the regulatory function of miRNAs in the IFN-γ signaling pathway, the functional role of miRNA-155 has been described in more detail.

miRNA-155 proceeding from the non-protein-coding transcript of the *BIC* gene RNA is required for the normal function of B, T, and DC [98. 99], and its expression is increased during B cell, T cell, macrophage, and DC activation [100]. miRNA-155 has been shown to regulate IFN-γ production in NK cells, while its disruption or knockdown suppressed IFN-γ induction of NK cells [101]. Additional studies reported that miRNA-155 also downregulates IFN-γ-R expression [102]. Furthermore, STAT1 upregulates miRNA-155, which in turn downregulates SOCS1, a negative inhibitor of JAK1 [103]. These findings illustrate that a single miRNA can regulate several target mRNAs of the IFN cascade and miRNAs can be regulated by a number of targets.

miRNA regulating components of IFN-γ signaling pathway mainly act as tumor-suppressive miRNAs. An antiproliferative effect of miRNA-375, which affects JAK2 protein expression, has been recently described [104, 105]. Furthermore, miRNA-135a expression was downregulated in gastric cancer cell lines, while its overexpression results in inhibition of gastric cancer cell proliferation by targeting JAK2 [106]. Thus, miRNA-135a may function as tumor suppressor by regulating JAK2 expression in gastric cancer cells [107]. Several studies confirmed other miRNAs targeting JAK2, including miRNA-216a, which is known to inhibit cell growth and promote apoptosis of pancreatic cancer cells by regulating JAK2/STAT3 signaling pathway [108, 109], as well as miRNA-101, which promotes apoptosis of breast cancer cells by targeting JAK2 [110]. Similar results were found for STAT1 and miRNA-145 [111]. miRNA-145 is reported to be downregulated in several cancers [112, 113] and has STAT1 as direct target [111]. Moreover, STAT1 is able to upregulate miRNA-29 family members in melanoma cells, which inhibit melanoma cell proliferation by downregulating CDK6 [114].

Further studies confirmed that miRNA-223 and miRNA-150 are equally involved in IFN-γ signaling, but their role in cancer cells is still controversially discussed. Both miRNA-150 and miRNA-223 could exert oncogenic or tumor-suppressive activity. In hepatocellular carcinoma, acute myeloid leukemia (AML) [115] and gastric mucosa-associated lymphoid tissue lymphoma miRNA-223 expression is repressed [116], while an upregulation of miRNA-223 has been recently described in T-cell acute lymphocytic leukemia (T-ALL) [117]. In this context, Moles and coworkers [118] demonstrated that both miRNA-223 and miRNA-150 target STAT1 3'-UTR and reduce STAT1 expression, which in turn results in reduced expression of IFN-γ-regulated genes. The expression of miRNA-150 is upregulated in $CD19^+$ B cells from chronic lymphocytic leukemia [119, 120], while in chronic myeloid leukemia [121, 122], ALL [123] and mantel cell carcinoma miRNA-150 is downregulated. Moreover, miRNA-150 is upregulated in adult T-cell leukemia/lymphoma cells. This discrepant expression pattern of miRNA-223 and miRNA-150 suggests that both miRNAs could act as oncogenic as well as tumor suppressor miRNAs, which are dependent on the cellular context.

6.5. Role of miRNAs in immune cell function

Cancer cells upregulate and downregulate different miRNAs in immune cells to limit the antitumor response. It is well known that tumor cells reprogram the myeloid compartment to evade the immune system and promote tumorigenesis. This might be partially mediated by alterations in the miRNA expression pattern. The miRNA-155 modulates the immune response mediated by T cells, NK cells, B cells, and antigen presenting cells, such as macrophages and DC [124]. Furthermore, miRNA-155 expression has been found to be downregulated in TAMs [125], but also in hepatocellular carcinoma. The restoration of miRNA-155 in macrophages leads to enhanced T-cell function by targeting the suppressor of cytokine signaling. Other miRNAs, like miRNA-142-3p, miRNA-125b, and miRNA-19a-3p, are often downregulated in TAMs, thereby limiting the tumor infiltration of macrophages and reducing the therapeutic effect of adoptive transfer. The restoration of miRNA-125b in macrophages enhances antitumor response by targeting the IFN-regulatory factor 4, which promotes the M2 macrophage phenotype [126].

Recently, miRNAs have been identified to play a role in MDSC that regulate immune suppression within the tumor microenvironment. miRNA array analysis identified a number of deregulated miRNAs, e.g., miRNA-494, which suppresses the antitumor $CD8^+$ T-cell responses due to response to TGF-β. miRNA-494 targets PTEN in MDSC, which is responsible for the enhanced immune suppression of $CD8^+$ T cells [127]. Furthermore, a number of other miRNAs are downregulated in MDSC [128], which promote the differentiation of myeloid cells and regulate immune-suppressive signaling pathways.

In addition, miRNAs have been demonstrated in tumor-infiltrating lymphocytes. The suppression of T-cell activity is due to different mechanisms, including the dysregulation of miRNA expression. In $CD4^+$ T cells from tumor bearing mice and tumor patients, the expression of miRNA-17-92 family members was reduced, while T cells derived from miRNA-17-9 transgenic mice demonstrated a superior type 1 phenotype [129]. Furthermore, the expression of miRNA-155 was shown to promote antitumor responses. miRNA-155 in combination with miRNA-146a could upregulate the IFN-γ production of T cells. Furthermore, cancer cells could regulate miRNAs in T cells in order to modulate antitumor T-cell responses. In order to escape immune surveillance, cancer cells alter the expression of transcription factors, surface receptors, soluble chemokines/cytokines, and miRNAs to support the immune system. The downregulation of miRNA-124 increases Treg infiltration and reduces cytokines production through an altered expression of STAT3, which represents a target of miRNA-124. In contrast, tumor-secreted miRNA-214 induces Treg. Regarding NK cells, the TGF-β-inducible miRNA-183 affects NK cell activity [130]. Thus, the regulation of miRNAs within the cancer cell alters the TME through manipulation.

7. Conclusion and future perspectives

Taken together, during the past years, the posttranscriptional control of gene expression by miRNAs has gained relevance as key regulator in a wide variety of physiological and pathophysiological processes due to the role of miRNA-mediated RNAi not only in differentiation, proliferation, apoptosis, immune responses but also in viral and bacterial infections as well as neoplastic transformation (Table 1). A deregulated expression of miRNAs has been often found in tumors of distinct origin, which have been classified into oncogenic or tumor-suppressive miRNAs known to play an essential role in cancer initiation and progression. Therefore, these miRNAs could act as potential biomarkers and therapeutic targets in cancer. *In silico* prediction analysis further proposed that many miRNAs could target different immune modulatory molecules expressed either on tumor cells or on different immune cell subpopulations.

As summarized, an emerging relevance of miRNAs in mounting the tumor immune escape by altering the communication between cancer cells, immune cells, and other components of the TME has been demonstrated. This leads to another level of complexity due to the involvement of miRNAs in the interaction between cancer cells and immune cells. These miRNAs might not only provide new insights into tumor growth and progression as well as antitumoral immune responses but also represent promising therapeutic targets for (immune) therapy. To date, many cancer-deregulated miRNAs have been identified in particular in cancer cells and also in components of the TMA. However, their role in modulating the antitumor immune responses has not yet been characterized in detail. Although the majority of the miRNA alterations detected are dedicated to cancer cells, there is already evidence that miRNAs of infiltrating immune cells also particularly influence tumorgenicity. The identification of further im-miRNAs as well as their functional characterization might lead to a plethora of novel candidate biomarkers for monitoring of immune responses, which might be also potentially used for targeted RNAi therapy.

miRNAs	target	biological impact of the miRNA					literature
		proliferation	invasion	apoptosis	angiogenesis	tumor suppressor/ oncogenic	
let-7c	JAK2	n.d.	n.d.	n.d.	n.d.	n.d.	[131]
miRNA-9	HLA-B, HLA-C, HLA-F, HLA-H, PSMB8, PSMB10, B2M, JAK1, IRF-1			controversially discussed			[54, 132]
miRNA-10b	MICB	up	up	down	up	oncogenic	[73, 76, 77]
miRNA-15a	FOXP3	down	down	up	down	tumor suppressor	[133-137]
miRNA-16	FOXP3	down	down	up	down	tumor suppressor	[133-135, 138, 139]
miRNA-17-5p	MICA	up	up	down	up	oncogenic	[73, 80, 83]
miRNA-20a	MICA, MICB	up	up	down	up	oncogenic	[73]
miRNA-24	B7-H2	n.d.	n.d.	n.d.	n.d.	n.d.	[140]
miRNA-25	MICA	up	up	down	up	oncogenic	[78, 81, 141, 142]
miRNA-29	STAT1, B7-H3	down	down	up	down	tumor suppressor	[114, 143]
miRNA-29b	IRF-1	down	down	up	n.d.	tumor suppressor	[144]
miRNA-29c	B7-H3	n.d.	n.d.	n.d.	n.d.	tumor suppressor	[93]
miRNA-34a	CD44, ULBP2	down	down	up	down	tumor suppressor	[73]
miRNA-34c	ULBP2	down	down	up	n.d.	tumor suppressor	[73]
miRNA-93	MICA	up	up	down	up	oncogenic	[73, 75]
miRNA-93	JAK1	down	down	n.d.	n.d.	tumor suppressor	[145]
miRNA-101	JAK2	down	down	up	n.d.	tumor suppressor	[110]
miRNA-106b	MICA	up	up	down	n.d.	oncogenic	[75, 79, 82, 146, 147]
miRNA-133a	HLA-G	down	down	up	n.d.	tumor suppressor	[73, 148, 149]
miRNA-135a	JAK2	down	n.d.	up	n.d.	tumor suppressor	[76, 106]
miRNA-140-5p	ULBP1	down	down	n.d.	n.d.	tumor suppressor	[73, 150]
miRNA-143	CD44	down	down	up	down	tumor suppressor	[151-155]
miRNA-145	CD44, JAK1, STAT1	down	down	up	down	tumor suppressor	[111, 156-160]
miRNA-146a	CD40-L	down	down	up	up	tumor suppressor	[161-165]
miRNA-148a	HLA-C, HLA-G	down	down	up	down	tumor suppressor	[68, 73, 166]
miRNA-148b	HLA-G	down	down	up	down	tumor suppressor	[73]
miRNA-150	STAT1			controversially discussed			[118, 121]
miRNA-152	HLA-G	down	down	up	down	tumor suppressor	[73]
miRNA155	CTLA4, STAT1	up	up	down	up	oncogenic	[167-172]
miRNA-187	B7-H3, ALDH1A3	down	down	up	n.d.	tumor suppressor	[94, 173]
miRNA-199a	CD44	down	down	up	down	tumor suppressor	[174-178]
miRNA-203	CD44, IRF-1	down	down	up	down	tumor suppressor	[179-184]
miRNA-216a	CD44, JAK2	down	down	up	down	tumor suppressor	[109, 128, 185, 186]
miRNA-219	JAK2	n.d.	n.d.	n.d.	n.d.	tumor suppressor	[187]
miRNA-221/222	STAT2, IRF-2, TIMP2	up	up	down	up	n.d. (oncogenic)	[188-191]
miRNA-223	STAT1			controversially discussed			[115, 117, 118]
miRNA-302c	MICA, MICB, ULBP2	down	n.d.	up	down	tumor suppressor	[85, 87]
miRNA-328	CD44	down	down	up	down	tumor suppressor	[192-195]
miRNA-330	CD44	down	down	up	n.d.	tumor suppressor	[196, 197]
miRNA-346	TAP1	n.d.	n.d.	n.d.	n.d.	n.d.	[65]
miRNA-373	CD44			controversially discussed			[198-200]
miRNA-376a	MICB, HLA-E	down	down	up	n.d.	tumor suppressor	[84, 86, 201]
miRNA-375	JAK2	down	down	n.d.	n.d.	tumor suppressor	[168, 202-204]
miRNA-383	IRF-1	down	n.d.	up	n.d.	tumor suppressor	[205]
miRNA-409-3p	ULBP1	down	down	n.d.	n.d.	tumor suppressor	[73]
miRNA-431	JAK1, STAT2	up	n.d.	n.d.	n.d.	oncogenic	[206]
miRNA-433-3p	MICB, ULBP1	down	down	n.d.	n.d.	tumor suppressor	[73]
miRNA-451	PSMB8	down	down	up	n.d.	tumor suppressor	[128]
miRNA-491	CD44	down	down	up	up	tumor suppressor	[207-209]
miRNA-512-3p	CD44	down	down	up	n.d.	tumor suppressor	[202, 210]
miRNA-513	PD-L1, B7-H1	n.d.	n.d.	n.d.	n.d.	n.d.	[89]
miRNA-520b	MICA	down	n.d.	n.d.	n.d.	n.d.	[73]
miRNA-520c	MICA, MICB, ULBP2, CD44			controversially discussed			[62, 211]
miRNA-570	PD-L1			controversially discussed			[212, 213]
miRNA-608	CD44	down	down	up	n.d.	tumor suppressor	[214, 215]
miRNA-650	ULBP1	up	up	n.d.	n.d.	oncogenic	[73]
miRNA-708	CD44			controversially discussed			[216, 217]

Table 1. Identified miRNAs involved in the tumor immune escape and their tumor–associated function. Controversially discussed miRNAs are found as tumor suppressors in some cancer types, while exhibiting oncogenic properties in other cancer types. n.d., no data.

8. Abbreviations

APC, antigen presenting cell; APM, antigen processing machinery; β_2-m, β_2-microglobulin; CDKN, cyclin-dependent kinase inhibitor; CTL, cytotoxic T lymphocyte; CXCL, chemokine (CXC motif) ligand; DC, dendritic cell; GAS, IFN-γ-activated sequence; HC, heavy chain; HLA, human leukocyte antigen; IFN, interferon; IL, interleukin; IRF, interferon regulatory factor; ISRE, IFN-stimulated response element; im-miRNA, immune modulatory miRNA; JAK, janus kinase; LMP, low molecular mass polypeptide; MAPK, MAP kinase; MDSC, myeloid-derived suppressor cell; MHC, major histocompatibility complex; MIC, major histocompatibility complex class I-related molecule; miRNA, microRNA; NK, natural killer cell; PD, programmed death; PDL, PD ligand; PLC, peptide loading complex; STAT, signal transducer and activator of transcription; SOCS, suppressor of cytokine signaling; TAF, tumor-associated fibroblast; TAM, tumor-associated macrophage; TAP, transporter associated with antigen processing; TGF, transforming growth factor; TLR, toll-like receptor; TME, tumor microenvironment; Treg, regulatory T cell; ULBP, human cytomegalovirus UL16-binding protein; UTR, untranslated region; and VEGF, vascular endothelial growth factor.

Acknowledgements

We would like to thank Sylvi Magdeburg for excellent secretarial help. This work was supported by a grant from the DFG SE585/22-1, GRK1591, GIF (I 1187-69), and Cancer Research Aid (110703).

Author details

Barbara Seliger*, Anne Meinhardt and Doerte Falke

*Address all correspondence to: barbara.seliger@uk-halle.de

Institute of Medical Immunology, Martin-Luther University Halle-Wittenberg, Germany

References

[1] Blum JS, Wearsch PA, Cresswell P. Pathways of antigen processing. Annu Rev Immunol. 2013;31:443. DOI: 10.1146/annurev-immunol-032712-095910.

[2] Ceeraz S, Nowak EC, Noelle RJ. B7 family checkpoint regulators in immune regulation and disease. Trends Immunol. 2013;34(11):556. DOI: 10.1016/j.it.2013.07.003.

[3] Maj T, Wei S, Welling T, Zou W. T cells and costimulation in cancer. Cancer J. 2013;19(6):473. DOI: 10.1097/PPO.0000000000000002.

[4] Wang S, Zhu G, Chapoval AI, Dong H, Tamada K, Ni J, Chen L. Costimulation of T cells by B7-H2, a B7-like molecule that binds ICOS. Blood. 2000;96(8):2808.

[5] Choi IH, Zhu G, Sica GL, Strome SE, Cheville JC, Lau JS, Zhu Y, Flies DB, Tamada K, Chen L. Genomic organization and expression analysis of B7-H4, an immune inhibitory molecule of the B7 family. J Immunol. 2003;171(9):4650.

[6] Sica GL, Choi IH, Zhu G, Tamada K, Wang SD, Tamura H, Chapoval AI, Flies DB, Bajorath J, Chen L. B7-H4, a molecule of the B7 family, negatively regulates T cell immunity. Immunity. 2003;18(6):849.

[7] Brandt CS, Baratin M, Yi EC, Kennedy J, Gao Z, Fox B, Haldeman B, Ostrander CD, Kaifu T, Chabannon C, Moretta A, West R, Xu W, Vivier E, Levin SD. The B7 family member B7-H6 is a tumor cell ligand for the activating natural killer cell receptor NKp30 in humans. J Exp Med. 2009;206(7):1495. DOI: 10.1084/jem.20090681.

[8] Pesce S, Tabellini G, Cantoni C, Patrizi O, Coltrini D, Rampinelli F, Matta J, Vivier E, Moretta A, Parolini S, Marcenaro E. B7-H6-mediated downregulation of NKp30 in NK cells contributes to ovarian carcinoma immune escape. Oncoimmunology. 2015;4(4):e1001224. DOI: 10.1080/2162402X.2014.1001224.

[9] Pestka S, Krause CD, Walter MR. Interferons, interferon-like cytokines, and their receptors. Immunol Rev. 2004;202:8. DOI: 10.1111/j.0105-2896.2004.00204.x.

[10] Trinchieri G. Type I interferon: friend or foe? J Exp Med. 2010;207(10):2053. DOI: 10.1084/jem.20101664.

[11] Fehniger TA, Shah MH, Turner MJ, VanDeusen JB, Whitman SP, Cooper MA, Suzuki K, Wechser M, Goodsaid F, Caligiuri MA. Differential cytokine and chemokine gene expression by human NK cells following activation with IL-18 or IL-15 in combination with IL-12: implications for the innate immune response. J Immunol. 1999;162(8):4511.

[12] Ealick SE, Cook WJ, Vijay-Kumar S, Carson M, Nagabhushan TL, Trotta PP, Bugg CE. Three-dimensional structure of recombinant human interferon-gamma. Science. 1991;252(5006):698.

[13] Platanias LC. Mechanisms of type-I- and type-II-interferon-mediated signalling. Nat Rev Immunol. 2005;5(5):375. DOI: 10.1038/nri1604.

[14] Boehm U, Klamp T, Groot M, Howard JC. Cellular responses to interferon-gamma. Annu Rev Immunol. 1997;15:749. DOI: 10.1146/annurev.immunol.15.1.749.

[15] Hu X, Chakravarty SD, Ivashkiv LB. Regulation of interferon and toll-like receptor signaling during macrophage activation by opposing feedforward and feedback in-

hibition mechanisms. Immunol Rev. 2008;226:41. DOI: 10.1111/j.1600-065X.2008.00707.x.

[16] Schroder K, Sweet MJ, Hume DA. Signal integration between IFNgamma and TLR signalling pathways in macrophages. Immunobiology. 2006;211(6-8):511. DOI: 10.1016/j.imbio.2006.05.007.

[17] Alexander WS, Starr R, Fenner JE, Scott CL, Handman E, Sprigg NS, Corbin JE, Cornish AL, Darwiche R, Owczarek CM, Kay TW, Nicola NA, Hertzog PJ, Metcalf D, Hilton DJ. SOCS1 is a critical inhibitor of interferon gamma signaling and prevents the potentially fatal neonatal actions of this cytokine. Cell. 1999;98(5):597.

[18] Dunn GP, Koebel CM, Schreiber RD. Interferons, immunity and cancer immunoediting. Nat Rev Immunol. 2006;6(11):836. DOI: 10.1038/nri1961.

[19] Liu B, Mink S, Wong KA, Stein N, Getman C, Dempsey PW, Wu H, Shuai K. PIAS1 selectively inhibits interferon-inducible genes and is important in innate immunity. Nat Immunol. 2004;5(9):891. DOI: 10.1038/ni1104.

[20] Draghiciu O, Lubbers J, Nijman HW, Daemen T. Myeloid derived suppressor cells-An overview of combat strategies to increase immunotherapy efficacy. Oncoimmunology. 2015;4(1):e954829. DOI: 10.4161/21624011.2014.954829.

[21] Giraldo NA, Becht E, Vano Y, Sautes-Fridman C, Fridman WH. The immune response in cancer: from immunology to pathology to immunotherapy. Virchows Arch. 2015;467(2):127. DOI: 10.1007/s00428-015-1787-7.

[22] Wolf D, Sopper S, Pircher A, Gastl G, Wolf AM. Treg(s) in Cancer: Friends or Foe? J Cell Physiol. 2015;230(11):2598. DOI: 10.1002/jcp.25016.

[23] Wu AA, Drake V, Huang HS, Chiu S, Zheng L. Reprogramming the tumor microenvironment: tumor-induced immunosuppressive factors paralyze T cells. Oncoimmunology. 2015;4(7):e1016700. DOI: 10.1080/2162402X.2015.1016700.

[24] Monu NR, Frey AB. Myeloid-derived suppressor cells and anti-tumor T cells: a complex relationship. Immunol Invest. 2012;41(6-7):595. DOI: 10.3109/08820139.2012.673191.

[25] Gabrilovich D. Mechanisms and functional significance of tumour-induced dendritic-cell defects. Nat Rev Immunol. 2004;4(12):941. DOI: 10.1038/nri1498.

[26] Ochoa AC, Zea AH, Hernandez C, Rodriguez PC. Arginase, prostaglandins, and myeloid-derived suppressor cells in renal cell carcinoma. Clin Cancer Res. 2007;13(2 Pt 2):721s. DOI: 10.1158/1078-0432.CCR-06-2197.

[27] Raber P, Ochoa AC, Rodriguez PC. Metabolism of L-arginine by myeloid-derived suppressor cells in cancer: mechanisms of T cell suppression and therapeutic perspectives. Immunol Invest. 2012;41(6-7):614. DOI: 10.3109/08820139.2012.680634.

[28] Saio M, Radoja S, Marino M, Frey AB. Tumor-infiltrating macrophages induce apoptosis in activated CD8(+) T cells by a mechanism requiring cell contact and mediated

by both the cell-associated form of TNF and nitric oxide. J Immunol. 2001;167(10): 5583.

[29] Curiel TJ, Coukos G, Zou L, Alvarez X, Cheng P, Mottram P, Evdemon-Hogan M, Conejo-Garcia JR, Zhang L, Burow M, Zhu Y, Wei S, Kryczek I, Daniel B, Gordon A, Myers L, Lackner A, Disis ML, Knutson KL, Chen L, Zou W. Specific recruitment of regulatory T cells in ovarian carcinoma fosters immune privilege and predicts reduced survival. Nat Med. 2004;10(9):942. DOI: 10.1038/nm1093.

[30] Valzasina B, Piconese S, Guiducci C, Colombo MP. Tumor-induced expansion of regulatory T cells by conversion of CD4+CD25- lymphocytes is thymus and proliferation independent. Cancer Res. 2006;66(8):4488. DOI: 10.1158/0008-5472.CAN-05-4217.

[31] Respa A, Bukur J, Ferrone S, Pawelec G, Zhao Y, Wang E, Marincola FM, Seliger B. Association of IFN-gamma signal transduction defects with impaired HLA class I antigen processing in melanoma cell lines. Clin Cancer Res. 2011;17(9):2668. DOI: 10.1158/1078-0432.CCR-10-2114.

[32] Schreiber RD, Old LJ, Smyth MJ. Cancer immunoediting: integrating immunity's roles in cancer suppression and promotion. Science. 2011;331(6024):1565. DOI: 10.1126/science.1203486.

[33] Whiteside TL, Mandapathil M, Szczepanski M, Szajnik M. Mechanisms of tumor escape from the immune system: adenosine-producing Treg, exosomes and tumor-associated TLRs. Bull Cancer. 2011;98(2):E25. DOI: 10.1684/bdc.2010.1294.

[34] Lin A, Yan WH. HLA-G expression in cancers: roles in immune evasion, metastasis and target for therapy. Mol Med. 2015. DOI: 10.2119/molmed.2015.00083.

[35] Carreno BM, Collins M. The B7 family of ligands and its receptors: new pathways for costimulation and inhibition of immune responses. Annu Rev Immunol. 2002;20:29. DOI: 10.1146/annurev.immunol.20.091101.091806.

[36] Khoury SJ, Sayegh MH. The roles of the new negative T cell costimulatory pathways in regulating autoimmunity. Immunity. 2004;20(5):529.

[37] Perez-Gracia JL, Labiano S, Rodriguez-Ruiz ME, Sanmamed MF, Melero I. Orchestrating immune check-point blockade for cancer immunotherapy in combinations. Curr Opin Immunol. 2014;27:89. DOI: 10.1016/j.coi.2014.01.002.

[38] Bubenik J. Tumour MHC class I downregulation and immunotherapy (Review). Oncol Rep. 2003;10(6):2005.

[39] Garrido F, Ruiz-Cabello F, Cabrera T, Perez-Villar JJ, Lopez-Botet M, Duggan-Keen M, Stern PL. Implications for immunosurveillance of altered HLA class I phenotypes in human tumours. Immunol Today. 1997;18(2):89.

[40] Kaplan DH, Shankaran V, Dighe AS, Stockert E, Aguet M, Old LJ, Schreiber RD. Demonstration of an interferon gamma-dependent tumor surveillance system in immunocompetent mice. Proc Natl Acad Sci U S A. 1998;95(13):7556.

[41] Dovhey SE, Ghosh NS, Wright KL. Loss of interferon-gamma inducibility of TAP1 and LMP2 in a renal cell carcinoma cell line. Cancer Res. 2000;60(20):5789.

[42] Rodriguez T, Mendez R, Del Campo A, Jimenez P, Aptsiauri N, Garrido F, Ruiz-Cabello F. Distinct mechanisms of loss of IFN-gamma mediated HLA class I inducibility in two melanoma cell lines. BMC Cancer. 2007;7:34. DOI: 10.1186/1471-2407-7-34.

[43] Gabathuler R, Reid G, Kolaitis G, Driscoll J, Jefferies WA. Comparison of cell lines deficient in antigen presentation reveals a functional role for TAP-1 alone in antigen processing. J Exp Med. 1994;180(4):1415.

[44] Seliger B, Wollscheid U, Momburg F, Blankenstein T, Huber C. Coordinate downregulation of multiple MHC class I antigen processing genes in chemical-induced murine tumor cell lines of distinct origin. Tissue Antigens. 2000;56(4):327.

[45] Street SE, Trapani JA, MacGregor D, Smyth MJ. Suppression of lymphoma and epithelial malignancies effected by interferon gamma. J Exp Med. 2002;196(1):129.

[46] Chin YE, Kitagawa M, Su WC, You ZH, Iwamoto Y, Fu XY. Cell growth arrest and induction of cyclin-dependent kinase inhibitor p21 WAF1/CIP1 mediated by STAT1. Science. 1996;272(5262):719.

[47] Vlkova V, Stepanek I, Hruskova V, Senigl F, Mayerova V, Sramek M, Simova J, Bieblova J, Indrova M, Hejhal T, Derian N, Klatzmann D, Six A, Reinis M. Epigenetic regulations in the IFNgamma signalling pathway: IFNgamma-mediated MHC class I upregulation on tumour cells is associated with DNA demethylation of antigen-presenting machinery genes. Oncotarget. 2014;5(16):6923.

[48] Winter J, Jung S, Keller S, Gregory RI, Diederichs S. Many roads to maturity: microRNA biogenesis pathways and their regulation. Nat Cell Biol. 2009;11(3):228. DOI: 10.1038/ncb0309-228.

[49] Baek D, Villen J, Shin C, Camargo FD, Gygi SP, Bartel DP. The impact of microRNAs on protein output. Nature. 2008;455(7209):64. DOI: 10.1038/nature07242.

[50] Bartel DP, Chen CZ. Micromanagers of gene expression: the potentially widespread influence of metazoan microRNAs. Nat Rev Genet. 2004;5(5):396. DOI: 10.1038/nrg1328.

[51] Krol J, Loedige I, Filipowicz W. The widespread regulation of microRNA biogenesis, function and decay. Nat Rev Genet. 2010;11(9):597. DOI: 10.1038/nrg2843.

[52] Ohtsuka M, Ling H, Doki Y, Mori M, Calin GA. MicroRNA processing and human cancer. J Clin Med. 2015;4(8):1651. DOI: 10.3390/jcm4081651.

[53] Neviani P, Fabbri M. Exosomic microRNAs in the tumor microenvironment. Front Med (Lausanne). 2015;2:47. DOI: 10.3389/fmed.2015.00047.

[54] Gao F, Zhao ZL, Zhao WT, Fan QR, Wang SC, Li J, Zhang YQ, Shi JW, Lin XL, Yang S, Xie RY, Liu W, Zhang TT, Sun YL, Xu K, Yao KT, Xiao D. miR-9 modulates the expression of interferon-regulated genes and MHC class I molecules in human nasopharyngeal carcinoma cells. Biochem Biophys Res Commun. 2013;431(3):610. DOI: 10.1016/j.bbrc.2012.12.097.

[55] Garaffo G, Conte D, Provero P, Tomaiuolo D, Luo Z, Pinciroli P, Peano C, D'Atri I, Gitton Y, Etzion T, Gothilf Y, Gays D, Santoro MM, Merlo GR. The Dlx5 and Foxg1 transcription factors, linked via miRNA-9 and -200, are required for the development of the olfactory and GnRH system. Mol Cell Neurosci. 2015;68:103. DOI: 10.1016/j.mcn.2015.04.007.

[56] Selcuklu SD, Donoghue MT, Rehmet K, de Souza Gomes M, Fort A, Kovvuru P, Muniyappa MK, Kerin MJ, Enright AJ, Spillane C. MicroRNA-9 inhibition of cell proliferation and identification of novel miR-9 targets by transcriptome profiling in breast cancer cells. J Biol Chem. 2012;287(35):29516. DOI: 10.1074/jbc.M111.335943.

[57] Bandres E, Agirre X, Bitarte N, Ramirez N, Zarate R, Roman-Gomez J, Prosper F, Garcia-Foncillas J. Epigenetic regulation of microRNA expression in colorectal cancer. Int J Cancer. 2009;125(11):2737. DOI: 10.1002/ijc.24638.

[58] Chen HC, Chen GH, Chen YH, Liao WL, Liu CY, Chang KP, Chang YS, Chen SJ. MicroRNA deregulation and pathway alterations in nasopharyngeal carcinoma. Br J Cancer. 2009;100(6):1002. DOI: 10.1038/sj.bjc.6604948.

[59] Liu S, Kumar SM, Lu H, Liu A, Yang R, Pushparajan A, Guo W, Xu X. MicroRNA-9 up-regulates E-cadherin through inhibition of NF-kappaB1-Snail1 pathway in melanoma. J Pathol. 2012;226(1):61. DOI: 10.1002/path.2964.

[60] Nass D, Rosenwald S, Meiri E, Gilad S, Tabibian-Keissar H, Schlosberg A, Kuker H, Sion-Vardy N, Tobar A, Kharenko O, Sitbon E, Lithwick Yanai G, Elyakim E, Cholakh H, Gibori H, Spector Y, Bentwich Z, Barshack I, Rosenfeld N. MiR-92b and miR-9/9* are specifically expressed in brain primary tumors and can be used to differentiate primary from metastatic brain tumors. Brain Pathol. 2009;19(3):375. DOI: 10.1111/j.1750-3639.2008.00184.x.

[61] Leucci E, Zriwil A, Gregersen LH, Jensen KT, Obad S, Bellan C, Leoncini L, Kauppinen S, Lund AH. Inhibition of miR-9 de-represses HuR and DICER1 and impairs Hodgkin lymphoma tumour outgrowth in vivo. Oncogene. 2012;31(49):5081. DOI: 10.1038/onc.2012.15.

[62] Liu P, Wilson MJ. miR-520c and miR-373 upregulate MMP9 expression by targeting mTOR and SIRT1, and activate the Ras/Raf/MEK/Erk signaling pathway and NF-kappaB factor in human fibrosarcoma cells. J Cell Physiol. 2012;227(2):867. DOI: 10.1002/jcp.22993.

[63] Ma L, Young J, Prabhala H, Pan E, Mestdagh P, Muth D, Teruya-Feldstein J, Reinhardt F, Onder TT, Valastyan S, Westermann F, Speleman F, Vandesompele J, Weinberg RA. miR-9, a MYC/MYCN-activated microRNA, regulates E-cadherin and cancer metastasis. Nat Cell Biol. 2010;12(3):247. DOI: 10.1038/ncb2024.

[64] Zhang H, Qi M, Li S, Qi T, Mei H, Huang K, Zheng L, Tong Q. microRNA-9 targets matrix metalloproteinase 14 to inhibit invasion, metastasis, and angiogenesis of neuroblastoma cells. Mol Cancer Ther. 2012;11(7):1454. DOI: 10.1158/1535-7163.MCT-12-0001.

[65] Bartoszewski R, Brewer JW, Rab A, Crossman DK, Bartoszewska S, Kapoor N, Fuller C, Collawn JF, Bebok Z. The unfolded protein response (UPR)-activated transcription factor X-box-binding protein 1 (XBP1) induces microRNA-346 expression that targets the human antigen peptide transporter 1 (TAP1) mRNA and governs immune regulatory genes. J Biol Chem. 2011;286(48):41862. DOI: 10.1074/jbc.M111.304956.

[66] Yin P, Peng R, Peng H, Yao L, Sun Y, Wen L, Wu T, Zhou J, Zhang Z. MiR-451 suppresses cell proliferation and metastasis in A549 lung cancer cells. Mol Biotechnol. 2015;57(1):1. DOI: 10.1007/s12033-014-9796-3.

[67] Celsi F, Catamo E, Kleiner G, Tricarico PM, Vuch J, Crovella S. HLA-G/C, miRNAs, and their role in HIV infection and replication. Biomed Res Int. 2013;2013:693643. DOI: 10.1155/2013/693643.

[68] Kulkarni S, Qi Y, O'HUigin C, Pereyra F, Ramsuran V, McLaren P, Fellay J, Nelson G, Chen H, Liao W, Bass S, Apps R, Gao X, Yuki Y, Lied A, Ganesan A, Hunt PW, Deeks SG, Wolinsky S, Walker BD, Carrington M. Genetic interplay between HLA-C and MIR148A in HIV control and Crohn disease. Proc Natl Acad Sci U S A. 2013;110(51):20705. DOI: 10.1073/pnas.1312237110.

[69] Kulkarni S, Savan R, Qi Y, Gao X, Yuki Y, Bass SE, Martin MP, Hunt P, Deeks SG, Telenti A, Pereyra F, Goldstein D, Wolinsky S, Walker B, Young HA, Carrington M. Differential microRNA regulation of HLA-C expression and its association with HIV control. Nature. 2011;472(7344):495. DOI: 10.1038/nature09914.

[70] O'Huigin C, Kulkarni S, Xu Y, Deng Z, Kidd J, Kidd K, Gao X, Carrington M. The molecular origin and consequences of escape from miRNA regulation by HLA-C alleles. Am J Hum Genet. 2011;89(3):424. DOI: 10.1016/j.ajhg.2011.07.024.

[71] Liu Y, Zhao JJ, Wang CM, Li MY, Han P, Wang L, Cheng YQ, Zoulim F, Ma X, Xu DP. Altered expression profiles of microRNAs in a stable hepatitis B virus-expressing cell line. Chin Med J (Engl). 2009;122(1):10.

[72] Kim S, Lee S, Shin J, Kim Y, Evnouchidou I, Kim D, Kim YK, Kim YE, Ahn JH, Riddell SR, Stratikos E, Kim VN, Ahn K. Human cytomegalovirus microRNA miR-US4-1 inhibits CD8(+) T cell responses by targeting the aminopeptidase ERAP1. Nat Immunol. 2011;12(10):984. DOI: 10.1038/ni.2097.

[73] Jasinski-Bergner S, Mandelboim O, Seliger B. The role of microRNAs in the control of innate immune response in cancer. J Natl Cancer Inst. 2014;106(10). DOI: 10.1093/jnci/dju257.

[74] Jasinski-Bergner S, Stoehr C, Bukur J, Massa C, Braun J, Huttelmaier S, Spath V, Wartenberg R, Legal W, Taubert H, Wach S, Wullich B, Hartmann A, Seliger B. Clinical relevance of miR-mediated HLA-G regulation and the associated immune cell infiltration in renal cell carcinoma. Oncoimmunology. 2015;4(6):e1008805. DOI: 10.1080/2162402X.2015.1008805.

[75] Choi N, Park J, Lee JS, Yoe J, Park GY, Kim E, Jeon H, Cho YM, Roh TY, Lee Y. miR-93/miR-106b/miR-375-CIC-CRABP1: a novel regulatory axis in prostate cancer progression. Oncotarget. 2015.

[76] Dong CG, Wu WK, Feng SY, Wang XJ, Shao JF, Qiao J. Co-inhibition of microRNA-10b and microRNA-21 exerts synergistic inhibition on the proliferation and invasion of human glioma cells. Int J Oncol. 2012;41(3):1005. DOI: 10.3892/ijo.2012.1542.

[77] Gabriely G, Teplyuk NM, Krichevsky AM. Context effect: microRNA-10b in cancer cell proliferation, spread and death. Autophagy. 2011;7(11):1384. DOI: 10.4161/auto.7.11.17371.

[78] Gong J, Cui Z, Li L, Ma Q, Wang Q, Gao Y, Sun H. MicroRNA-25 promotes gastric cancer proliferation, invasion, and migration by directly targeting F-box and WD-40 Domain Protein 7, FBXW7. Tumour Biol. 2015. DOI: 10.1007/s13277-015-3510-3.

[79] Li KK, Xia T, Ma FM, Zhang R, Mao Y, Wang Y, Zhou L, Lau KM, Ng HK. miR-106b is overexpressed in medulloblastomas and interacts directly with PTEN. Neuropathol Appl Neurobiol. 2015;41(2):145. DOI: 10.1111/nan.12169.

[80] Lu Y, Thomson JM, Wong HY, Hammond SM, Hogan BL. Transgenic over-expression of the microRNA miR-17-92 cluster promotes proliferation and inhibits differentiation of lung epithelial progenitor cells. Dev Biol. 2007;310(2):442. DOI: 10.1016/j.ydbio.2007.08.007.

[81] Semo J, Sharir R, Afek A, Avivi C, Barshack I, Maysel-Auslender S, Krelin Y, Kain D, Entin-Meer M, Keren G, George J. The 106b approximately 25 microRNA cluster is essential for neovascularization after hindlimb ischaemia in mice. Eur Heart J. 2014;35(45):3212. DOI: 10.1093/eurheartj/eht041.

[82] Shen G, Jia H, Chen D, Zhang J. [Effects of miR-106b expression on the proliferation of human hepatocellular carcinoma cells]. Zhonghua Zhong Liu Za Zhi. 2014;36(7):489.

[83] Yang X, Du WW, Li H, Liu F, Khorshidi A, Rutnam ZJ, Yang BB. Both mature miR-17-5p and passenger strand miR-17-3p target TIMP3 and induce prostate tumor growth and invasion. Nucleic Acids Res. 2013;41(21):9688. DOI: 10.1093/nar/gkt680.

[84] Formosa A, Markert EK, Lena AM, Italiano D, Finazzi-Agro E, Levine AJ, Bernardini S, Garabadgiu AV, Melino G, Candi E. MicroRNAs, miR-154, miR-299-5p, miR-376a,

miR-376c, miR-377, miR-381, miR-487b, miR-485-3p, miR-495 and miR-654-3p, mapped to the 14q32.31 locus, regulate proliferation, apoptosis, migration and invasion in metastatic prostate cancer cells. Oncogene. 2014;33(44):5173. DOI: 10.1038/onc.2013.451.

[85] Lin SL, Chang DC, Ying SY, Leu D, Wu DT. MicroRNA miR-302 inhibits the tumorigenicity of human pluripotent stem cells by coordinate suppression of the CDK2 and CDK4/6 cell cycle pathways. Cancer Res. 2010;70(22):9473. DOI: 10.1158/0008-5472.CAN-10-2746.

[86] Zehavi L, Avraham R, Barzilai A, Bar-Ilan D, Navon R, Sidi Y, Avni D, Leibowitz-Amit R. Silencing of a large microRNA cluster on human chromosome 14q32 in melanoma: biological effects of mir-376a and mir-376c on insulin growth factor 1 receptor. Mol Cancer. 2012;11:44. DOI: 10.1186/1476-4598-11-44.

[87] Zhu K, Pan Q, Jia LQ, Dai Z, Ke AW, Zeng HY, Tang ZY, Fan J, Zhou J. MiR-302c inhibits tumor growth of hepatocellular carcinoma by suppressing the endothelial-mesenchymal transition of endothelial cells. Sci Rep. 2014;4:5524. DOI: 10.1038/srep05524.

[88] Yamazaki T, Akiba H, Koyanagi A, Azuma M, Yagita H, Okumura K. Blockade of B7-H1 on macrophages suppresses CD4+ T cell proliferation by augmenting IFN-gamma-induced nitric oxide production. J Immunol. 2005;175(3):1586.

[89] Gong AY, Zhou R, Hu G, Li X, Splinter PL, O'Hara SP, LaRusso NF, Soukup GA, Dong H, Chen XM. MicroRNA-513 regulates B7-H1 translation and is involved in IFN-gamma-induced B7-H1 expression in cholangiocytes. J Immunol. 2009;182(3):1325.

[90] Tamura H, Dan K, Tamada K, Nakamura K, Shioi Y, Hyodo H, Wang SD, Dong H, Chen L, Ogata K. Expression of functional B7-H2 and B7.2 costimulatory molecules and their prognostic implications in de novo acute myeloid leukemia. Clin Cancer Res. 2005;11(16):5708. DOI: 10.1158/1078-0432.CCR-04-2672.

[91] Roth TJ, Sheinin Y, Lohse CM, Kuntz SM, Frigola X, Inman BA, Krambeck AE, McKenney ME, Karnes RJ, Blute ML, Cheville JC, Sebo TJ, Kwon ED. B7-H3 ligand expression by prostate cancer: a novel marker of prognosis and potential target for therapy. Cancer Res. 2007;67(16):7893. DOI: 10.1158/0008-5472.CAN-07-1068.

[92] Sun Y, Wang Y, Zhao J, Gu M, Giscombe R, Lefvert AK, Wang X. B7-H3 and B7-H4 expression in non-small-cell lung cancer. Lung Cancer. 2006;53(2):143. DOI: 10.1016/j.lungcan.2006.05.012.

[93] Nygren MK, Tekle C, Ingebrigtsen VA, Makela R, Krohn M, Aure MR, Nunes-Xavier CE, Perala M, Tramm T, Alsner J, Overgaard J, Nesland JM, Borgen E, Borresen-Dale AL, Fodstad O, Sahlberg KK, Leivonen SK. Identifying microRNAs regulating B7-H3 in breast cancer: the clinical impact of microRNA-29c. Br J Cancer. 2014;110(8):2072. DOI: 10.1038/bjc.2014.113.

[94] Zhao J, Lei T, Xu C, Li H, Ma W, Yang Y, Fan S, Liu Y. MicroRNA-187, down-regulated in clear cell renal cell carcinoma and associated with lower survival, inhibits cell growth and migration though targeting B7-H3. Biochem Biophys Res Commun. 2013;438(2):439. DOI: 10.1016/j.bbrc.2013.07.095.

[95] Reinsbach S, Nazarov PV, Philippidou D, Schmitt M, Wienecke-Baldacchino A, Muller A, Vallar L, Behrmann I, Kreis S. Dynamic regulation of microRNA expression following interferon-gamma-induced gene transcription. RNA Biol. 2012;9(7):978. DOI: 10.4161/rna.20494.

[96] Fiorucci G, Chiantore MV, Mangino G, Romeo G. MicroRNAs in virus-induced tumorigenesis and IFN system. Cytokine Growth Factor Rev. 2015;26(2):183. DOI: 10.1016/j.cytogfr.2014.11.002.

[97] Kohanbash G, Okada H. MicroRNAs and STAT interplay. Semin Cancer Biol. 2012;22(1):70. DOI: 10.1016/j.semcancer.2011.12.010.

[98] Rodriguez A, Vigorito E, Clare S, Warren MV, Couttet P, Soond DR, van Dongen S, Grocock RJ, Das PP, Miska EA, Vetrie D, Okkenhaug K, Enright AJ, Dougan G, Turner M, Bradley A. Requirement of bic/microRNA-155 for normal immune function. Science. 2007;316(5824):608. DOI: 10.1126/science.1139253.

[99] Thai TH, Calado DP, Casola S, Ansel KM, Xiao C, Xue Y, Murphy A, Frendewey D, Valenzuela D, Kutok JL, Schmidt-Supprian M, Rajewsky N, Yancopoulos G, Rao A, Rajewsky K. Regulation of the germinal center response by microRNA-155. Science. 2007;316(5824):604. DOI: 10.1126/science.1141229.

[100] Tili E, Croce CM, Michaille JJ. miR-155: on the crosstalk between inflammation and cancer. Int Rev Immunol. 2009;28(5):264. DOI: 10.1080/08830180903093796.

[101] Trotta R, Chen L, Ciarlariello D, Josyula S, Mao C, Costinean S, Yu L, Butchar JP, Tridandapani S, Croce CM, Caligiuri MA. miR-155 regulates IFN-gamma production in natural killer cells. Blood. 2012;119(15):3478. DOI: 10.1182/blood-2011-12-398099.

[102] Banerjee A, Schambach F, DeJong CS, Hammond SM, Reiner SL. Micro-RNA-155 inhibits IFN-gamma signaling in CD4+ T cells. Eur J Immunol. 2010;40(1):225. DOI: 10.1002/eji.200939381.

[103] Kutty RK, Nagineni CN, Samuel W, Vijayasarathy C, Hooks JJ, Redmond TM. Inflammatory cytokines regulate microRNA-155 expression in human retinal pigment epithelial cells by activating JAK/STAT pathway. Biochem Biophys Res Commun. 2010;402(2):390. DOI: 10.1016/j.bbrc.2010.10.042.

[104] Ding L, Xu Y, Zhang W, Deng Y, Si M, Du Y, Yao H, Liu X, Ke Y, Si J, Zhou T. MiR-375 frequently downregulated in gastric cancer inhibits cell proliferation by targeting JAK2. Cell Res. 2010;20(7):784. DOI: 10.1038/cr.2010.79.

[105] Xu Y, Jin J, Liu Y, Huang Z, Deng Y, You T, Zhou T, Si J, Zhuo W. Snail-regulated MiR-375 inhibits migration and invasion of gastric cancer cells by targeting JAK2. PLoS One. 2014;9(7):e99516. DOI: 10.1371/journal.pone.0099516.

[106] Navarro A, Diaz T, Martinez A, Gaya A, Pons A, Gel B, Codony C, Ferrer G, Martinez C, Montserrat E, Monzo M. Regulation of JAK2 by miR-135a: prognostic impact in classic Hodgkin lymphoma. Blood. 2009;114(14):2945. DOI: 10.1182/blood-2009-02-204842.

[107] Wu H, Huang M, Cao P, Wang T, Shu Y, Liu P. MiR-135a targets JAK2 and inhibits gastric cancer cell proliferation. Cancer Biol Ther. 2012;13(5):281. DOI: 10.4161/cbt.18943.

[108] Hou BH, Jian ZX, Cui P, Li SJ, Tian RQ, Ou JR. miR-216a may inhibit pancreatic tumor growth by targeting JAK2. FEBS Lett. 2015;589(17):2224. DOI: 10.1016/j.febslet.2015.06.036.

[109] Wang S, Chen X, Tang M. MicroRNA-216a inhibits pancreatic cancer by directly targeting Janus kinase 2. Oncol Rep. 2014;32(6):2824. DOI: 10.3892/or.2014.3478.

[110] Wang L, Li L, Guo R, Li X, Lu Y, Guan X, Gitau SC, Wang L, Xu C, Yang B, Shan H. miR-101 promotes breast cancer cell apoptosis by targeting Janus kinase 2. Cell Physiol Biochem. 2014 (b);34(2):413. DOI: 10.1159/000363010.

[111] Gregersen LH, Jacobsen AB, Frankel LB, Wen J, Krogh A, Lund AH. MicroRNA-145 targets YES and STAT1 in colon cancer cells. PLoS One. 2010;5(1):e8836. DOI: 10.1371/journal.pone.0008836.

[112] Akao Y, Nakagawa Y, Naoe T. MicroRNA-143 and -145 in colon cancer. DNA Cell Biol. 2007;26(5):311. DOI: 10.1089/dna.2006.0550.

[113] Ozen M, Creighton CJ, Ozdemir M, Ittmann M. Widespread deregulation of microRNA expression in human prostate cancer. Oncogene. 2008;27(12):1788. DOI: 10.1038/sj.onc.1210809.

[114] Schmitt MJ, Philippidou D, Reinsbach SE, Margue C, Wienecke-Baldacchino A, Nashan D, Behrmann I, Kreis S. Interferon-gamma-induced activation of signal transducer and activator of transcription 1 (STAT1) up-regulates the tumor suppressing microRNA-29 family in melanoma cells. Cell Commun Signal. 2012;10(1):41. DOI: 10.1186/1478-811X-10-41.

[115] Mi S, Lu J, Sun M, Li Z, Zhang H, Neilly MB, Wang Y, Qian Z, Jin J, Zhang Y, Bohlander SK, Le Beau MM, Larson RA, Golub TR, Rowley JD, Chen J. MicroRNA expression signatures accurately discriminate acute lymphoblastic leukemia from acute myeloid leukemia. Proc Natl Acad Sci U S A. 2007;104(50):19971. DOI: 10.1073/pnas.0709313104.

[116] Liu TY, Chen SU, Kuo SH, Cheng AL, Lin CW. E2A-positive gastric MALT lymphoma has weaker plasmacytoid infiltrates and stronger expression of the memory B-

cell-associated miR-223: possible correlation with stage and treatment response. Mod Pathol. 2010;23(11):1507. DOI: 10.1038/modpathol.2010.139.

[117] Kumar V, Palermo R, Talora C, Campese AF, Checquolo S, Bellavia D, Tottone L, Testa G, Miele E, Indraccolo S, Amadori A, Ferretti E, Gulino A, Vacca A, Screpanti I. Notch and NF-kB signaling pathways regulate miR-223/FBXW7 axis in T-cell acute lymphoblastic leukemia. Leukemia. 2014;28(12):2324. DOI: 10.1038/leu.2014.133.

[118] Moles R, Bellon M, Nicot C. STAT1: A novel target of miR-150 and miR-223 is involved in the proliferation of HTLV-I-transformed and ATL cells. Neoplasia. 2015;17(5):449. DOI: 10.1016/j.neo.2015.04.005.

[119] Mraz M, Chen L, Rassenti LZ, Ghia EM, Li H, Jepsen K, Smith EN, Messer K, Frazer KA, Kipps TJ. miR-150 influences B-cell receptor signaling in chronic lymphocytic leukemia by regulating expression of GAB1 and FOXP1. Blood. 2014;124(1):84. DOI: 10.1182/blood-2013-09-527234.

[120] Papakonstantinou N, Ntoufa S, Chartomatsidou E, Papadopoulos G, Hatzigeorgiou A, Anagnostopoulos A, Chlichlia K, Ghia P, Muzio M, Belessi C, Stamatopoulos K. Differential microRNA profiles and their functional implications in different immunogenetic subsets of chronic lymphocytic leukemia. Mol Med. 2013;19:115. DOI: 10.2119/molmed.2013.00005.

[121] Machova Polakova K, Lopotova T, Klamova H, Burda P, Trneny M, Stopka T, Moravcova J. Expression patterns of microRNAs associated with CML phases and their disease related targets. Mol Cancer. 2011;10:41. DOI: 10.1186/1476-4598-10-41.

[122] Morris VA, Zhang A, Yang T, Stirewalt DL, Ramamurthy R, Meshinchi S, Oehler VG. MicroRNA-150 expression induces myeloid differentiation of human acute leukemia cells and normal hematopoietic progenitors. PLoS One. 2013;8(9):e75815. DOI: 10.1371/journal.pone.0075815.

[123] Xu L, Liang YN, Luo XQ, Liu XD, Guo HX. [Association of miRNAs expression profiles with prognosis and relapse in childhood acute lymphoblastic leukemia]. Zhonghua Xue Ye Xue Za Zhi. 2011;32(3):178.

[124] Mashima R. Physiological roles of miR-155. Immunology. 2015;145(3):323. DOI: 10.1111/imm.12468.

[125] Squadrito ML, Etzrodt M, De Palma M, Pittet MJ. MicroRNA-mediated control of macrophages and its implications for cancer. Trends Immunol. 2013;34(7):350. DOI: 10.1016/j.it.2013.02.003.

[126] Chaudhuri AA, So AY, Sinha N, Gibson WS, Taganov KD, O'Connell RM, Baltimore D. MicroRNA-125b potentiates macrophage activation. J Immunol. 2011;187(10):5062. DOI: 10.4049/jimmunol.1102001.

[127] Liu Y, Lai L, Chen Q, Song Y, Xu S, Ma F, Wang X, Wang J, Yu H, Cao X, Wang Q. MicroRNA-494 is required for the accumulation and functions of tumor-expanded

myeloid-derived suppressor cells via targeting of PTEN. J Immunol. 2012;188(11): 5500. DOI: 10.4049/jimmunol.1103505.

[128] Chen S, Zhang Y, Kuzel TM, Zhang B. Regulating tumor myeloid-derived suppressor cells by microRNAs. Cancer Cell Microenviron. 2015;2(1). DOI: 10.14800/ccm.637.

[129] Sasaki K, Kohanbash G, Hoji A, Ueda R, McDonald HA, Reinhart TA, Martinson J, Lotze MT, Marincola FM, Wang E, Fujita M, Okada H. miR-17-92 expression in differentiated T cells—implications for cancer immunotherapy. J Transl Med. 2010;8:17. DOI: 10.1186/1479-5876-8-17.

[130] Donatelli SS, Zhou JM, Gilvary DL, Eksioglu EA, Chen X, Cress WD, Haura EB, Schabath MB, Coppola D, Wei S, Djeu JY. TGF-beta-inducible microRNA-183 silences tumor-associated natural killer cells. Proc Natl Acad Sci U S A. 2014;111(11):4203. DOI: 10.1073/pnas.1319269111.

Chapter 4

Long Noncoding RNAs are Frontier Breakthrough of RNA World and RNAi-based Gene Regulation

Utpal Bhadra, Debabani Roy Chowdhury, Tanmoy Mondal and Manika Pal Bhadra

Additional information is available at the end of the chapter

http://dx.doi.org/10.5772/61975

Abstract

General complexities in versatile animals are not always proportional to their genome size. A notable example is that the salamander genome size is 15-fold larger than that of human, which mostly contains unfolded "junk DNA." A vast portion of this non-protein-coding unfolded DNA undergoes transcriptional regulation and produces a large number of long noncoding RNAs (lncRNAs). LncRNAs play key roles in gene expression and therapies of different human diseases. Recently, novel lncRNAs and their function on the silencing or activation of a particular gene(s) are regularly being discovered. Another important component of gene regulation is high packing of chromatin, which is composed of mainly repetitive sequences with negligible coding potential. In particular, an epigenetic marker determines the state of the gene associated with it, whether the gene will be expressed or silenced. Here, we elaborately discuss the biogenesis pathway of lncRNAs as well as their mechanism of action and role in gene silencing and regulation, including RNA interference. Moreover, several lncRNAs are the common precursors of small regulatory RNAs. It is thus becoming increasingly clear that lncRNAs can function via numerous paradigms as key regulatory molecules in different organisms.

Keywords: Transcriptional silencing, long noncoding RNA, cancer, neurological disorder, *Drosophila*

1. Introduction

Since the earliest days of molecular biology, RNA-mediated gene regulation was known to the researchers, and it was first suggested that noncoding RNA (ncRNA) might have a role in gene regulation by interacting with promoters [1, 2]. After more than four decades of research, the discovery of RNA interference (RNAi) has revolutionized our perception of the mechanism of gene regulation, organization of chromosomes, and epigenetic regulations. Important clues to ncRNA regulatory mechanisms came from homology-dependent gene silencing in plants, which can be initiated by transgenes and recombinant viruses [3]. Studies on the nematode *Caenorhabditis elegans*, the fruit fly *Drosophila melanogaster* [4], fungi mainly yeast, mammalian cells, and plants revealed transcriptional silencing mechanisms involving RNAi, chromatin, and its various modifications [3]. RNAi operates mainly posttranscriptionally; however, its components are associated with transcriptional gene silencing and heterochromatin formation, too [5].

Recent findings have made it clear that transcriptional gene silencing (TGS), posttranscriptional gene silencing (PTGS), and chromatin modifications are utilized by eukaryotic cells to bring about endogenous gene regulation, chromosome organization, and nuclear clustering. The RNA interference mechanisms mainly target the transposable elements, which are abundant and perhaps a defining component of heterochromatin. The role of ncRNA in dosage compensation, inactivation of X chromosome, genomic imprinting, polycomb silencing, and blocking of interactions between enhancers and promoters by chromatin insulators is well proven. Although the studies strongly point towards the involvement of RNAi, its role has not been demonstrated directly [6].

The non-protein-coding transcripts longer than 200 nucleotides are known as long noncoding RNAs to differentiate superficially this class of ncRNAs from microRNAs, short interfering RNAs, piwi-interacting RNAs, small nucleolar RNAs, etc [7]. LncRNAs have emerged as important regulators of cell physiology and pathology. Different studies have come up with an increasing number of lncRNAs showing tissue-specific expression; however, the exact mechanism of action of only a few lncRNAs has been elucidated *in vivo* [8–14]. The biological functions and mechanisms of action of the majority of lncRNAs still remain unknown. LncRNAs can interact with a wide range of molecules and can form RNA-RNA, RNA-DNA, or RNA-protein complexes through specific RNA functional domains [15], resulting in extensive functional diversities. Recent research focuses on lncRNAs and divulges the association of lncRNAs with epigenetic machinery to control chromatin structure, nuclear clustering, and gene expression. The studies reveal that lncRNAs may act together with many histone- and DNA-modifying enzymes to modify the histones or DNA. In addition, a recent discovery of a cardioprotective lncRNA showed a targeting mechanism through ATP-dependent chromatin remodeling factors [16], indicating an extensive role of lncRNAs in chromatin structure and regulation. The mechanisms of how lncRNAs control chromatin by covalent modifications are extensively reviewed in the literature [17–20].

The study of lncRNAs has taken the center stage for the researchers working with epigenetic regulations, and there is a report of a new lncRNA regulating a disease, or transcriptome studies come up with a new class of noncoding RNA, or we are introduced to hitherto unknown mechanisms by which an lncRNA regulates a particular gene almost on a weekly basis. These are all possible due to the introduction of many advanced, high-throughput genomic technologies such as microarrays and next-generation sequencing (NGS). There are a huge number of reported lncRNAs that are not derived from protein-coding genes, and in spite of this vast number of reports on lncRNA, we have just started getting a clear picture about how lncRNAs function, how many different types of lncRNAs exist, and how many of the reported lncRNAs are biologically important.

2. The C-value enigma and junk DNA

It has long been known that developmental complexity or size of an animal does not correspond with C-value or the amount of DNA in the haploid genome [21–23]. The lower animal in the evolution ladder, salamander, has a genome size 15 times larger than that of humans [21], and this discrepancy is known as the "C-value paradox" [23]. Since the introns were discovered, we started to presume that the C-value paradox was now solved [24]. We are almost sure that humans have about 25,000–35,000 protein-coding genes unlike the overestimates of 50,000–100,000 from the initial days of the Human Genome Project [25]. The remaining huge amount of noncoding DNA was termed as "junk DNA" [24, 26] due to the presence of transposons, pseudogenes, and simple repeats, which occupies about 50–70% of the human genome [27]. C-value enigma poses a discrepancy in genome size and number of protein-coding genes. Phylogenetically close genera may vary in C-value by around four- to five fold [28].

In spite of their "junk" status, scientists were always curious to study them and even realized that "being junk doesn't mean it is entirely useless" [26]. It was hypothesized that the junk DNA might be useful in chromosomal pairing, genome integrity, gene regulation, mRNA processing, and serving as a reservoir for evolutionary innovation. We are now pleasantly surprised at their foresight. In the 1970s, it was already thought that noncoding RNA products, such as rRNAs, tRNAs do not make up the whole transcribed genome.

The scale of "pervasive transcription," however, was not fully appreciated until the late 1990s and early 2000s. After the arrival of whole genome technologies, from microarray hybridization and deep sequencing analysis techniques, it was recently shown that 70–90% of our genome is transcribed at some point during embryogenesis [29]. Some recently identified transcripts may be present at as low as 0.0006 copies per cell [30]. Another concern is that tiling microarrays can come up with false positives, low dynamic range, resolution, and low concordance between studies [31]. The existence of noncoding transcription in intergenic regions is evident from correlations with chromatin signatures, such as DNase1 hypersensitivity, and histone modifications such as H3K9ac, H3K4me3, and H3K36me3 [31]. Although these studies report novel and conserved lncRNAs, that is not enough to explain the function of 70–90% of the genome and biological functionality of the ncRNAs. In 1969, Britten and Davidson presented a model for regulation of gene expression in eukaryotic cells where ncRNAs have important roles as regulatory intermediaries to convey signals from sensory to receptor elements [1]. Some of the first examples of gene-specific regulatory roles of lncRNAs were revealed with the discovery of lncRNAs involved in epigenetic regulation, such as H19 [32] and X-inactive specific transcript (Xist) [33, 34].

3. Stand-alone lncRNAs

These lncRNAs are located as separate units and do not overlap protein-coding genes. Some of these are known as lincRNAs for large intergenic (or intervening) noncoding RNAs (lincRNAs) [35]. Many of the lincRNAs were identified through chromatin signatures for actively transcribed genes (H3K4me3 at the promoter and H3K36me3 along the transcribed length). Many of the characterized lncRNAs are transcribed by RNA Pol II, polyadenylated, and spliced and have an average length of 1 kb.

4. Natural antisense transcripts

In this study, transcription occurs in the antisense strand of annotated transcription units; about 70% of sense transcripts have reported antisense counterparts [36]. The overlap between these sense/antisense pairs can be a complete sequence, but natural antisense transcripts are mostly found to be enriched around the 5′ promoter or 3′ terminator ends of the sense transcript. The most extensively studied example of sense/antisense pairing is Xist/Tsix (lncRNA antisense to Xist), with two RNAs that control X chromosome inactivation [37]. In addition, many imprinted regions contain coding/noncoding sense/antisense pairs, such as Kcnq1 (potassium channel, voltage-gated KQT-like subfamily Q, member 1)/Kcnq1ot1 (Kcnq1 overlapping transcript 1) [38] and Igf2r (insulin-like growth factor 2 receptor)/Air (antisense Igf2r RNA) [39]. These pairs are generally less spliced or polyadenylated when compared to mRNAs or stand-alone lncRNAs.

5. Long intronic ncRNAs

Introns have long been known to contain small ncRNAs such as small nucleolar RNAs (snoRNAs) and microRNAs (miRNAs). However, by large-scale transcriptomic or computational analyses, many long transcripts have been reported to be encoded within the introns of known genes [40]. Although they have differential expression patterns and respond to the environmental stimuli differently, only a few have been extensively studied to date. One such example is cold-assisted intronic noncoding RNA (COLDAIR) that has been implicated in plant vernalization, which is located in the first intron of the flowering repressor locus FLC [41].

6. Identification of long noncoding RNAs

LncRNAs are identified by transcripts that map to genomic regions outside the boundaries of protein-coding genes. It is difficult to ascertain the function of a transcript that overlaps a protein-coding gene using targeted knockout or knockdown approaches. Thus, most experimental investigations of lncRNAs have been focused on those that are located in intron sequences. It is also very difficult to ascertain whether an lncRNA locus is entirely intergenic because lncRNA transcripts are often incomplete and they can originate from a protein-coding gene's promoter or enhancer on either strand [42]. Tiling microarray technique is often useful to detect intergenic transcripts [43]. However, controversial results were found here and these experiments can be ruled out [31]. Early lncRNA collections relied primarily on sequenced cDNA and EST clones [44]. More recently, RNA-Seq has come up with a number of lncRNAs derived from whole transcriptome sequencing. RNA-Seq generates millions of 35–100 nt sequences read in parallel, and it has been confirmed that a large chunk of intergenic sequences are transcribed into lncRNAs [45]. The high-throughput and impartial nature of this technique is being utilized for the detailed assessment of the contribution of lncRNAs to a variety of tissue and/or species under different conditions.

To accurately distinguish noncoding from coding transcripts, sophisticated approaches have been developed. For example, the Coding Potential Calculator [46] takes into account six features of a transcript, including the proportion of the transcript enclosed by the candidate peptide-encoding region, and the sequence similarity to known proteins. An evolutionary approach, followed in phyloCSF, predicts ncRNAs when their sequence differences among species do not show preference as to whether they disrupt or not putatively encode peptides [47].

Experimentally determined transcripts always are relied on more than predicted ones. The availability of large proteomic databases can be utilized to investigate whether a specific RNA molecule is translated into a protein. *In vitro* translation assays have been used, too, but they do not necessarily reflect *in vivo* biology. A true lncRNA should not bind with translation machinery, and this approach is also adopted in the identification of candidate lncRNA. However, a study has reported that 50% of a set of putative lncRNAs are ribosome associated [48], leaving in doubt whether this test is accurate in separating coding from noncoding transcripts. To assign an lncRNA, an experimental determination of the function of a transcript will be necessary. Nevertheless, some transcripts possess both RNA- and coding-sequence-dependent functions [49] and demarcating them will be difficult. A computational or experimental method has not yet been developed that discriminates accurately between coding and noncoding transcripts. For the time being, we can rely on *in silico* screens for the protein-coding potential of putative lncRNAs but be aware that these will contain false-positive predictions, too, especially for genes that encode short polypeptides.

Although many genomes contain a substantial number of lncRNA loci, we still do not know the proportion and number of these that are biologically functional. Because the functional mechanisms of most noncoding transcripts or transcript regions are unknown, it is difficult to design point mutation or deletion experiments and their results are difficult to interpret. Even RNAi techniques are not being helpful to assign the functionality of the ncRNAs.

7. Mechanisms of action

We do not know yet the mechanistic detail of the enormous number of reported lncRNAs. However, a few that have been thoroughly studied provide clues regarding how lncRNAs might carry out gene regulation (Figure 1). In addition, many lncRNAs blur the line of different categories and employ several different mechanisms. The discovery of new lncRNAs and more thorough characterization of those already known will reveal additional modes of action.

It has been found that a major role of lncRNA is to recruit regulatory proteins for the regulation of chromatin states [50]. This kind of lncRNAs may act in *cis*, on adjacent or nearby genes, or they might act in *trans*, regulating genes located in distant domains or chromosomes. Polycomb repressive complex 2 (PRC2) interacts with a large number of lncRNAs [51–54]. The *Drosophila* polycomb proteins, first discovered as homeotic gene, express during development [55, 56]. These include enhance of zeste homolog 2 (Ezh2, catalytic subunit in PRC2), which is a key H3K27 methyltransferase, and the Pc/Chromobox (Cbx) family proteins in PRC1, chromodomain-containing proteins that can bind trimethylated H3K27 [55, 56]. Observed interactions of polycomb proteins with lncRNAs suggest that polycomb recruitment is RNA directed in mammals. HOX transcript antisense RNA (HOTAIR) in the homeobox (HOX) C cluster is reported to repress transcription of HOXD in *trans* through interaction with PRC2 [57]. Xist RNA-containing repeat A (RepA) has been found to recruit PRC2 [58]. RepA targets PRC2 to the Xist promoter resulting in Xist up-regulation. The interesting fact is that RepA/Xist interaction with PRC2 may be blocked by the antisense Tsix transcript, also interacting with PRC2 and competitively inhibiting the painting of Xist on inactive X chromosome [58].

Other epigenetic complexes interact with lncRNAs as well, such as the H3K9 methyltransferase G9a interacting with the imprinted lncRNA Air [59]. Kcnq1ot1 has been hypothesized to recruit both PRC2 and G9a to the promoter of Kcnq1 [60] acting as a scaffold. On the other hand, antisense ncRNA in the INK4 locus (ANRIL), associated with p15/INK4 (inhibitors of CDK4 family) B-p16/INK4A-p14/ARF tumor suppressor gene cluster, interacts with both the PRC1 component Cbx7 and the PRC2 component Suz1 [61, 62]. HOTAIR also interacts with the lysine-specific demethylase 1 (LSD1)/corepressor protein of LSD1 (CoREST)/repressor for element 1-silencing transcription factor (REST) complex in addition to PRC2 to prevent gene activation [63].

LncRNAs can also act by recruiting factors involved in gene activation. Such factors from the HOXA (homeotic gene A cluster), two lncRNAs, Mistral (Mira), and HOXA transcript at the distal tip (HOTTIP) have been involved in recruiting the mixed lineage leukemia (MLL) complex in *cis* regulation [64, 65].

An H3K4 trimethylase, myeloid/lymphoid or mixed-lineage leukemia (MLL), is a member of the Trithorax group of developmentally important gene-activating proteins in flies [66]. Using 3C or chromosome conformation capture technique, it was found that multiple loci, which are 40 kb apart in the HOXA cluster, are in close physical proximity, enabling MLL to regulate their expression. Other than histone modifications, lncRNAs also impact epigenetic regulation by modulating DNA methylation at CpG dinucleotides, which has an important role in the stable repression of genes [67]. During embryogenesis, methylation markers are first to be found on previously unmethylated DNA by the DNA (cytosine-5-)-methyltransferase 3α (Dnmt3a) and 3β (Dnmt3b) and later maintained through DNA replication by Dnmt1. Tsix might be converted to Xist by utilizing Dnmt3a activity to methylate and finally silence the Xist promoter [68, 69]. In the same way, Kcnq1ot1 may recruit Dnmt1 [70].

http://dx.doi.org/10.5772/61975

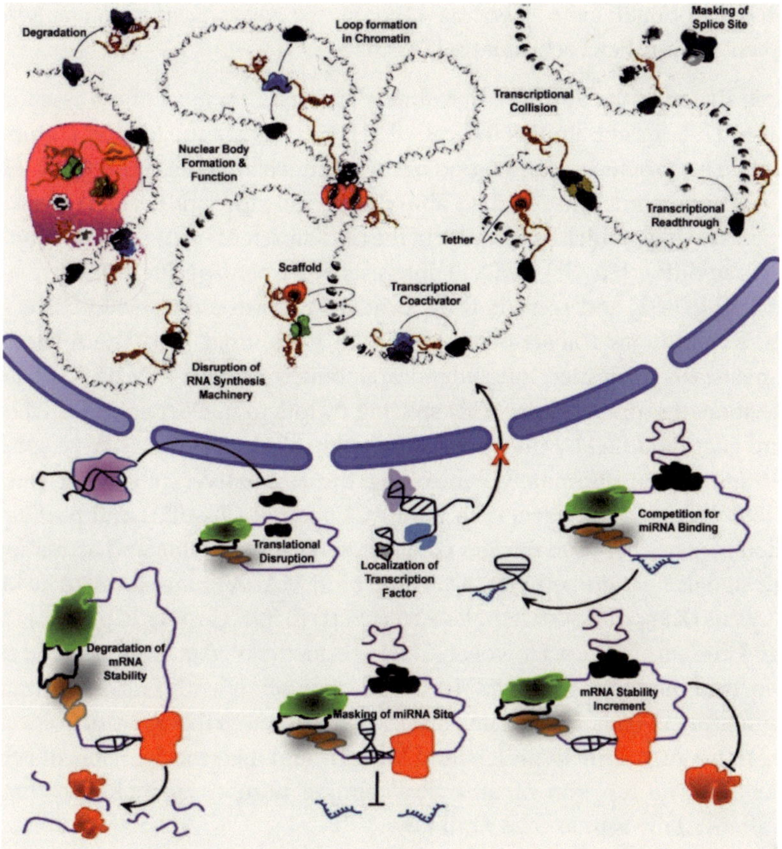

Figure 1. Mechanisms of lncRNA function (modified from Kung et al. [129]).

LncRNA-directed methylation has also been implicated in the regulation of rDNA. Ribosomal DNA exists in the genome as tandem repeat units [71]. Each unit encodes a polycistronic transcript consisting various rRNAs, and each unit is separated by intergenic spacers (IGSs) transcribed by RNA Pol I [72]. Recently, it was reported that IGS transcripts undergo processing into 150- to 300-nt fragments called promoter (p)RNAs, which act as scaffolds to recruit poly (ADP ribose)-polymerase-1 (PARP1) [73], the ATP-dependent nucleolar chromatin remodeling complex (NoRC) [74], and Dnmt3b [75]. A conserved hairpin structure is formed by pRNA that binds both PARP1 and the TIP5 subunit of NoRC, leading to TIP5 conformation change resulting in the recruitment of NoRC to the nucleolus, where rDNA is located [74, 76]. The interesting fact is that the recruitment of Dnmt3b by pRNA is dependent on DNA:RNA triplexing, possibly via Hoogsteen base pairing, between the 5′ end of pRNA and the rDNA promoter [75]. The DNA:RNA triplex formation might be a general mechanism by which lncRNAs recruit *trans* factors to specific DNA loci. LncRNAs are intrinsically bound to chromatin during transcription and transcribed from a single locus in the genome, so they have a direct allele- and locus-specific control in *cis* unlike transcription factors. The length of lncRNAs is also suitable to reach out and capture epigenetic marks. This *cis*-acting mechanism resembles transcriptional gene silencing seen in the yeast *Schizosaccharomyces pombe* in assembling centromeric heterochromatin [77, 78].

The nucleus is always in the dynamic state and is the center for most of the essential functions of an organism [79]. Recent studies indicate that lncRNAs are the key regulators of nuclear compartments. The structure and function of several nuclear bodies seem to be controlled by RNA. One example is nuclear-enriched abundant transcript 1 (NEAT1) that maintains the stability of paraspeckles, which participate in the nuclear retention of mRNAs after adenosine-to-inosine hyperediting [80, 81]. NEAT1 interacts with paraspeckle proteins, such as p54/NONO and PSP [80–82] and recruits these proteins to form paraspeckles. This is an active process where continuous transcription of NEAT1 is required [84]. The related molecules, NEAT2 or metastasis-associated lung adenocarcinoma transcript 1 (MALAT1), are involved in the localization of serine/arginine (SR) splicing factors to nuclear speckles where they can be stored and later modified by phosphorylation [85]. MALAT1 directs these splicing factors to sites of transcription, ultimately controlling the alternative splicing of certain mRNA precursors [86]. MALAT1 interacts with the PRC1 subunit Cbx4/Pc2 and participates in the transportation of genes between nuclear compartments for silencing and activation. Extracellular growth signals help unmethylated Cbx4 to bind MALAT1 and localize its target genes, along with Lysine (K)-specific demethylase 1A (LSD1) to interchromatin granules that usually cluster around nuclear speckles. However, Cbx4 gets methylated in the absence of extracellular signal and instead binds another lncRNA TUG1, then binds with Ezh2, and translocates to silencing compartments called polycomb bodies [87]. Although these recent observations have started to open up an avenue to understand lncRNA and their mechanisms of action, we are still way behind. The function of an overwhelming number of lncRNAs that are being discovered almost daily is unknown until now.

8. Epigenetic regulation

The two most abundant modes of action of lncRNAs are the modulation of chromatin by recruiting histone proteins and transcription factors within specific chromatin-modifying complexes. A very good example of recruitment of specific histones is X chromosome inactivation (XCI), which is caused by "Xist" as described in the earlier section [58]. A similar event is genomic imprinting, where genes are expressed from the allele of only one parent. One of the first and best studied lncRNAs is H19, which is mutually imprinted with insulin-like growth factor 2 (Igf2). This lncRNA is highly expressed, but its deletion has no phenotypic outcome, and it is anticipated to function as a microRNA precursor [88]. Other lncRNAs (e.g., Air, Kcnq1ot1, and HOTAIR) show modulatory activities both in *cis* or in *trans* and regulating gene expression through partnering with chromatin-modifying complexes [70, 89]. Specifically, HOTAIR is a *trans*-acting lncRNA that serves as a scaffold for two histone modification complexes: it binds both to PRC2 and to LSD1 [63]. In the *Arabidopsis* plant, it was found that different environmental conditions are able to induce the transcription of related NATs (i.e., COOLAIR) that eventually silence a flower repressor locus, flowering locus c (FLC) [90]. Recently, it was discovered that lncRNA, namely COLDAIR, bearing minor differences from

http://dx.doi.org/10.5772/61975

COOLAIR (transcribed in the sense direction relative to FLC mRNA transcription), interacts on its own with PRC2 and targets it to FLC [41]. Other *trans*-acting lncRNAs have different functions, some of which remain incompletely defined. There are several poorly defined *trans*-acting lncRNAs, such as the p21-associated ncRNA DNA damage activated (PANDA), which is induced upon DNA damage in a p53-dependent manner and it controls the expression of proapoptotic genes [91].

9. Transcriptional regulation

The discovery and characterization of promoter-associated RNAs opened up a new understanding on how genes are regulated during transcription. These RNAs are localized within the promoter and consist of various sizes of RNA molecules [92]. The long ones are found at a single-gene level and are associated with the modification of DNA methylation and demethylation patterns [93] as mentioned earlier. Interestingly, long (antisense) pRNAs generally form double-stranded molecules that are processed into endo-siRNAs, and since they have sequence complementarity with the promoter, they induce transcriptional gene silencing [20, 94–96] or activation [97–99].

LncRNAs sometimes affect transcription by acting as coregulators or by regulating the association and activity of coregulators. One example is embryonic ventral forebrain-2 (Evf-2) that functions as a coactivator for the homeobox transcription factor distal-less homeobox 2 (Dlx2) [100].

10. Posttranscriptional regulation

lncRNAs not only have a role in transcription but also they function in splicing, mRNA stability, and translation. Antisense lncRNA sometimes bind to the sense RNA, conceal the splice sites, and thereby modify the balance between splice variants. Antisense transcript RevErbAα modifies the splicing of thyroid hormone receptor alpha genes (TRα) TRα1 and TRα2 mRNAs [101].

The terminal differentiation-induced ncRNA (TINCR) associates with Staufen 1 but not with the complex between TINCR-NA, which is a differentiation factor [102].

LncRNAs have also been implicated in translational regulation. An example is the antisense for PU1 mRNA. Its translation is inhibited by an antisense polyadenylated lncRNA with a half-life longer than the original transcript [103]. Another example is the lncRNA Uchl1, which is controlled by mammalian target of rapamycin (mTOR) pathway, shuttles from the nucleus to the cytoplasm, and controls the translation of the ubiquitin carboxy-terminal hydrolase L1 (UCHL1) mRNA by promoting its association with polysomes [104].

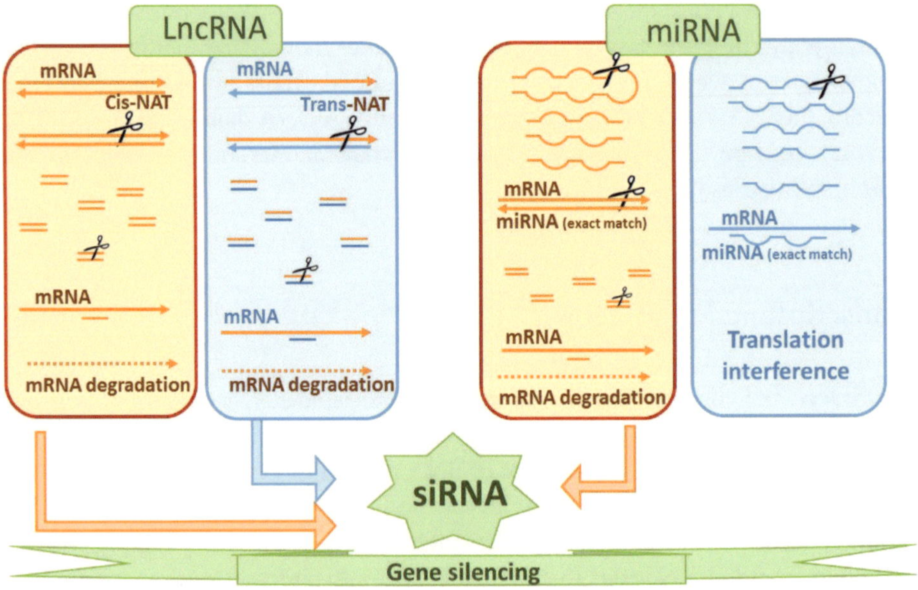

Figure 2. Posttranscriptional gene silencing by lncRNA and miRNA (adapted from Gomes et al. [130]).

11. Role of lncRNAs in cancer and other human diseases

The genome-wide association studies identify several cancer risk loci outside of protein-coding regions. Of 301 single-nucleotide polymorphisms currently linked to cancer, only 12 (3.3%) modify the amino acid sequence of the protein, and most of the loci are located in the introns (40%) or intergenic regions (44%) [105]. These facts and the observations that miRNA and lncRNAs are involved in differentiation and development point towards the fact that alterations in their expression profiles could be correlated with cancer development. Reports suggested that lncRNAs have tissue-specific expression and is found to be deregulated in distinct types of cancers. For example, overexpression of miR-155 was reported in hematopoietic, breast, lung, and colon cancers [106], whereas miR-21 is overexpressed in glioblastoma [107]. In addition, lymphoproliferative disorders were found in transgenic mice overexpressing miR-17-92 [108]. Incidences of lung, colon, and gastric cancers were found to be correlated with the overexpression of miR-17-92 cluster [109]. LncRNAs have been associated with cancer development likewise. The lncRNA MALAT1 is up-regulated in several cancer types, resulting in an increase in cell proliferation and migration in lung and colorectal cancer cells [105]. The role of MALAT1 in controlling alternative splicing of pre-mRNAs [86] can be deduced from this. A more recent study indicates that MALAT1 may also participate in the regulation of gene expression by a mechanism other than alternative splicing in lung metastasis [110].

Other studies have shown that miRNA and lncRNAs both can function as tumor suppressor genes or oncogenes. The tumor suppressor gene p53 regulates the three gene members of the

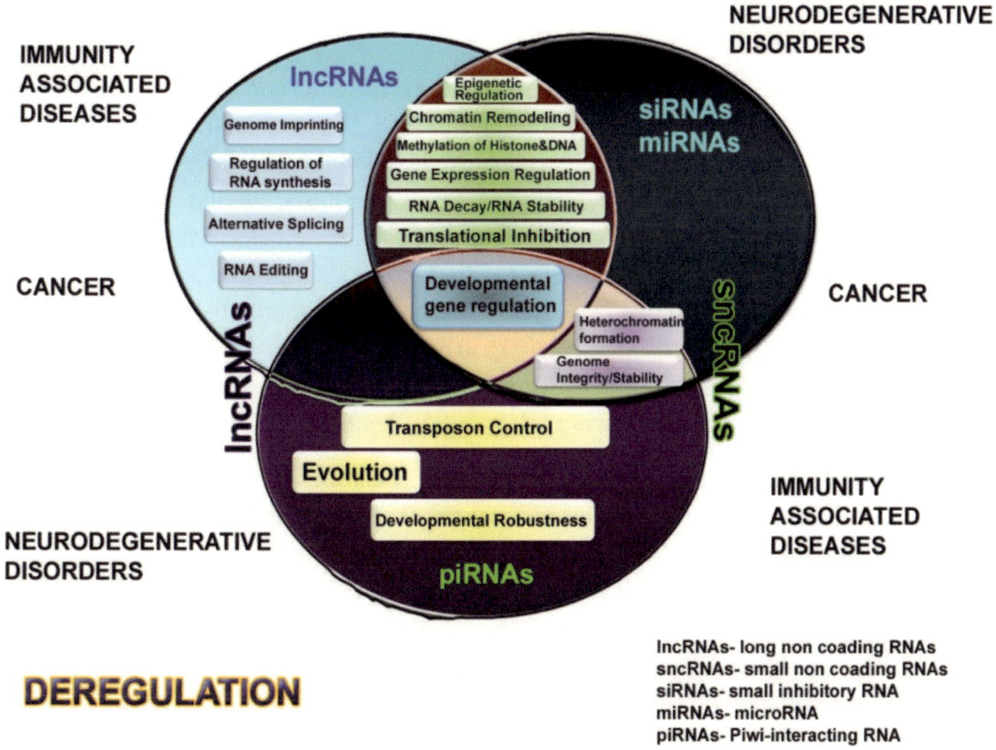

Figure 3. Relationship among various noncoding RNAs and different disorders caused by them (adapted from Gomes et al. [130].

miR-34 family. Curiously, the microRNA-34 (miR-34) activation resembles p53 activity, such as the induction of cell cycle arrest and promotion of apoptosis, and p53-mediated apoptosis becomes defective in the absence of miR-34 [111].

LncRNAs that recruit epigenetic modifiers to specific loci such as ANRIL, XIST, HOTAIR, and KCNQ1OT1 are found to have altered expression in a variety of cancers [112]. Another lncRNA called TERRA binds telomerase, inhibiting its activity *in vitro* [113], and is observed to be down-regulated in many cancer cells, linking it with the longevity of cancer cells.

Chromatin remodeling by lncRNA is linked to other diseases such as facioscapulohumeral muscular dystrophy (FSHD) [97], lethal lung developmental disorder [114], and the HELLP syndrome, a pregnancy-associated disease [114] in addition to cancer. The HELLP stands for H = hemolysis (breakdown of red blood cells), EL = elevated liver enzymes (liver function), and LP = low platelet counts (platelets help the blood clot). These examples directly link lncRNA and miRNAs in cancer biology and other human diseases and indicate the involvement of a complex interplay among their biogenesis pathways, their regulatory mechanisms, and their targets.

12. Dosage compensation and X inactivation

X chromosome inactivation (XCI) occurs in females during embryogenesis, where either the maternal or paternal X chromosome is randomly silenced. The molecular mechanisms of XCI are not yet fully understood. However, it is known that a 500-kb stretch of DNA at Xq13 known as the X-inactivation centre (XIC) is the site for initiation of X inactivation. There are several lncRNAs, including X-inactive specific transcript (Xist), its antisense transcript Tsix, X-inactivation intergenic transcription elements (Xite), Jpx transcript, and Xist activator (Jpx), and others play pivotal roles in XCI [115]. Xist was one of the first to be identified and best studied lncRNAs. It is a ~17-kb transcript (~19 kb in humans) expressed from the future inactive X chromosome (Xi) [116]. Tsix is a ~40-kb antisense transcript to Xist. It negatively regulates Xist. Recent studies indicate that Xite is a transcriptional enhancer of Tsix [115], and likewise, Jpx RNA appears to help in Xist expression [117].

When two homologous X chromosomes are brought at close proximity, Tsix and Xite initiate the inactivation process by counting, and this is associated with the presence of RNA polymerase II (RNAPII) [118, 119]. The chromatin insulator CTCF, which binds to Tsix and Xite genomic loci [120], play an important role. The transcription factor OCT4 is then hypothesized to bind with Tsix promoters of one of the X chromosomes, which then converts to active X chromosome (Xa) due to increased transcription of Tsix [120]. Thereafter, Dnmt3a is recruited to the Xa and establishes stable silencing of Xist on the Xa [115, 118].

13. LncRNA in genomic imprinting

In mammals, genomic imprinting is an epigenetic marker in a way that their expression occurs specifically in parental origin manner. This occurs during early gametogenesis in nearly 1% of protein-coding genes. To date, we have identified around 150 imprinted genes in mice. Imprinted genes are often located in clusters of size from a few kilobases to 2 to 3 Mb. LncRNAs are present in all the identified and elucidated imprinted clusters as their partners. The expression of lncRNAs is reciprocally linked with corresponding protein-coding genes [121–123].

Genomic imprinting mainly happens by chromatin insulators [124–126] and lncRNAs [38, 127]. LncRNAs repress flanking gene promoters in *cis* action (Kcnq1ot1 and Airn lncRNAs [115]). However, several reports indicate that lncRNAs function as a major force in the regulation of parent-of-origin-specific expression. Today, we know that the human genome contains more than 58,648 lncRNA expressed genes compared to only 21,313 protein-coding genes [128]. The majority of the lncRNAs act by interacting with chromatin-modifying complexes such as PRC2, G9a, hnRNPK, and SWI/SNF, recruiting them sequentially to silence genes in *cis* or *trans* action [57, 60].

14. Perspectives

LncRNA has diversified tentacles for functions. Those include an alteration of transcriptional profiles, controlling of protein expression, complex structural or organizational roles, RNA processing or RNA editing and role of being the precursor of small RNAs. Because a very small fraction of lncRNA have been molecularly characterized to date, many more yet to be discovered that fit into this diversified functional paradigms. Future work will definitely ask many more questions about the interplay of lncRNA transcripts and whether it is sufficient to have fundamental sequence of events or not. Many lncRNAs play intermediate roles in *cis* regulation that gets represented in ectopic expression in *trans* regulation.

Most recent challenges are to identify how the molecular function of each type of lncRNA results in different diseases of the organism. LncRNA appears to expose numerous developmental events such as the generation of photoreceptor cells in retina development, control of cell surveillance, cell cycle progression of mammary gland development, and finally generation of knockout animal development. Many lncRNAs are not eliminated as transcriptional noise in the genome but are useful for normal developmental processes.

LncRNA has a tremendous impact on disease development due to its flawless miscegenation. In tumor formation, the expression of lncRNAs is very important. They function like specific markers of tumor formation. However, the exact mechanism by which tumor initiation, formation, and progression would occur is not fully understood. It is true that the interplay and significant role of lncRNA in different disease research is really an unexplored area, which is eventually determining the new therapeutic targets. Recently, it was found that lncRNA may form β-amyloid plaques in Alzheimer's disease. This possibility suggested that noncoding transcript might serve as an attractive drug target for Alzheimer's disease.

Most conventionally, genetic information may run through protein-coding sequences, but it is now found that transcription is pervasive through the nucleic acid content of eukaryotic genome, which generated a numerous number of lncRNA, which are possibly the key regulators of protein-coding sequences. We anticipate that many more surprises are yet to be explored in the coming decades. Therefore, future research might provide more pleasant but unexpected surprises in the lncRNA function.

15. Conclusion

The above description exhibits a brief survey of the current status of knowledge regarding the identification, localization, functions, and mechanisms of actions of lncRNAs related to different human diseases. A fraction of genomic nucleic acid is transcribed to protein, but an overwhelming majority of the genome sectors of the organisms contain lncRNA with unknown functional efficacy. Some are nuclear or cytoplasmic and are highly overexpressed, and others are rarely detected. Truly, it is impossible to discern the important criteria such as stability, conservation, and time of expression related to human diseases. LncRNA in the Xic is only found in placental mammals and is not conserved in other mammals. However, this limited conservation might not be essential in other higher animals. The true test for real function lies in the mechanism, genetic pathway, and tissue-specific activity for each lncRNA. The genome of an organism is not always streamlined by the natural selection. Thus, here, we really tried to avoid the speculative statements about localization, function, and dissecting mechanism regarding long noncoding RNA. Truly, we have just begun to scratch the skin of LncRNA in the human body. The lncRNA world is so galactically vast that we have an enormous task to completely learn about it. We feel that additional discoveries of lncRNA may provide a real exciting phase in the study of RNA world.

Acknowledgements

We thank the lab members and Sohini Bose for the extensive discussion in the subjects and help in writing. This work is sponsored by the CSIR Net work grant (BSC-0121) of UB and DBT grant to M.P.B. (GAP 0362). DRC work supported by DST (GAP0432) grant.

Author details

Utpal Bhadra[1*], Debabani Roy Chowdhury[1], Tanmoy Mondal[2] and Manika Pal Bhadra[2]

*Address all correspondence to: utpal@ccmb.res.in

1 Functional Genomics and Gene Silencing Group, Centre for Cellular and Molecular Biology, Hyderabad, India

2 Centre for Chemical Biology, Indian Institute of Chemical Technology, Hyderabad, India

References

[1] Britten RJ, Davidson. Gene regulation for higher cells: A theory. Science. 1969;165(3891):349–357. DOI: 10.1126/science.165.3891.349.

[2] Jacob F, Monod J. Genetic regulatory mechanisms in the synthesis of proteins. J Mol Biol. 1961;3(3):318–356. DOI: 10.1016/S0022-2836(61)80072-7

[3] Matzke MA, Birchler JA. RNAi-mediated pathways in the nucleus. Nat Rev Genet. 2005;6(1):24–35. DOI: 10.1038/nrg1500

[4] Pal-Bhadra M, Bhadra U, Birchler JA. Cosuppression in *Drosophila*: Gene silencing of alcohol dehydrogenase by white-Adh transgenes is polycomb dependent. Cell. 1997;90(3):479–490. DOI: 10.1016/S0092-8674(00)80508-5

[5] Wassenegger M. The role of the RNAi machinery in heterochromatin formation. Cell. 2005;122(1):13–16. DOI: 10.1016/j.cell.2005.06.034

[6] Zaratiegui M, Irvine DV, Martienssen RA. Noncoding RNAs and gene silencing. Cell. 2007;128(4):763–776. DOI: 10.1016/j.cell.2007.02.016

[7] Perkel JM. Visiting "Noncodarnia". Biotechniques. 2013;54(6):301–304. DOI: 10.2144/000114037

[8] Bassett AR, Akhtar A, Barlow DP, Bird AP, Brockdorff N, Duboule D, et al. Considerations when investigating lncRNA function *in vivo*. Elife. 2014;3:e03058. DOI: 10.7554/eLife.03058

[9] Esteller M. Non-coding RNAs in human disease. Nat Rev Genet. 2011;12(12):861–874. DOI: 10.1038/nrg3074

[10] Li L, Chang HY. Physiological roles of long noncoding RNAs: Insight from knockout mice. Trends Cell Biol. 2014;24(10):594–602. DOI: 10.1016/j.tcb.2014.06.003

[11] Maass PG, Luft FC, Bahring S. Long non-coding RNA in health and disease. J Mol Med (Berl). 2014;92(4):337–346. DOI: 10.1007/s00109-014-1131-8

[12] Ponting CP, Oliver PL, Reik W. Evolution and functions of long noncoding RNAs. Cell. 2009;136(4):629–641. DOI: 10.1016/j.cell.2009.02.006

[13] Wapinski O, Chang HY. Long noncoding RNAs and human disease. Trends Cell Biol. 2011;21(6):354–361. DOI: 10.1016/j.tcb.2011.04.001

[14] Mercer TR, Dinger ME, Mattick JS. Long non-coding RNAs: Insights into functions. Nat Rev Genet. 2009;10(3):155–159. DOI: 10.1038/nrg2521

[15] Quinn JJ, Ilik IA, Qu K, Georgiev P, Chu C, Akhtar A, et al. Revealing long noncoding RNA architecture and functions using domain-specific chromatin isolation by RNA purification. Nat Biotechnol. 2014;32(9):933–940. DOI: 10.1038/nbt.2943

[16] Han P, Li W, Lin CH, Yang J, Shang C, Nurnberg ST, et al. A long noncoding RNA protects the heart from pathological hypertrophy. Nature. 2014;514(7520):102–106. DOI: 10.1038/nature13596

[17] Han P, Chang CP. Long non-coding RNA and chromatin remodeling. RNA Biol. 2015;12(10):1–5. DOI: 10.1080/15476286.2015.1063770

[18] Rinn JL. lncRNAs: Linking RNA to chromatin. Cold Spring Harb Perspect Biol. 2014;6(8). DOI: 10.1101/cshperspect.a018614

[19] Rinn JL, Chang HY. Genome regulation by long noncoding RNAs. Annu Rev Biochem. 2012;81:145–166. DOI: 10.1146/annurev-biochem-051410-092902.

[20] Devaux Y, Zangrando J, Schroen B, Creemers EE, Pedrazzini T, Chang CP, et al. Long noncoding RNAs in cardiac development and ageing. Nat Rev Cardiol. 2015;12(7):415–425. DOI: 10.1038/nrcardio.2015.55

[21] Gall JG. Chromosome structure and the C-value paradox. J Cell Biol. 1981;91(3 Pt 2): 3s–14s. 1981;91(3):3–14.

[22] Mirsky AE, Ris H. The deoxyribonucleic acid content of animal cells and its evolutionary significance. J Gen Physiol. 1951;34(4):451–462.

[23] Thomas CA Jr. The genetic organization of chromosomes. Annu Rev Genet. 1971;5:237–256. DOI: 10.1146/annurev.ge.05.120171.001321

[24] Ohno S. So much "junk" DNA in our genome. Brookhaven Symp Biol. 1972;23:366–370.

[25] Pertea M, Salzberg SL. Between a chicken and a grape: Estimating the number of human genes. Genome Biol. 2010;11(5):206–212. DOI: 10.1186/gb-2010-11-5-206

[26] Comings DE. The structure and function of chromatin. Adv Hum Genet. 1972;3:237–431.

[27] de Koning AP, Gu W, Castoe TA, Batzer MA, Pollock DD. Repetitive elements may comprise over two-thirds of the human genome. PLoS Genet. 2011;7(12):e1002384. DOI: 10.1371/journal.pgen.1002384

[28] Ricroch A, Yockteng R, Brown SC, Nadot S. Evolution of genome size across some cultivated *Allium* species. Genome. 2005;48(3):511–520. DOI: 10.1139/g05-017

[29] Djebali S, Davis CA, Merkel A, Dobin A, Lassmann T, Mortazavi A, et al. Landscape of transcription in human cells. Nature. 2012;489(7414):101–108. DOI: 10.1038/nature11233

[30] Mercer TR, Gerhardt DJ, Dinger ME, Crawford J, Trapnell C, Jeddeloh JA, et al. Targeted RNA sequencing reveals the deep complexity of the human transcriptome. Nat Biotechnol. 2011;30(1):99–104. DOI: 10.1038/nbt.2024

[31] van Bakel H, Nislow C, Blencowe BJ, Hughes TR. Most "dark matter" transcripts are associated with known genes. PLoS Biol. 2010;8(5):e1000371. DOI: 10.1371/journal.pbio.1000371

[32] Brannan CI, Dees EC, Ingram RS, Tilghman SM. The product of the H19 gene may function as an RNA. Mol Cell Biol. 1990;10(1):28–36. DOI: 10.1128/MCB.10.1.28

[33] Brockdorff N, Ashworth A, Kay GF, McCabe VM, Norris DP, Cooper PJ, et al. The product of the mouse Xist gene is a 15 kb inactive X-specific transcript containing no conserved ORF and located in the nucleus. Cell. 1992;71(3):515–526. DOI: 10.1016/0092-8674(92)90519-I

[34] Brown CJ, Hendrich BD, Rupert JL, Lafreniere RG, Xing Y, Lawrence J, et al. The human XIST gene: Analysis of a 17 kb inactive X-specific RNA that contains conserved repeats and is highly localized within the nucleus. Cell. 1992;71(3):527–542. DOI: 10.1016/0092-8674(92)90520-M

[35] Cabili MN, Trapnell C, Goff L, Koziol M, Tazon-Vega B, Regev A, et al. Integrative annotation of human large intergenic noncoding RNAs reveals global properties and specific subclasses. Genes Dev. 2011;25(18):1915–1927. DOI: 10.1101/gad.17446611

[36] Faghihi MA, Wahlestedt C. Regulatory roles of natural antisense transcripts. Nat Rev Mol Cell Biol. 2009;10(9):637–643. DOI: 10.1038/nrm2738

[37] Lee JT, Davidow LS, Warshawsky D. Tsix, a gene antisense to Xist at the X-inactivation centre. Nat Genet. 1999;21(4):400–404. DOI: 10.1038/7734

[38] Kanduri C, Thakur N, Pandey RR. The length of the transcript encoded from the Kcnq1ot1 antisense promoter determines the degree of silencing. EMBO J. 2006;25(10):2096–2106. DOI: 10.1038/sj.emboj.7601090

[39] Lyle R, Watanabe D, te Vruchte D, Lerchner W, Smrzka OW, Wutz A, et al. The imprinted antisense RNA at the Igf2r locus overlaps but does not imprint Mas1. Nat Genet. 2000;25(1):19–21. DOI: 10.1038/75546

[40] Rearick D, Prakash A, McSweeny A, Shepard SS, Fedorova L, Fedorov A. Critical association of ncRNA with introns. Nucleic Acids Res. 2011;39(6):2357–2366. DOI: 10.1093/nar/gkq1080

[41] Heo JB, Sung S. Vernalization-mediated epigenetic silencing by a long intronic noncoding RNA. Science. 2011;331(6013):76–79. DOI: 10.1126/science.1197349

[42] Taft RJ, Kaplan CD, Simons C, Mattick JS. Evolution, biogenesis and function of promoter-associated RNAs. Cell Cycle. 2009;8(15):2332–2338. DOI: 10.4161/cc.8.15.9154

[43] Bertone P, Stolc V, Royce TE, Rozowsky JS, Urban AE, Zhu X, et al. Global identification of human transcribed sequences with genome tiling arrays. Science. 2004;306(5705):2242–2246. DOI: 10.1126/science.1103388

[44] Okazaki Y, Furuno M, Kasukawa T, Adachi J, Bono H, Kondo S, et al. Analysis of the mouse transcriptome based on functional annotation of 60,770 full-length cDNAs. Nature. 2002;420(6915):563–573. DOI: 10.1038/nature01266

[45] Derrien T, Johnson R, Bussotti G, Tanzer A, Djebali S, Tilgner H, et al. The GENCODE v7 catalog of human long noncoding RNAs: Analysis of their gene structure, evolution, and expression. Genome Res. 2012;22(9):1775–1789. DOI: 10.1101/gr. 132159.111

[46] Kong L, Zhang Y, Ye ZQ, Liu XQ, Zhao SQ, Wei L, et al. CPC: Assess the protein-coding potential of transcripts using sequence features and support vector machine. Nucleic Acids Res. 2007:35(Web Server issue):W345–W349. DOI: 10.1093/nar/gkm391

[47] Lin MF, Jungreis I, Kellis M. PhyloCSF: A comparative genomics method to distinguish protein coding and non-coding regions. Bioinformatics. 2011;27(13):i275–i282. DOI: 10.1093/bioinformatics/btr209

[48] Wilson BA, Masel J. Putatively noncoding transcripts show extensive association with ribosomes. Genome Biol Evol. 2011;3:1245–1252. DOI: 10.1093/gbe/evr099

[49] Dinger ME, Pang KC, Mercer TR, Mattick JS. Differentiating protein-coding and noncoding RNA: Challenges and ambiguities. PLoS Comput Biol. 2008;4(11):e1000176. DOI: 10.1371/journal.pcbi.1000176

[50] Campos EI, Reinberg D. Histones: Annotating chromatin. Annu Rev Genet. 2009;43:559–599. DOI: 10.1146/annurev.genet.032608.103928

[51] Khalil AM, Guttman M, Huarte M, Garber M, Raj A, Rivea Morales D, et al. Many human large intergenic noncoding RNAs associate with chromatin-modifying complexes and affect gene expression. Proc Natl Acad Sci U S A. 2009;106(28):11667–11672. DOI: 10.1073/pnas.0904715106

[52] Kanhere A, Viiri K, Araujo CC, Rasaiyaah J, Bouwman RD, Whyte WA, et al. Short RNAs are transcribed from repressed polycomb target genes and interact with polycomb repressive complex-2. Mol Cell. 2010;38(5):675–688. DOI: 10.1016/j.molcel.2010.03.019

[53] Zhao J, Ohsumi TK, Kung JT, Ogawa Y, Grau DJ, Sarma K, et al. Genome-wide identification of polycomb-associated RNAs by RIP-seq. Mol Cell. 2010;40(6):939–953. DOI: 10.1016/j.molcel.2010.12.011

[54] Guil S, Soler M, Portela A, Carrere J, Fonalleras E, Gomez A, et al. Intronic RNAs mediate EZH2 regulation of epigenetic targets. Nat Struct Mol Biol. 2012;19(7):664–670. DOI: 10.1038/nsmb.2315

[55] Schwartz YB, Pirrotta V. Polycomb silencing mechanisms and the management of genomic programmes. Nat Rev Genet. 2007;8(1):9–22. DOI: 10.1038/nrg1981

[56] Sparmann A, van Lohuizen M. Polycomb silencers control cell fate, development and cancer. Nat Rev Cancer. 2006;6(11):846–856. DOI: 10.1038/nrc1991

[57] Rinn JL, Kertesz M, Wang JK, Squazzo SL, Xu X, Brugmann SA, et al. Functional demarcation of active and silent chromatin domains in human HOX loci by noncoding RNAs. Cell. 2007;129(7):1311–1323. DOI: 10.1016/j.cell.2007.05.022

[58] Zhao J, Sun BK, Erwin JA, Song JJ, Lee JT. Polycomb proteins targeted by a short repeat RNA to the mouse X chromosome. Science. 2008;322(5902):750–756. DOI: 10.1126/science.1163045

[59] Nagano T, Mitchell JA, Sanz LA, Pauler FM, Ferguson-Smith AC, Feil R, et al. The Air noncoding RNA epigenetically silences transcription by targeting G9a to chromatin. Science. 2008;322(5908):1717–1720. DOI: 10.1126/science.1163802

[60] Pandey RR, Mondal T, Mohammad F, Enroth S, Redrup L, Komorowski J, et al. Kcnq1ot1 antisense noncoding RNA mediates lineage-specific transcriptional silenc-

ing through chromatin-level regulation. Mol Cell. 2008;32(2):232–246. DOI: 10.1016/j.molcel.2008.08.022

[61] Yap KL, Li S, Munoz-Cabello AM, Raguz S, Zeng L, Mujtaba S, et al. Molecular interplay of the noncoding RNA ANRIL and methylated histone H3 lysine 27 by polycomb CBX7 in transcriptional silencing of INK4a. Mol Cell. 2010;38(5):662–674. DOI: 10.1016/j.molcel.2010.03.021

[62] Kotake Y, Nakagawa T, Kitagawa K, Suzuki S, Liu N, Kitagawa M, et al. Long noncoding RNA ANRIL is required for the PRC2 recruitment to and silencing of p15(INK4B) tumor suppressor gene. Oncogene. 2011;30(16):1956–1962. DOI: 10.1038/onc.2010.568

[63] Tsai MC, Manor O, Wan Y, Mosammaparast N, Wang JK, Lan F, et al. Long noncoding RNA as modular scaffold of histone modification complexes. Science. 2010;329(5992):689–693. DOI: 10.1126/science.1192002

[64] Bertani S, Sauer S, Bolotin E, Sauer F. The noncoding RNA Mistral activates Hoxa6 and Hoxa7 expression and stem cell differentiation by recruiting MLL1 to chromatin. Mol Cell. 2011;43(6):1040–1046. DOI: 10.1016/j.molcel.2011.08.019

[65] Wang KC, Yang YW, Liu B, Sanyal A, Corces-Zimmerman R, Chen Y, et al. A long noncoding RNA maintains active chromatin to coordinate homeotic gene expression. Nature. 2011;472(7341):120–124. DOI: 10.1038/nature09819

[66] Schuettengruber B, Martinez AM, Iovino N, Cavalli G. Trithorax group proteins: Switching genes on and keeping them active. Nat Rev Mol Cell Biol. 2011;12(12):799–814. DOI: 10.1038/nrm3230

[67] Law JA, Jacobsen SE. Establishing, maintaining and modifying DNA methylation patterns in plants and animals. Nat Rev Genet. 2010;11(3):204–220. DOI: 10.1038/nrg2719

[68] Sado T, Hoki Y, Sasaki H. Tsix defective in splicing is competent to establish Xist silencing. Development. 2006;133(24):4925–4931. DOI: 10.1242/dev.02670

[69] Sun BK, Deaton AM, Lee JT. A transient heterochromatic state in Xist preempts X inactivation choice without RNA stabilization. Mol Cell. 2006;21(5):617–628. DOI: 10.1016/j.molcel.2006.01.028

[70] Mohammad F, Mondal T, Guseva N, Pandey GK, Kanduri C. Kcnq1ot1 noncoding RNA mediates transcriptional gene silencing by interacting with Dnmt1. Development. 2010;137(15):2493–2499. DOI: 10.1242/dev.048181

[71] McStay B, Grummt I. The epigenetics of rRNA genes: From molecular to chromosome biology. Annu Rev Cell Dev Biol. 2008;24:131–157. DOI: 10.1146/annurev.cellbio.24.110707.175259

[72] Mayer C, Schmitz KM, Li J, Grummt I, Santoro R. Intergenic transcripts regulate the epigenetic state of rRNA genes. Mol Cell. 2006;22(3):351–361. DOI: 10.1016/j.molcel.2006.03.028

[73] Guetg C, Scheifele F, Rosenthal F, Hottiger MO, Santoro R. Inheritance of silent rDNA chromatin is mediated by PARP1 via noncoding RNA. Mol Cell. 2012;45(6):790–800. DOI: 10.1016/j.molcel.2012.01.024

[74] Mayer C, Neubert M, Grummt I. The structure of NoRC-associated RNA is crucial for targeting the chromatin remodelling complex NoRC to the nucleolus. EMBO Rep. 2008;9(8):774–780. DOI: 10.1038/embor.2008.109

[75] Schmitz KM, Mayer C, Postepska A, Grummt I. Interaction of noncoding RNA with the rDNA promoter mediates recruitment of DNMT3b and silencing of rRNA genes. Genes Dev. 2010;24(20):2264–2269. DOI: 10.1101/gad.590910

[76] Guetg C, Lienemann P, Sirri V, Grummt I, Hernandez-Verdun D, Hottiger MO, et al. The NoRC complex mediates the heterochromatin formation and stability of silent rRNA genes and centromeric repeats. EMBO J. 2010;29(13):2135–2146. DOI: 10.1038/emboj.2010

[77] Cam HP, Chen ES, Grewal SI. Transcriptional scaffolds for heterochromatin assembly. Cell. 2009;136(4):610–614. DOI: 10.1016/j.cell.2014.11.052

[78] Moazed D. Small RNAs in transcriptional gene silencing and genome defence. Nature. 2009;457(7228):413–420. DOI: 10.1038/nature07756

[79] Mao YS, Zhang B, Spector DL. Biogenesis and function of nuclear bodies. Trends Genet. 2011;27(8):295–306. DOI: 10.1016/j.tig.2011.05.006

[80] Chen LL, Carmichael GG. Altered nuclear retention of mRNAs containing inverted repeats in human embryonic stem cells: Functional role of a nuclear noncoding RNA. Mol Cell. 2009;35(4):467–478. DOI: 10.1016/j.molcel.2009.06.027

[81] Sunwoo H, Dinger ME, Wilusz JE, Amaral PP, Mattick JS, Spector DL. MEN epsilon/beta nuclear-retained non-coding RNAs are up-regulated upon muscle differentiation and are essential components of paraspeckles. Genome Res. 2009;19(3):347–359. DOI: 10.1101/gr.087775.108

[82] Clemson CM, Hutchinson JN, Sara SA, Ensminger AW, Fox AH, Chess A, et al. An architectural role for a nuclear noncoding RNA: NEAT1 RNA is essential for the structure of paraspeckles. Mol Cell. 2009;33(6):717–726. DOI: 10.1016/j.molcel.2009.01.026

[83] Sasaki YT, Ideue T, Sano M, Mituyama T, Hirose T. MENepsilon/beta noncoding RNAs are essential for structural integrity of nuclear paraspeckles. Proc Natl Acad Sci U S A. 2009;106(8):2525–2530. DOI: 10.1073/pnas.0807899106

[84] Mao YS, Sunwoo H, Zhang B, Spector DL. Direct visualization of the co-transcriptional assembly of a nuclear body by noncoding RNAs. Nat Cell Biol. 2011;13(1):95–101. DOI: 10.1038/ncb2140

[85] Bernard D, Prasanth KV, Tripathi V, Colasse S, Nakamura T, Xuan Z, et al. A long nuclear-retained non-coding RNA regulates synaptogenesis by modulating gene expression. EMBO J. 2010;29(18):3082–3093. DOI: 10.1038/emboj.2010.199

[86] Tripathi V, Ellis JD, Shen Z, Song DY, Pan Q, Watt AT, et al. The nuclear-retained noncoding RNA MALAT1 regulates alternative splicing by modulating SR splicing factor phosphorylation. Mol Cell. 2010;39(6):925–938. DOI: 10.1016/j.molcel.2010.08.011

[87] Yang L, Lin C, Liu W, Zhang J, Ohgi KA, Grinstein JD, et al. ncRNA- and Pc2 methylation-dependent gene relocation between nuclear structures mediates gene activation programs. Cell. 2011;147(4):773–778. DOI: 10.1016/j.cell.2011.08.054

[88] Cai X, Cullen BR. The imprinted H19 noncoding RNA is a primary microRNA precursor. RNA. 2007;13(3):313–316. DOI: 10.1261/rna.351707

[89] Hung T, Chang HY. Long noncoding RNA in genome regulation: Prospects and mechanisms. RNA Biol. 2010;7(5):582–585. DOI: 10.4161/rna.7.5.13216

[90] Swiezewski S, Liu F, Magusin A, Dean C. Cold-induced silencing by long antisense transcripts of an *Arabidopsis* polycomb target. Nature. 2009;462(7274):799–802. DOI: 10.1038/nature08618

[91] Hung T, Wang Y, Lin MF, Koegel AK, Kotake Y, Grant GD, et al. Extensive and coordinated transcription of noncoding RNAs within cell-cycle promoters. Nat Gene. 2011;43(7):621–629. DOI: 10.1038/ng.848

[92] Yan BX, Ma JX. Promoter-associated RNAs and promoter-targeted RNAs. Cell Mol Life Sci. 2012;69(17):2833–2842. DOI: 10.1007/s00018-012-0953-1

[93] Imamura T, Yamamoto S, Ohgane J, Hattori N, Tanaka S, Shiota K. Non-coding RNA directed DNA demethylation of Sphk1 CpG island. Biochem Biophys Res Commun. 2004;322(2):593–600. DOI: 10.1016/j.bbrc.2004.07.159

[94] Morris KV, Chan SW, Jacobsen SE, Looney DJ. Small interfering RNA-induced transcriptional gene silencing in human cells. Science. 2004;305(5688):1289–1292. DOI: 10.1126/science.1101372

[95] Napoli S, Pastori C, Magistri M, Carbone GM, Catapano CV. Promoter-specific transcriptional interference and c-myc gene silencing by siRNAs in human cells. EMBO J. 2009;28(12):1708–1719. DOI: 10.1038/emboj.2009

[96] Hawkins PG, Santoso S, Adams C, Anest V, Morris KV. Promoter targeted small RNAs induce long-term transcriptional gene silencing in human cells. Nucleic Acids Res. 2009;37(9):2984–2995. DOI: 10.1093/nar/gkp127

[97] Place RF, Li LC, Pookot D, Noonan EJ, Dahiya R. MicroRNA-373 induces expression of genes with complementary promoter sequences. Proc Natl Acad Sci U S A. 2008;105(5):1608–1613. DOI: 10.1073/pnas.0707594105

[98] Li LC, Okino ST, Zhao H, Pookot D, Place RF, Urakami S, et al. Small dsRNAs induce transcriptional activation in human cells. Proc Natl Acad Sci U S A. 2006;103(46): 17337–17342. DOI: 10.1073/pnas.0607015103

[99] Janowski BA, Younger ST, Hardy DB, Ram R, Huffman KE, Corey DR. Activating gene expression in mammalian cells with promoter-targeted duplex RNAs. Nat Chem Biol. 2007;3(3):166–173. DOI: 10.1038/nchembio860

[100] Panganiban G, Rubenstein JL. Developmental functions of the Distal-less/Dlx homeobox genes. Development. 2002;129(19):4371–4386.

[101] Hastings ML, Ingle HA, Lazar MA, Munroe SH. Post-transcriptional regulation of thyroid hormone receptor expression by *cis*-acting sequences and a naturally occurring antisense RNA. J Biol Chem. 2000;275(15):11507–11513. DOI: 10.1074/jbc.275.15.11507

[102] Kretz M, Siprashvili Z, Chu C, Webster DE, Zehnder A, Qu K, et al. Control of somatic tissue differentiation by the long non-coding RNA TINCR. Nature. 2013;493(7431):231–235. DOI: 10.1038/nature11661

[103] Faghihi MA, Modarresi F, Khalil AM, Wood DE, Sahagan BG, Morgan TE, et al. Expression of a noncoding RNA is elevated in Alzheimer's disease and drives rapid feed-forward regulation of beta-secretase. Nat Med. 2008;14(7):723–730. DOI: 10.1038/nm1784

[104] Carrieri C, Cimatti L, Biagioli M, Beugnet A, Zucchelli S, Fedele S, et al. Long non-coding antisense RNA controls Uchl1 translation through an embedded SINEB2 repeat. Nature. 2012;491(7424):454–457. DOI: 10.1038/nature11508

[105] Cheetham SW, Gruhl F, Mattick JS, Dinger ME. Long noncoding RNAs and the genetics of cancer. Br J Cancer. 2013;108(12):2419–2425. DOI: 10.1038/bjc.2013.233

[106] Faraoni I, Antonetti FR, Cardone J, Bonmassar E. miR-155 gene: A typical multifunctional microRNA. Biochim Biophys Acta. 2009;1792(6):497–505. DOI: 10.1016/j.bbadis.2009.02.013

[107] Chan JA, Krichevsky AM, Kosik KS. MicroRNA-21 is an antiapoptotic factor in human glioblastoma cells. Cancer Res. 2005;65(14):6029–6033. DOI: 10.1158/0008-5472.CAN-05-0137

[108] Xiao C, Srinivasan L, Calado DP, Patterson HC, Zhang B, Wang J, et al. Lymphoproliferative disease and autoimmunity in mice with increased miR-17-92 expression in lymphocytes. Nat Immunol. 2008;9(4):405–414. DOI: 10.1038/ni1575

[109] Concepcion CP, Bonetti C, Ventura A. The microRNA-17-92 family of microRNA clusters in development and disease. Cancer J. 2012;18(3):262–267. DOI: 10.1097/PPO.0b013e318258b60a

[110] Gutschner T, Hammerle M, Eissmann M, Hsu J, Kim Y, Hung G, et al. The noncoding RNA MALAT1 is a critical regulator of the metastasis phenotype of lung cancer cells. Cancer Res. 2013;73(3):1180–1189. DOI: 10.1158/0008-5472.CAN-12-2850

[111] He L, He X, Lim LP, de Stanchina E, Xuan Z, Liang Y, et al. A microRNA component of the p53 tumour suppressor network. Nature. 2007;447(7148):1130–1134. DOI: 10.1038/nature05939

[112] Gutschner T, Diederichs S. The hallmarks of cancer: A long non-coding RNA point of view. RNA Biol. 2012;9(6):703–719. DOI: 10.4161/rna.20481

[113] Redon S, Reichenbach P, Lingner J. The non-coding RNA TERRA is a natural ligand and direct inhibitor of human telomerase. Nucleic Acids Res. 2010;38(17):5797–5806. DOI: 10.1093/nar/gkq296

[114] Szafranski P, Dharmadhikari AV, Brosens E, Gurha P, Kolodziejska KE, Zhishuo O, et al. Small noncoding differentially methylated copy-number variants, including lncRNA genes, cause a lethal lung developmental disorder. Genome Res. 2013;23(1): 23–33. DOI: 10.1101/gr.141887.112

[115] Kanduri C. Long noncoding RNA and epigenomics. Adv Exp Med Biol. 2011;722:174–195. DOI: 10.1007/978-1-4614-0332-6_11

[116] Brown CJ, Ballabio A, Rupert JL, Lafreniere RG, Grompe M, Tonlorenzi R, et al. A gene from the region of the human X inactivation centre is expressed exclusively from the inactive X chromosome. Nature. 1991;349(6304):38–44. DOI: 10.1038/349038a0

[117] Lee JT. Epigenetic regulation by long noncoding RNAs. Science. 2012;338(6113):1435–1439. DOI: 10.1126/science.1231776

[118] Caley DP, Pink RC, Trujillano D, Carter DR. Long noncoding RNAs, chromatin, and development. Sci World J. 2010;10:90–102. DOI: 10.1100/tsw.2010.7

[119] Zakharova IS, Shevchenko AI, Zakian SM. Monoallelic gene expression in mammals. Chromosoma. 2009;118(3):279–290. DOI: 10.1007/s00412-009-0206-8

[120] Umlauf D, Fraser P, Nagano T. The role of long non-coding RNAs in chromatin structure and gene regulation: Variations on a theme. Biol Chem. 2008;389(4):323–331. DOI: 10.1515/BC.2008.047

[121] Mohammad F, Mondal T, Kanduri C. Epigenetics of imprinted long noncoding RNAs. Epigenetics. 2009;4(5):277–286. DOI: 10.4161/epi.4.5.9242

[122] Lee JT, Bartolomei MS. X-inactivation, imprinting, and long noncoding RNAs in health and disease. Cell. 2013;152(6):1308–1323. DOI: 10.1016/j.cell.2013.02.016

[123] Sleutels F, Barlow DP. The origins of genomic imprinting in mammals. Adv Genet. 2002;46:119–163. DOI: 10.1016/S0065-2660(02)46006-3

[124] Kanduri C, Fitzpatrick G, Mukhopadhyay R, Kanduri M, Lobanenkov V, Higgins M, et al. A differentially methylated imprinting control region within the Kcnq1 locus harbors a methylation-sensitive chromatin insulator. J Biol Chem. 2002;277(20): 18106–18110.

[125] Kanduri C, Holmgren C, Pilartz M, Franklin G, Kanduri M, Liu L, et al. The 5′ flank of mouse H19 in an unusual chromatin conformation unidirectionally blocks enhancer-promoter communication. Curr Biol. 2000;10(8):449–457. DOI: 10.1016/S0960-9822(00)00442-5

[126] Kanduri C, Pant V, Loukinov D, Pugacheva E, Qi CF, Wolffe A, et al. Functional association of CTCF with the insulator upstream of the H19 gene is parent of origin-specific and methylation-sensitive. Curr Biol. 2000;10(14):853–856. DOI: 10.1016/S0960-9822(00)00597-2

[127] Sleutels F, Zwart R, Barlow DP. The non-coding air RNA is required for silencing autosomal imprinted genes. Nature. 2002;415(6873):810–813. DOI: 10.1038/415810a

[128] Iyer MK, Niknafs YS, Malik R, Singhal U, Sahu A, Hosono Y, et al. The landscape of long noncoding RNAs in the human transcriptome. Nat Genet. 2015;47(3):199–208. DOI: 10.1038/ng.3192

[129] Kung JTY, Colognori D, Lee JT. Long noncoding RNAs: Past, present and future. Genetics. 2013;193:651–659. DOI: 10.1534/genetics.112.146704

[130] Gomes AQ, Nolasco S, Soares H. Non-coding RNAs: Multi-tasking molecules in the cell. Int J Mol Sci. 2013;14(8):16010–16039. DOI: 10.3390/ijms140816010

Section 3

RNA Interference Methods and its Alternatives

Chapter 5

Noncanonical Synthetic RNAi Inducers

O.V. Gvozdeva and E.L. Chernolovskaya

Additional information is available at the end of the chapter

http://dx.doi.org/10.5772/61685

Abstract

This review focuses on current strategies of development of noncanonical synthetic RNA interference (RNAi) inducers with structural modifications for promoting better gene silencing with low risk of side effects. A particular focus is on longer RNA duplexes 25–30 nucleotides (nt) in length that mimic Dicer substrates to improve interaction of RNAi inducers with RNAi machinery. Various design strategies of efficient Dicer substrate small-interfering RNA (siRNA) are described. It was found that the length, chemical modifications, and overhang structure influence the gene silencing activity and RNA-induced silencing complex (RISC) assembly. Special attention is paid to the long double-stranded RNA duplexes that induce effective gene silencing in Dicer-dependent or Dicer-independent mode. Some structural variants of shorter siRNAs, including hairpin and dumbbell siRNAs and fork-siRNA (fsiRNA) with several nucleotide substitutions at the 3′ end of the sense strand, are also analyzed. These structural modifications provide efficiently increased gene silencing of targets with unfavorable duplex thermodynamic asymmetry. Recent data remove the length and structure limits for the design of RNAi effectors, and add another example in the list of novel RNAi-inducing molecules differing from the classical siRNA, which is discussed in this chapter.

Keywords: RNAi, siRNA, fsiRNA, dsiRNA, tsiRNA, structural modifications, mechanism of action

1. Introduction

RNA interference is a conserved mechanism of a sequence-specific posttranscriptional gene silencing triggered by double-stranded RNAs homologous to the silenced gene [1, 2]. Long double-stranded RNA(dsRNAs) are cleaved in the cell by RNase III class endonuclease Dicer into short fragments 21–22 nucleotides (nt) in length with 2–3-nt 3′ overhangs at both ends [3, 4]. These fragments (small-interfering RNAs, siRNAs) enter RNA-induced silencing complex (RISC) and associate with core proteins belonging to Argonaute (AGO) family [5]. AGO unwinds the duplex and cuts one of the strands in the middle, and then this strand (designated as "passenger") dissociates from the complex and is degraded by cellular ribonucleases. The other strand (designated as "guide") remains in activated RISC and recognizes the cellular mRNA complementary to the guide strand. The configuration of the complex determines which strand remains in the complex and which strand leaves and degrades. Active RISC complex containing the guide strand binds to the complementary mRNA and induces its cleavage. When the cleaved mRNA is released, RISC is recycled for a new round of cleavage [4, 6]. The details of the RNAi mechanism are well reviewed in literature [7–9].

Synthetic small-interfering RNAs have become an advanced and powerful tool for specific gene silencing and could be considered as promising class of therapeutics for the treatment of diseases associated with overexpression of specific genes [10–12]. However, therapeutic applications of canonical non-modified siRNAs are limited by their sensitivity to ribonucleases, possibility of unfavorable guide strand selection, and activation of innate immune system by siRNA containing immunostimulatory motives in the sequence, which can lead to poor gene silencing efficiency [13, 14]. Different structural variations of the RNAi inducers together with chemical modification were developed to overcome these problems.

This review focuses on current strategies of development of siRNA structural modifications for promoting better gene silencing with low risk of side effects, with particular focus on longer siRNA duplexes 25–30 nt in length that mimic Dicer substrates (Dicer substrate siRNA (dsiRNA)) [15–20]. Special attention has been paid to the long double-stranded RNA duplexes, which induced effective gene silencing and did not require Dicer-mediated processing of the substrate into smaller units: trimer RNA (tsiRNA) with 63 nt in length and tripartite-interfering RNA (tiRNA) with 38 nt in length [21, 22]. Applications of some structure variations of shorter siRNAs and the potential of different synthetic RNAi inducers in different applications have also been reviewed and summarized.

2. Dicer substrate interfering RNAs

Long dsRNAs homologous to the targeted mRNA were successfully used for silencing of gene expression in nonmammalian species [1, 4]. Early attempts to use long dsRNAs in mammalian cells triggering of RNAi failed due to activation of innate immune system by dsRNA [15]. Although activation of innate immunity may be beneficial for the therapy in some cases, uncontrolled induction of the interferon response results in global changes in gene expression profile and, in some cases, in cells death [23–25]. It was found that chemically synthesized 21-mer RNA duplexes with 2-nt 3′ overhangs at both ends, which directly mimic the products produced by Dicer, efficiently suppressed gene expression in mammalian cells [4, 26]. These duplexes, referred to as canonical siRNAs, are widely used in biomedical research [11]. Later, it was found that RNA duplexes, smaller than 30 nt in length but longer than siRNAs, were significantly more efficient than canonical siRNAs and did not induce interferon response in a variety of cell lines [15]. It was established experimentally that 27-mer duplexes possess maximal silencing activity, longer duplexes demonstrated reduced silencing activity, and 40–

45-mer duplexes were inactive. At the same time, 27-mer duplexes, named as Dicer substrate siRNA (dsiRNA), were efficiently cleaved by Dicer producing a variety of 21-nt-long distinct products. High potency of 27-mer duplexes initially was explained by the formation of siRNA pool containing functional siRNAs with extremely high silencing activity. Some of 27-mer duplexes were significantly more potent at nanomolar or picomolar concentrations than the specific 21-mer siRNA selected according to the current computational algorithms [15]. However, further experiments demonstrated that none of the synthetic 21-nt siRNAs, included in the corresponding set to all possible products of Dicer processing of 27-mer duplexes, demonstrated the same level of silencing activity as 27-mers at low concentrations [15].

Based on the earlier observations that Dicer participates both in the cleavage of dsRNAs and in the incorporation of the products of cleavage into RISC complex in *Drosophila melanogaster*, it has been suggested that Dicer could participate in direct loading of siRNA into RISC and in RISC assembly [16, 27]. It has been experimentally proved that dsiRNAs form the RISC loading complex (RLC) in vitro more efficiently than the canonical 21-mer siRNA duplexes [18]. Because Dicer does not form complexes with 21-base pair (bp) duplexes, it was assumed that Dicer facilitates RLC formation after dsRNA cleavage without dissociation from the cleavage product. These findings become a basis for the development of a new class of RNAi inducers [16, 17, 28].

The silencing activity of dsiRNA depends on its structure. At the first step of recognition, PAZ (Piwi Argonaut and Zwille) domain of Dicer predominantly "anchors" two ribonucleotides on 3′ overhangs because those blunt 27-mer duplexes are not good substrates for Dicer. PAZ domain plays a vital role in the orientation of bound RNA in the active site of the enzyme and determines the cleavage position on RNA for AGO protein. Unlike 21-mer siRNA, where two-base 3′-deoxynucleotide overhangs are often used regardless of their complementarity to the target mRNA sequence (mostly dTdT), the overhang sequences are important for the properties of dsiRNA. Incorporation of deoxynucleotides at the 3′ ends of dsiRNA strands has an adverse effect on dsiRNA processing [19]. The sequence of 3′ terminal overhangs could control dicing polarity and strand selection into RISC. Thus, Dicer preferentially binds with purine/purine (GG, AA) nucleotides [19]. Protruding nucleotides added to the 3′ terminal of the antisense strand facilitate its preferential loading into RISC [19]. Hence, asymmetric duplexes with one 2-nt 3′ overhang and DNA residues on the blunt end of the duplex provide a single favorable PAZ binding site and reduce heterogeneity of cleavage products (Figure 1) [16–18, 29, 30].

The stability of dsiRNA in physiological fluids is extremely an important factor for its applications in vivo [31]. Although dsRNAs are more stable in comparison with single-stranded RNAs and 21-bp siRNA, they still rapidly degrade in the serum [32]. It was found that bonds with 3′ pyrimidine nucleotides are cleaved faster than bonds with 3′ purines. Kubo and his colleagues demonstrated that degradation rate of dsiRNAs correlated with the amount of pyrimidines at the 3′ end [31]. At the same time, degradation rate of dsiRNAs also correlates with the presence of AU-rich domains that might be related to low thermal stability, easy dissociation, and faster cleavage by both endo- and exonucleases. Chemical modifications can improve nuclease stability and reduce off-target effects [33–36]. Fluorescein modification of 3′

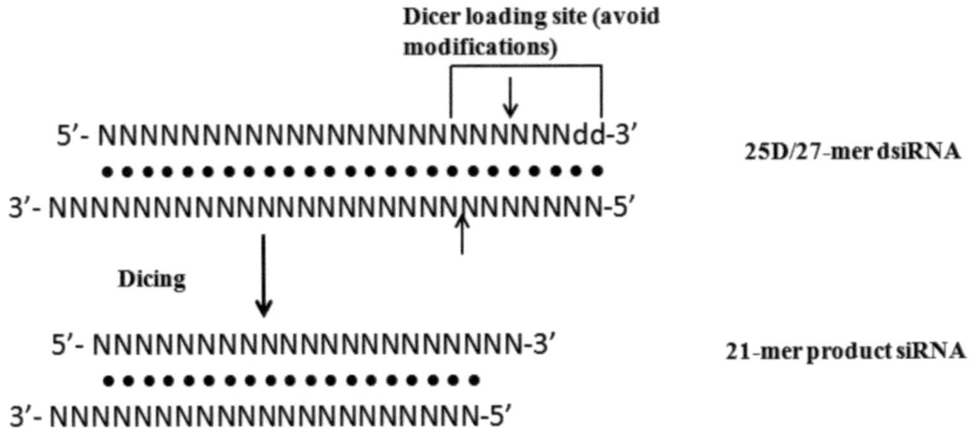

Figure 1. The scheme of dsiRNA design (according to [17]). N – ribonucleic acids, d - deoxyribonucleic acids, short arrows – the site of Dicer cleavage.

end of 27-mer RNA duplexes significantly reduces RNAi activity because 3′ ends are important for interaction with Dicer and should be available for the proper recognition [15]. On the other hand, dsiRNAs with chemical modifications of the 5′ end possess high nuclease stability and RNAi activity in the cell-cultured medium. Thus, 5′-end amino-modified dsiRNA demonstrated improved RNAi activity and stability in the cell-cultured medium [31].

Incorporation of 2′-O-methyl modifications is an efficient and inexpensive method to improve nuclease resistance of synthetic RNA duplexes [33, 37–40]. However, dsiRNA duplexes with modifications of all or the majority of nucleotides in both sense and antisense strands are practically inactive, because extensive modification blocks the cleavage of duplex by Dicer [17]. Limiting the modifications to incorporation of only 9–11 modified bases into the antisense strand and avoiding modifications in the site of Dicer cleavage prevents this undesired effect [17]. Mass spectrometry analysis of in vitro dicing reactions showed that modified duplexes produce a mixture of 21- and 22-nt species, whereas unmodified duplexes are processed only into 21-mer species. If modifications were spaced further away from the dicing site, a preferential accumulation of 21-mer species was observed [17]. However, it was noted that in some cases, usually, a good modification pattern may decrease the silencing activity of dsiRNA. This phenomenon has been related to the newly unidentified sites in the sequence context of some chemically modified dsiRNAs, contributing to impairment of dsiRNAs silencing effect [17]. These observations could explain differences in the efficiency of various dsiRNAs and made possible the creation of the modification patterns compatible with dicing.

Accumulation of experimental data revealed that 27–30-bp dsRNAs, including dsiRNA and, in some cases, even 21-bp siRNA, could stimulate innate immune system and induce interferon response in certain cell types [23]. Toll-like receptors (TLRs) 7 and 8 appear to be the main molecules responsible for the immune recognition of siRNA and dsiRNA, whereas toll-like receptor 3 recognizes longer than 30-bp dsRNA [41, 42]. Activation of innate immune system through TLRs results in the production of interferon α, tumor necrosis factors α, and interleukins IL6 and IL12 [42]. Immunostimulatory properties of siRNA are sequence dependent; TLR7 and TLR8 receptors recognize GU-rich sequences of siRNA [43]. Moreover, several immunostimulatory motifs of siRNA enriched in GU nucleotides were identified [44, 45]. It is recommended to avoid these motives in siRNA and dsiRNA design; unfortunately, not all immunostimulatory motifs have been discovered that complicate the design procedure. Earlier, it was demonstrated that chemical modifications involving 2′ position of the ribose ring in siRNA could block the immune response [46]. Incorporation of 2′-O-methyl U and G bases into siRNA significantly reduced immunostimulatory activity of siRNA in vitro and in vivo, containing immune-stimulating motives in the sequence [41]. Moreover, the effective suppression of immunostimulatory activity could be reached by using only a small percentage of modified nucleotides (<10%). Collingwood and his colleagues [17] applied this approach to dsiRNA and demonstrated that limited 2′-O-methyl modifications of uridine and guanosine into antisense strand of dsiRNA efficiently prevent induction of innate immune response in different cell lines.

Another option to reduce nonspecific effects of dsiRNA is to use enzymatically produced pools of Dicer substrate RNA [20]. Dicer from the protozoan parasite *Giardia intestinalis* was used to obtain enzymatically produced dsiRNAs. It cuts long dsRNA into fragments from 25 to 27 nt in length. The sequences-related side effects were decreased in the pool of enzymatically produced dsiRNAs due to the low concentration of individual dsiRNAs with undesirable sequence.

In the cases when silencing of more than one gene is required, the transfection of siRNA mixture is used. Co-transfection of different siRNAs may result in different knockdown efficiency of individual targets due to competition between siRNAs for RISC loading depending on the thermodynamic asymmetry of the duplexes [30]. Therefore, preliminary testing is required to assess the degree of competition between various siRNAs. Competition between RNAi inducers aimed at different mRNAs could be avoided by using Dicer substrate RNA. Entry of dsiRNAs into RNAi pathway is not limited by RISC loading step, and discrimination of canonical siRNAs based on RISC incorporation is reduced. These beneficial properties of dsiRNAs can provide an effective tool for targeting multiple mRNAs.

Currently, siRNAs have become a powerful tool for effective suppression of expression of target genes in vitro and in vivo applications. Moreover, several compounds are already used in clinical trials. However, the examples of Dicer substrate RNAs usage in vivo are fewer in number. Several studies use dsiRNA to silence therapeutically relevant genes in vivo (Table 1). Frequently, cancer-related genes and genes of viruses [50, 51, 56–59] are chosen as targets for dsiRNAs [47–49]. Several researchers used *TNFα* gene as a target for the treatment of inflammatory and autoimmune diseases [52–54]. Murine models are the most popular animal models among various studies that used dsiRNA in vivo [47–54]; however, there are studies where other animal models, for example, rats, were used [53, 55]. An exciting example of dsiRNA application was described by Doré-Savard and his colleagues, who demonstrated, for the first time, the efficient suppression of target genes in central nervous system (CNS) of rats by dsiRNA [55]. In this study, 27-mer dsiRNAs were used to reduce expression of neurotensin receptor-2 (NTS2) involved in ascending nociception. dsiRNAs were formulated with cationic lipid i-Fect and used in intrathecal spinal cord injection. Extremely low doses of dsiRNA (0.005 mg/kg) efficiently silenced NTS2 mRNA and protein levels for 3–4 days. It is known that administration of high doses of non-modified siRNA increases the risk of activation of innate immune system, especially when siRNA is used together with cationic lipids. Low doses of highly active dsiRNAs could minimize this adverse effect. No apparent toxicity and other off-target effects were found during the experiment [55]. The dose–response experiments performed in another study [28] also show that 27-mer Dicer substrate RNA provide improved gene silencing when used at lower concentrations [28]. The silencing activity of canonical 21-mer siRNAs was compared with that of dsiRNA at 1 and 5 nM concentrations. The 27-mer dsiRNA displayed more potent gene silencing at 1 nM concentration, while at 5 nM concentration, the difference in silencing was less pronounced [28].

Experimental system	**Structure**	**Target (gene)**	**Disease**	**Concentration/dose**	**Biological effect**	**Reference**
MDA-MB-435 cells	25D/27-mer	*cdc20* (mouse)	Breast cancer	20 nM	>80% cell growth inhibition	[47]
Mice				2 μg/mouse	Tumor growth inhibition after second injection	
Huh7.5 cells	25D/27-mer	5' UTR and coding regions of hepatitis C virus: *NS3, NS4B, NS5A, NS5B*	Hepatitis C virus infection	5 nM	99.5% inhibition in luciferase assay	[57]
PC-3 cells	25D/27-mer	*HSP27* (human)	Prostate cancer	50 nM	>50% reduction of both mRNA and protein	[48]
Mice		*Hsp27* (mouse)		3 mg/kg	>50% reduction of both mRNA and protein	
HAE cells obtained from bronchi and lungs	25D/27-mer 2′OMe	*N* gene of respiratory syncytial virus (RSV)	Respiratory syncytial virus infection	250 nM	> 100-fold decrease of viral titer	[57]
Hela cells	25D/27-mer 2′OMe	*CTNNB1* (human)	Liver cancer	1 nM	>90% mRNA level reduction	[49]
Mice		*Ctnnb1* (mouse)		5 mg/kg	Significant reduction of tumor weight	
AY-27 cells	25D/27-mer	*Mki-67* (rat)	Bladder cancer	10 nM	50% mRNA reduction	[53]
LLC-MK2 cells	25D/27-mer	*N, D,L* genes of human	Human metapneum	0.65 nM	50% reduction in plaque assay	[50]

Experimental system	Structure	Target (gene)	Disease	Concentration/dose	Biological effect	Reference
		metapneumovirus (hMPV)	ovirus infection			
Mice				4 mg/kg	Reduction of virus titers in lungs of infected mice	
RAW264.7 cells	25D/27-mer	*Tnf* (mouse)	Inflammatory diseases (sepsis model)	5 nM	>50% reduction of the number of TNFα positive cells	[52]
Mice				10 mg/dose	4-fold reduction of the number of TNFα positive peritoneal macrophages	
keratocytes from rabbit corneal stroma	25/27-mer	*JKAMP* (rabbit)	Corneal wound healing	10 nM	70% - *JNK1* mRNA level reduction 50% - *JNK2* mRNA level reduction	[58]
CCRF-CEM cells	25/27-mer	*TNPO3* *CD4* (human) *Tet/rev* (viral)	HIV-1	50 nM	50% *TNPO3* mRNA level reduction 75% *CD4* mRNA level reduction 60% *Tet/re* mRNA level reduction	[51]
Mice				0.15 mg/kg	Prolonged antiviral effect	
Kupffer cells	25D/27-mer	*Tnf* (rat)	Inflammatory diseases	10 nM	80% reduction of TNFα level after LPS stimulation	[53]
Rat				100 μg/kg	50% reduction of TNFα level in blood	
CHSE-214 cells (fish)	25/27-mer	*N* gene of hemorrhagic septicemia virus (HSV)	Hemorrhagic septicemia virus infection	15 nM	99% mRNA level reduction	[59]
Murine peritoneal macrophages	25/27-mer 2′OMe	*Tnf* (mouse)	Rheumatoid arthritis	50 nM	66% protein level reduction	[54]
Mice				5 μg/dose	Block the development of inflammation after second dose	
NTS2 cells	25D/27-mer	*Ntsr2* (rat)	Pain states	10 nM	>90% mRNA level reduction	[55]

Experimental system	Structure	Target (gene)	Disease	Concentration/dose	Biological effect	Reference
Rat				0.005 mg/kg	86% and 62% mRNA level reduction in lumbar dorsal root ganglia and in spinal cord, respectively	

Table 1. Application of dsiRNA for silencing of disease-related genes (summarized from PubMed). 25/27-mer – dsiRNAs with 25 - base sense strand and 27 – base antisense strand; 25D – 2 bases at the 3′-end are substituted with DNA; 2'OMe – 2′ – O methyl modifications as described in [17].

In another study, potent 2′-O-methyl modified dsiRNAs targeted to β-catenin were designed [49]. It is known that β-catenin acts as the transcription factor and its overexpression causes the development of several types of cancer, including liver cancer. At the first step, large-scale screening of 488 dsiRNAs for in vitro mRNA knockdown activity was performed to choose the most efficient dsiRNAs for targeting β-catenin. Then, the absence of immunostimulatory activity attributed to selected dsiRNA was confirmed using the assay based on the ability of an oligonucleotide to induce the production of antibodies to the PEGylated components of the lipid nanoparticles containing oligonucleotides. dsiRNA was administered to mice intravenously twice a week during 3 weeks after implanting Hep 3B tumor cells. dsiRNAs induced strong β-catenin mRNA knockdown and efficient tumor inhibition. Other examples of dsiRNAs applications as potential therapeutics for inhibition of the disease-related overexpressed genes in vivo and in vitro have been summarized in Table 1.

Beneficial properties of dsiRNAs make these structures popular inhibitors of target genes. At first, dsiRNAs induce more potent silencing of the target genes at lower concentrations than canonical siRNAs. The next advantage of dsiRNAs is longevity of silencing: In some cases, it lasts up to 10 days. Then, the usage of dsiRNAs enables to minimize off-target effects such as toxicity and heterogeneity of processed products. An additional benefit is the high potency of dsiRNAs in silencing of multiple mRNAs where canonical siRNAs due to competition during RISC loading step appear to be less effective. The main disadvantage of dsiRNA is the higher cost of synthesis in comparison with canonical siRNA. However, low dosage of dsiRNA used in experiments eliminates this drawback. On the other hand, dsiRNAs share with siRNAs the same problems in therapeutic applications. The major challenge lies in the delivery of these structures into desired cells, tissues, and organs. To overcome this problem, various approaches are developed; however, this question has not been completely answered yet. Nevertheless, dsiRNA as potent inducers of RNAi offers promising strategies for efficient therapy.

3. Interfering RNA with noncanonical duplex structure

Different variations of siRNA duplex structures were proposed to improve their silencing activity. Here we will consider three types of the most frequently used siRNAs with structural

http://dx.doi.org/10.5772/61685

modifications of duplexes: short hairpin RNAs (shRNAs)/microRNA (miRNA) mimics, dumbbell RNAs, and fork-siRNA (Figure 2).

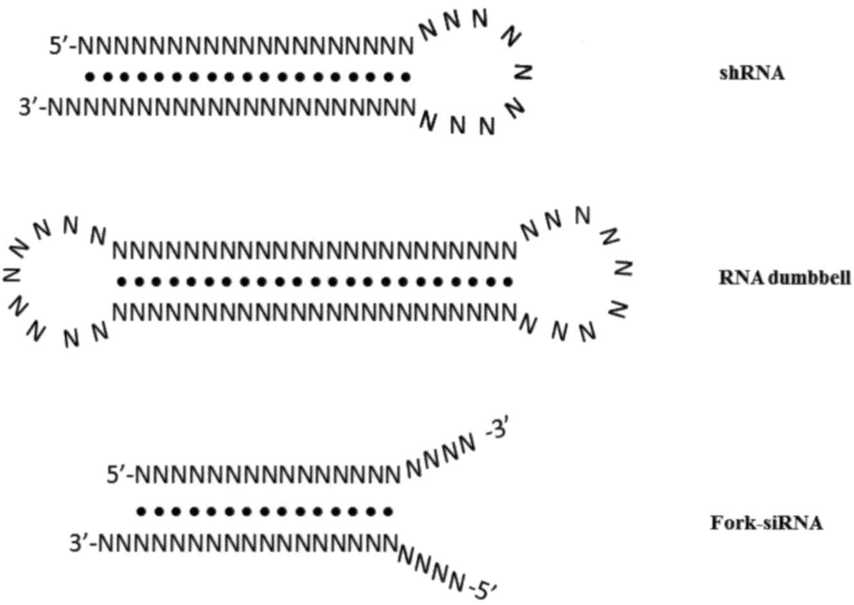

Figure 2. The different types of interfering RNAs with non-canonical duplex structures.

The identification of a large class of endogenous regulatory RNA molecules – microRNAs (miRNAs) arouse interest in constructing the similar synthetic structures for efficient silencing of target genes. miRNA precursors are generated in the cell as long primary transcripts that are cleaved in nucleus by RNase III class nuclease Drosha [60–62]. Then, they are exported to the cytoplasm and cleaved by Dicer, which is active at processing of complex hairpin structures [63]. It is known that Dicer substrates more effectively enter RISC complex than canonical siRNA and induce more potent RNAi [15–17, 28]. Moreover, shRNAs could interact with particular chaperones that promote recognition of shRNA by Dicer [64]. miRNAs form imperfect complementary complexes containing bulges with 3′ untranslated region of the target mRNA, wherein the position of the loops defines the mechanism of action: target cleavage or the block of translation. In the first case, synthetic miRNA mimics have no advantages over shRNA, and in the second case, they do not act in a catalytic mode. Therefore, synthetic miRNA applications are restricted to exploring the miRNA-regulated pathways involved in the natural processes, or development of replacement therapy for the diseases associated with mutation in specific miRNA. The use of shRNA seems to be more promising.

Although long dsRNA hairpins are prepared synthetically, enzymatically, or endogenously expressed, plasmid or viral vectors could be used in nonmammalian organisms. Long RNA hairpins cannot be applied in mammals for the specific gene silencing because they also induce interferon response in mammals via the same mechanism used by long RNA duplexes [3, 65, 66]. Therefore, length of hairpin RNAs for application in this type of species is limited by 30 bp. shRNAs expressed by different vectors under control of RNA polymerase III and CMV promoters were proved to efficiently trigger RNAi [67, 68].

Applications of viral vector-based expression of shRNAs are limited because of some obstacles such as possibility of insertional mutagenesis, malignant transformation, and host immune response [69]. At the same time, an application of plasmid vectors is safe, but inefficient delivery into cells limits its use only for experimental purposes, where antibiotic resistance genes included in the vector is used for the selection. In contrast to expressed shRNA, synthetic shRNA seems to be more attractive for RNAi-based therapies. It was found that chemically synthesized short hairpin RNAs (shRNAs) with 19–29-base-pair stem, at least 4-nucleotide loop and 2-nucleotide 3′ overhangs are more potent inducers of RNAi than the canonical small-interfering RNAs targeted to the same sequence in mRNA [64, 70–73]. Two main types of shRNAs with opposite positions of the loops were designed (Figure 3). The right loop structures (R-shRNAs) have sense strand at the 5′ end of the hairpin, whereas the left loop shRNAs (L-shRNAs) have antisense strand at the 5′ end of the hairpin (Figure 3) [71–74]. The majority of studies were carried out using R-hand loop structure.

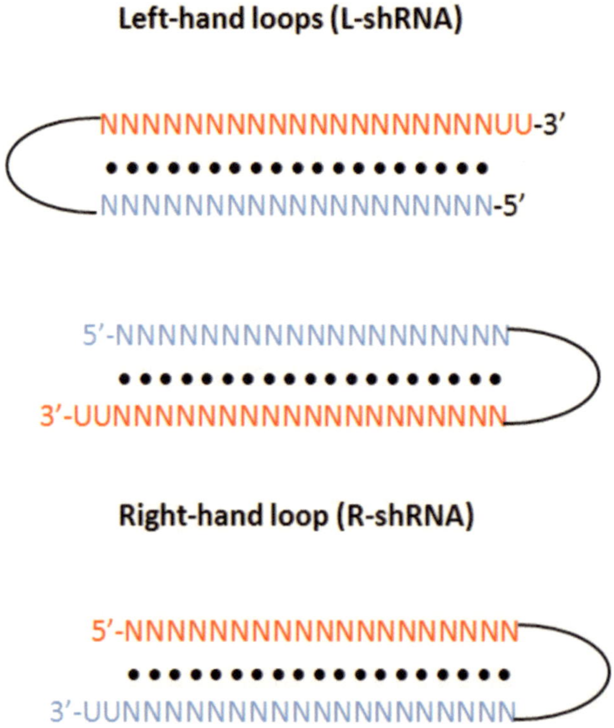

Figure 3. General structures of L-shRNAs and R-shRNA (according to [71]). Red color: sense strand, blue color: antisense strand.

It was clearly demonstrated that the silencing activity of shRNAs depends on stem length, loop length, sequence, and terminal overhangs [70]. Dicer efficiently cleaves shRNA with certain minimum stem of 19 nt in length forming 22-nt products starting from the free 3′ end of the RNA.

Correct 3′ overhangs increase the efficacy and specificity of processing, whereas blunt-end shRNAs produce a set of products [64]. In the case of endogenously expressing regulatory RNAs, 3′ UU overhangs of miRNA precursors generated by Drosha cleavage determine subsequent proper recognition and processing by Dicer [75]. Synthetic shRNA with similar overhangs and mimicking the products of Drosha preprocessing is used. The presence of a 3′-UU overhang improves silencing activity of 19-mer shRNAs as 3′-UU overhangs might provide additional site for PAZ domain of Dicer [70].

The loop length also plays a crucial role in the silencing activity of shRNAs. Thus, it was found that 29-nt stem and 4-nt loop inhibited the target gene expression more efficiently as compared with shRNA with 19-nt stem and loop [76, 70]. In contrast, when 9-nt loop was used for 19-nt stem shRNA, it demonstrated more potent silencing of target genes than longer shRNA with the 4-nt loop. Brummelkamp and his colleagues also demonstrated that shRNAs with 19-nt stem and 9-nt loops possessed the maximum silencing activity as compared with shRNAs with 7-nt loops, while shRNA with 5-nt loops were inactive [68]. All observed differences in the silencing activities of shRNA, divergent in the length of the stem and loop, were more pronounced under low or intermediate concentrations. The silencing activity of different shRNAs, used at high concentrations, did not depend substantially on the loop length [70].

These results may be explained by the fact that the loop length influences the efficiency of processing by Dicer. [64]. Indeed, 4-nt loops of shRNA with 19-nt stem have poorer conformation flexibility at the junction between the duplex stem and a single strand of the loop. As short loops are set close or at the Dicer cleavage site, the restriction-associated conformational changes made shRNAs stems poor substrates for Dicer. Therefore, shRNAs with short loops and 19-nt stem enter RISC complex in the later stages and remain not processed by Dicer [64]. It was suggested that another single-strand-specific ribonuclease, independent from Dicer, cleaved this type of shRNA. On the other hand, shRNAs with 19-nt stem and longer loops (9–10 nt) are efficiently processed by Dicer [76].

The potency of 19-nt stem shRNAs, targeted to the same sequence, depends on the position of the loop. Right (R)-shRNAs 19 nt in length are significantly less active than left (L)-shRNAs of the same length [71, 72]. However, the position of the loop (left or right) in longer shRNAs did not affect their activity. It was suggested that low potency of R-shRNA form is related to the fact that 5′ end of the antisense strand must be readily available for the efficient binding of AGO2 in the RISC complex. Otherwise, the 5′ end of sense strand would enter RISC and the target mRNA would not be cleaved. [77]. L-shRNAs with a short loop of 1–2 nt in length could be active. Moreover, L-shRNAs without any loop, where sense strand is directly connected with antisense strand, may be also active. In this case, the sense strand is shorter than antisense strand and the loop is formed by 3′ end of the antisense strand [71].

Moreover, the nature of nucleotides in 3′ overhang does not influence the activity of L-shRNA and 3′ overhangs could be substituted for deoxyribonucleotides [71]. The high efficiency of L-shRNAs may be explained by the high energy of binding of antisense strand with AGO2 due to availability of 5′ end of antisense strand in L-shRNA, dominated over the influence of overhangs and loop length. [71].

shRNAs have similar but not identical sequence preferences with siRNAs. Thus, the functional shRNAs have mainly AU nucleotides at position 9 and GC nucleotides at position 11, while these preferences are less significant in functional siRNA. At the same time, the functional shRNAs have the similar thermodynamic asymmetry as functional siRNAs. The computer algorithms for selection of potent shRNAs have been developed [76].

Short hairpin RNAs are a little more resistant to nucleases than siRNAs due to the protection of one end; however, shRNAs still quickly degrade in biological fluids [78]. The elegant method to stabilize non-modified RNA strands was described by Abe et al. [79]. Abe and his colleagues constructed dumbbell-shaped RNA structures and demonstrated their potency as RNAi inducers with stability in the biological fluids [79]. Dumbbell-shaped RNAs were designed by analogy with DNA dumbbells consisted of double-helical stem and closed by two hairpin loops. Dumbbell-shaped RNA structures are used as models for the analysis of local structures in DNA [80]. Local unwinding of duplexes facilitates enzymatic cleavage by nucleases. Two loops at the both ends of dumbbell RNA stabilize the duplex and limit its enzymatic cleavage [79, 81]. Dumbbell structures get processed by Dicer much more slowly in comparison with their linear analogues due to inefficient recognition by Dicer. The rate of processing depends on the stem length, too. For example, dumbbell RNAs with 27-bp-stem length were processed more quickly than the same sequence with 15–19-bp stem length. RNA dumbbells with 23-bp stems and 9-nt loops were found to be the most active. Indeed, 9-nt loops are commonly used in shRNAs as the most effective hairpin loops [67]. The stem length was optimized to keep high potency and reduce interferon response. Silencing activity of these dumbbell RNAs was significantly higher than that induced by linear counterparts and was retained for longer period even at lower concentrations [81]. The introduction of deoxynucleotides into the loop of dumbbell RNAs further significantly increases shRNA stability in biological fluids without loss of silencing activity. Moreover, the loop of dumbbell RNAs can be modified by carriers such as aptamers and peptides [81]. All benefits of dumbbell RNAs make them new potent RNAi inducers. The main disadvantage of these structures is the high cost of their synthesis in comparison with canonical siRNAs. At the same time, the low dosage and prolonged silencing effect can reduce expenses. The detailed scheme of RNA dumbbell synthesis is described by Abe and his colleagues [82].

Another type of RNAi inducer, fork-siRNA, was first introduced by Hohjoh [83]. Fork-siRNAs contain base substitutions in the 3′ end of the sense strand of siRNA, resulting in destabilization of the duplex [83–85]. The effect of fork-siRNAs is explained by the fact that thermodynamic asymmetry of the duplexes determines the orientation of siRNA in RISC. Thermodynamic stability of the terminal regions of the duplex defines which strand is cleaved and dissociated during RISC activation, and another strand remains in the activated RISC and guides target mRNA recognition and cleavage [86]. Antisense strand of siRNA must be included in activated RISC for efficient gene silencing, if activated RISC contains the sense strand no silencing occur.

The selection of active siRNAs may be complicated if a target mRNA is mutated or is a chimerical gene. To address this issue, the favorable asymmetry can be achieved by the introduction of several base substitutions at the 3′ end of the sense strand. Mismatches at the 3′ end of the sense strand, resulting in the formation of unpaired or destabilized regions, increase the silencing activity of siRNA with low or moderate concentrations [83]. The number of mismatches in fork-siRNA also plays a crucial role in its silencing activity [85]. Fork-siRNAs with one to two mismatches at the 3′ end possess silencing activity similar to that of canonical siRNAs, indicating that this number of mismatches is not enough for the efficient silencing. Fork-siRNA with four mismatches is the most potent, whereas fork-siRNA with six mismatches possesses reduced silencing activity [85].

An optimal number of mismatches depend on the overall thermodynamic stability of the duplex. Computational algorithms for siRNA sequence selection determine the recommended range of T_m difference between the terminal regions, and four mismatches could work for sequences within the range. On the other hand, mismatches in the 3′ part of the sense strand and long unpaired ends increase the sensitivity of fork-siRNA to nucleases. Consequently, the application of non-modified fork-siRNAs in vivo is limited by the fact that they have reduced stability in biological fluids due to the increased degradation by nucleases [83, 85]. To solve this problem, the algorithm for designing nuclease-resistant fork-siRNAs that contain 2′-O-methyl modifications in nuclease-sensitive sites was developed, which allows obtaining fork-siRNAs whose stability is comparable to that of canonical siRNAs [85].

Thereby, fork-siRNAs may improve unfavorable asymmetry of siRNA with low or moderate silencing activity, especially when the selection of functional siRNA is restricted by the sequence content of the corresponding mRNA. It makes sense to use them for silencing of uneasy or precisely located targets.

4. Short noncanonical RNA

siRNA shorter than canonical siRNA could also induce efficient silencing of target genes in mammalian cells acting via RNAi mechanism [87–90]. Short siRNAs have some benefits as inducers of RNAi such as reduction of immune response and decreased cost of the synthesis [76]. Various strategies have been used to design the minimal length for inducing RNA interference. As A-form helix of RNA plays an essential role for inducing RNAi, Chiu and Rana [91] found minimal length of dsRNA A-form helical structure required to enter active RISC complex. They demonstrated that siRNA with 16 bp in length and 2-nt 3′ overhangs representing ~ 1.5 helical turns efficiently assembles into catalytically active RISC and was sufficient for silencing of target genes. Indeed, 16-mer siRNAs were more potent in comparison to 19-mer siRNAs, while 15-mer siRNAs silenced gene expression at lower efficacy than 16-mer siRNAs, and 14–13-mer siRNAs were practically inactive [87]. It was demonstrated that the mechanism of target cleavage was different: cleavage sites in 16-mer siRNAs were shifted to

3 nt in comparison with 19-mer siRNAs (Figure 4). The 16-bp siRNAs induced the silencing faster than canonical siRNA due to the higher efficacy of RISC formation [87, 91]. Moreover, asymmetric duplexes with 3′ overhang on the antisense strand only demonstrated reduced off-target silencing in comparison with symmetric duplexes of the same length due to preferential incorporation of the guide strand into the RISC complex [91]. Thus, considering the benefits of 16-mer siRNAs, they possess high potential for using in biomedical studies, but new examples of their use are not available.

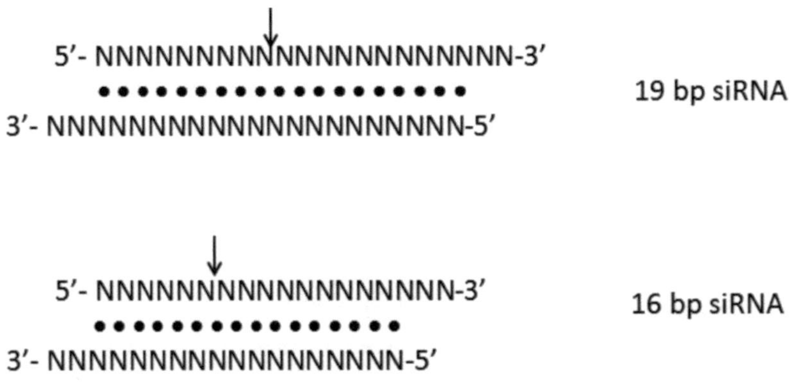

Figure 4. The mechanism of Dicer cleavage for 19 bp siRNA and short siRNA 16 bp in length. Arrows indicate cleavage sites defined by the 5′-end of guide strand (according to [87]).

Antisense siRNA also have been proposed as RNAi triggers. The sense strand of siRNA duplex is degraded and antisense strand remains in the active RISC to target complementary mRNA. Early studies demonstrated that 5′-phosohorylated antisense siRNAs with 22–40 nt in length were able to induce gene silencing in *Caenorhabditis elegans* [92, 93]. Several studies investigated the possibility of using antisense strand of siRNA 19–29 nt in length for transient knockdown of target genes in mammalian cells [88–90]. Antisense siRNA entered the RISC complex and provided mRNA cleavage but with lower efficiency in comparison with canonical siRNA. Antisense siRNA and canonical siRNA possess similar mRNA target position effects, cleavage fragment production, and tolerance to mutational and chemical modifications. However, antisense siRNA modified at 3′ end by fluorescein group or deoxyribose showed reduced silencing activity compared with canonical siRNA, where silencing activity remained at the same level in spite of 3′ modifications [89]. Moreover, the velocity of mRNA degradation induced by antisense siRNA is higher than that provided by canonical siRNA, but the duration of silencing effect is shorter. Thus, it was assumed that antisense siRNA induces RNAi through similar pathways as double-stranded siRNA but enters the pathway at the intermediate stage [89].

The differences in the silencing activity between antisense and canonical siRNAs may be explained by the low intracellular stability of the single-stranded RNA and by low efficacy of association with RISC [89]. Among the advantages of siRNAs, a lower price of synthesis and no side effects associated with the induction of interferon response should be considered [88].

Partial boranophosphate backbone (BP) modifications were designed to increase the stability and the silencing activity of the antisense siRNA [88]. BP-modified antisense siRNAs possess silencing activity comparable to unmodified double-stranded siRNAs. Partial 2′-O-methyl modification was used for the stabilization of antisense RNA, the activity resulting in single-stranded siRNA was comparable with the activity of double-stranded siRNA when used in high or intermediate concentrations, where in low concentration, canonical siRNAs were more active [85].

Overall, in spite of lower silencing activity compared with canonical siRNA, antisense siRNA may be used in specific situations, for instance, to eliminate off-target silencing of genes in the case when the sense strand has substantial homology to nontarget genes [88].

5. Long-interfering RNAs

Long dsRNAs >30 nt in length efficiently silence the expression of target gene in nonmammalian cells [1, 4]. The early attempts to use the similar structures for efficient knockdown of target genes in mammalian cells failed due to activation of interferon response [4, 94]. Later, various design strategies have been developed to prevent the induction of interferon response and construct new potent RNAi inducers [21, 95, 96]. Depending on the architecture of duplexes, all long dsRNAs may be divided into linear and branched structures.

Partial 2′-O-methyl modification effectively prevents the activation of interferon response by Dicer-substrate RNAs [17]; therefore, it was proposed to use similar approach for longer linear duplexes [21]. Longer siRNAs containing the sequence of canonical siRNAs repeated two and three times are called dimer (42 nt in length) and trimer (63 nt in length) small-interfering RNA. Selective 2′-O-methyl modifications were introduced into nuclease-sensitive sites of both sense and antisense strands of dimer and trimer siRNAs, the modifications in the sites of potential Dicer cleavage were omitted. Selectively modified dimer and trimer siRNAs, unlike the unmodified ones, did not induce interferon response in cultured cells. The trimers (called tsiRNA) were significantly more active at lower dose-equivalent (per moles of 21 bp) concentrations than their canonical analogues but the silencing effect develops more slowly [21] and acts in a Dicer-independent mode, presumably via direct RISC loading. Although the Dicer cleavage sites were free from modifications, modifications in flanking regions of tsiRNAs could inhibit the Dicer cleavage. The observed mechanism may be associated with a specific pattern of modification, used by the authors, which cannot be excluded such that the change in the pattern will allow the tsiRNA to be processed by Dicer and act through a canonical mechanism.

Targeting single mRNA by RNAi inducer for therapeutic purposes has several limitations: (1) the presence of mutation in the target site reduces the efficiency of silencing, which is especially important for viral genes, and (2) signal pathways involved in cancer cell growth contain duplications of regulatory elements and bypass regulatory pathways [97–99]. Thus, simultaneous inhibition of several genes seems to be an effective strategy. Co-transfection of several siRNAs may be not effective due to competition between siRNAs [30]. Therefore, long linear synthetic siRNAs targeted two or more genes hold great promise in these cases.

Peng and his colleagues designed long linear siRNA at least 30 nt in length (multi-siRNAs) for dual-gene silencing [95]. To avoid undesired interferon response and improve RNAi potency, 2′-O-methyl modifications and gap in either sense or antisense strands were used. 2′-O-methyl modifications were introduced into every second nucleotide of both strands. The gap divided the complementary strand into two equal segments. It was demonstrated that multi-siRNAs with the gap provided more efficient simultaneous silencing of two target genes in comparison with corresponding single-target siRNAs (Figure 5). Interestingly, the simultaneous silencing of two target genes by long siRNA without gap was ineffective. It was supposed that the gap may provide sites for Dicer or facilitate Dicer processing. Because the Dicer substrates have preference in RISC loading, multi-siRNAs could possess more efficient silencing activity than canonical siRNAs [16, 18]. The experiments demonstrated that silencing effects of multi-siRNA was eliminated when AGO2 was downregulated confirming the action through the same RNAi pathway as canonical siRNAs [95]. However, further experiments are required to clarify the exact mechanism of increased activity of these siRNAs.

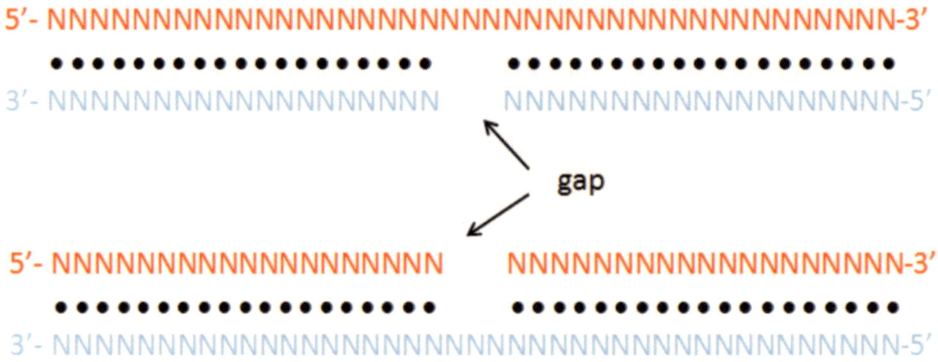

Figure 5. Design of long linear duplexes with gap in either sense or antisense strands. Red color: sense strand, blue color: antisense strand.

Long unmodified siRNAs up to 42 nt in length were used for silencing of gene expression in some specific cell lines without the induction of interferon response [96–101]. For example, direct fusion of two 17- and 19-bp long non-modified siRNAs resulted in efficient silencing of two target genes [96]. Two RNAs were merged "head-to-head" in a way that the 5'-ends of both antisense strands would look outside from the duplex allowing efficient and stereospecific AGO2 binding and efficient silencing of both targets [96]. Heterologous duplexes merged "head-to-tail" of antisense strands demonstrated reduced silencing activity [96]. Similar results were obtained for tandem siRNAs of 40–42 nt in length consisting of 21+21 and 21+23 units [101] as well as 40-nt long duplexes [100]. These results may be explained by the fact that the induction of interferon response depends on the cell type [23]. Indeed, some cell lines may possess reduced immune-sensitivity to the siRNA treatment and the results obtained on the cell cultures cannot be unacceptable for in vivo experiments.

Another class of long siRNAs are various branched structures (Figure 6). Initially, branched oligonucleotides were applied to study mRNA splicing [102–104]. Then diverse branched structures were used as building blocks for self-assembling nanostructures [105–107]. Moreover, nanostructures of different shapes and sizes have been proposed as an effective delivery system for siRNA, ribozymes, etc. [106, 107]. Recently, it has been demonstrated that branched small RNA structures may also be effective RNAi inducers. Thus, these duplexes can simultaneously inhibit two or more genes and possess improved silencing activity and intracellular delivery properties [96–109]. Different strategies are developed to form branches. Symmetric doubler phosphoramidites are used to construct branches with two or four strands [108]. In another variant, trebler phosphoramidite structure with extended short DNA linker is used as a core for branched small RNA with three arms [110]. Direct annealing was used to design RNAs with three and four arms [111, 109]. However, base pairing close to the junction region may be disturbed and single-stranded nuclease-sensitive region may be formed.

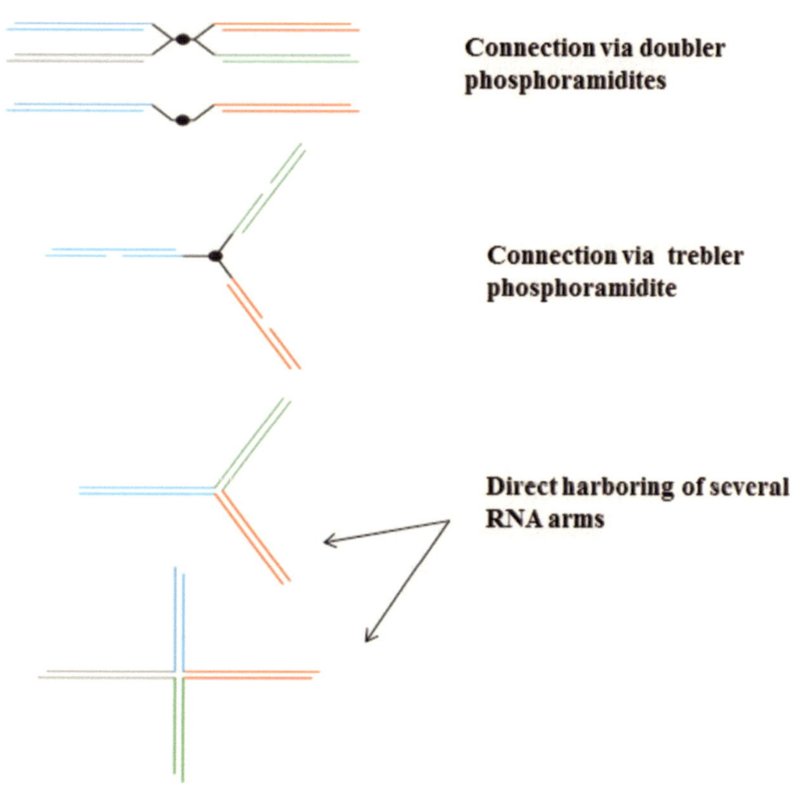

Figure 6. The architecture of various multi-target branched siRNAs. Different colors indicate siRNA units targeted to various genes.

Chang and his colleagues introduced tripartite RNA structure without any linker containing three 19-bp-duplex regions obtained by annealing of three 38-nt single-stranded RNAs [111]. The 5′ end of each antisense strand was directed outside, making seed regions of all antisense strands accessible for AGO2 loading. Single-stranded regions near the strand junction were defended by 2′-O-methyl modifications affecting six nucleotides. It was demonstrated that tripartite small RNA more efficiently silences the expression of three target genes in comparison with a mixture of corresponding canonical siRNAs due to a more efficient intracellular delivery by Lipofectamine [111]. Specifically, tripartite small RNA was not processed by Dicer possibly due to the influence of 2′-O-methyl modifications introduced into the single-stranded region of tripartite RNA [111]. Similar structures without any modifications, designed by another group of scientists, were efficiently processed by Dicer into 20-nt products [109]. On the other hand, tripartite small RNA without any modifications was unstable in biological fluids and quickly degraded.

Tetramer RNA consisted of four arms 23 bp in length proved to be more stable and also acts in a Dicer-dependent mode. Both trimer and tetramer siRNAs provided prolonged RNAi effect and efficiently inhibited the expression of three or four genes simultaneously. The influence of the structures on the interferon response was not reported [109].

Overall, long linear and branched siRNAs could be efficiently used for simultaneous inhibition of multiple genes. Selective 2′-O-methyl modifications and specific elements of the structure (gaps, nonnucleotide insertions) could reduce undesired interferon response. The application of long RNAi inducers is restricted by the complexity of the design (in the case of branched molecules) and the higher cost of synthesis in comparison with canonical siRNAs; however, recent advances in the synthesis of oligoribonucleotide allows overcoming these problems. Long linear and branched siRNAs could be useful for the development of anticancer and antiviral therapeutics targeting multiple genes.

6. Conclusion

Small-interfering RNAs provide universal and effective method for the silencing of target genes because almost all genes could be targeted by siRNAs. A large number of diseases, associated with hyperexpression of certain genes or expression of their chimeric or mutated variants, could be treated by inhibition of gene expression; therefore, siRNA has a great potential as a new therapeutic drug. Different design strategies have been used to improve properties of siRNAs and reduce off-target effects. Structural modifications can expand the boundaries of siRNA applications.

At present, synthetic siRNAs structurally mimicking the Dicer substrates (dsiRNAs) are widely used as potent RNAi inducers. The use of dsiRNA may prevent the development of undesired toxicity associated with off-target effects of both the inducer and the transfection reagent or any type of carrier due to the lower effective concentrations and the increase in the longevity of silencing. Therefore, application of dsiRNAs is considered to be extremely promising in anticancer and antiviral therapeutics as well as for the treatment of chronic diseases where multiple administrations are necessary to reach the desired silencing effect. Chemical modification patterns compatible with Dicer processing were designed and successfully applied for prevention of undesired stimulation of immune system and for acquiring nuclease resistance. Single-stranded structured synthetic siRNAs, such as Dicer-processed short hairpin RNA and dumbbell RNA, possess all benefits as Dicer substrates and exhibit additional flexibility in fine-tuning of the stability, kinetics, and silencing duration. Long RNAi inducers, acting in a Dicer-dependent or Dicer-independent mode, effectively silence target genes at low concentrations. Multi-target siRNAs have a great promise in the treatment of complex diseases such as cancer and immune-inflammatory disorders or viral infections [108]. Long linear or branched structures with selective chemical or structural modifications could successfully inhibit the expression of several genes without undesired off-target effects. Currently, however, the complexity and high cost of the synthesis restrict the biomedical application of long small RNAs. Some structural modifications in siRNAs have specific applications. Fork-siRNA are successfully being used for the silencing of genes with restricted selection of sequence content such as chimeric or point-mutated genes.

siRNAs with various structural modifications find a wide application in biomedical research and therapeutics. Some of them have already been used in clinical trials. The great success was achieved in the multi-target therapy that may increase treatment effectiveness. However, the therapeutics applications are limited by the inefficient delivery of these compounds into organs, tissues, and cells. Problem of low bioavailability of siRNA in vivo could be overcome by two ways: the better delivery and the higher activity. Future expansion of the repertoire of RNAi inducers contributes to resolving of both challenges. Although many approaches are developed, more efforts are still needed to improve safety and efficiency of siRNA in vivo.

Acknowledgements

This work was supported by the Russian Scientific Foundation under the grant #14-14-00697.

Author details

O.V. Gvozdeva and E.L. Chernolovskaya

*Address all correspondence to: elena_ch@niboch.nsc.ru

Laboratory of Nucleic Acids Biochemistry, Institute of Chemical Biology and Fundamental Medicine SB RAS, Novosibirsk, Russia

References

[1] Fire A, Xu S, Montgomery MK, Kostas SA, Driver SE, and Mello C. Potent and specific genetic interference by double-stranded RNA in *Caenorhabditis elegans*. Nature. 1998; 391: 806–811. DOI: 10.1038/35888.

[2] Sharp PA. RNAi and double-strand RNA. Genes Dev. 1999; 13: 139–141. DOI: is not available.

[3] Bernstein E, Caudy AA, Hammond SM, Hannon GJ. Role for a bidentate ribonuclease in the initiation step of RNA interference. Nature. 2001; 409: 363–366. DOI: 10.1038/35053110.

[4] Elbashir SM, Harborth J, Lendeckel W, Yalcin A, Weber K, Tuschl T. Duplexes of 21-nucleotide RNAs mediate RNA interference in cultured mammalian cells. Nature. 2001; 411: 494–498.

[5] Hammond SM, Bernstein E, Beach D, Hannon GJ. An RNA-directed nuclease mediates post-transcriptional gene silencing in Drosophila cells. Nature. 2000; 404: 293–296. DOI: 10.1038/35078107.

[6] Robb GB, Brown KM, Khurana J, Rana TM. Specific and potent RNAi in the nucleus of human cells. Nat Struct Mol Biol. 2005; 12: 133–137. DOI: 10.1038/nsmb886.

[7] Jinek M, Doudna JA. A three-dimensional view of the molecular machinery of RNA interference. Nature. 2009; 457: 405–412. DOI: 10.1038/nature07755.

[8] Ipsaro JJ, Joshua-Tor L. From guide to target: molecular insights into eukaryotic RNA-interference machinery. Nat Struct Mol Biol. 2015; 22: 20–28. DOI: 10.1038/nsmb.2931.

[9] Wilson RC, Doudna JA. Molecular mechanisms of RNA interference. Annu Rev Biophys. 2013; 42: 217–239. DOI: 10.1146/annurev-biophys-083012-130404.

[10] Soutschek J, Akinc A, Bramlage B, Charisse K, Constien R, Donoghue M, Elbashir S, Geick A, Hadwiger P, Harborth J, John M, Kesavan V, Lavine G, Pandey RK, Racie T, Rajeev KG, Rohl I, Toudjarska I, Wang G, Wuschko S, Bumcrot D, Koteliansky V, Limmer S, Manoharan M, Vornlocher HP. Therapeutic silencing of anendogenous gene by systemic administration of modified siRNAs. Nature. 2004; 432: 173–178. DOI: 10.1038/nature03121.

[11] Videira M, Arranja A, Rafael D, Gaspar R. Preclinical development of siRNA therapeutics: towards the match between fundamental science and engineered systems. Nanomedicine. 2014; 10: 689–702. DOI: 10.1016/j.nano.2013.11.018.

[12] Castanotto D, Rossi JJ. The promises and pitfalls of RNA-interference-based therapeutics. Nature. 2009; 457: 426–433. DOI: 10.1038/nature07758.

[13] Deng Y, Wang CC, Choy KW, Du Q, Chen J, Wang Q, Li L, Chung TK, Tang T. Therapeutic potentials of gene silencing by RNA interference: principles, challenges, new strategies. Gene. 2014; 538: 217–227. DOI: 10.1038/nature07758.

[14] Guo P, Coban O, Snead NM, Trebley J, Hoeprich S, Guo S, Shu Y. Engineering RNA for targeted siRNA delivery and medical application. Adv Drug Deliv Rev. 2010; 62: 650–666. DOI: 10.1016/j.addr.2010.03.008.

[15] Kim DH, Behlke MA, Rose SD, Chang MS, Choi S, Rossi JJ. Synthetic dsRNA Dicer substrates enhance RNAi potency and efficacy. Nat Biotechnol. 2005; 23: 222–226. DOI: 10.1038/nbt1051.

[16] Rose SD, Kim DH, Amarzguioui M, Heidel JD, Collingwood MA, Davis ME, Rossi JJ, Behlke MA. Functional polarity is introduced by Dicer processing of short substrate RNAs. Nucleic Acids Res. 2005; 33: 4140–4156. DOI: 10.1093/nar/gki732.

[17] Collingwood MA, Rose SD, Huang L, Hillier C, Amarzguioui M, Wiiger MT, Soifer HS, Rossi JJ, Behlke MA. Chemical modification patterns compatible with high potency Dicer-substrate small interfering RNAs. Oligonucleotides. 2008; 18: 187–200. DOI: 10.1089/oli.2008.0123.

[18] Snead NM, Wu X, Li A, Cui Q, Sakurai K, Burnett JC, Rossi JJ. Molecular basis for improved gene silencing by Dicer substrate interfering RNA compared with other siRNA variants. Nucleic Acids Res. 2013; 41: 6209–6221. DOI: 10.1093/nar/gkt200.

[19] Zhou J, Song MS, Jacobi AM, Behlke MA, Wu X, Rossi JJ. Deep sequencing analyses of DsiRNAs reveal the influence of 3′ terminal overhangs on dicing polarity, strand selectivity, RNA editing of siRNAs. Mol Ther Nucleic Acids, 2012; 1: e17. DOI: 10.1038/mtna.2012.6.

[20] Romanovskaya A, Paavilainen H, Nygårdas M, Bamford DH, Hukkanen V, Poranen MM. Enzymatically produced pools of canonical and Dicer-substrate siRNA molecules display comparable gene silencing and antiviral activities against herpes simplex virus. PLoS One. 2012; 7: e51019. DOI: 10.1371/journal.pone.0051019.

[21] Gvozdeva OV, Dovydenko IS, Venyaminova AG, Zenkova MA, Vlassov VV, Chernolovskaya EL. 42- and 63-bp anti-MDR1-siRNAs bearing 2′-OMe modifications in nuclease-sensitive sites induce specific and potent gene silencing. FEBS Lett. 2014; 588: 1037–4156. DOI: 10.1016/j.febslet.2014.02.015.

[22] Chang CI, Lee TY, Yoo JW, Shin D, Kim M, Kim S, Lee DK. Branched, tripartite-interfering RNAs silence multiple target genes with long guide strands. Nucleic Acid Ther. 2012; 22: 30–39. DOI: 10.1089/nat.2011.0315.

[23] Reynolds A, Anderson EM, Vermeulen A, Fedorov Y, Robinson K, Leake D, Karpilow J, Marshall WS, Khvorova A. Induction of the interferon response by siRNA is cell type and duplex length-dependent. RNA. 2006; 1: 988–993. DOI: 10.1261/rna.2340906.

[24] Sioud M, Furset G. Molecular basis for the immunostimulatory potency of small interfering RNAs. J Biomed Biotechnol. 2006; 4: 1–4. DOI: 10.1155/JBB/2006/23429.

[25] Schlee M, Hornung V, Hartmann G. siRNA and isRNA: two edges of one sword. Mol Ther. 2006; 14: 463–470. DOI: 10.1016/j.ymthe.2006.06.001.

[26] Elbashir SM, Harborth J, Weber K, Tuschl T. Analysis of gene function in somatic mammalian cells using small interfering RNAs. Methods. 2002; 26: 199–213. DOI: 10.1016/S1046-20230200023-3.

[27] Sontheimer EJ. Assembly and function of RNA silencing complexes. Nat Rev Mol Cell Biol. 2005; 6: 127–138. DOI: 10.1038/nrm1568.

[28] Hefner E, Clark K, Whitman C, Behlke MA, Rose SD, Peek AS, Rubio T. Increased potency and longevity of gene silencing using validated Dicer substrates. J Biomol Tech. 2008; 19: 231–237.

[29] Amarzguioui M, Rossi JJ. Principles of Dicer substrate D-siRNA design and function. Methods Mol Biol. 2006; 442: 3–10. DOI: 10.1007/978-1-59745-191-8_1.

[30] Tanudji M, Machalek D, Arndt GM, Rivory L. Competition between siRNA duplexes: impact of RNA-induced silencing complex loading efficiency and comparison between conventional-21 bp and Dicer-substrate siRNAs. Oligonucleotides. 2010; 20: 27–32. DOI: 10.1089/oli.2009.0195.

[31] Kubo T, Zhelev Z, Ohba H, Bakalova R. Modified 27-nt dsRNAs with dramatically enhanced stability in serum and long-term RNAi activity. Oligonucleotides. 2007; 17: 445–464. DOI: 10.1089/oli.2007.0096.

[32] Turner JJ, Jones SW, Moschos SA, Lindsay MA, Gait MJ. MALDI-TOF mass spectral analysis of siRNA degradation in serum confirms an RNAse A-like activity. Mol Biosyst. 2007; 3: 43–50. DOI: 10.1039/b611612d.

[33] Chiu YL, Rana TM. siRNA function in RNAi: a chemical modification analysis. RNA. 2003; 9: 1034–1048. DOI:10.1261/rna.5103703.

[34] Manoharan M. RNA interference and chemically modified small interfering RNAs. Curr Opin Chem Biol. 2004; 8: 570–579. DOI:10.1016/j.cbpa.2004.10.007.

[35] Watts JK, Deleavey GF, Damha MJ. Chemically modified siRNA: tools and applications. Drug Discov Today. 2008; 13: 842–855. DOI: 10.1016/j.drudis.2008.05.007.

[36] Behlke MA. Chemical modification of siRNAs for in vivo use. Oligonucleotides. 2008; 18: 305–319. DOI: 10.1016/j.drudis.2008.05.007.

[37] Amarzguioui M, Holen T, Babaie E, Prydz H. Tolerance for mutations and chemical modifications in a siRNA. Nucleic Acids Res. 2003; 31: 589–595. DOI: 10.1093/nar/gkg147.

[38] Czauderna F, Fechtner M, Dames S, Aygün H, Klippel A, Pronk GJ, Giese K, Kaufmann J. Structural variations and stabilizing modifications of synthetic siRNAs in mammalian cells. Nucleic Acids Res. 2003; 31: 2705–2716. DOI: 10.1093/nar/gkg393.

[39] Harborth J, Elbashir SM, Vandenburgh K, Manninga H, Scaringe SA, Weber K, Tuschl T. Sequence, chemical, and structural variation of small interfering RNAs and

short hairpin RNAs and the effect on mammalian gene silencing. Antisense Nucleic Acid Drug Dev. 2003; 13: 83–105. DOI: 10.1089/108729003321629638.

[40] Choung S, Kim YJ, Kim S, Park HO, Choi YC. Chemical modification of siRNAs to improve serum stability without loss of efficacy. Biochem Biophys Res Commun. 2006; 342: 919–927. DOI: 10.1016/j.bbrc.2006.02.049.

[41] Robbins M, Judge A, Liang L, McClintock K, Yaworski E, MacLachlan I. 2'- O-methyl-modified RNAs act as TLR7 antagonists. Mol Ther. 2007; 15: 1663–1669. DOI: 10.1038/sj.mt.6300240.

[42] Cekaite L, Furset G, Hovig E, Sioud M. Gene expression analysis in blood cells in response to unmodified and 2'-modified siRNAs reveals TLR-dependent and independent effects. J Mol Biol. 2006; 365: 90–108. DOI: 10.1016/j.jmb.2006.09.034.

[43] Heil F, Hemmi H, Hochrein H, Ampenberger F, Kirschning C, Akira S, Lipford G, Wagner H, Bauer S. Species-specific recognition of single-stranded RNA via toll-like receptor 7 and 8. Science. 2004; 303: 1526–1529. DOI: 10.1126/science.1093620.

[44] Judge AD, Sood V, Shaw JR, Fang D, McClintock K, MacLachlan I. Sequence-dependent stimulation of the mammalian innate immune response by synthetic siRNA. Nat Biotechnol. 2005; 23: 457–462. DOI: 10.1038/nbt1081.

[45] Hornung V, Guenthner-Biller M, Bourquin C, Ablasser A, Schlee M, Uematsu S, Noronha A, Manoharan M, Akira S, de Fougerolles A, Endres S, Hartmann G. Sequence-specific potent induction of IFN-alpha by short interfering RNA in plasmacytoid dendritic cells through TLR7. Nat Med. 2005; 11: 263–270. DOI: 10.1038/nm1191.

[46] Morrissey DV, Lockridge JA, Shaw L, Blanchard K, Jensen K, Breen W, Hartsough K, Machemer L, Radka S, Jadhav V, Vaish N, Zinnen S, Vargeese C, Bowman K, Shaffer CS, Jeffs LB, Judge A, MacLachlan I, Polisky B. Potent and persistent in vivo anti-HBV activity of chemically modified siRNAs. Nat Biotechnol. 2005; 23: 1002–1007. DOI: 10.1038/nbt1122.

[47] Parmar MB, Aliabadi HM, Mahdipoor P, Kucharski C, Maranchuk R, Hugh JC, Uludağ H. Targeting cell cycle proteins in breast cancer cells with siRNA by using lipid-substituted polyethylenimines. Front Bioeng Biotechnol. 2015; 16: 1–14. DOI: 10.3389/fbioe.2015.00014.

[48] Liu X, Liu C, Chen C, Bentobji M, Cheillan FA, Piana JT, Qu F, Rocchi P, Peng L. Targeted delivery of Dicer-substrate siRNAs using a dual targeting peptide decorated dendrimer delivery system. Nanomedicine. 2014; 10: 1627–1636. DOI: 10.1016/j.nano.2014.05.008.

[49] Dudek H, Wong DH, Arvan R, Shah A, Wortham K, Ying B, Diwanji R, Zhou W, Holmes B, Yang H, Cyr WA, Zhou Y, Shah A, Farkiwala R, Lee M, Li Y, Rettig GR, Collingwood MA, Basu SK, Behlke MA, Brown BD. Knockdown of β-catenin with

Dicer-substrate siRNAs reduces liver tumor burden in vivo. Mol Ther. 2013; 22: 92–101. DOI: 10.1038/mt.2013.233.

[50] Darniot M, Schildgen V, Schildgen O, Sproat B, Kleines M, Ditt V, Pitoiset C, Pothier P, Manoha C. RNA interference in vitro and in vivo using DsiRNA targeting the nucleocapsid N mRNA of human metapneumovirus. Antiviral Res. 2012; 93: 364–373. DOI: 10.1016/j.antiviral.2012.01.004.

[51] Zhou J, Song MS, Jacobi AM, Behlke MA, Wu X, Rossi JJ. Deep sequencing analyses of DsiRNAs reveal the influence of 3' terminal overhangs on dicing polarity, strand selectivity, and RNA editing of siRNAs. Mol Ther Nucleic Acids. 2012; 1: e17. DOI: 10.1038/mtna.2012.6.

[52] Lundberg P, Yang HJ, Jung SJ, Behlke MA, Rose SD, Cantin EM. Protection against TNFα-dependent liver toxicity by intraperitoneal liposome delivered DsiRNA targeting TNFα in vivo. J Control Release. 2012; 160: 194–199. DOI: 10.1016/j.jconrel.2011.10.034.

[53] Pichu S, Krishnamoorthy S, Zhang B, Jing Y, Shishkov A, Ponnappa BC. Dicer-substrate siRNA inhibits tumor necrosis factor alpha secretion in Kupffer cells in vitro: in vivo targeting of Kupffer cells by siRNA-liposomes. Pharmacol Res. 2012; 65: 48–55. DOI: 10.1016/j.phrs.2011.09.001.

[54] Howard KA, Paludan SR, Behlke MA, Besenbacher F, Deleuran B, Kjems J. Chitosan/siRNA nanoparticle-mediated TNF-alpha knockdown in peritoneal macrophages for anti-inflammatory treatment in a murine arthritis model. Mol Ther. 2009; 17: 162–168. DOI: 10.1038/mt.2008.220.

[55] Doré-Savard L, Roussy G, Dansereau MA, Collingwood MA, Lennox KA, Rose SD, Beaudet N, Behlke MA, Sarret P. Central delivery of Dicer-substrate siRNA: a direct application for pain research. Mol Ther. 2008; 16: 1331–1339. DOI: 10.1038/mt.2008.98.

[56] Carneiro B, Braga AC, Batista MN, Harris M, Rahal P. Evaluation of canonical siRNA and Dicer substrate RNA for inhibition of hepatitis C virus genome replication – a comparative study. PLoS One. 2015; 10: e0117742. DOI: 10.1371/journal.pone.0117742.

[57] Krishnamurthy S, Behlke MA, Apicella MA, McCray PB. Jr, Davidson BL. Platelet activating factor receptor activation improves siRNA uptake and RNAi responses in well-differentiated airway epithelia. Mol Ther Nucleic Acids. 2014; 15: e175. DOI: 10.1038/mtna.2014.26.

[58] Chen J, Wong-Chong J, SundarRaj N. FGF-2- and TGF-β1-induced downregulation of lumican and keratocan in activated corneal keratocytes by JNK signaling pathway. Invest Ophthalmol Vis Sci. 2011; 52: 8957–8964. DOI: 10.1167/iovs.11-8078.

[59] Bohle H, Lorenzen N, Schyth BD. Species specific inhibition of viral replication using dicer substrate siRNAs DsiRNAs targeting the viral nucleoprotein of the fish patho-

genic rhabdovirus viral hemorrhagic septicemia virus VHSV. Antiviral Res. 2011; 187–194. DOI: 10.1016/j.antiviral.2011.03.174.

[60] Lee RC, Ambros V. An extensive class of small RNAs in *Caenorhabditis elegans*. Science. 2001; 294: 862–864. DOI: 10.1126/science.1065329.

[61] Lau NC, Lim LP, Weinstein EG, Bartel DP. An abundant class of tiny RNAs with probable regulatory roles in *Caenorhabditis elegans*. Science. 2001; 294: 858–862. DOI: 10.1126/science.1065062.

[62] Lagos-Quintana M, Rauhut R, Lendeckel W, Tuschl T. Identification of novel genes coding for small expressed RNAs. Science. 2001; 294: 853–858. DOI: 10.1126/science.1064921.

[63] Hutvágner G, McLachlan J, Pasquinelli AE, Bálint E, Tuschl T, Zamore PD. A cellular function for the RNA-interference enzyme Dicer in the maturation of the let-7 small temporal RNA. Science. 2001; 293: 894–898. DOI: 10.1126/science.1062961.

[64] Siolas D, Lerner C, Burchard J, Ge W, Linsley PS, Paddison PJ, Hannon GJ, Cleary MA. Synthetic shRNAs as potent RNAi triggers. Nat Biotechnol. 2005; 23: 227–231. DOI: 10.1038/nbt1052.

[65] Svoboda P, Stein P, Schultz RM. RNAi in mouse oocytes and preimplantation embryos: effectiveness of hairpin dsRNA. Biochem Biophys Res Commun. 2001; 287: 1099–1104. DOI: 10.1006/bbrc.2001.5707.

[66] Sharp PA. RNA interference – 2001. Genes Dev. 2001; 15: 485–490. DOI: 10.1101/gad.880001.

[67] Brummelkamp TR, Bernards R, Agami R. A system for stable expression of short interfering RNAs in mammalian cells. Science.2002; 296: 550–553. DOI: 10.1126/science.1068999.

[68] Paddison PJ, Caudy AA, Bernstein E, Hannon GJ, Conklin DS. Short hairpin RNAs shRNAs induce sequence-specific silencing in mammalian cells. Genes Dev. 2002; 16: 948–958. DOI: 10.1101/gad.981002.

[69] Thomas CE, Ehrhardt A, Kay MA. Progress and problems with the use of viral vectors for gene therapy. Nat Rev Genet. 2003; 4: 346–358. DOI: 10.1038/nrg1066.

[70] Vlassov AV, Korba B, Farrar K, Mukerjee S, Seyhan AA, Ilves H, Kaspar RL, Leake D, Kazakov SA, Johnston BH. shRNAs targeting hepatitis C: effects of sequence and structural features, and comparison with siRNA. Oligonucleotides. 2007; 17: 223–236. DOI: 10.1089/oli.2006.0069.

[71] Ge Q, Ilves H, Dallas A, Kumar P, Shorenstein J, Kazakov SA, Johnston BH. Minimal-length short hairpin RNAs: the relationship of structure and RNAi activity. RNA. 2010; 16: 106–117. DOI: 10.1261/rna.1894510.

[72] McManus MT, Petersen CP, Haines BB, Chen J, Sharp PA. Gene silencing using micro-RNA designed hairpins. RNA. 2010; 8: 842–850. DOI: 10.1017.S1355838202024032.

[73] Harborth J, Elbashir SM, Vandenburgh K, Manninga H, Scaringe SA, Weber K, Tuschl T. Sequence, chemical, and structural variation of small interfering RNAs and short hairpin RNAs and the effect on mammalian gene silencing. Antisense Nucleic Acid Drug Dev. 2003; 13: 83–105. DOI: 10.1089/108729003321629638.

[74] Wang Q, Contag CH, Ilves H, Johnston BH, Kaspar RL. Small hairpin RNAs efficiently inhibit hepatitis C IRES-mediated gene expression in human tissue culture cells and a mouse model. Mol Ther. 2005; 12: 562–568. DOI: 10.1016/j.ymthe.2005.04.014.

[75] Song JJ, Liu J, Tolia NH, Schneiderman J, Smith SK, Martienssen RA, Hannon GJ, Joshua-Tor L. The crystal structure of the Argonaute2 PAZ domain reveals an RNA binding motif in RNAi effector complexes. Nat Struct Biol. 2003; 10: 1026–1032. DOI: 10.1038/nsb1016.

[76] Li L, Lin X, Khvorova A, Fesik SW, Shen Y. Defining the optimal parameters for hairpin-based knockdown constructs. RNA. 2007; 13: 1765–1774. DOI: 10.1038/nsb1016.

[77] Nykänen A, Haley B, Zamore PD. ATP requirements and small interfering RNA structure in the RNA interference pathway. Cell. 2001; 107: 309–321. DOI: 10.1016/S0092-86740100547-5.

[78] Tsui NB, Ng EK, Lo YM. Stability of endogenous and added RNA in blood specimens, serum, and plasma. Clin Chem. 2002; 48: 1647–1657. DOI: is not available.

[79] Abe N, Abe H, Ito Y. Dumbbell-shaped nanocircular RNAs for RNA interference. J Am Chem Soc. 2007; 129: 15108–15109. DOI: 10.1021/ja0754453.

[80] Erie DA, Jones RA, Olson WK, Sinha NK, Breslauer KJ. Melting behavior of a covalently closed, single-stranded, circular DNA. Biochemistry. 1989; 28: 268–273. DOI: is not available.

[81] Abe N, Abe H, Nagai C, Harada M, Hatakeyama H, Harashima H, Ohshiro T, Nishihara M, Furukawa K, Maeda M, Tsuneda S, Ito Y. Synthesis, structure, and biological activity of dumbbell-shaped nanocircular RNAs for RNA interference. Bioconjug Chem. 2011; 22: 2082–2092. DOI: 10.1021/bc2003154.

[82] Abe N, Abe H, Ito Y. Synthesis of dumbbell-shaped cyclic RNAs for RNA interference. Curr Protoc Nucleic Acid Chem. 2012; 16: 1–11. DOI: 0.1002/0471142700.nc1604s48.

[83] Hohjoh H. Enhancement of RNAi activity by improved siRNA duplexes. FEBS Lett. 2004; 557: 193–198. DOI: 10.1016/S0014-57930301492-3.

[84] Ohnishi Y, Tokunaga K, Hohjoh H. Influence of assembly of siRNA elements into RNA-induced silencing complex by fork-siRNA duplex carrying nucleotide mis-

matches at the 3'- or 5'-end of the sense-stranded siRNA element. Biochem Biophys Res Commun. 2005; 329: 516–521. DOI: 10.1016/j.bbrc.2005.02.012.

[85] Petrova Kruglova NS, Meschaninova MI, Venyaminova AG, Zenkova MA, Vlassov VV, Chernolovskaya EL. 2'-O-methyl-modified anti-MDR1 fork-siRNA duplexes exhibiting high nuclease resistance and prolonged silencing activity. Oligonucleotides. 2010; 20: 297–308. DOI: 10.1089/oli.2010.0246.

[86] Khvorova A, Reynolds A, Jayasena SD. Functional siRNAs and miRNAs exhibit strand bias. Cell. 2003; 115: 209–216. DOI:10.1016/S0014-57930301492-3.

[87] Chu CY, Rana TM. Potent RNAi by short RNA triggers. RNA. 2008; 14: 1714–1719. DOI: 10.1261/rna.1161908.

[88] Hall AH, Wan J, Spesock A, Sergueeva Z, Shaw BR, Alexander KA. High potency silencing by single-stranded boranophosphate siRNA. Nucleic Acids Res. 2006; 34: 2773–2781. DOI: 10.1093/nar/gkl339.

[89] Holen T, Amarzguioui M, Babaie E, Prydz H. Similar behavior of single-strand and double-strand siRNAs suggests they act through a common RNAi pathway. Nucleic Acids Res. 2003; 31: 2401–2407. DOI: 10.1093/nar/gkg338.

[90] Martinez J, Patkaniowska A, Urlaub H, Lührmann R, Tuschl T. Single-stranded antisense siRNAs guide target RNA cleavage in RNAi. Cell. 2002; 110: 563–574. DOI: 10.1016/S0092-86740200908-X.

[91] Chiu YL, Rana TM. RNAi in human cells: basic structural and functional features of small interfering RNA. Mol Cell. 2002; 10: 549–561. DOI: 10.1016/S1097-27650200652-4.

[92] Chang CI, Yoo JW, Hong SW, Lee SE, Kang HS, Sun X, Rogoff HA, Ban C, Kim S, Li CJ, Lee DK. Asymmetric shorter-duplex siRNA structures trigger efficient gene silencing with reduced nonspecific effects. Mol Ther. 2009; 17: 725–732. DOI: 10.1038/mt.2008.298.

[93] Tijsterman M, Ketting RF, Plasterk RH. The genetics of RNA silencing. Annu Rev Genet. 2002; 36: 489–519. DOI: 10.1146/annurev.genet.36.043002.091619.

[94] Stark GR, Kerr IM, Williams BR, Silverman RH, Schreiber RD. How cells respond to interferons. Annu Rev Biochem. 1998; 67: 227–264. DOI: 10.1146/annurev.biochem.67.1.227.

[95] Peng W, Chen J, Qin Y, Yang Z, Zhu YY. Long double-stranded multiplex siRNAs for dual genes silencing. Nucleic Acid Ther. 2013; 23: 281–288. DOI: 10.1089/nat.2013.0416.

[96] Chang CI, Kang HS, Ban C, Kim S, Lee DK. Dual-target gene silencing by using long, synthetic siRNA duplexes without triggering antiviral responses. Mol Cells. 2009; 27: 689–695. DOI: 10.1007/s10059-009-0093-0.

[97] Boden D, Pusch O, Lee F, Tucker L, Ramratnam B. Human immunodeficiency virus type 1 escape from RNA interference. J Virol. 2003; 77: 11531–11535. DOI: 10.1128/JVI.77.21.11531-11535.2003.

[98] Das AT, Brummelkamp TR, Westerhout EM, Vink M, Madiredjo M, Bernards R, Berkhout B. Human immunodeficiency virus type 1 escapes from RNA interference-mediated inhibition. J Virol. 2004; 78: 2601–2605. DOI: 10.1128/JVI.78.5.2601-2605.2004.

[99] Menendez JA, Vellon L, Mehmi I, Oza BP, Ropero S, Colomer R, Lupu, R. Inhibition of fatty acid synthase FAS suppresses HER2/neu erbB-2 oncogene overexpression in cancer cells. Proc Natl Acad Sci 2004; 10715–10720. DOI: 10.1073/pnas.0403390101.

[100] Vickers TA, Lima WF, Nichols JG, Crooke, ST. Reduced levels of Ago2 expression result in increased siRNA competition in mammalian cells. Nucleic Acids Res. 2007; 6598–6610. DOI: 10.1093/nar/gkm663.

[101] Shin D, Lee H, Kim SI, Yoon Y, Kim M. Optimization of linear double-stranded RNA for the production of multiple siRNAs targeting hepatitis C virus. RNA 2009; 15: 898–910. DOI: 10.1261/rna.1268209.

[102] Damha MJ, Ogilvie KK. Synthesis and spectroscopic analysis of branched RNA fragments: messenger RNA splicing intermediates. J Org Chem. 1998; 16: 3710–3722. DOI: 10.1021/jo00251a010.

[103] Grøtli M, Eritja R, Sproat B. Solid-phase synthesis of branched RNA and branched DNA/RNA chimeras. Tetrahedron, 1997; 33: 11317–11346. DOI: 10.1016/S0040-40209700731-X.

[104] Carriero S, Damha MJ. Inhibition of pre-mRNA splicing by synthetic branched nucleic acids. Nucleic Acids Res. 2003; 31: 6157–6167. DOI:10.1093/nar/gkg824.

[105] Jasinski DL, Khisamutdinov EF, Lyubchenko YL, Guo P. Physicochemically tunable polyfunctionalized RNA square architecture with fluorogenic and ribozymatic properties. ACS Nano. 2014; 8: 7620–7629. DOI: 10.1021/nn502160s.

[106] Guo P. Rolling circle transcription of tandem siRNA to generate spherulitic RNA nanoparticles for cell entry. Mol Ther Nucleic Acids. 2012; 1: e36. DOI: 10.1038/mtna.2012.31.

[107] Shu Y, Pi F, Sharma A, Rajabi M, Haque F, Shu D, Leggas M, Evers BM, Guo P. Stable RNA nanoparticles as potential new generation drugs for cancer therapy. Adv Drug Deliv Rev. 2013; 66: 74–89. DOI: 10.1016/j.addr.2013.11.006.

[108] Aviñó A, Ocampo SM, Perales JC, Eritja R. Branched RNA: a new architecture for RNA interference. J Nucleic Acids. 2014; 2011: 1–7. DOI: 10.4061/2011/586935.

[109] Nakashima Y, Abe H, Abe N, Aikawa K, Ito Y. Branched RNA nanostructures for RNA interference. Chem Commun Camb. 2011; 47: 8367–8369. DOI: 10.1039/c1cc11780g.

[110] Chang CI, Lee TY, Yoo JW, Shin D, Kim M, Kim S, Lee DK. Branched, tripartite-interfering RNAs silence multiple target genes with long guide strands. Nucleic Acid Ther. 2012; 22: 30–39. DOI: 10.1089/nat.2011.0315.

[111] Chang CI, Lee TY, Kim S, Sun X, Hong SW, Yoo JW, Dua P, Kang HS, Kim S, Li CJ, Lee DK. Enhanced intracellular delivery and multi-target gene silencing triggered by tripodal RNA structures. J Gene Med. 2012; 14: 138–146. DOI: 10.1002/jgm.1653.

Chapter 6

Microinjection-Based RNA Interference Method in the Water Flea, *Daphnia pulex* and *Daphnia magna*

Kenji Toyota, Shinichi Miyagawa, Yukiko Ogino and Taisen Iguchi

Additional information is available at the end of the chapter

http://dx.doi.org/10.5772/61485

Abstract

It is well known that most daphnid species have several attractive life history characteristics such as cyclical parthenogenesis, environmental sex determination, and predator-induced defense formation. Recent advances in high-throughput omics technologies make it easy to obtain a huge number of potential candidate factors involved in environmental stimuli-triggered phenotypic alterations. Furthermore, our group has developed a microinjection system to introduce foreign materials such as nucleotides and chemicals into the early-stage (one-cell stage) egg of *Daphnia pulex* and *Daphnia magna*. Consequently, we established a microinjection-based RNAi system that allows arbitrary gene functions to be investigated. However, this microinjection system does not seem to have pervaded in the daphnid research community due to its low throughput and high level of skills required. In this chapter, we review the microinjection method and its RNAi system in water fleas, *D. pulex* and *D. magna*, providing some technical tips and making challenging proposals for the development of novel high-throughput RNAi methods. Finally, we provide an overview of recently developed gene functional analysis methods such as overexpression and genome-editing systems.

Keywords: *Daphnia pulex*, *Daphnia magna*, genome editing, microinjection, RNAi-related gene

1. Introduction

The cladoceran crustacean water fleas are representative zooplankton ubiquitously found in freshwater habitats around the world [1]. Among them, species of the family Daphniidae, particularly genus *Daphnia*, have been well studied. All age classes of daphnids are principle consumers of algae and thus play an important role in the food web in freshwater ecosystems. In addition to this ecological significance, over the last decade, daphnids have drawn considerable attention as a good indicator organism for aquatic toxicology and have thus been used in ecotoxicological studies [2]. Moreover, for over 100 years, they have shown various adaptive phenotypic alterations in response to external environmental stimuli, including environmental sex determination (ESD) [3, 4], cyclical parthenogenesis, in which the mode of reproduction changes between parthenogenesis and sexual reproduction [3, 4], and inducible defense, which is a predator-triggered alteration of body shape [5, 6]. The acquisition of such sophisticated life history strategies has enabled daphnids to prosper around the world. These environmental stimuli-triggered phenomena in daphnid species have attracted many scientists involved in ecological, developmental, and evolutionary biology [4, 7–12]. Although recent progress in sequencing technology facilitates the deciphering of genome and transcriptome information using 'nonmodel organisms', analytical methods for arbitrary gene functions are still insufficiently developed. In studies involving daphnids, the whole-genome sequencing project of *D. pulex* has been completed [12]. Furthermore, a microinjection system using early-stage embryos has been established, allowing gene functional analyses, including RNA interference (RNAi), to be possible in daphnids [13, 14]. Even though this microinjection-based experimental method can be used in two representative daphnid species, *D. pulex* and *D. magna*, some experimental aspects are different between them due to the difference in size of their early-stage embryos.

This chapter introduces *Daphnia* species as attractive models for eco-evo-devo studies and summarizes technical methods and tips for microinjection-based RNAi in *D. pulex* and *D. magna*. Finally, we review recent advances in the application of microinjection methods in daphnids such as genome editing and transgenesis.

1.1. Life cycle

Daphnids produce offspring either by parthenogenesis or by sexual reproduction in response to external environmental conditions. This mode of reproduction is referred to as cyclical parthenogenesis. They have a short generation period that lasts approximately 1 week under constant laboratory conditions, and their lifetime spans over 2 months or as much as 1 year when reared under colder temperatures [15]. Under optimal growing conditions, daphnids parthenogenetically produce offspring that expand their population consisting almost exclusively of females. This results in the exponential growth of genetically identical clone clusters. Mother daphnids produce several dozen eggs in their own brood chamber as a clutch just a few minutes after molting. Embryonic development occurs in the brood chamber. Subsequently, neonates are released to the outside just before the mother molts. Then individual mothers in the parthenogenetic phase repeat molting, spawning, and the release of neonates throughout their lifetime (Figure 1, parthenogenetic phase).

On the other hand, when environmental conditions deteriorate, for instance, a short day-length, lower temperature, food shortage, overcrowding, and the presence of predators, males are induced by parthenogenesis and are, therefore, genetically identical to their sisters and mother [4, 7–9, 16, 17] (Figure 1, sexual reproductive phase). In other words, an individual parthenogenetic mother has the potential to produce female and male offspring in response to changes in external environmental conditions. After copulation, sexual eggs, referred to as resting eggs that are enclosed in an ephippium (modified carapace that is darkly pigmented by melanin), are produced. Resting eggs can tolerate extreme conditions such as drying, freezing, and digestion by fish and can remain viable for over 100 years [18]. When favorable conditions are restored, female neonates hatch out from resting eggs and reinitiate the parthenogenetic phase, thus building up a new population (Figure 1, sexual reproductive phase).

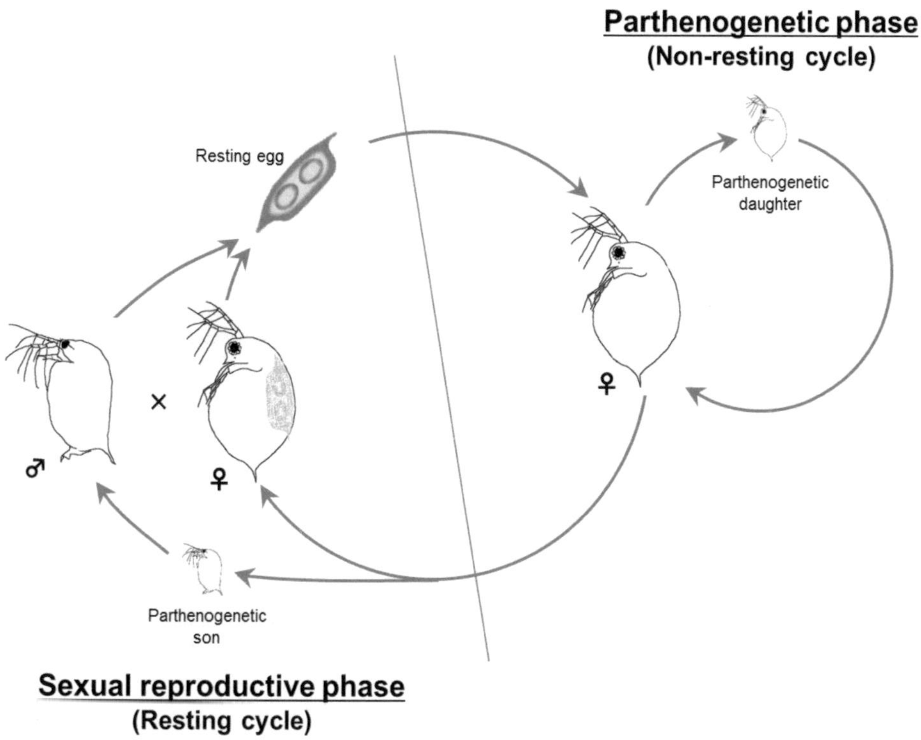

Figure 1. Schematic drawing of cyclical parthenogenesis in daphnids.

1.2. *Daphnia* as model species for ecological, evolutionary and developmental biology: eco-evo-devo

Although several details are still controversial, recent molecular phylogenetic analyses of the Arthropoda have revealed that the Crustacea clade is not monophyletic and is divided into at least three clades (Ostracoda, Malacostraca, and Branchiopoda) that include daphnids (Figure 2). Also, the current phylogenetic hypothesis supports the notion that Branchiopoda and Hexapoda form a sister group (Figure 2). This suggests that a growing body of findings involving daphnids has accumulated and can contribute to our understanding of the evolutionary and developmental aspects of Arthropoda, connecting knowledge between well-studied Hexapoda and more primitive Arthropoda clades.

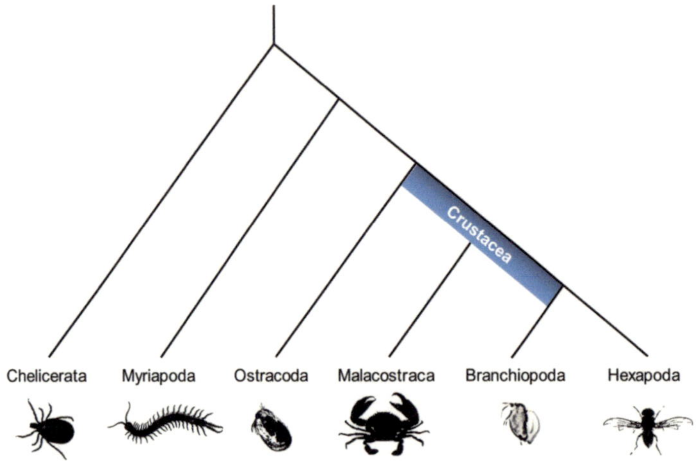

Figure 2. Phylogenetic tree of the Arthropoda. The branching pattern is based on Oakley *et al.* [19] with some modifications [20].

D. pulex and *D. magna have* long been used in ecological, evolutionary, developmental, and ecotoxicological studies as representative model daphnid species for the following reasons: *D. pulex* is ubiquitously widespread around the world, including Japan (Figure 3A), and shows striking phenotypic alterations in response to predator-released chemicals, forming 'neckteeth' [5]; *D. magna* has a huge body size among cladoceran species (maximum length of approximately 10 mm, Figure 3B); they are easy to maintain and rear under laboratory conditions; they propagate rapidly because of their short generation time and reproductive cycle; embryonic development can be observed *in vitro*; male offspring can be induced by administration of juvenile hormone agonists [21, 22]. In addition, individuals within a single strain are most likely genetically identical due to the diploidy of the parthenogenetic eggs that are maintained by mitosis-like meiosis, which skips a part of the first meiosis [23], allowing the environmental effects on their physiological and developmental processes to be investigated under a constant genetic background. Furthermore, we established a reliable induction system for environmental sex determination (ESD) studies using the *D. pulex* WTN6 strain, in which the sex of the offspring can be controlled by changing the day-length conditions in which long-day (14 h light:10 h dark) and short-day (10 h light:14 h dark) conditions can induce female and male offspring, respectively [17], and for inducible defense in several *D. pulex* strains where the incidence and number of neckteeth vary in response to different concentrations of *Chaoborus* kairomone [24].

In addition to the aforementioned advantages, useful experimental tools are available, for example, embryonic developmental staging [25, 26], whole-mount *in situ* hybridization and immunostaining using developing embryos [27], immunofluorescence and fluorescence *in situ* hybridization (FISH) [28], an expressed sequence tags (ESTs) database [29], and genetic linkage maps [30–32]. Furthermore, the whole-genome sequencing of *D. pulex* is complete [12, 32], although that of *D. magna* is still ongoing (https://wiki.cgb.indiana.edu/display/magna/Home). In addition, recent growing omics and bioinformatics technology enables daphnid researchers to investigate cells, tissues, and organisms from a multilevel perspective such as the transcriptome [12, 33–35], proteome [36], or metabolome [37]. Thus, various excellent experimental tools and an increasingly huge accumulation of omics data make *D. pulex* and *D. magna* attractive model organisms for studying the molecular mechanisms underlying phenotypic alterations that depend on external environmental conditions. These reliable induction systems of focal phenotypes are indispensable for analyzing their physiological and developmental mechanisms.

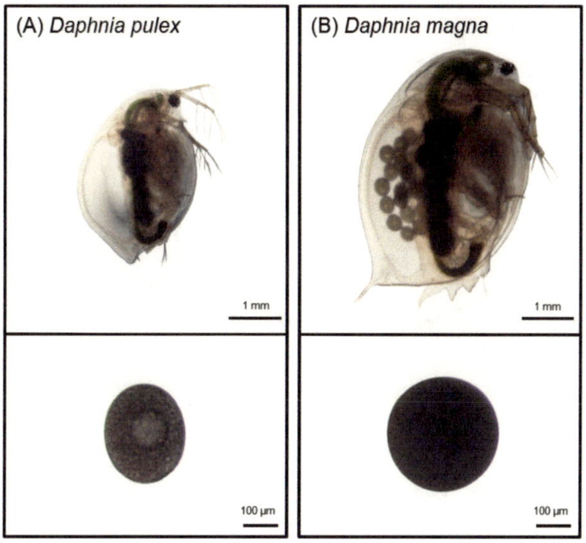

Figure 3. *Daphnia pulex* (A) and *D. magna* (B). Upper and lower parts indicate the adult and embryo just after ovulation, respectively.

2. Microinjection-based RNA interference (RNAi) in daphnid species

As mentioned above, recent high-throughput sequencing technologies have enabled biologists to use nonmodel organisms to easily access genomic information. However, the development of experimental methods for gene functional analysis still hampers their reverse genetics approach. To date, the RNAi method in *D. pulex* and *D. magna* has been established by a microinjection method using early-stage embryos. Although our previous reports described detailed methodology for microinjection and the tips, tricks, and traps associated with this methodology [13, 14], there are slight differences for each daphnid species. Furthermore, descriptions of genes involved in the RNAi machinery is insufficient. Therefore, we comparatively summarize the tips to manipulate the microinjection methods in detail prior to focusing on the current status of daphnid RNAi. We then introduce the gene repertoires involved in the RNAi mechanism in *D. pulex* and *D. magna* genomes.

2.1. Microinjection system

The daphnid microinjection system uses parthenogenetic eggs just after ovulation into the mother's brood chamber. The individual mother begins to lay eggs into the brood chamber a few minutes after releasing neonates and molting. To obtain many healthy eggs, eggs from 2 to 6-week-old daphnids should be collected.

There are two major technical issues in microinjection of daphnids. One is the rapid hardening of the egg membrane just after ovulation [38], which is caused by enzymatic activity of peroxidase. The second problem is a substantial difference between the internal and external osmotic pressures of the egg. The former issue hampers the penetration of the egg membrane by a needle while the latter causes the leakage of egg components after injection. To overcome these problems, Kato et al. [13] and Hiruta et al. [14] established improved protocols for microinjection in *D. magna* and *D. pulex*, respectively. They succeeded in the transient inhibition of the egg membrane hardening by ice-cold treatment just after ovulation. They also found the best culture conditions after injection by increasing external osmotic pressures: M4 medium [39] with 80-mM sucrose in *D. magna* [13] and a 2% agar plate covered with 60-mM sucrose dissolved in M4 media in *D. pulex* [14].

In addition, since the fineness of the needle is critical for the success of microinjection, we next describe a detailed preparation method. A glass needle is made from a glass capillary tube (GD-1; Narishige, Tokyo, Japan) by a micropipette puller (P-97/IVF; Sutter Instrument, Novato, CA, USA). The programmed P-97 parameters are as follows: heat: 845; pull: 50; velocity: 120; time: 200; pressure: 500. The value of the 'heat' parameter required for the ramp test is based on the manufacturer's protocol because this value depends on a combination of the filament and the glass capillary. In our case, using a combination of a regular P-97 filament and a GD-1 glass capillary, the 'heat' parameter value ranges between 845 and 870.

Based on the aforementioned information, we describe next the manipulation procedure of microinjection using daphnids eggs.

1. The setting of tools for microinjection and surgery are shown in Figure 4A-C. A glass Petri dish is prepared by placing two cover glasses side by side with M4-sucrose at ambient temperature.

2. The synthesized double-strand RNA (dsRNA) is mixed with an equal amount of 2-mM Chromeo 494 fluorescent dye (Active Motif Chromeon GmbH, Tegernheim, Germany), which is used as a visible marker for injection. When using *D. pulex* eggs, it is possible to confirm whether injection has succeeded by visual observation since the eggs are more transparent than *D. magna* eggs (Figure 3). A visible marker is thus not essential.

3. The dsRNA solution (1.0–1.5 μL) is loaded into the needle. The tip of the needle is then manually cut off using forceps under a stereomicroscope.

4. Mother daphnids just before molting (brood chamber is empty) are collected and observed until spawning begins. They are transferred to ice-cold M4-sucrose medium just before spawning is complete (4–5 eggs remain in each ovary).

http://dx.doi.org/10.5772/61485

5. Eggs are surgically obtained from the mother daphnid and placed in ice-cold M4-sucrose medium.

6. One to three eggs are immobilize by placing them at the edge of the left cover glass and are injected by using a microinjector (Femtojet, Eppendorf, Hauppauge, NY, USA) and a micromanipulator (MN-153, Narishige, Tokyo, Japan ; Figure 4D–F). The right cover glass is used as a holder when the needle is not withdrawn from the egg. Microinjections can be carried out within 1 h after ovulation.

7. The injected eggs are transferred into a plastic 6-well plate with 80-mM M4-sucrose medium for *D. magna* [13] or a 2% agar plate on a 6-well plate with 60-mM M4-sucrose medium for *D. pulex* [14] (Figure 4G) and subsequently incubated under constant temperature (18–20°C).

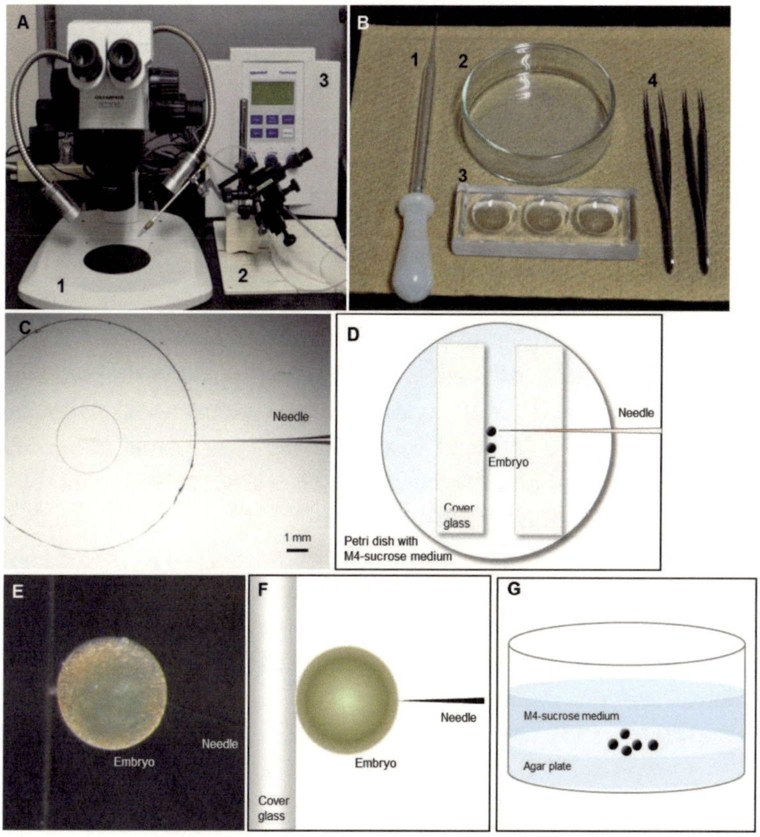

Figure 4. Microinjection of daphnid egg. (A) Experimental equipment. 1: stereomicroscope; 2: micromanipulator (MN-153, Narishige, Tokyo, Japan); 3: electronic microinjector (Femtojet, Eppendorf, Hauppauge, NY, USA). (B) Tools for surgical manipulation. 1: Pasteur pipet (Thomas Scientific, Swedesboro, NJ, USA); 2: glass dish with two cover glasses; 3: plate for blood test; 4: forceps (Dumoxel #5 Biologie). (C) A glass needle is made from a glass capillary tube (GD-1; Narishige, Tokyo, Japan). (D) Overview illustration of microinjection field. (E, F) Magnified view and illustration of microinjection using *D. pulex* egg. (G) Schematic illustration of embryo incubation after injection.

2.2. RNAi machinery in daphnid species

The well-known natural role of RNAi in organisms is the innate immune system against viruses and transposable elements [40]. Using this phenomenon, RNAi induction has been developed as an innovative method for gene functional analysis by exogenous application of dsRNA in *Caenorhabditis elegans* [41]. The dsRNA is first recognized by Dicer protein and cut off into short 21–24 nucleotides referred to as short interfering RNAs (siRNA). These are then invariably incorporated into large Argonaute-containing effector complexes known as RNA-induced silencing complexes (RISCs), after which one-side strand of the dsRNA is cleaved and degraded. Finally, the active Argonaute-containing RISC cleaves the target RNA sequence with the complementary sequence to siRNA [40, 42]. In addition to this core machinery of the RNAi pathway, many eukaryotes have the potential to amplify an amount of siRNA by a host-encoded RNA-dependent RNA polymerase (RdRp). However, RdRp orthologs have not been identified from the Arthropoda genome including *D. pulex* except for the tick genome [42].

In the *D. pulex* and *D. magna* genomes, there are three Dicer and Argonaute paralogs, but the *D. magna* genome contains two copies of Dicer. Previous studies have shown that Dicer paralogs are categorized into two clusters corresponding to the microRNA (miRNA) pathway (Dicer-1) and the siRNA pathway (Dicer-2) [42, 43]. The miRNA is also a short 21–25 RNA, which is generated from a hairpin in pre-mRNA, and plays an important role in translational repression associated with RISC [44]. Phylogenetic analyses found that all Dicer paralogs of *D. pulex* and *D. magna* were classed into the Dicer-1 group [45] (Figure 5A). Moreover, we successfully recruited three Argonaute paralogs from the genome of each daphnid and constructed a phylogenetic tree (Figure 5B). Previous studies revealed that Argonaute family members are key components in different RNA silencing pathways and are categorized into two subfamilies, Argonaute and PIWI (P-element induced wimpy testis). Argonaute subfamily members have been found in widespread taxa, including yeast, plants, and animals and have been identified as Argonaute-1 and Argonaute-2, which are involved in miRNA and siRNA pathways, respectively. In contrast, the PIWI subfamily has been identified only in animals as Argonaute-3, which is involved in PIWI-interacting RNA (piRNA) pathways [42, 46, 47]. Four Argonaute family members were found from *D. pulex* and *D. magna* genome sequences in this study, although only two paralogs have already been previously reported [43]. Phylogenetic analysis revealed that both paralogs fall into the Arogonaute-1 clade of the Argonaute subfamily, whereas each one paralog was categorized into Argonaute-3 and PIWI clades of the PIWI subfamily (Figure 5B). The number of Argonaute family members found in daphnids seems to be as conserved as in insect species [42, 48], although no Argonaute-2 paralogs have yet been identified. Taken together, our results suggest that the genomes of daphnids might lack the Dicer-2 and Argonaute-2 orthologs, which are factors responsible for regulating the siRNA-inducing transcriptional gene-silencing pathway. In other words, our data imply that the RNAi machinery of daphnid species might be distinct from the equivalent well-studied mechanism in insects. To understand the full picture of the RNAi machinery of daphnid species, further studies that examine domain sequence similarity and gene functional analysis will be required.

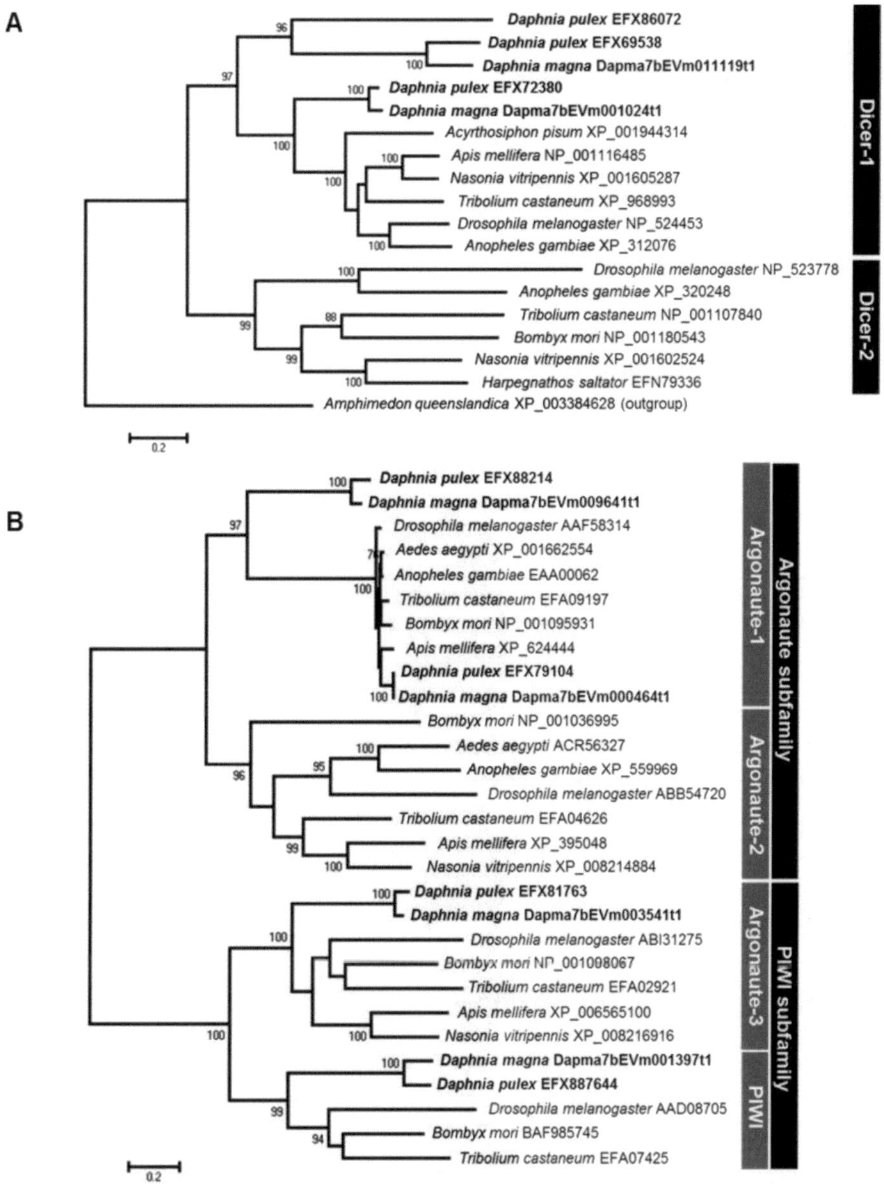

Figure 5. Phylogenetic trees of Dicer (A) and Argonaute (B). Amino acid sequences were aligned by ClustalW, and the maximum likelihood trees were constructed from these alignments using the JTT model with bootstrap analyses of 1000 replicates along with complete deletion options (818 and 597 amino acid positions were used, respectively) by MEGA6 [49]. Branches with bootstrap support >70% are indicated by numbers at nodes. Both *D. pulex* and *D. magna* are indicated in bold. To obtain the predicted sequences encoding the *D. magna* orthologs of RNAi-related genes, protein sequences of *D. pulex* were used in BLAST searches querying *D. magna* Genome BLAST (http://arthropods.eugenes.org/EvidentialGene/daphnia/daphnia_magna/BLAST/). The SID protein sequences of *D. pulex* were retrieved from wFleaBase (http://wfleabase.org/). Phylogenetic trees were constructed based on data from McTaggart et al. [43] with some modifications.

2.3. Future challenges for development of high-throughput RNAi method in daphnids

Despite the availability of a microinjection-based RNAi method in daphnids, as demonstrated by knocking down genes responsible for morphogenesis (*distal-less* and *eyeless*) [13, 14, 50], sexual differentiation (*doublesex1*) [51], endocrine system (*ecdysteroid-phosphate phosphatase*) [52], and neurogenesis (*single-minded homolog*) [53], this method has several experimental limitations. For example, microinjection can only be performed using an early stage (1-cell stage) egg, suggesting that this system cannot be used to perform a functional analysis of genes that act during the adult stage and is unsuitable for large-scale experiments. Moreover, specialized and skillful technical training is necessary to master the microinjection technique in daphnids. To overcome those technical hurdles, we introduce two potential ideas to establish more high-throughput and user-friendly methods for the study of daphnids. One is electroporation, which is a physical transfection method that uses an electrical pulse to increase the permeability of cell membranes, allowing nucleic acids and/or chemicals to be introduced into cells. Recent innovation of the electroporation system has enabled the establishment of rapid functional analysis in various organisms [54–56]. Indeed, our group has successfully developed an *in vivo* electroporation system for the introduction of foreign DNA into neonatal *D. magna* within 6 hours after release from the mother's brood chamber [57]. Therefore, it might be possible to apply this system for RNAi using various stages of daphnids.

The second method is a feeding (oral delivery) RNAi system, which was first developed in *C. elegans* [58]. The feeding RNAi system is the most convenient and inexpensive method for high-throughput screening since bacteria produce the designed dsRNA that are fed to host animals. This system has so far been applied in various insects [59] and decapod crustaceans [60–62]. Unlike the time-consuming and troublesome microinjection method that can only be performed in the early egg stage in daphnids, the alternative feeding RNAi method may potentially be applied for manipulating a wide range of genes in many individuals at the same time.

3. Extended microinjection-based applications

The microinjection system can be widely applied for the development of not only RNAi but also other attractive methods for gene functional analysis. Indeed, several microinjection-based functional methods have been developed in daphnid species. First, a transient overexpression system for arbitrary genes or reporter constructs was established by microinjection of synthesized mRNA bearing the 5′ cap structure and the 3′ poly(A) tail [51] and a DNA reporter construct [63]. These methods allow for a gain-of-function analysis, although only one example has shown that the phenotype induced by transient overexpression was only observed in the first instar juvenile [51]. However, the aforementioned overexpression and RNAi system in daphndis suffer from several drawbacks such as incomplete gain- or loss-of-function, transient effect, and limited analyzable stages.

To overcome these limitations, a transgenic *D. magna* line was established by using microinjected GFP or DsRED reporter plasmid, although the success rate was quite low (0.67%) [64,

http://dx.doi.org/10.5772/61485

65]. Furthermore, genome editing with engineered endonucleases is rapidly growing as a stable experimental method for generating heritable mutations in not only well-known in model organisms but also in nonmodel organisms. There are three representative methods: zinc-finger nucleases (ZFNs), transcription activator-like effector nucleases (TALENs), and clustered regularly interspaced short palindromic repeats (CRISPR/Cas9) systems [66]. In order to perform targeted mutagenesis in the *D. pulex* and *D. magna* genomes, TALEN and CRISPR/Cas9 systems have been established by microinjection of these engineered nucleases [50, 65, 67]. Taken together, these genome-editing techniques will enable scientists to accurately define arbitrary gene functions in daphnid species in future studies.

4. Conclusion

Recent growing innovations in high-throughput omics technologies (e.g., genomics, transcriptomics, proteomics, and metabolomics) enable us to obtain comprehensive profiles of a huge amount of candidate factors responsible for unique life history features of daphnids [12, 34, 68]. In order to investigate an arbitrary gene function, the establishment of an experimental method for gene functional analysis has been enthusiastically addressed by researchers using nonmodel organisms, even in the postgenomic era. In this chapter, we summarized (1) the experimental procedure with several tips for a microinjection system in *D. pulex* and *D. magna,* (2) information about genes responsible for their RNAi machinery, (3) potential concepts for novel user-friendly high-throughput RNAi systems in daphnids, and (4) other microinjection-based applications in daphnids. Further studies involved in the development of novel experimental methods and investigation of a wide range of gene functions can lead to a better understanding of the overview of the attractive environmental stimuli-dependent phenomenon in daphnids.

Acknowledgements

We thank members of the Iguchi laboratory for helpful advice and comments. Our work benefits from, and contributes to, the *Daphnia* Genomics Consortium. This work was supported by a JSPS Research Fellowship for Young Scientists to KT (No. 12J05579), a Sasakawa Scientific Research Grant from the Japan Science Society to KT, a Saito Ho-on Kai Scientific Research Grant from the Saito Gratitude Foundation to KT, grants from the Ministry of Education, Culture, Sports, Science, and Technology (TI), the Ministry of the Environment of Japan (TI), a Grant from the National Institute for Basic Biology (TI), and the Research Council of Norway (project 221455), Adverse Outcome Pathways for Endocrine Disruption in *Daphnia magna,* a conceptual approach for mechanistically based risk assessment (TI).

Author details

Kenji Toyota, Shinichi Miyagawa, Yukiko Ogino and Taisen Iguchi*

*Address all correspondence to: taisen@nibb.ac.jp

Okazaki Institute for Integrative Bioscience, National Institute for Basic Biology, and National Institutes of Natural Sciences, Higashiyama, Myodaiji, Okazaki, Aichi, Japan

References

[1] Dieter E. Ecology, Epidemiology, and Evolution of Parasitism in *Daphnia*. Bethesda (MD): National Library of Medicine (US), National Center for Biotechnology Information.; 2005.

[2] Iguchi T., Watanabe H., Katsu Y. Toxicogenomics and ecotoxicogenomics for studying endocrine disruption and basic biology. General and Comparative Endocrinology. 2007;153:25–29. DOI:10.1016/j.ygcen.2007.01.013

[3] Grosvenor G. H., Smith G. The life-cycle of *Moina rectirostris*. Quarterly Journal of Microscopical Science. 1913;2(58):511–522.

[4] Smith G. The life-cycle of Cladocera, with remarks on the physiology of growth and reproduction in crustacea. Proceedings of the Royal Society of London. Series B: Biological Sciences. 1915;88(605):418–435.

[5] Tollrian R. Predator-induced morphological defenses: costs, life history shifts, and maternal effects in *Daphnia pulex*. Ecology. 1995;76(6):1691–1705. DOI: 10.2307/1940703

[6] Wesenberg-Lund C. Von dem Abhiingigkeitsverhaltnis zwischen dem Bau der. Planktonorganismen nnd dem spezifischen Gewicht des Siifiwassers. Biologisches Zentralblatt. 1900;20:644–656.

[7] Banta A. M., Brown L. A. Control of sex in Cladocera. II. The unstable nature of the excretory products involved in male production. Physiological Zoology. 1929;2(1): 93–98.

[8] Hobæk A., Larsson P. Sex determination in *Daphnia magna*. Ecology. 1990;71(6):2255–2268. DOI: 10.2307/1938637

[9] Kleiven O. T., Larsson P., Hobæk A. Sexual reproduction in *Daphnia magna* requires three stimuli. Oikos. 1992;65(2):197–206. DOI: 10.2307/3545010

[10] Eads B. D., Andrews J., Colbourne J. K. Ecological genomics in *Daphnia*: stress responses and environmental sex determination. Heredity. 2008;100:184–190. DOI: 10.1038/sj.hdy.6800999

[11] Gilbert S. F., Epel D. Ecological Developmental Biology: Integrating Epigenetics, Medicine, and Evolution. Sinauer Associates, USA; 2009. DOI: 10.1093/icb/icp106

[12] Colbourne J. K., Pfrender M. E., Gilbert D., Thomas W. K., Tucker A., Oakley T. H., et al. The ecoresponsive genome of *Daphnia pulex*. Science. 2011;331(6017):555–561. DOI: 10.1126/science.1197761

[13] Kato Y., Shiga Y., Kobayashi K., Tokishita S., Yamagata H., Iguchi T., et al. Development of an RNA interference method in the cladoceran crustacean *Daphnia magna*. Development Genes and Evolution. 2011;220:337–345. DOI: 10.1007/s00427-011-0353-9

[14] Hiruta C., Toyota K., Miyakawa H., Ogino Y., Miyagawa S., Tatarazako N., et al. Development of a microinjection system for RNA interference in the water flea *Daphnia pulex*. BMC Biotechnology. 2013;13:96. DOI: 10.1186/1472-6750-13-96

[15] Gliwicz M., Slusarczyk A., Slusarczyk M. Life history synchronization in a long-lifespan single-cohort *Daphnia* population in a fishless alpine lake. Oecologia. 2001;128:368–378. DOI: 10.1007/s004420100673

[16] Pijanowska J., Stolpe G. Summer diapause in *Daphnia* as a reaction to the presence of fish. Journal of Plankton Research. 1996;18(8):1407–1412. DOI: 10.1093/plankt/18.8.1407

[17] Toyota K., Miyakawa H., Hiruta C., Furuta K., Ogino Y., Shinoda T., et al. Methyl farnesoate synthesis is necessary for the environmental sex determination in the water flea *Daphnia pulex*. Journal of Insect Physiology. 2015;80:22–30. DOI: 10.1016/j.jinsphys.2015.02.002

[18] Caceres C. E. Interspecific variation in the abundance, production, and emergence of *Daphnia* diapuasing eggs. Ecology. 1998;79(5):1699–1710. DOI: 10.2307/176789

[19] Oakley T. H., Wolfe J. M., Lindgren A. R., Zaharoff A. K. Phylotranscriptomics to bring the understudied into the fold: monophyletic ostracoda, fossil placement, and pancrustacean phylogeny. Molecular Biology and Evolution. 2013;30(1):215–233. DOI: 10.1093/molbev/mss216

[20] Miyakawa H., Toyota K., Sumiya E., Iguchi T. Comparison of JH signaling in insects and crustaceans. Current Opinion in Insect Science. 2014;1:81–87. DOI: 10.1016/j.cois.2014.04.006

[21] Olmstead A. W., LeBlanc G. A. Juvenoid hormone methyl farnesoate is a sex determinant in the crustacean *Daphnia magna*. Journal of Experimental Zoology. 2002;293:736–739. DOI: 10.1002/jez.10162

[22] Tatarazako N., Oda S., Watanabe H., Morita M., Iguchi T. Juvenile hormone agonists affect the occurrence of male *Daphnia*. Chemosphere. 2003;53:827–833. DOI: 10.1016/S0045-6535(03)00761-6

[23] Hiruta C., Nishida C., Tochinai S. Abortive meiosis in the oogenesis of parthenogenetic *Daphnia pulex*. Chromosome Research. 2010;18:833–840. DOI: 10.1007/s10577-010-9159-2

[24] Miyakawa H., Sugimoto N., Kohyama T. I., Iguchi T., Miura T. Intra-specific variations in reaction norms of predator-induced polyphenism in the water flea *Daphnia pulex*. Ecological Research. 2015;30(4):705–713. DOI: 10.1007/s11284-015-1272-4

[25] Threlkeld S. T. Estimating cladoceran birth rates: the importance egg mortality and the egg age distribution. Limnology and Oceanography. 1979;24(4):601–611. DOI: 10.1023/A:1003915431746

[26] Hiruta C., Toyota K., MIyakawa H., Sumiya E., Iguchi T. Sexual reproduction is a key element in the life history strategy of water fleas, *Daphnia magna* and *Daphnia pulex*: casting a spotlight on male induction and its morphology. In: *Daphnia*: Biology and Mathematics Perspectives. Nova; 2014. p. 261–278.

[27] Sagawa K., Yamagata H., Shiga Y. Exploring embryonic germ line development in the water flea, *Daphnia magna*, by zinc-finger-containing VASA as a marker. Gene Expression Patterns. 2005;5:669–678. DOI: 10.1016/j.modgep.2005.02.007

[28] Tsuchiya D., Eads B. D., Zolan M. E. Methods for meiotic chromosome preparation, immunofluorescence, and fluorescence in situ hybridization in *Daphnia pulex*. Methods in Molecular Biology. 2009;558:235–249. DOI: 10.1007/978-1-60761-103-5_14

[29] Watanabe H., Tatarazako N., Oda S., Nishide H., Uchiyama I., Morita M., et al. Analysis of expressed sequence tags of the water flea *Daphnia magna*. Genome. 2005;48(4):606–609. DOI: 10.1139/G05-038

[30] Cristescu M. E. A., Colbourne J. K., Radivojac J., Lynch M. A microsatellite-based genetic linkage map of the waterflea, *Daphnia pulex*: On the prospect of crustacean genomics. Genomics. 2006;88:415–430. DOI: 10.1016/j.ygeno.2006.03.007

[31] Routtu J., Jansen B., Colson I., Meester L. D., Ebert D. The first-generation *Daphnia magna* linkage map. BMC Genomics. 2010;11:508. DOI: 10.1186/1471-2164-11-508

[32] Xu S., Ackerman M. S., Long H., Bright L., Spitze K., Ramsdell J. S., et al. A male-specific genetic map of the microcrustacean *Daphnia pulex* based on single sperm whole-genome sequencing. Genetics. 2015;201:31–38. DOI: 10.1534/genetics.115.179028

[33] Eads B. D., Colbourne J.K., Bohuski E., Andrews J. Profiling sex-biased gene expression during parthenogenetic reproduction in *Daphnia pulex*. BMC Genomics. 2007;8:464. DOI: :10.1186/1471-2164-8-464

[34] Toyota K., Miyakawa H., Yamaguchi K., Shigenobu S., Ogino Y., Tatarazako N., et al. NMDA receptor activation upstream of methyl farnesoate signaling for short day-induced male offspring production in the water flea, *Daphnia pulex*. BMC Genomics. 2015;16:186. DOI: :10.1186/s12864-015-1392-9

[35] Toyota K., Kato Y., Miyakawa H., Yatsu R., Mizutani T., Ogino Y., et al. Molecular impact of juvenile hormone agonists on neonatal *Daphnia magna*. Journal of Applied Toxicology. 2014;34:537–544. DOI: 10.1002/jat.2922

[36] Fröhlich T., Arnold G. J., Fritsch R., Mayr T., Laforsch C. LC-MS/MS-based proteome profiling in *Daphnia pulex* and *Daphnia longicephala*: the *Daphnia pulex* genome database as a key for high throughput proteomics in *Daphnia*. BMC Genomics. 2009;10:171. DOI: 10.1186/1471-2164-10-171

[37] Poynton H. C., Taylor N. S., Hicks J., Scanlan L., Loguinov A. V., Vulpe C., et al. Metabolomics of microliter hemolymph samples enables an improved understanding of the combined metabolic and transcriptional responses of *Daphnia magna* to cadmium. Environmental Science and Technology. 2011;45:3710–3717. DOI: : 10.1021/es1037222

[38] Zaffagnini F. Reproduction in *Daphnia*. Memorie dell' Istituto Italiano di Idrobiologia. 1987;45:245–284.

[39] Elendt B. P., Bias W. R. Trace nutrient deficiency in *Daphnia magna* cultured in standard medium for toxicity testing: effects of the optimization of culture conditions on life history parameters of *D. magna*. Water Research. 1990;24(9):1157–1167. DOI: 10.1016/0043-1354(90)90180-E

[40] Ding S. W., Voinnet O. Antiviral immunity directed by small RNAs. Cell. 2007;130:413–426. DOI: 10.1016/j.cell.2007.07.039

[41] Fire A., Xu S. Q., Montgomery M. K., Kostas S. A., Driver S. E., Mello C. C. Potent and specific genetic interference by double-stranded RNA in *Caenorhabditis elegans*. Nature. 1998;391:806–811. DOI:10.1038/35888

[42] Obbard D. J., Gordon K. H. J., Buck A. H., Jiggins F. M. The evolution of RNAi as a defence against viruses and transposable elements. Philosophical Transactions of the Royal Society of London B. 2009;364:99–115. DOI: 10.1098/rstb.2008.0168

[43] McTaggart S. J., Conlon C., Colbourne J. K., Blaxter M. L., Little T, J. The components of the *Daphnia pulex* immune system as revealed by complete genome sequencing. BMC Genomics. 2009;10:175. DOI: 10.1186/1471-2164-10-175

[44] He L., Hannon G. J. MicroRNAs: small RNAs with a big role in gene regulation. Nature Reviews Genetics. 2004;5:522–531. DOI: 10.1038/nrg1379

[45] Gao Z., Wang M., Blair D., Zheng Y., Dou Y. Phylogenetic analysis of the endoribonuclease dicer family. PLoS One. 2014;9(4):e95350. DOI: 10.1371/journal.pone.0095350

[46] Zhou R., Hotta I., Denli A. M., Hong R., Perrimon N., Hannon G. J. Comparative analysis of argonaute-dependent small RNA pathways in *Drosophila*. Molecular Cell. 2008;32:592–599. DOI: 10.1016/j.molcel.2008.10.018

[47] Jinek M., Doudna J. A. A three-dimensional view of the molecular machinery of RNA interference. Nature. 2009;457(22):405–412. DOI: 10.1038/nature07755

[48] Wang G. H., Jiang L., Zhu L., Cheng T. C. Niu W. H. Yan Y. F., et al. Characterization of Argonaute family members in the silkworm, *Bombyx mori*. Insect Science. 2013;20:78–91. DOI: 10.1111/j.1744-7917.2012.01555

[49] Tamura K., Stecher G., Peterson D., Filipski A., Kumar S. MEGA6: molecular evolutionary genetics analysis version 6.0. Molecular Biology and Evolution. 2013;30(12): 2725–2729. DOI: 10.1093/molbev/mst197

[50] Nakanishi T., Kato Y., Matsuura T., Watanabe H. CRISPR/Cas-mediated targeted mutagenesis in *Daphnia magna*. PLoS One. 2014;9(5):e98363. DOI: 10.1371/journal.pone.0098363

[51] Kato Y., Kobayashi K., Watanabe H., Iguchi T. Environmental sex determination in the branchiopod crustacean *Daphnia magna*: deep conservation of a *Doublesex* gene in the sex-determining pathway. PLoS Genetics. 2011;7(3):e1001345. DOI: 10.1371/journal.pgen.1001345

[52] Asada M., Kato Y., Matsuura T., Watanabe H. Early embryonic expression of a putative ecdysteroid-phosphate phosphatase in the water flea, *Daphnia magna* (Cladocera: Daphniidae). Journal of Insect Science. 2014;14(181):ieu043. DOI: 10.1093/jisesa/ieu043

[53] Morita S., Shiga Y., Tokishita S., Ohta T. Analysis of spatiotemporal expression and function of the single-minded homolog in the branchiopod crustacean *Daphnia magna*. Gene. 2015;555:335–345. DOI: 10.1016/j.gene.2014.11.028

[54] Ando T., Fujiwara H. Electroporation-mediated somatic transgenesis for rapid functional analysis in insects. Development. 2013;140(2):454–458. DOI: 10.1242/dev.085241

[55] Hashimoto M., Takemoto T. Electroporation enables the efficient mRNA delivery into the mouse zygotes and facilitates CRISPR/Cas9-based genome editing. Scientific Reports. 2015;5:11315. DOI: 10.1038/srep11315

[56] Nomura T., Yamashita W., Gotoh H., Ono K. Genetic manipulation of reptilian embryos: toward an understanding of cortical development and evolution. Frontiers in Neuroscience. 2015;9(45). DOI: 10.3389/fnins.2015.00045

[57] Kato Y., Kobayashi K., Watanabe H., Iguchi T. Introduction of foreign DNA into the water flea, *Daphnia magna*, by electroporation. Ecotoxicology. 2010;19:589–592. DOI: 10.1007/s10646-010-0460-9

[58] Timmons L., Fire A. Specific interference by ingested dsRNA. Nature. 1998;395:854. DOI: 10.1038/27579

[59] Huvenne H., Smagghe G. Mechanisms of dsRNA uptake in insects and potential of RNAi for pest control: A review. Journal of Insect Physiology. 2010;56:227–235. DOI: 10.1016/j.jinsphys.2009.10.004

[60] Sun P. S., Venson Jr. N. C., Calderon F. R. O., Esaki D. M. Evaluation of methods for DNA delivery into shrimp zygotes of *Penaeus* (*Litopenaeus*) *vannamei*. Aquaculture. 2005;243(1–4):19–26. DOI: 10.1016/j.aquaculture.2004.09.037

[61] Sarathi M., Simon M. C., Venkatesan C., Hameed A. S. S. Oral administration of bacterially expressed VP28dsRNA to protect *Penaeus monodon* from white spot syndrome virus. Marine Biotechnology. 2008;10(3):242–249. DOI: 10.1007/s10126-007-9057-6

[62] Treerattrakool S., Chartthai C., Phromma-in N., Panyim S., Udomkit A. Silencing of gonad-inhibiting hormone gene expression in *Penaeus monodon* by feeding with GIH dsRNA-enriched *Artemia*. Aquaculture. 2013;404–405:116–121. DOI: 10.1016/j.aquaculture.2013.04.024

[63] Asada M., Kato Y., Matsuura T., Watanabe H. Visualization of ecdysteroid activity using a reporter gene in the crustacean, *Daphnia*. Marine Environmental Research. 2014;93:118–122. DOI: 10.1016/j.marenvres.2013.11.005

[64] Kato Y., Matsuura T., Watanabe H. Genomic integration and germline transmission of plasmid injected into crustacean *Daphnia magna* eggs. PLoS One. 7;9:e45318. DOI: 10.1371/journal.pone.0045318

[65] Naitou A., Kato Y., Nakanishi T., Matsuura T., Watanabe H. Heterodimeric TALENs induce targeted heritable mutations in the crustacean *Daphnia magna*. Biology Open. 2015. DOI: 10.1242/bio.20149738

[66] Sakuma T., Woltjen K. Nuclease-mediated genome editing: at the front-line of functional genomics technology. Development Growth and Differentiation. 2014;56:2–13. DOI: 10.1111/dgd.12111

[67] Hiruta C., Ogino Y., Sakuma T., Toyota K., Miyagawa S., Yamamoto T., et al. Targeted gene disruption by use of transcription activator-like effector nuclease (TALEN) in the water flea *Daphnia pulex*. BMC Biotechnology. 2014;14:95. DOI: 10.1186/s12896-014-0095-7

[68] Miyakawa H., Sato M., Colbourne J. K., Iguchi T. Ionotropic glutamate receptors mediate inducible defense in the water flea Daphnia pulex. PLoS One. 10;3:e0121324. DOI: 10.1371/journal.pone.0121324

Chapter 7

ER-targeted Intrabodies Mediating Specific *In Vivo* Knockdown of Transitory Proteins in Comparison to RNAi

Oliver Backhaus and Thomas Böldicke

Additional information is available at the end of the chapter

http://dx.doi.org/10.5772/62103

Abstract

In animals and mammalian cells, protein function can be analyzed by nucleotide sequence-based methods such as gene knockout, targeted gene disruption, CRISPR/Cas, TALEN, zinc finger nucleases, or the RNAi technique. Alternatively, protein knockdown approaches are available based on direct interference of the target protein with the inhibitor.

Among protein knockdown techniques, the endoplasmic reticulum (ER) intrabodies are potent molecules for protein knockdown *in vitro* and *in vivo*. These molecules are increasingly used for protein knockdown in living cells and transgenic mice. ER intrabody knockdown technique is based on the retention of membrane proteins and secretory proteins inside the ER, mediated by recombinant antibody fragments. In contrast to nucleotide sequence-based methods, the intrabody-mediated knockdown acts only on the posttranslational level.

In this review, the ER intrabody technology has been compared with the RNAi technique on the molecular level. The generation of intrabodies and RNAi has also been discussed. Specificity and off-target effects (OTE) of these molecules as well as the therapeutic potential of ER intrabodies and RNAi have been compared.

Keywords: Knockdown techniques, intracellular antibodies, ER intrabodies, RNA interference, off-target effects

1. Introduction

For the study of protein function in animals and mammalian cells, DNA-based methods such as gene knockout, targeted gene disruption, CRISPR/Cas, TALEN, zinc finger nucleases [1], as well as the RNAi technique [2] were proven and reliable tools. Besides the RNAi technique, approaches with miRNA are also very attractive [3]. Silencing of target mRNA can be achieved using siRNA, miRNA, or shRNA (Box 1).

Box 1

siRNA

Small interfering RNA (siRNA) are small pieces of double-stranded (ds) RNA, usually about 21 nt long, with 2-nt-long 3′ overhangs at each end. They can be applied for the interference with the protein translation by binding to the messenger RNA (mRNA), whereby promoting the degradation or destabilization of the mRNA.

shRNA

shRNAs form hairpin structures, which consist of a stem region of paired antisense and sense strands, connected by unpaired nucleotides building a loop. They are converted into siRNAs by the same RNAi machinery that processes miRNAs.

miRNA

MicroRNAs are small RNA molecules, encoded in the genome of plants and animals. These highly conserved, ~21-mer RNAs regulate the expression of genes by binding to the 3' untranslated regions (3'-UTR) of specific mRNAs.

Protein knockdown is possible with small molecule inhibitors including peptides, neutralizing and intracellular antibodies, and allosteric modulators [4–8]. In addition, aptamers and intramers, in general short single-stranded DNA or RNA oligonucleotides are also potent molecules for specific inhibition of small molecules, peptides, proteins, or even whole living cells [9].

Currently, RNAi is the most often used gene-silencing technique in functional genomics [2]. In this article, we described an emerging protein knockdown technology using intracellular antibodies (intrabodies) targeted to the ER and compared the advantages and disadvantages of this promising technique with the RNAi technology. We tried to make scientists, who are interested in protein research or have very specific protein-related questions, familiar with the ER intrabody technology [10]. The molecular mechanisms of both methods are different. RNAi-mediated knockdown is based on the interference of siRNA with mRNA (Figure 1), whereas the protein knockdown by ER intrabodies is exerted upon binding of a recombinant antibody fragment to its specific antigen inside the ER [10] (Figure 2).

Intrabodies are recombinant antibody fragments targeted to a cell expressing the specific antigen. Intracellular binding of the intrabody to the antigen results in inhibition of antigen function. Moreover, intrabodies can specifically be targeted to subcellular compartments such

http://dx.doi.org/10.5772/62103

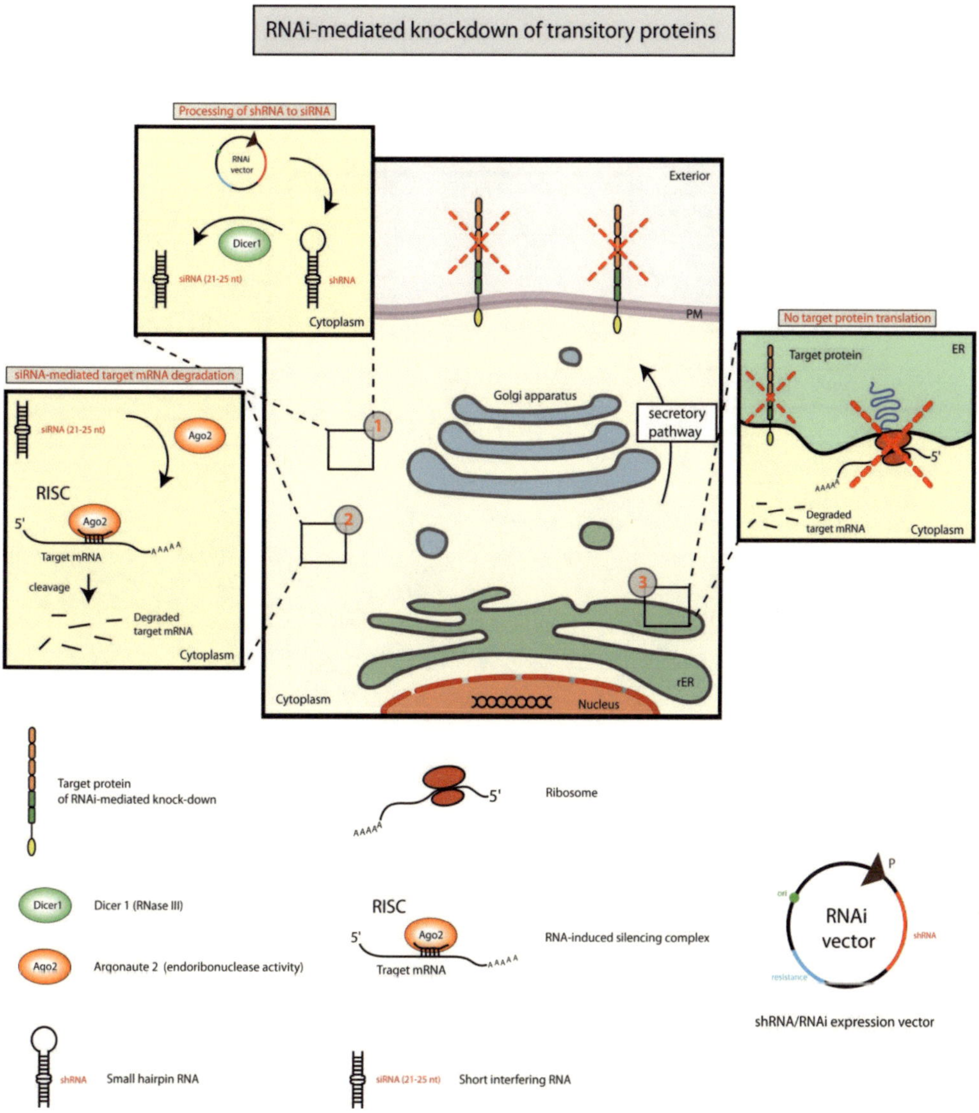

Figure 1. Principle of the knockdown of transitory proteins using the RNA interference technique. For knockdown of the mRNA of transitory proteins, transfection with a specific shRNA-expressing plasmid is sufficient. Although by using the RNA interference technology all kinds of proteins could be targeted, only knockdown of transitory proteins is illustrated. (1) Specific shRNA is transcribed and processed by the RNase III Dicer-1 enzyme in mammalian cells in order to form the mature siRNA. (2) The Argonaute 2 protein (Ago2) is loaded with the siRNA and forms together with additional proteins the RNA-induced silencing complex (RISC), which is a multiprotein complex consisting of effector (Argonaute proteins), accessory proteins, and si/miRNA. During the loading of the Argonaute protein, one strand of the siRNA duplex is discarded. Next, the RISC complex associates with its target mRNA via complementary base pairing of the siRNA and the target mRNA. In many cases, the recognition site comprises the 3′ untranslated regions (UTR) of the mRNA. Finally, target binding leads to mRNA degradation or translational inhibition [11]. mRNA degradation is mediated through the endonuclease activity of the Argonaute proteins. (3) As a result of mRNA knockdown, the target protein is not expressed on the cell surface [11].

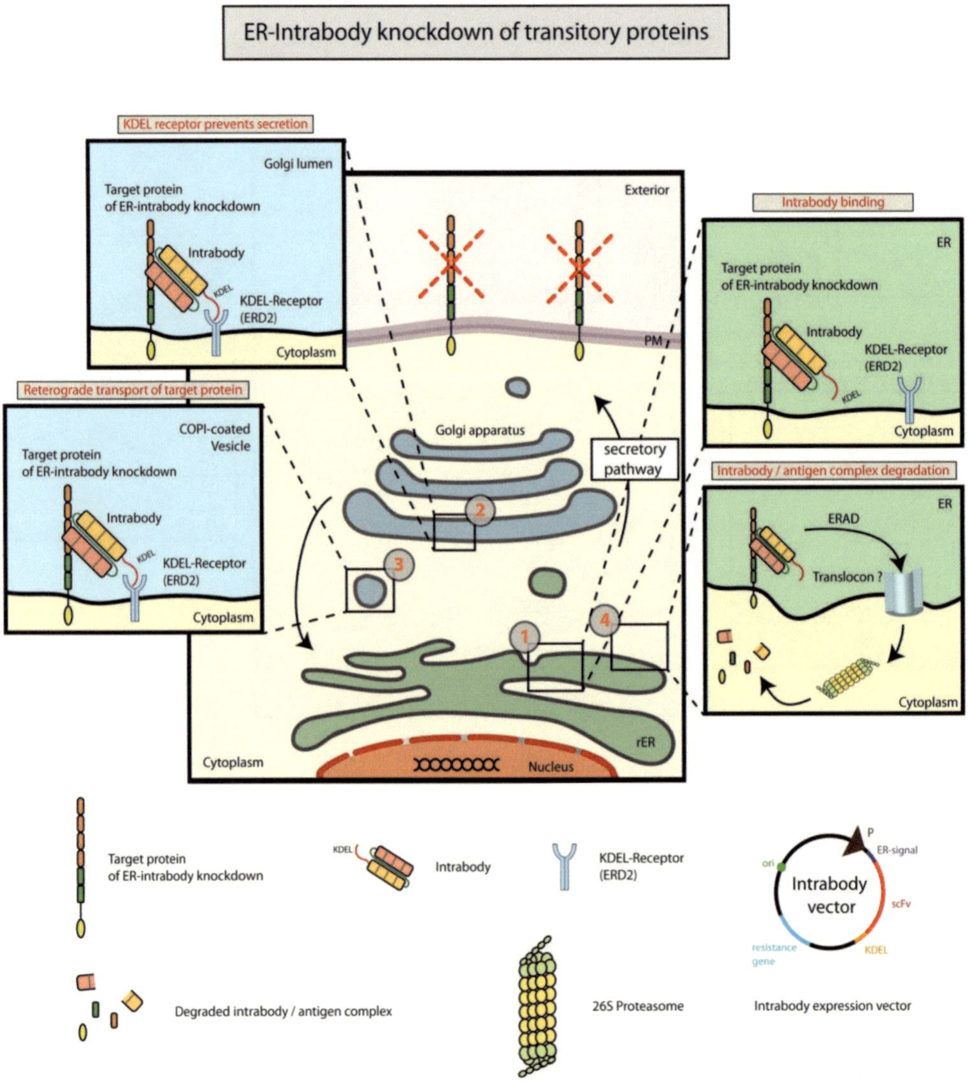

Figure 2. Principle of the specific knockdown of transitory proteins with endoplasmic reticulum (ER)-retained intrabodies. In wild-type cells, transitory proteins are transported through the ER and can be further processed (e.g., glycosylated) in the Golgi apparatus. These proteins could reside in the secretory cell compartments, secreted through the plasma membrane (PM), or become integrated in the PM as a membrane protein. For functional inhibition of these proteins, transfection with an ER intrabody expressing plasmid is sufficient. The intrabody construct consists of an N-terminal secretion sequence for the translocation in the ER (leader sequence) and the C-terminal retention signal (KDEL). (1) The intrabody inside of the ER binds to the target protein. This complex of antibody and target protein is further processed and transported through the secretory pathway. (2) In the cis-cisterna of the Golgi stack, the hERD2 receptor binds to the KDEL sequence and (3) initiates the retrograde transport back to the ER compartment. This continuous binding of the intrabody and retrograde transport prevents the target protein to reach its localization where it normally acts. (4) The accumulated intrabody–antigen complex in the ER might be transported into the cytoplasm, where it is marked for degradation by the 26S proteasome [12, 13]. Böldicke and Burgdorf have shown that an anti-toll-like receptor 2 (TLR2) ER intrabody is degraded by the proteasome (unpublished data).

http://dx.doi.org/10.5772/62103

as the nucleus, cytoplasm, mitochondria, or ER [10] (Box 2). Currently, the most used and promising intrabodies are the ER intrabodies, because of the correct folding in the oxidative environment of the ER [14]. This contrasts with cytosolic intrabodies, in which disulfide bridges are not formed in the reducing environment of the cytoplasm [15, 16].

Box 2

Intrabodies are intracellularly expressed recombinant antibody fragments, which specifically inhibit the function of target proteins produced in the same cell [10].

ER Intrabodies retain their corresponding antigen inside the ER by inhibiting the translocation of the antigen to the cell compartment where it normally acts.

Cytosolic Intrabodies are expressed in the cytoplasm. They inactivate their targets or interfere with the binding of the target protein to its corresponding binding partner.

The effect of ER intrabodies is based on retention of proteins passing the secretory pathway. Secretory proteins, membrane proteins, and even Golgi or endosomal-located proteins can be targeted [17–19], which cannot be reached by classical antibodies, due to the extracellular presence. Successful functional knockdown was achieved for oncogenic receptors, viral proteins for preventing virus assembly, cellular virus receptors to block virus entry, and receptors of the immune system as well as of the nervous system [20–24].

The format of expressed intrabodies is, in general, the single-chain variable fragment (scFv) or less common the antigen-binding fragment (Fab) [25]. The only prerequisite of ER intrabodies is the efficient binding to the antigen, and the method to select and generate an ER intrabody is greatly simplified by phage display. On the contrary, functional cytoplasmic intrabodies have to inactivate the antigen or have to interfere with the binding of the target protein to its corresponding binding partner [10].

The starting material for construction of an ER intrabody is an scFv or Fab, which can be obtained by amplification of the variable domains from a hybridoma clone [26], or scFv fragments can be selected from phage or yeast display [27, 28].

Early attempts using the intrabody approach failed frequently due to the lack of reliable techniques for the identification of the correct functional antibody sequence from a hybridoma clone. The genes of the variable domains for construction of recombinant antibody fragments can be amplified from hybridoma clones using mixtures of consensus primers [29]. This approach was used in the beginning. As hybridoma cells could secrete several different antibodies, it was sometimes difficult to isolate the correct functional sequences of the variable domains. Presently, with reliable protein sequencing techniques, next generation of DNA sequencing and optimized consensus primer sequences, the functional antibody DNA can much better be identified. Furthermore, optimized strategies for amplification of the correct functional antibody sequence are available [30–32].

In the case of using *in vitro* display systems, like phage or yeast cell surface display, the selected scFv fragment has only to be cloned into the ER-targeting vector. For preliminary characterization of the intrabody function, co-transfection of the intrabody expression plasmid with the corresponding antigen expression plasmid into HEK 293 cells is sufficient and followed by co-immunoprecipitation and immunofluorescence analysis [33].

In contrast to the ER intrabody technology, the advantage of the RNAi is that it can be applied for almost every mRNA and also non-coding RNAs. Here, we further compared the RNAi with the intrabody technology, regarding specificity, off-target effects, and therapeutic approaches.

2. Intracellular intrabodies versus RNA interference

2.1. Generation of ER intrabodies

The prerequisite for generating intrabodies is the availability of a hybridoma antibody clone or scFv/Fab fragments selected from *in vitro display* systems [10]. Starting from a hybridoma clone, the variable domains of the heavy and light chain are amplified by PCR from the cDNA. This can be achieved by (1) PCR amplification using consensus primer [29, 34–36], (2) rapid amplification of cDNA ends (RACE) [30], (3) PCR amplification using adaptor-ligated cDNA [31], or (4) inverse PCR with constant region heavy chain and light chain primer, amplifying the corresponding antibody sequence from circularized double-stranded cDNA [32] (Figure 3 A).

In most cases, using consensus primers is a fast and efficient approach for amplification of the correct functional antibody sequence from a hybridoma clone. However, less-common non-consensus antibody sequences cannot be amplified and primer mismatching could be a problem. Approaches (no. 2–4 shown in Figure 3) for amplifying the variable antibody domains are more time-consuming; however, the correct functional antibody gene sequence can be obtained. The variable domains are compiled by assembly PCR, linking both variable domains together by a short flexible linker sequence, for example $(Gly_4Ser)_3$, resulting in the scFv fragment. Next, the scFv fragment will be cloned into the ER targeting vector, providing the ER signal sequence, an myc tag for detection of intrabody, and the KDEL retention sequence localized at the C-terminus of the intrabody gene [26].

Following the *in vitro* display pipeline, an scFv fragment or Fab fragment selected by phage or yeast cell surface display can directly be cloned into the ER targeting vector. Most recombinant antibody fragments in the scFv or Fab format are selected by phage display or also the frequently used yeast cell surface display [27, 28, 41]. Other *in vitro* display systems are bacterial, mammalian cell surface display, or ribosome display [42–44]. Cytoplasmic intrabodies are generated from hybridoma clones or scFv/Fab fragments from *in vitro* display libraries in a similar way and cloned into an appropriate cytosolic targeting vector [10]. The main difference in comparison to ER intrabodies is that cytosolic intrabodies have to demonstrate neutralizing activity, and furthermore stable folding antibody fragments have to be selected [10].

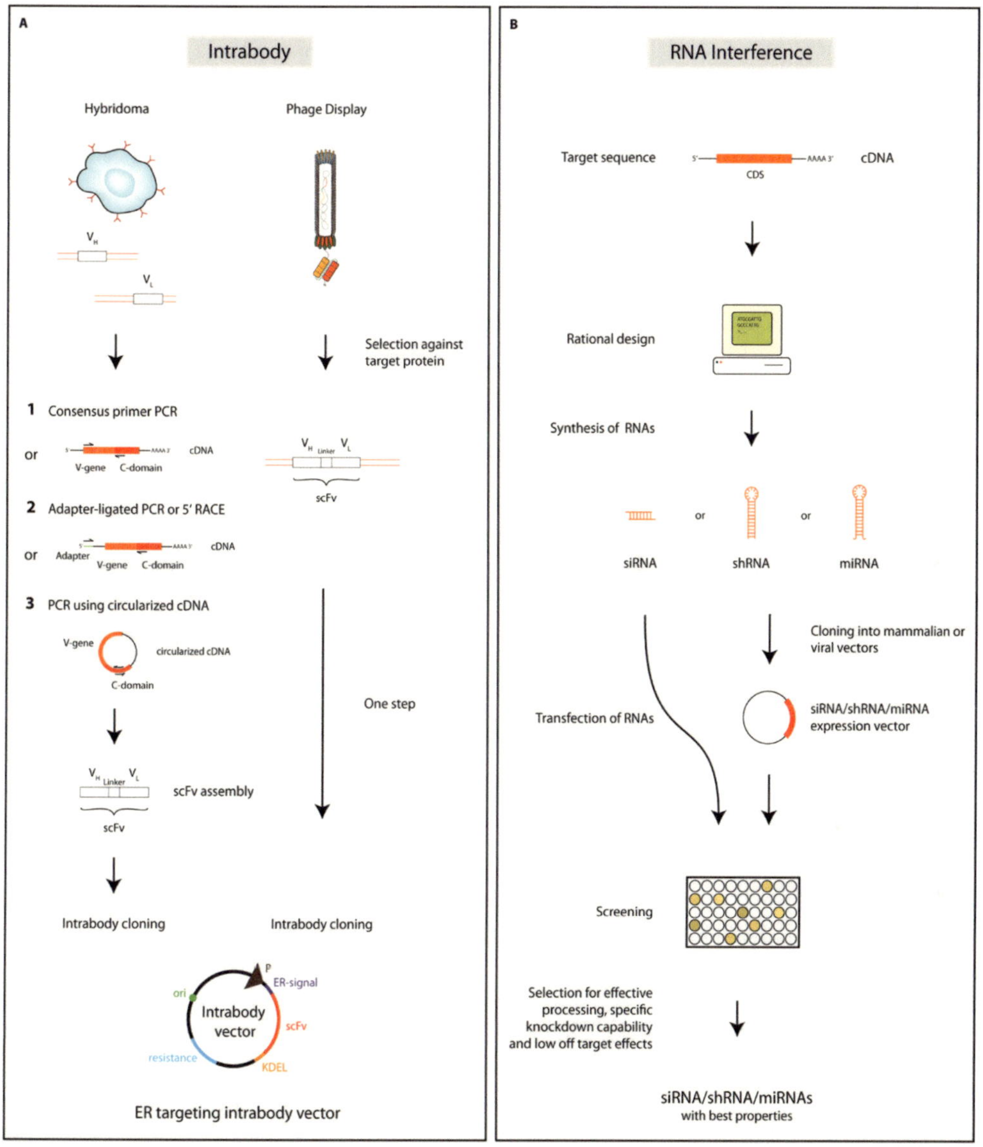

Figure 3. Generation of intrabody and RNA interference knockdown constructs. (**A**) Generation of intrabody knockdown vectors. The scFv fragment could be either cloned from hybridoma cell lines or selected from huge human naive phage display libraries. The antibody variable domain of the light chain (VL) and heavy chain (VH) is amplified from cDNA using consensus primer mixtures (1), 5′ adapter-ligated PCR or rapid amplification of cDNA ends (RACE) (2) or with constant domain-specific primer from circularized cDNA (3). The antibody VL and VH genes are assembled as scFv by fusing both domains with a flexible $(Gly_4Ser)_3$-linker sequence and cloned into the ER targeting intrabody vector. The scFvs are cloned between an upstream secretion signal and a downstream retention sequence (KDEL). Using the phage display system, selected scFvs can directly be cloned into the intrabody vector in one cloning step. Shown is an ER-targeting vector. (**B**) Generation of siRNA/shRNA/miRNA knockdown vectors. Rational *in silico* design of siRNA, shRNA, or miRNA mimics using software algorithms like those mentioned in Ref. [37] or in Ref. [38], a recent publication, deduced from the target cDNA. The algorithms are designed to select appropriated sequences by means of empiric criteria. Main criteria are an siRNA length of 19–21 nucleotides (nt) in conjunction with 2 nt overhangs at

their 3′ ends, as well as thermodynamic properties of target mRNA hybridization. Rational design can be expanded by testing *in silico* the potential off-target effects of the designed sequences by using genome-wide enrichment of seed sequence matches (GESS) [39] or Haystack [40]. Designed sequences are chemically synthesized and cloned into appropriate mammalian or viral knockdown expression vectors. Alternatively, siRNA can be used for direct cell transfection. The siRNA/shRNA/miRNA sequences originated from rational design are screened for effective processing, specific knockdown capabilities, and potential off-target effects. Corresponding clones are selected, and for most applications 3–4 different targeting sequences were chosen and theses libraries are used for the RNA interference knockdown. ER: endoplasmic reticulum, CDS: coding DNA sequence, p:promoter.

2.2. Generation of siRNA, miRNA, and shRNA

In order to generate siRNAs for a specific target, only the mRNA information about the target sequence is needed [45] (Figure 3 B). siRNA-mediated mRNA knockdown can be performed in several ways. In general, cells can directly be transfected with siRNA, using transfection reagents like lipofectamine. Cells can also be transfected using siRNA/shRNA/miRNA-expressing plasmids or viral vectors. Long-lasting gene silencing can be achieved with shRNAs expressed from stably transfected plasmids or from integrated retro- or lentiviral vectors [46]. Several approaches exist for RNA interference-mediated knockdown, the principle workflow of *in silico* design, screening, and selection of siRNA/shRNA/miRNA, with best knockdown properties shown in Figure 3 B. Currently, software algorithms mentioned in Ref. [37] or [38] can help to find the appropriate knockdown sequences of 19–21 nt length siRNA by analysis of the optimal thermodynamic properties of mRNA hybridization. Potential off-target effects can be reduced by *in silico* optimization with GESS [39] or Haystack [40]. Resulting siRNA/shRNA/miRNA sequences are tested for effective processing, specific knockdown capability, and low off-target effects.

2.3. Stability

Intrabodies are stably expressed inside the ER [14], whereas most cytosolic intrabodies are not correctly folded [15, 16]. On the other hand, siRNA can be cleaved by nucleases, present in the blood serum and cellular cytoplasm.

2.4. Specificity and Off-Target Effects (OTE)

For the knockdown of distinct target proteins, the specificity of the process is crucial. Otherwise, the resulting phenotypes of the induced knockdown experiment might be superimposed with off-target effects. The specificity of the RNAi and the ER intrabody knockdown technique is the main difference between them.

Intrabodies, which are also known as intracellular antibodies, are generated from monoclonal antibodies (mAbs) and phage or yeast antibody repertoires. Intrabodies are very specific to their targets due to antibody–antigen interactions.

The high specificity of ER intrabodies has been demonstrated for the specific knockdown of members of the TLRs. The knockdown of toll-like receptor 2 (TLR2) and TLR9, which functions as a part of the innate immunity and recognizes pathogen-associated molecular patterns (PAMP), did not influence the expression of other TLRs. The developed anti-TLR2 intrabody

http://dx.doi.org/10.5772/62103

did not inhibit TLR3-, TLR4-, and TLR9-driven signal transduction [33] and the anti-TLR9 intrabody did not inhibit TLR3-, TLR4-, TLR7-, and TLR8-driven signaling, respectively [18].

Stress response induction in the endoplasmic reticulum (ER), due to the accumulation of retained and partially unfolded target proteins upon intrabody–antigen complex formation, was analyzed by measuring the unfolded protein response (UPR) for an overexpressed anti-p75NTR ER intrabody and could not be proven [24]. No off-target effects of expressed intrabodies are known yet, particularly any activation of the immune system.

On the other hand, unspecific silencing is a major problem using RNAi-mediated gene silencing, due to the expression of short-interfering RNA sequences, such as miRNA, siRNA, shRNA, or dsRNA [47]. The short seed region of these silencing RNAs recognizes and hybridizes with 2–8 nt to the target mRNA. Even with specific alignment software, it is practically impossible to exclude any possible transcript, which aligns with the target seed sequence, because statistically the chance is high to have the same sequence or secondary structure in other non-target mRNA transcripts too. However, at least software algorithms such as GESS [39] and Haystack [40] are able to predict potential off-targeted genes. By computer-aided optimization of the miRNA, siRNA, or shRNA, the OTEs can be reduced to a minimum.

siRNA can bind to TLR3, TLR7, and TLR8, resulting in secretion of type I interferon and pro-inflammatory cytokines [48–50]. Aberrant expression of up to more than 1000 genes has also been described [51].

Fortunately, some progress has been made in the repression of the RNAi-induced immune response. When siRNA is *in vitro* transcribed by the T7 polymerase, a 5′-triphosphate group is added. The 5′ triphosphate is recognized by the innate immunity, and it activates the type I interferon response. This can be prevented by chemical synthesis of siRNA, which misses the 5′-triphosphate group. Furthermore, the siRNA molecules can be modified by adding 2′-O-methyl groups, in order to reduce the recognition by toll-like receptors (TLRs) [52]. Interestingly, this modification additionally hampers degradation of the siRNA by RNases, leading to an increase in serum half-life [53]. Finally, strong destabilizing unlocked nucleic acids (UNAs), which were altered to have an acyclic ribose, also reduce the recognition by TLRs [54].

The specific suppression of one allele in heterozygous genes is of concern in dominantly inherited genetic disorders. Huntington's disease (HD) is caused by a dominant mutation of the huntingtin protein (Htt) and an excellent target for the examination of allele-specific knockdown of the mutated Htt, with high therapeutic potential. Huntington's disease is based on a long stretch of CAG triplets on one disease-caused allele [55]. Most of the patients are heterozygous for the *htt* gene mutation and 48% of the American and European HD patients are heterozygous at a single nucleotide polymorphism (SNP) site, making this genetic disease a *bono fide* target for specific protein knockdown. Approaches to inhibit the appearance of Huntington's disease is silencing of wild type and mutant Htt or silencing of only the disease-causing allele.

Although it was found in HD mice that co-silencing of wild type and mutant Htt provides therapeutic benefit, nothing is known of such a long-term suppression of huntingtin [56]. Thus, the effect and safety over decades have yet to be proven in clinical trials. Therefore, there is still a need for high allele-specific inhibition of the mutant Htt protein, which is toxic due to an expanded polyglutamine (polyQ) motif (CAG motif). Targeting of the CAG motif is not selective for the mutant allele and affected both alleles. Genotyping of the Huntington's disease patients resulted in three single nucleotide polymorphisms (SNP) in huntingtin [57]. Therefore, an alternative strategy when using RNAi is targeting a single nucleotide mutation localized in the disease-caused sequence [58]. Furthermore, targeting of the mutant huntingtin SNPs or the expanded CAG motif by designed artificial miRNAs was recently demonstrated *in vitro*, using an allele-specific reporter system and *in vivo* in a transgenic mouse model [59].

For the RNAi technique, it is possible to discriminate between very similar targets with a specific reduction on the RNA and protein level [58, 60, 61]. However, there are still some concerns and limitations. The RNAi-mediated allele-specific knockdown may result in a broad off-targeting and therefore has to be further evaluated in appropriate preclinical model systems [62]. Using both target strategies, CAG motif and prevalent mutant SNPs, in the case of huntingtin, the wild-type allele is also affected by the knockdown, and the knockdown ratio between the wild type and mutant allele remains unsatisfactory. Furthermore, the shift to *in vivo* delivery systems can have a substantial impact on the specificity, as was demonstrated in the mouse model [59]. Next, a limited expression of the miRNA vectors is important to avoid saturation of the miRNA processing machinery, as the selectivity seems to be reduced when miRNAs are highly expressed *in vivo* [59].

Different alleles can also be targeted and discriminated using specific intracellular antibodies (intrabodies) and represent a valuable alternative to RNA interference. Intrabodies targeting, for example, huntingtin have to recognize an epitope common in most disease-associated huntingtin SNP forms, which also has to be different in the translated amino acid between the mutant and wild-type allele. Alternatively, they could target the expanded polyglutamine (polyQ) motif associated with misfolding and aggregation [63]. Furthermore, cytoplasmic intrabodies have been developed, which efficiently inhibited aggregation of mutant HD [64]. Interestingly, a disulfide bond-free single-domain intracellular antibody with high affinity was developed after affinity maturation [65] from a specific anti-HD scFv fragment, demonstrating the power of antibody engineering.

For the allele-specific knockdown, the intrabody technology utilizes the high specificity of monoclonal antibodies, with no or low concerns about off-target effects and activation of the immune system. In the case of huntingtin, no RNAi approach was able to discriminate effectively between the wild-type and mutant expanded polyglutamine stretch [59]. Here, intracellular antibodies could, in principle, recognize different conformational epitopes formed by polyglutamine and might be able to discriminate between the length of the polyQ motifs [63]. However, in the case of the cytoplasmic huntingtin protein, it is more difficult to generate and select cyto-intrabodies, due to the reducing environment of the cytoplasm. In general, the allele-specific knockdown strategy should be also applied with ER intrabodies.

The kind of mismatches introduced into siRNAs or artificial miRNAs, in order to increase allele specificity for preference of the mutant allele, can differ. Purine-to-purine mismatches, for example, are more effective than purine-to-pyrimidine mismatches. This limitation can be overcome by introduction of a second mismatch, preferentially into the seed or cleavage region of the siRNA/miRNA [59]. Using a set of SNP sites, common in disease-associated alleles, might enable reaching many patients [57], but it is hard to access the whole population. For those genotypes that could not be cured by using mutant SNP-targeting siRNA, intrabody-mediated protein knockdown, recognizing a prevalent mutant epitope could be superior. Whereby, in the case of SNPs due to the posttranslational targeting, the intrabody technology demonstrates one of its weaknesses. Discrimination between mutant and wild-type SNP could only be achieved when the mutant SNP induces a change of the encoded amino acid. In addition, mutant SNPs in introns and untranslated regions (UTR) cannot be addressed, as it is in the case of HD.

Features	Intrabodies	siRNA, shRNA, miRNA
Requirements	Monoclonal antibody or scFv/Fab selected by phage or yeast cell surface display	Sequence of the mRNA
Very high specificity to the antigen	+	Off-target effects
Stability	Stable in the ER	Susceptibility to nucleases
Inhibition of post-translational modifications	+	-
Inhibition of splice variants	+	+
Inhibition of several protein isoforms with one intrabody or siRNA	+	+
Targeting of specific protein domains	+	+
High-throughput screening	-	+
In vivo knockdown	+	+

Table 1. Intrabodies versus siRNA

2.5. High-throughput screening

Oligonucleotide and cDNA microarrays can be applied for simultaneous quantitative monitoring of gene expression of thousands of genes [66]. A combination of cDNA microarrays and

RNA interference was used to validate upregulated genes, playing an important role in cancer development [67]. In this case, a pre-screening with cDNA microarrays is performed followed by silencing of selected upregulated mRNAs using RNAi. This might also be possible with intrabodies.

Although high-throughput RNAi screening is very useful in order to validate new genes involved in cancer pathogenesis or infection processes [68, 69], such high-throughput screening is not possible with intrabodies.

2.6. Therapeutic potential of siRNA and ER intrabodies

The therapeutic potential of siRNA and ER intrabodies has been shown in different mouse models [70–73]. It has been shown that siRNA protected mice from fulminant hepatitis [74], viral infection [75], sepsis [76], tumor growth [77], and macular degeneration [78]. In these mouse models, synthetic siRNA was delivered systemically, peritoneally, or subretinally.

Furthermore, in an Alzheimer's and spinocerebellar ataxia disease-related mouse model, RNAi suppresses the expression of amyloid-β peptide or ataxia, respectively [79, 80]. In these mouse models, target-specific RNAi was virally delivered using adeno-associated virus or Herpes simplex virus. Interestingly, the knockdown of angiopoietin-2 mRNA in a mouse model with pancreatic carcinoma and xenotransplantation suppresses metastasis and downregulates metalloproteinase-2 [81].

Many ER intrabodies have shown therapeutic potential against relevant targets in cancer, infection, and brain diseases, for example, ErbB-2, EGFR, VEGFR-2, Tie-2, VEGFR-2 × Tie-2, metalloproteinases MMP-2, MMP-9, E7 oncoprotein of human papillomavirus, CCR5, TLR2, TLR9, and amyloid-β protein [18, 33, 82–90]. Nevertheless, only four of these antigens have been applied in xenograft tumor mouse models so far, using an anti-Tie intrabody [85], a bispecific VEGFR-2 × Tie-2 intrabody [86], an anti-amyloid-β protein intrabody in an Alzheimer's disease mouse model [90], and an anti-E7 oncoprotein intrabody in a mouse infection model with human papillomavirus [89]. Intrabody delivery was performed via adenovirus, adeno-associated virus, and retrovirus, respectively.

2.6.1. *Transgenic mice*

Transgenic RNAi mouse against p120-Ras GTPase-activating protein [91] and cytokine-activated IκB kinase 1 (IKK1) has been established [92]. Furthermore, RNAi transgenic mice and non-germline genetically engineered RNAi cancer mouse models were established [93]. In contrast to constitutive RNAi transgenic mice, generation of conditional RNAi in mice is also possible [94].

Recently, two transgenic ER intrabody mice have been generated against VCAM and gelsolin [71, 72]. In addition, a transgenic mouse expressing an anti-EVH1 intrabody has been published [73]. However, the inhibitory results obtained with these mice have been criticized because the intrabody was directed to the secretory pathway, but confusingly recognized a cytosolic protein [95]. Interestingly, the transgenic VCAM intrabody mouse was viable in contrast to the lethal knockout mice generated by targeted homologous recombination [96]. The intrabody mice were deficient in VCAM-1 cell surface expression.

2.6.2. Clinical approaches

Different clinical approaches have been performed with siRNA. RNAi-based clinical trials are ongoing (phase I–III) [62, 97]. For example, a Bevasiranib RNAi targeting VEGF has been applied to heal macular degeneration [98] and RNAi targeting the RSV nucleocapsid SPC3649 has shown significant anti-viral activity [99].

In comparison to the RNAi, only one example of an ER intrabody targeting erbB-2 has been applied in a clinical phase I study [82]. As demonstrated, none of the patients treated in this study exhibited a dramatic clinical benefit.

Both methods share the limitations of viral and non-viral delivery methods. Using integrating vectors, insertional mutagenesis is still the main problem [100]. Concerning non-viral delivery methods, lipid-based and peptide polymer-based delivery systems have been applied [101]. However, for some diseases like HD, the non-neurotropic feature of many delivery systems and the lack of passing the blood–brain barrier (BBB) remain problematic.

Cell- and tissue-specific targeting is also always a concern; however, transductional and transcriptional targeting is promising [102]. Tissue-specific carrier for siRNA includes aptamers, antibodies, peptides, proteins, and oligonucleotide agonists [101]. Referring to ER intrabodies, the use of mRNA in clinical approaches is promising [103].

2.7. Other features

Intrabodies are able to inhibit posttranslational modifications, such as phosphorylation sites [104, 105]. This is not possible using RNAi. Besides the high specificity of intrabodies, this is an important advantage of intrabodies over RNAi.

Recently, single-stranded siRNA was used to suppress the spliced variants of proteins [106]. This might also be possible with specific intrabodies (Table 1). In addition, targeting of specific protein domains and isomers of a protein might also be feasible. For example, miRNA suppresses specifically an oncogenic isoform [107]. Intriguingly, the suppression of different protein isoforms with only one intrabody or one siRNA, recognizing a common epitope within all isoforms, might be possible, for example, the knockdown of all interferon alpha isoforms (13 different subtypes in human).

2.8. miRNA

It is known that miRNA influences tumorigenesis [3], and therefore miRNA and combined miRNA/siRNA pharmacological approaches are attractive [108]. miRNA has been applied in cancer mouse models as for lymphoid malignancies [109]. Furthermore, important studies using miRNA has been performed for diagnosis, prognosis, and prediction of cancer [108]. One of the most developed microRNA-based candidates is MRX34, a miR-34 mimetic that restores the function of miR-34 in cancer cells [110], which is applied in an ongoing multicenter phase I clinical trial. The repression of expression of several potential miR-34 target oncogenes was demonstrated [111]. Finally, miRNAs can be used to reprogram somatic cells into pluripotent stem cells [112]. However, siRNA and miRNA share the same silencing machinery and microRNA causes also off-target effects [113].

3. Conclusions and perspectives

siRNA and ER intrabody technology are both efficient knockdown techniques. siRNA is acting on the mRNA level, whereas ER intrabodies are acting on the protein level. The strength of the RNAi technology results from the possibility that nearly all mRNAs of a cell can be targeted. Currently, the knockdown of proteins mediated by intrabodies is most promising with ER intrabodies, because they are correctly folded inside the ER and can be generated more easily than in the past. Because of the availability of many new scFv fragments, generated by research consortia, one cloning step is sufficient to convert selected scFv fragments into ER intrabodies.

Stable cytosolic intrabodies have to be selected with considerable effort. Two approaches are successful and reliable: the intracellular antibody capture technology, based on an antigen-dependent two-hybrid system [114] and single-domain antibodies [115], which are stably folded in a reducing environment for inhibition of cytoplasmic proteins. Single-domain antibodies comprise only one V region, the variable domain of the heavy or light chain. Most successfully applied are camelid single-domain antibodies (V_HHs) [115–118]. Alternatively, human VL and VH domains are also potent molecules and their successful construction is ongoing [119, 120].

The number of ER intrabodies will increase due to the fact that international research consortia as the "Affinomics" initiative [121] in the European Union and similar initiatives in the United States have already generated several thousands of recombinant antibodies, including the V-region genes, which can be used to build up a new repertoire of intrabodies. Using this pipeline, the duration for development of intrabodies is similar to that of siRNA/shRNA/miRNAs. In the future, scFvs against very valuable disease-related targets have to be provided.

The main advantage of intrabodies is their specificity, no off-target effects, and posttranslational modification inhibition. The specificity of an intrabody can be estimated by immunoassays such as ELISA, flow cytometry, and immunoprecipitation. On the contrary, the specificity and off-target effects of RNAi are often more difficult to predict.

Conferring to *in vivo* application, RNAi has been currently applied predominantly in phase 1 and 2 studies [62, 97]. In the future, the success of clinical approaches using RNAi and ER intrabodies is dependent on the development of safe viral vectors and the development of non-viral vectors possessing high transfection efficiency [122].

Two attractive applications of RNAi, hardly to perform with ER intrabodies, are genome-wide screening [68, 69] and reprogramming of somatic cells into pluripotent stem cells [112].

Thus, the ER intrabody approach has demonstrated its huge potential for *in vitro* and *in vivo* analysis of protein function [10]. The ER intrabody technique can complement the RNAi technique in cases where siRNA, shRNA, and miRNA molecules demonstrate unwanted unspecificity and off-target effects.

Acknowledgements

The authors thank Prof. Peter Müller for critical reading of the manuscript.

Author details

Oliver Backhaus and Thomas Böldicke*

*Address all correspondence to: thomas.boeldicke@helmholtz-hzi.de

Helmholtz Centre for Infection Research, Department of Structural and Functional Protein Research, Braunschweig, Germany

References

[1] Carroll D. Genome engineering with targetable nucleases. Annu Rev Biochem. 2014;83:409–39. DOI: 10.1146/annurev-biochem-060713-035418

[2] Dorsett Y, Tuschl T. siRNAs: applications in functional genomics and potential as therapeutics. Nat Rev Drug Discov. 2004;3:318–29. DOI: 10.1038/nrd1345

[3] Croce CM. Causes and consequences of microRNA dysregulation in cancer. Nat Rev Genet. 2009;10:704–14. DOI: 10.1038/nrg2634

[4] Roskoski R, Jr. A historical overview of protein kinases and their targeted small molecule inhibitors. Pharmacol Res. 2015; 100:1-23. DOI: 10.1016/j.phrs.2015.07.010

[5] Lobato MN, Rabbitts TH. Intracellular antibodies and challenges facing their use as therapeutic agents. Trends Mol Med. 2003;9:390–96. DOI: 10.1016/S1471-4914(03)00163-1

[6] Meng G, Rutz M, Schiemann M, Metzger J, Grabiec A, Schwandner R, et al. Antagonistic antibody prevents toll-like receptor 2-driven lethal shock-like syndromes. J Clin Invest. 2004;113:1473–81. DOI: 10.1172/JCI20762

[7] Neduva V, Russell RB. Peptides mediating interaction networks: new leads at last. Curr Opin Biotechnol. 2006;17:465–71. DOI: 10.1016/j.copbio.2006.08.002

[8] Christopoulos A, Kenakin T. G protein-coupled receptor allosterism and complexing. Pharmacol Rev. 2002;54:323–74. DOI: 10.1124/pr.54.2.323

[9] Breaker RR. Natural and engineered nucleic acids as tools to explore biology. Nature. 2004;432:838–45. DOI: 10.1038/nature03195

[10] Marschall AL, Dübel S, Böldicke T. Specific in vivo knockdown of protein function by intrabodies. MAbs. 2015; 7(6):1010-35. DOI: 10.1080/19420862.2015.1076601

[11] Zhou R, Rana TM. RNA-based mechanisms regulating host-virus interactions. Immunol Rev. 2013;253:97–111. DOI: 10.1111/imr.12053

[12] Cardinale A, Filesi I, Biocca S. Aggresome formation by anti-Ras intracellular scFv fragments. The fate of the antigen-antibody complex. Eur J Biochem. 2001;268:268–77. DOI: 10.1046/j.1432-1033.2001.01876.x

[13] Paganetti P, Calanca V, Galli C, Stefani M, Molinari M. Beta-site specific intrabodies to decrease and prevent generation of Alzheimer's Abeta peptide. J Cell Biol. 2005;168:863–68. DOI: 10.1083/jcb.200410047

[14] van Anken E, Braakman I. Versatility of the endoplasmic reticulum protein folding factory. Crit Rev Biochem Mol Biol. 2005;40:191–228. DOI: 10.1080/10409230591008161

[15] Biocca S, Ruberti F, Tafani M, Pierandrei-Amaldi P, Cattaneo A. Redox state of single chain Fv fragments targeted to the endoplasmic reticulum, cytosol and mitochondria. Biotechnology (N Y). 1995;13:1110–15

[16] Wörn A, Plückthun A. Stability engineering of antibody single-chain Fv fragments. J Mol Biol. 2001;305:989–1010. DOI: 10.1006/jmbi.2000.4265

[17] Böldicke T. Blocking translocation of cell surface molecules from the ER to the cell surface by intracellular antibodies targeted to the ER. J Cell Mol Med. 2007;11:54–70. DOI: 10.1111/j.1582-4934.2007.00002.x

[18] Reimer E, Somplatzki S, Zegenhagen D, Hanel S, Fels A, Bollhorst T, et al. Molecular cloning and characterization of a novel anti-TLR9 intrabody. Cell Mol Biol Lett. 2013;18:433–46. DOI: 10.2478/s11658-013-0098-8

[19] Zehner M, Marschall AL, Bos E, Schloetel JG, Kreer C, Fehrenschild D, et al. The translocon protein sec61 mediates antigen transport from endosomes in the cytosol for cross-presentation to CD8(+) T cells. Immunity. 2015;42:850–63. DOI: 10.1016/j.immuni.2015.04.008

[20] Wheeler YY, Kute TE, Willingham MC, Chen SY, Sane DC. Intrabody-based strategies for inhibition of vascular endothelial growth factor receptor-2: effects on apoptosis, cell growth, and angiogenesis. FASEB J. 2003;17:1733–35. DOI: 10.1096/fj.02-0942fje

[21] Liao W, Strube RW, Milne RW, Chen SY, Chan L. Cloning of apoB intrabodies: specific knockdown of apoB in HepG2 cells. Biochem Biophys Res Commun. 2008;373:235–40. DOI: 10.1016/j.bbrc.2008.06.020

[22] Steinberger P, Andris-Widhopf J, Buhler B, Torbett BE, Barbas CF, 3rd. Functional deletion of the CCR5 receptor by intracellular immunization produces cells that are refractory to CCR5-dependent HIV-1 infection and cell fusion. Proc Natl Acad Sci U S A. 2000;97:805–10. DOI: 10.1073/pnas.97.2.805

[23] Intasai N, Tragoolpua K, Pingmuang P, Khunkaewla P, Moonsom S, Kasinrerk W, et al. Potent inhibition of OKT3-induced T cell proliferation and suppression of CD147 cell surface expression in HeLa cells by scFv-M6-1B9. Immunobiology. 2008;214(6): 410-21 DOI: 10.1016/j.imbio.2008.12.006

[24] Zhang C, Helmsing S, Zagrebelsky M, Schirrmann T, Marschall AL, Schungel M, et al. Suppression of p75 neurotrophin receptor surface expression with intrabodies influences Bcl-xL mRNA expression and neurite outgrowth in PC12 cells. PLoS One. 2012;7:e30684. DOI: 10.1371/journal.pone.0030684

[25] Frenzel A, Hust M, Schirrmann T. Expression of recombinant antibodies. Front Immunol. 2013;4:217: 1-20. DOI: 10.3389/fimmu.2013.00217

[26] Böldicke T, Somplatzki S, Sergeev G, Mueller PP. Functional inhibition of transitory proteins by intrabody-mediated retention in the endoplasmatic reticulum. Methods. 2012;56:338–50. DOI: 10.1016/j.ymeth.2011.10.008

[27] Bradbury AR, Sidhu S, Dubel S, McCafferty J. Beyond natural antibodies: the power of in vitro display technologies. Nat Biotechnol. 2011;29:245–54. DOI: 10.1038/nbt. 1791

[28] Boder ET, Wittrup KD. Yeast surface display for screening combinatorial polypeptide libraries. Nat Biotechnol. 1997;15:553–57. DOI: 10.1038/nbt0697-553

[29] Toleikis L, Frenzel A. Cloning single-chain antibody fragments (ScFv) from hyrbidoma cells. Methods Mol Biol. 2012;907:59–71. DOI: 10.1007/978-1-61779-974-7_3

[30] Ruberti F, Cattaneo A, Bradbury A. The use of the RACE method to clone hybridoma cDNA when V region primers fail. J Immunol Methods. 1994;173:33–39

[31] Ladiges W, Osman GE. Molecular characterization of immunoglobulin genes. In: Howard GC, Bethell DR (eds). Basic Methods in Antibody Production and Characterization. CRC Press Ltd, Bocuraton, Florida. 2000:169–91

[32] Herrmann T, Grosse-Hovest L, Otz T, Krammer PH, Rammensee HG, Jung G. Construction of optimized bispecific antibodies for selective activation of the death receptor CD95. Cancer Res. 2008;68:1221–27. DOI: 10.1158/0008-5472.CAN-07-6175

[33] Kirschning CJ, Dreher S, Maass B, Fichte S, Schade J, Koster M, et al. Generation of anti-TLR2 intrabody mediating inhibition of macrophage surface TLR2 expression

and TLR2-driven cell activation. BMC Biotechnol. 2010;10:31. DOI: 10.1186/1472-6750-10-31

[34] Dübel S, Breitling F, Fuchs P, Zewe M, Gotter S, Welschof M, et al. Isolation of IgG antibody Fv-DNA from various mouse and rat hybridoma cell lines using the polymerase chain reaction with a simple set of primers. J Immunol Methods. 1994;175:89–95. DOI: 10.1016/0022-1759(94)90334-4

[35] Nam CH, Moutel S, Teillaud JL. Generation of murine scFv intrabodies from B-cell hybridomas. Methods Mol Biol. 2002;193:301–27. DOI: 10.1385/1-59259-283-X:301

[36] Pope AR, Embleton MJ, Mernaugh R. Construction and use of antibody gene repertoires. In: McCafferty J, Hoogenboom HR, Chiswell DJ (eds). Antibody Engineering: A Practical Approach. Oxford University Press, New York, USA. 1996; pp 1-40.

[37] Reynolds A, Leake D, Boese Q, Scaringe S, Marshall WS, Khvorova A. Rational siRNA design for RNA interference. Nat Biotechnol. 2004;22:326–30. DOI: 10.1038/nbt936

[38] Thang BN, Ho TB, Kanda T. A semi-supervised tensor regression model for siRNA efficacy prediction. BMC Bioinformatics. 2015;16:80. DOI: 10.1186/s12859-015-0495-2

[39] Sigoillot FD, Lyman S, Huckins JF, Adamson B, Chung E, Quattrochi B, et al. A bioinformatics method identifies prominent off-targeted transcripts in RNAi screens. Nat Methods. 2012;9:363–66. DOI: 10.1038/nmeth.1898

[40] Buehler E, Khan AA, Marine S, Rajaram M, Bahl A, Burchard J, et al. siRNA off-target effects in genome-wide screens identify signaling pathway members. Sci Rep. 2012;2:428: 1-6. DOI: 10.1038/srep00428

[41] Hust M, Frenzel A, Tomszak F, Kügler J, Dübel S. Antibody Phage Display. Handbook of Therapeutic Antibodies 3rd ed, Wiley-VCH, Weinheim. 2014:43–76. DOI: 10.1002/9783527682423.ch3

[42] Beerli RR, Bauer M, Buser RB, Gwerder M, Muntwiler S, Maurer P, et al. Isolation of human monoclonal antibodies by mammalian cell display. Proc Natl Acad Sci U S A. 2008;105:14336–41. DOI: 10.1073/pnas.0805942105

[43] Samuelson P, Gunneriusson E, Nygren PA, Stahl S. Display of proteins on bacteria. J Biotechnol. 2002;96:129–54. DOI: 10.1016/S0168-1656(02)00043-3

[44] Zhao XL, Chen WQ, Yang ZH, Li JM, Zhang SJ, Tian LF. Selection and affinity maturation of human antibodies against rabies virus from a scFv gene library using ribosome display. J Biotechnol. 2009;144:253–58. DOI: 10.1016/j.jbiotec.2009.09.022

[45] Boudreau RL, Davidson BL. Generation of hairpin-based RNAi vectors for biological and therapeutic application. Methods Enzymol. 2012;507:275–96. DOI: 10.1016/B978-0-12-386509-0.00014-4

[46] Sandy P, Ventura A, Jacks T. Mammalian RNAi: a practical guide. Biotechniques. 2005;39:215–24. DOI: 05392RV01 [pii]

[47] Behlke MA. Chemical modification of siRNAs for in vivo use. Oligonucleotides. 2008;18:305–19. DOI: 10.1089/oli.2008.0164

[48] Judge AD, Sood V, Shaw JR, Fang D, McClintock K, MacLachlan I. Sequence-dependent stimulation of the mammalian innate immune response by synthetic siRNA. Nat Biotechnol. 2005;23:457–62. DOI: 10.1038/nbt1081

[49] Sledz CA, Holko M, de Veer MJ, Silverman RH, Williams BR. Activation of the interferon system by short-interfering RNAs. Nat Cell Biol. 2003;5:834–39. DOI: 10.1038/ncb1038

[50] Jackson AL, Linsley PS. Noise amidst the silence: off-target effects of siRNAs? Trends Genet. 2004;20:521–24. DOI: 10.1016/j.tig.2004.08.006

[51] Persengiev SP, Zhu X, Green MR. Nonspecific, concentration-dependent stimulation and repression of mammalian gene expression by small interfering RNAs (siRNAs). Rna. 2004;10:12–18. DOI: 10.1261/rna5160904

[52] Morrissey DV, Lockridge JA, Shaw L, Blanchard K, Jensen K, Breen W, et al. Potent and persistent in vivo anti-HBV activity of chemically modified siRNAs. Nat Biotechnol. 2005;23:1002–07. DOI: 10.1038/nbt1122

[53] Kittler R, Pelletier L, Ma C, Poser I, Fischer S, Hyman AA, et al. RNA interference rescue by bacterial artificial chromosome transgenesis in mammalian tissue culture cells. Proc Natl Acad Sci U S A. 2005;102:2396–401. DOI: 10.1073/pnas.0409861102

[54] Bramsen JB, Pakula MM, Hansen TB, Bus C, Langkjaer N, Odadzic D, et al. A screen of chemical modifications identifies position-specific modification by UNA to most potently reduce siRNA off-target effects. Nucleic Acids Res. 2010;38:5761–73. DOI: 10.1093/nar/gkq341

[55] Kim SD, Fung VS. An update on Huntington's disease: from the gene to the clinic. Curr Opin Neurol. 2014;27:477–83. DOI: 10.1097/WCO.0000000000000116

[56] Boudreau RL, McBride JL, Martins I, Shen S, Xing Y, Carter BJ, et al. Nonallele-specific silencing of mutant and wild-type huntingtin demonstrates therapeutic efficacy in Huntington's disease mice. Mol Ther. 2009;17:1053–63. DOI: 10.1038/mt.2009.17

[57] Pfister EL, Kennington L, Straubhaar J, Wagh S, Liu W, DiFiglia M, et al. Five siRNAs targeting three SNPs may provide therapy for three-quarters of Huntington's disease patients. Curr Biol. 2009;19:774–78. DOI: 10.1016/j.cub.2009.03.030

[58] Hu J, Liu J, Corey DR. Allele-selective inhibition of huntingtin expression by switching to an miRNA-like RNAi mechanism. Chem Biol. 2010;17:1183–88. DOI: 10.1016/j.chembiol.2010.10.013

[59] Monteys AM, Wilson MJ, Boudreau RL, Spengler RM, Davidson BL. Artificial miRNAs targeting mutant huntingtin show preferential silencing in vitro and in vivo. Mol Ther Nucleic Acids. 2015;4:e234. DOI: 10.1038/mtna.2015.7

[60] Martinez LA, Naguibneva I, Lehrmann H, Vervisch A, Tchenio T, Lozano G, et al. Synthetic small inhibiting RNAs: efficient tools to inactivate oncogenic mutations and restore p53 pathways. Proc Natl Acad Sci U S A. 2002;99:14849–54. DOI: 10.1073/pnas.222406899

[61] Brummelkamp TR, Bernards R, Agami R. Stable suppression of tumorigenicity by virus-mediated RNA interference. Cancer Cell. 2002;2:243–47. DOI: http://dx.doi.org/10.1016/S1535-6108(02)00122-8

[62] Davidson BL, McCray PB, Jr. Current prospects for RNA interference-based therapies. Nat Rev Genet. 2011;12:329–40. DOI: 10.1038/nrg2968

[63] Legleiter J, Lotz GP, Miller J, Ko J, Ng C, Williams GL, et al. Monoclonal antibodies recognize distinct conformational epitopes formed by polyglutamine in a mutant huntingtin fragment. J Biol Chem. 2009;284:21647–58. DOI: 10.1074/jbc.M109.016923

[64] Wolfgang WJ, Miller TW, Webster JM, Huston JS, Thompson LM, Marsh JL, et al. Suppression of Huntington's disease pathology in Drosophila by human single-chain Fv antibodies. Proc Natl Acad Sci U S A. 2005;102:11563–68. DOI: 10.1073/pnas.0505321102

[65] Colby DW, Chu Y, Cassady JP, Duennwald M, Zazulak H, Webster JM, et al. Potent inhibition of huntingtin aggregation and cytotoxicity by a disulfide bond-free single-domain intracellular antibody. Proc Natl Acad Sci U S A. 2004;101:17616–21. DOI: 10.1073/pnas.0408134101

[66] Schena M, Shalon D, Davis RW, Brown PO. Quantitative monitoring of gene expression patterns with a complementary DNA microarray. Science. 1995;270:467–70. DOI: 10.1126/science.270.5235.467

[67] Williams NS, Gaynor RB, Scoggin S, Verma U, Gokaslan T, Simmang C, et al. Identification and validation of genes involved in the pathogenesis of colorectal cancer using cDNA microarrays and RNA interference. Clin Cancer Res. 2003;9:931–46

[68] Taylor J, Woodcock S. A perspective on the future of high-throughput RNAi screening: will CRISPR cut out the competition or can RNAi help guide the way? J Biomol Screen. 2015; 20(8):1040-51. DOI: 10.1177/1087057115590069

[69] Gao S, Yang C, Jiang S, Xu XN, Lu X, He YW, et al. Applications of RNA interference high-throughput screening technology in cancer biology and virology. Protein Cell. 2014;5:805–15. DOI: 10.1007/s13238-014-0076-6

[70] Rytlewski JA, Beronja S. RNAi in the mouse: rapid and affordable gene function studies in a vertebrate system. Wiley Interdiscip Rev Dev Biol. 2015;4:45–57. DOI: 10.1002/wdev.164

[71] Van Overbeke W, Wongsantichon J, Everaert I, Verhelle A, Zwaenepoel O, Loonchanta A, et al. An ER-directed gelsolin nanobody targets the first step in amyloid formation in a gelsolin amyloidosis mouse model. Hum Mol Genet. 2015;24:2492–507. DOI: 10.1093/hmg/ddv010

[72] Marschall AL, Single FN, Schlarmann K, Bosio A, Strebe N, van den Heuvel J, et al. Functional knock down of VCAM1 in mice mediated by endoplasmatic reticulum retained intrabodies. MAbs. 2014; 6(6):1394-401. DOI: 10.4161/mabs.34377

[73] Sato M, Iwaya R, Ogihara K, Sawahata R, Kitani H, Chiba J, et al. Intrabodies against the EVH1 domain of Wiskott-Aldrich syndrome protein inhibit T cell receptor signaling in transgenic mice T cells. FEBS J. 2005;272:6131–44. DOI: 10.1111/j.1742-4658.2005.05011.x

[74] Song E, Lee SK, Wang J, Ince N, Ouyang N, Min J, et al. RNA interference targeting Fas protects mice from fulminant hepatitis. Nat Med. 2003;9:347–51. DOI: 10.1038/nm828

[75] McCaffrey AP, Nakai H, Pandey K, Huang Z, Salazar FH, Xu H, et al. Inhibition of hepatitis B virus in mice by RNA interference. Nat Biotechnol. 2003;21:639–44. DOI: 10.1038/nbt824

[76] Sorensen DR, Leirdal M, Sioud M. Gene silencing by systemic delivery of synthetic siRNAs in adult mice. J Mol Biol. 2003;327:761–66. DOI: 10.1016/S0022-2836(03)00181-5

[77] Verma UN, Surabhi RM, Schmaltieg A, Becerra C, Gaynor RB. Small interfering RNAs directed against beta-catenin inhibit the in vitro and in vivo growth of colon cancer cells. Clin Cancer Res. 2003;9:1291–300

[78] Reich SJ, Fosnot J, Kuroki A, Tang W, Yang X, Maguire AM, et al. Small interfering RNA (siRNA) targeting VEGF effectively inhibits ocular neovascularization in a mouse model. Mol Vis. 2003;9:210–16

[79] Hong CS, Goins WF, Goss JR, Burton EA, Glorioso JC. Herpes simplex virus RNAi and neprilysin gene transfer vectors reduce accumulation of Alzheimer's disease-related amyloid-beta peptide in vivo. Gene Ther. 2006;13:1068–79. DOI: 10.1038/sj.gt.3302719

[80] Xia H, Mao Q, Eliason SL, Harper SQ, Martins IH, Orr HT, et al. RNAi suppresses polyglutamine-induced neurodegeneration in a model of spinocerebellar ataxia. Nat Med. 2004;10:816–20. DOI: 10.1038/nm1076

[81] Zhang ZX, Zhou J, Zhang Y, Zhu DM, Li DC, Zhao H. Knockdown of angiopoietin-2 suppresses metastasis in human pancreatic carcinoma by reduced matrix metalloproteinase-2. Mol Biotechnol. 2013;53:336–44. DOI: 10.1007/s12033-012-9532-9

[82] Alvarez RD, Barnes MN, Gomez-Navarro J, Wang M, Strong TV, Arafat W, et al. A cancer gene therapy approach utilizing an anti-erbB-2 single-chain antibody-encoding adenovirus (AD21): a phase I trial. Clin Cancer Res. 2000;6:3081–87

[83] Jannot CB, Beerli RR, Mason S, Gullick WJ, Hynes NE. Intracellular expression of a single-chain antibody directed to the EGFR leads to growth inhibition of tumor cells. Oncogene. 1996;13:275–82

[84] Böldicke T, Weber H, Mueller PP, Barleon B, Bernal M. Novel highly efficient intrabody mediates complete inhibition of cell surface expression of the human vascular endothelial growth factor receptor-2 (VEGFR-2/KDR). J Immunol Methods. 2005;300:146–59. DOI: 10.1016/j.jim.2005.03.007

[85] Popkov M, Jendreyko N, McGavern DB, Rader C, Barbas CF, 3rd. Targeting tumor angiogenesis with adenovirus-delivered anti-Tie-2 intrabody. Cancer Res. 2005;65:972–81

[86] Jendreyko N, Popkov M, Rader C, Barbas CF, 3rd. Phenotypic knockout of VEGF-R2 and Tie-2 with an intradiabody reduces tumor growth and angiogenesis in vivo. Proc Natl Acad Sci U S A. 2005;102:8293–98. DOI: 10.1073/pnas.0503168102

[87] Wang W, Zhou J, Xu L, Zhen Y. Antineoplastic effect of intracellular expression of a single-chain antibody directed against type IV collagenase. J Environ Pathol Toxicol Oncol. 2000;19:61–68

[88] Swan CH, Buhler B, Steinberger P, Tschan MP, Barbas CF, 3rd, Torbett BE. T-cell protection and enrichment through lentiviral CCR5 intrabody gene delivery. Gene Ther. 2006;13:1480–92. DOI: 10.1038/sj.gt.3302801

[89] Accardi L, Paolini F, Mandarino A, Percario Z, Di Bonito P, Di Carlo V, et al. In vivo antitumor effect of an intracellular single-chain antibody fragment against the E7 oncoprotein of human papillomavirus 16. Int J Cancer. 2014;134:2742–47. DOI: 10.1002/ijc.28604

[90] Sudol KL, Mastrangelo MA, Narrow WC, Frazer ME, Levites YR, Golde TE, et al. Generating differentially targeted amyloid-beta specific intrabodies as a passive vaccination strategy for Alzheimer's disease. Mol Ther. 2009;17:2031–40. DOI: doi: 10.1038/mt.2009.174

[91] Kunath T, Gish G, Lickert H, Jones N, Pawson T, Rossant J. Transgenic RNA interference in ES cell-derived embryos recapitulates a genetic null phenotype. Nat Biotechnol. 2003;21:559–61. DOI: 10.1038/nbt813

[92] Moreno-Maldonado R, Murillas R, Navarro M, Page A, Suarez-Cabrera C, Alameda JP, et al. RNAi-mediated knockdown of IKK1 in transgenic mice using a transgenic construct containing the human H1 promoter. Sci World J. 2014: 1-11. DOI: 10.1155/2014/193803

[93] Livshits G, Lowe SW. Accelerating cancer modeling with RNAi and nongermline genetically engineered mouse models. Cold Spring Harb Protoc. 2013: 1-23. DOI: 10.1101/pdb.top069856

[94] Kleinhammer A, Wurst W, Kuhn R. Constitutive and conditional RNAi transgenesis in mice. Methods. 2011;53:430–36. DOI: 10.1016/j.ymeth.2010.12.015

[95] Cardinale A, Biocca S. Can intrabodies targeted to the secretory compartment interact with a cytosolic protein? A comment on the article by Sawahata et al. "Cytoplasmic expression and specific binding of the VH/VL single domain intrabodies in transfected NIH3T3 cells", Exp. Mol. Pathol. 2008 Nov 27; Epub ahead of print. Exp Mol Pathol. 2009;86:138. DOI: 10.1016/j.yexmp.2009.01.002

[96] Kwee L, Baldwin HS, Shen HM, Stewart CL, Buck C, Buck CA, et al. Defective development of the embryonic and extraembryonic circulatory systems in vascular cell adhesion molecule (VCAM-1) deficient mice. Development. 1995;121:489–503

[97] Deng Y, Wang CC, Choy KW, Du Q, Chen J, Wang Q, et al. Therapeutic potentials of gene silencing by RNA interference: principles, challenges, and new strategies. Gene. 2014;538:217–27. DOI: 10.1016/j.gene.2013.12.019

[98] Do DV, Nguyen QD, Shah SM, Browning DJ, Haller JA, Chu K, et al. An exploratory study of the safety, tolerability and bioactivity of a single intravitreal injection of vascular endothelial growth factor Trap-Eye in patients with diabetic macular oedema. Br J Ophthalmol. 2009;93:144–49. DOI: 10.1136/bjo.2008.138271

[99] DeVincenzo J, Lambkin-Williams R, Wilkinson T, Cehelsky J, Nochur S, Walsh E, et al. A randomized, double-blind, placebo-controlled study of an RNAi-based therapy directed against respiratory syncytial virus. Proc Natl Acad Sci U S A. 2010;107:8800–05. DOI: 10.1073/pnas.0912186107

[100] Wirth T, Parker N, Yla-Herttuala S. History of gene therapy. Gene. 2013;525:162–69. DOI: 10.1016/j.gene.2013.03.137

[101] Lares MR, Rossi JJ, Ouellet DL. RNAi and small interfering RNAs in human disease therapeutic applications. Trends Biotechnol. 2010;28:570–79. DOI: 10.1016/j.tibtech.2010.07.009

[102] Waehler R, Russell SJ, Curiel DT. Engineering targeted viral vectors for gene therapy. Nat Rev Genet. 2007;8:573–87. DOI: 10.1038/nrg2141

[103] Dolgin E. Business: the billion-dollar biotech. Nature. 2015;522:26–28. DOI: 10.1038/522026a

[104] Koo MY, Park J, Lim JM, Joo SY, Shin SP, Shim HB, et al. Selective inhibition of the function of tyrosine-phosphorylated STAT3 with a phosphorylation site-specific intrabody. Proc Natl Acad Sci U S A. 2014;111:6269–74. DOI: 10.1073/pnas.1316815111

[105] Paz K, Brennan LA, Iacolina M, Doody J, Hadari YR, Zhu Z. Human single-domain neutralizing intrabodies directed against Etk kinase: a novel approach to impair cel-

lular transformation. Mol Cancer Ther. 2005;4:1801–09. DOI: 10.1158/1535-7163.MCT-05-0174

[106] Liu J, Hu J, Hicks JA, Prakash TP, Corey DR. Modulation of splicing by single-stranded silencing RNAs. Nucleic Acid Ther. 2015;25:113–20. DOI: 10.1089/nat.2014.0527

[107] Liang WC, Wang Y, Xiao LJ, Wang YB, Fu WM, Wang WM, et al. Identification of miRNAs that specifically target tumor suppressive KLF6-FL rather than oncogenic KLF6-SV1 isoform. RNA Biol. 2014;11:845–54. DOI: 10.4161/rna.29356

[108] Pichler M, Calin GA. MicroRNAs in cancer: from developmental genes in worms to their clinical application in patients. Br J Cancer. 2015; 113(4):569-73. DOI: 10.1038/bjc.2015.253

[109] Zanesi N, Pekarsky Y, Trapasso F, Calin G, Croce CM. MicroRNAs in mouse models of lymphoid malignancies. J Nucleic Acids Investig. 2010;1:36–40. DOI: 10.4081/jnai.2010.e8

[110] Navarro F, Lieberman J. miR-34 and p53: new Insights into a complex functional relationship. PLoS One. 2015;10:e0132767. DOI: 10.1371/journal.pone.0132767

[111] Hong et al. Oral presentation at the Annual Meeting of the American Association for Cancer Research. 2015; Philadelphia

[112] Underbayev C, Kasar S, Yuan Y, Raveche E. MicroRNAs and induced pluripotent stem cells for human disease mouse modeling. J Biomed Biotechnol. 2012; 2012: 1-7 DOI: 10.1155/2012/758169

[113] Jackson AL, Linsley PS. Recognizing and avoiding siRNA off-target effects for target identification and therapeutic application. Nat Rev Drug Discov. 2010;9:57–67. DOI: 10.1038/nrd3010

[114] Visintin M, Settanni G, Maritan A, Graziosi S, Marks JD, Cattaneo A. The intracellular antibody capture technology (IACT): towards a consensus sequence for intracellular antibodies. J Mol Biol. 2002;317:73–83. DOI: 10.1006/jmbi.2002.5392

[115] Muyldermans S. Nanobodies: natural single-domain antibodies. Annu Rev Biochem. 2013;82:775–97. DOI: 10.1146/annurev-biochem-063011-092449

[116] Van Impe K, Bethuyne J, Cool S, Impens F, Ruano-Gallego D, De Wever O, et al. A nanobody targeting the F-actin capping protein CapG restrains breast cancer metastasis. Breast Cancer Res. 2013;15:R116. DOI: 10.1186/bcr3585

[117] Staus DP, Wingler LM, Strachan RT, Rasmussen SG, Pardon E, Ahn S, et al. Regulation of beta2-adrenergic receptor function by conformationally selective single-domain intrabodies. Mol Pharmacol. 2014;85:472–81. DOI: 10.1124/mol.113.089516

[118] Verheesen P, de Kluijver A, van Koningsbruggen S, de Brij M, de Haard HJ, van Ommen GJ, et al. Prevention of oculopharyngeal muscular dystrophy-associated aggre-

gation of nuclear polyA-binding protein with a single-domain intracellular antibody. Hum Mol Genet. 2006;15:105–11. DOI: 10.1093/hmg/ddi432

[119] Kim DS, Song HN, Nam HJ, Kim SG, Park YS, Park JC, et al. Directed evolution of human heavy chain variable domain (VH) using in vivo protein fitness filter. PLoS One. 2014;9:e98178. DOI: 10.1371/journal.pone.0098178

[120] Kim DY, To R, Kandalaft H, Ding W, van Faassen H, Luo Y, et al. Antibody light chain variable domains and their biophysically improved versions for human immunotherapy. MAbs. 2014;6:219–35. DOI: 10.4161/mabs.26844

[121] Taussig M (Project Coordinator). EC FP7 Collaborative Project "Affinomics". 2015. Available from: www.affinomics.org.

[122] Cejka D, Losert D, Wacheck V. Short interfering RNA (siRNA): tool or therapeutic? Clin Sci (Lond). 2006;110:47–58. DOI: 10.1042/cs20050162

Section 4

RNA Interference for Disease Therapy

Chapter 8

RNAi Therapeutic Potentials and Prospects in CNS Disease

Kyoung Joo Cho and Gyung Whan Kim

Additional information is available at the end of the chapter

http://dx.doi.org/10.5772/62896

Abstract

Over the past 20 years, RNA interference (RNAi) technology has provided a new regulatory paradigm in biology. This technique can efficiently suppress target genes of interest in mammalian cells. Small non-coding RNAs play important roles in gene regulation, including both in post-transcriptional and in translational regulation. For *in vivo* experiments, continuous development has resulted in successful new ways of designing, identifying, and delivering small interfering RNAs (siRNAs). Proof-of-principle studies *in vivo* have clearly demonstrated that both viral and non-viral delivery methods can provide selective and potent target gene suppression without any clear toxic effects. There are also the persistent problems with off-target effects (OTEs), competition with cellular RNAi components, and effective delivery *in vivo*. Although recent researches and trials from a large number of animal model studies have confirmed that most OTEs are not dangerous, other important issues need to be addressed before RNAi-based drugs are ready for clinical use. Currently, RNAi may be harnessed as a new therapeutic modality for brain diseases. Finally, there are already several RNAi-based human clinical trials in progress. It is hoped that this technology will have also effective applications in human central nervous system (CNS)-related disease.

Keywords: RNAi therapy, brain, neurodegenerative disease, allele-specific, neurovascular

1. Introduction

During developmental stage and in response to internal and external cellular stresses, small RNA molecules regulate gene expression [1]. Specialized ribonucleases and RNA-binding proteins govern the production and action of small regulatory RNAs [2]. In most eukaryotic cells, RNA interference (RNAi) is a regulatory mechanism using small double-stranded RNA (dsRNA) molecules to direct homology-dependent control of gene activity [3, 4]. Small size [20–30 nucleotide (nt)] non-coding RNAs and associated proteins regulate the expression of genetic information [5]. The discovery of RNAi phenomenon widened our understanding of gene regulation and revealed related pathways in small RNAs [6]. As it processes, RNAi has been finding widespread in plants [7] and animals [8]. Each small RNA associates with an Argonaute (AGO) family protein to form a sequence-specific complex. After then, gene-silencing ribonucleo-protein complex with specificity conferred by base pairing between the small RNA (guide RNA) and its target mRNA [5]. The pathway is well known as the RNA-induced silencing complex (RISC), which gives a target mRNA silencing by degradation or transcriptional regression [2]. Small interfering RNAs (siRNAs) loaded into RISC are double-stranded, and AGO-2, which having an active catalytic domain in human, cleaves and releases the "passenger" strand. RISC is activated with a single-stranded "guide RNA" molecule to impose the specificity recognizing the target by intermolecular base pairing [9].

MicroRNAs (miRNAs) are other endogenous substrates for the RNAi machinery, but the cellular origins of miRNA and siRNA are distinct. miRNAs are derived from the genome, whereas siRNAs may be endogenous or arise through viral infection or other exogenous sources [2]. Typically, miRNAs are initially expressed in the nucleus with a transcript as long as primary miRNA (pri-miRNA), and the transcripts are at least over 1000 nt. Pri-miRNAs are processed by the microprocessor complex (histone deacetylase proteins) consisting in Drosha-DGCR8 [DiGeorge critical region 8 (a double cysteine-ligated Fe (III) heme protein)—DGCR8] in the nucleus [10, 11]. They are cleaved in the nucleus into 60–70 base pair (bp) hairpins, which are consisted in single-stranded 5′- and 3′-terminal overhangs and about 10-nt distal loops [12]. In cytoplasm, the loop is further processed by the RNAse III Dicer, and one strand is loaded onto RISC. The mature miRNAs bind to the 3′ UTR of target mRNAs and then degrade the target [13]. Despite their differing origins, these RNA processing pathways converge once either type of RNA assembles into the RISC.

With development of an efficient delivery system in various diseases, RNAi has been an emerging therapeutic approach for *in vivo* studies with specific synthetic siRNAs against each disease. It should be considered as novel and interesting therapeutic challenge with the major concern how to administer the siRNAs with specific, efficient, and targeted way. Despite some hurdles for applying to clinical challenges such as anatomical barriers, drug stability and availability, various delivery routes, and different genetic backgrounds, an application of siRNAs has become extremely attractive in development of new drugs. Currently, one of the important challenges in siRNA bioinformatics is target prediction, when there is still no proper tool with certain drug design grade. Besides specific challenges in siRNA therapeutics, an efficient delivery method, targeting a specific tissue or cell, is another fundamental challenge.

This chapter introduced two of main themes. The first is the possibilities of therapeutics using RNAi principles and technique. The second is the challenges with siRNAs or miRNAs specifically in the area of brain disease. In addition, this chapter provided some prospects of siRNAs or miRNAs on disease prognosis, progress, and therapeutics in the present and future.

2. Principles of RNAi therapy

As far as it is true that siRNA has promising benefits, and, concomitantly, siRNA has still some of technological barriers to be widely used in clinical therapy, which generally due to the lack of efficient delivery tools. To success with siRNA therapies, an effective and safe carrier system is required that would overcome the inherent defects of siRNA and achieve maximum gene-silencing effect. There are many approaches that are being developed to achieve the efficient delivery of siRNA. In that, non-viral vectors have advantages of reproducibility, low immunogenicity, and relatively low production cost [14]; therefore, non-viral vectors made siRNA to be a potential therapeutic and nucleic acid–based drugs, such as plasmid DNAs or antisense oligonucleotides (ASOs) [15].

2.1. Advantages of RNAi

Theoretically, all disease-associated genes could be amenable to antisense-mediated RNAi suppression. RNAi can be a strategy for silencing of virtually all annotated protein-encoding genes in the human genome in large scale. The high specificity of siRNA lets targeting of disease-specific alleles that differ from the normal allele by only one or few nucleotide substitutions. This high fidelity and specificity of siRNAs are useful for targeting for some oncogenes, too.

The first advantage is the powerfulness of RNAi when compared with other antisense strategies, such as antisense DNA oligonucleotides and ribozymes [16]. It is important fact that the effector molecules work at much lower concentration than any other antisense oligomers or ribozymes, suggesting that RNAi has higher potency. This is a critical point to set therapeutics.

The second is efficacy. The efficacy is generally presented by the half level of maximal inhibition or the value of IC50 against target site. The efficacy level is crucial for determining thermodynamic stability [17], targeted gene accessibility [18], or structure [18] of designed siRNA. For designing siRNA, the most important thing is end stability that is different from each end and is also meaning asymmetry and consistent with selected miRNA [19]. However, to date, our knowledge of siRNA and the selection of targets are incomplete and being explored. The identification of "hyperfunctional" siRNAs, functioning at sub-nanomolar concentration, remains an elusive task.

2.2. Basic strategies for targeting-specific molecules

RNAi can be triggered by two different pathways: (1) a RNA-based approach, where the 21-nt long duplexed siRNA effectors are delivered to target cells, and (2) a DNA-based strategy, where the siRNA effectors are produced by intracellular processing of longer RNA hairpin transcripts [3]. DNA-based strategy is based on short hairpin RNA (shRNA) synthesis in nucleus and transportation to the cytoplasm through miRNA machinery, which subsequently is processed by Dicer. Although the direct use of siRNA effectors is simple and effective way for gene silencing, the effect is transient. Therefore, it is costly for clinical usage due to the need of multiple large-scale application. In contrast, DNA-based RNAi drugs have the potential and stably introduced for application in a gene therapy. In principle, DNA-based RNAi allows a single treatment of viral vector that delivers shRNA genes to the targeted cells/or tissues.

2.3. Delivery routes for targeting

The effective delivery of siRNAs acts to be significant step in accelerating RNAi-based treatments. The instability of RNA and the relatively inefficient encapsulation process of siRNA remain critical issues toward the clinical translation of RNAi as a therapeutic tool. There are several obstacles for extracellular introduction of siRNA to deliver the target. Under normal physiological condition, the introduced molecules ought to have a positive charge to diffuse to cell membrane [20]. It is the simplest way of naked nucleotides or transfecting siRNAs to deliver into cells [21]. Another technique is microinjection and electroporation for direct delivery, but it has higher level of cellular toxicity [22]. The delivery routes can be intra-peritoneal, intra-vascular, intra-muscular, intra-splenic, intra-cranial, and intra-tumoral injection. In addition, siRNAs can be delivered through subretinal, subcutaneous, mucosal, topical application, and oral ingestion to improve delivery [22]. However, these transfection processes should be optimized for siRNA concentration, cell density, and ratio of transfection reagent to siRNA [23]. Carriers for delivery of siRNA with cationic environment surrounding of siRNAs can be liposomes and dendrimers. These carriers reduce the nuclease activity and improve siRNA delivery into cells [24].

Microsponge is one of the mediators for siRNA delivery. Carrier and cargo combine and self-assemble into nanoscale pleated sheets of hairpin RNA. Subsequently, this complex forms sponge-like microspheres [25]. The complex of siRNA and microsponges consists in cleavable RNA strands, and the stable hairpin RNA converts into working siRNA once cells uptake the complex. Therefore, it can provide a protection for siRNA during delivery and transport it to the cytoplasm. Single microsponge complex can deliver more than half a million copies of siRNA when uptaken into a cell [25].

2.4. Stabilizing the siRNA delivery

The stability of the siRNA complexes, penetrating into target cells without stimulating immune responses, is one of the limiting factors and the major bottleneck for developing siRNA therapeutic tools. It restricts the delivery of siRNA macromolecular complexes to the desired cell types, tissues, or organs. Usually, siRNAs do not easily penetrate the cellular membrane because of their negative charge and macromolecular size. Manipulation of nucleotide bases is needed to increase stability and protein interactions, which can harness to increase the structural improvement of siRNAs [26]. The delivery systems for siRNA consist of four main methods, namely naked, lipid-based, peptide-based, and polymer-based delivery [27]. Basically, polymer-based methods are similar to lipid-based methods in targeting, except some special triggers, such as temperature, pH, or pulse release [28].

Initial efforts to improve stability addressed above were focused on incorporating chemical modifications into the sugar backbone or bases of siRNA duplexes [29]. The modified siRNA molecules increased stability, which effectively lowered the dose to achieve measurable and reproducible gene silencing [30]. Several modifications were introduced. The thio (–SH), hydroxyl (–OH), or iodo (–I) can modify bases in specific sites or utilize the pseudouracil base in siRNA, which would augment potency of naked siRNA [31]. There are three most popular chemical modification sites on siRNA structure containing the phosphodiester backbone, ribose 2′-hydroxyl group (R-2′-OH), and ribose ring. Endogenous cellular endonucleases can easily digest phosphodiester bond in RNA backbone [32]. Alternative modification is oxygen bridges of RNA backbone that can be replaced with phosphorothioate, although it would increase toxicity and reduce silencing activity [33, 34]. Another alternative is boranophosphate linkages. These are more nuclease resistant and less toxic compared to phosphorothioate [35]. Phosphonoacetate linkages are other candidates [36]. The linkage is completely resistant to nuclease and is electrochemically neutral when they are esterified [36, 37]. Another modification is 2′-*O*-methoxyethyl (2′-*O*-MOE), 2′-*O*-alkyl, and other bulky groups. These modifications can improve anti-nuclease shield of siRNA that simultaneously makes them less tolerable when they are positioned on 3′ overhangs [38]. Despite disturbing thermodynamic asymmetry of siRNA by addition of 2′-aminoethyl at 3′ end of passenger strand, this modification improves efficiency of target silencing [39].

On the other hand, alterations in sugar compartment of nucleotides reduced flexibility and nuclease sensitivity of siRNA structure [39, 40]. Binding of ribose 2′O into 1′C with methylene bridges, which finally produces oxetane, forms a locked conformation nucleic acid (locked nucleic acid—LNA) [41]. *In vivo* nuclease resistance of this structure is enhanced [42]. In contrast to LNA, derivatives of RNA without C2′–C3′ sugar bonds (unlocked nucleic acid—UNA) destabilize a sequence structure [43]. Substitution of pentose with hexose monosaccharides, such as cyclohexenyl, anitrol, and arabinose, was applied to develop CeNA, ANA, and 2′-F-ANA [44], subsequently resulting in enhanced stability of siRNA *in vivo* [45]. During systemic delivery, however, internal modifications failed to improve central nervous system (CNS) entry and uptake. Researchers put new efforts to move toward using liposomes, nanoparticles, and cell-penetrating peptides (CPPs), among others, to stabilize and navigate siRNAs into and throughout the brain [46].

2.4.1. Liposomes

Generally, liposomes are classified into three classes: multilmellar vesicle (0.5~20 μm), small unilamellar vesicles (25~100 nm), and large unilamellar vesicles (100~500 nm) [47]. Liposomes are developed for passive or active targeting mechanisms in different complexes of liposome and other interacting molecules, namely lipoplex (cationic liposome-pDNA complex), liposome polycationic DNA, mannose liposome, and so on [48, 49]. The siRNA with mannose (Man)-coated liposomes would be useful for treatment of some cancers, especially liver and brain cancers [50].

2.4.2. Dendrimers

Dendrimers are hyper-branched, tree-shaped, and 3-D structures [51]. Dendrimer can utilize broad spectrum, and the broad range of functional groups makes it possible to introduce dendrimers with extensive applications. There are different classes of cationic and anionic dendrimers, such as polyamidoamine (PAMAM), polypropylene imine (PPI), and polyethylene glycol (PEG)-grafted carbosilane [52]. Specific dendritic polymers like PAMAM have been widely utilized in *in vivo* drug delivery [53]. Conjugation of Tat peptide (GRKKRRQRRRPQ) with PAMAM-G5 can efficiently inhibit multi-drug resistance-1 (MDR-1) gene expression *in vitro* [51]. Capping poly-l-lysine (PLL) dendrimers with methotrexate enhances stability and decreases toxicity [54].

2.4.3. Cationic polymers

Cationic polymers include chitosan, gelatin, cationic dextran, cationic cellulose, and cationic cyclodextrin and some synthetic biocompatible polyethyleneimine (PEI), PLL, poly(amidoamine)s (PAAs), poly(amino-co-ester), and poly(2-*N*,*N*-dimethylaminoethylmethacrylate). Moreover, they are less immunogenic response because these polymers are natural biodegradable [55].

2.4.4. Cationic peptides

CPPs are cationic peptides. CPPs interact covalently or non-covalently through disulfide or electrostatic–hydrogen interactions with siRNAs [56]. Viral protein (VP22) [57], MPG (a peptide vector) [58], amphipathic peptide [59], and poly-arginine [60] were reported the same abilities. In addition, small cationic polypeptides (poly His, Lys, and Arg) coat and neutralize siRNA helping to pass through membrane [61].

2.4.5. Nanoparticles

For systemic delivery, a targeted nanocarrier-siRNA complex has been used. There are some studies that have experimentally condensed DNA or RNA into cancer-targeted nanoparticles with PEI, PLL, and cyclodextrin-containing polymers [62]. PEI–PEG–arginine–glycine–aspartic acid (RGD) fusion was used to inhibit vascular endothelial growth factor receptor-2 (VEGFR-2) expression [63]. Angiogenesis can be inhibited by downregulation or silencing of VEGFR-2 expression [64]. PEGylation of nanoparticles causes "muco-inert" properties, which enhances diffusion process through mucus and peptidoglycan barriers [65].

2.4.6. Aptamer

siRNAs can be coupled with aptamers or oligodeoxynucleotide through a disulfide bond. This releases actively into targeted cells siRNAs before cytosolic uptake. Conjugate of aptamer siRNA has suggested a novel therapeutics with widespread applications in medicine [66].

2.5. Limitations

2.5.1. Competition with endogenous RNAs

In human brain diseases and normal brain development, RNAi potentiates the important role in normal neuronal function, although it is underestimated. When exogenous shRNA is introduced into the neuron, it might be considered whether the RNAi machinery perturbs normal physiologic condition of the system. Bioactive drugs that rely on cellular processing to exert their action face the risk of saturating such pathways and hence perturb the natural system. Sometimes, ectopically introduced RNAi does not trigger the silencing process because siRNA/shRNA activity may depend on the endogenous miRNA to achieve efficient target silencing. Mice that received liver-directed associate adeovirus (AAV)-encoded shRNAs were damaged in liver with dose-dependent manner. Within 2 months, the mice were killed by introducing high doses of AAV-encoded shRNAs. It was interpreted that the liver-specific miRNA was unexpectedly down-regulated by introducing shRNA [67]. The enhanced expression of Exportin 5, the nuclear export component, increased RNAi efficacy, which was shown by competition assay [68].

2.5.2. *Stimulation of innate immune responses*

RNAi therapy is importantly considered because of its potential for generating an adverse immune response, particularly in neurodegenerative diseases with affected brain. It has been already known as "heightened state of alert" to start chronic pro-inflammatory signaling cascades [30]. All evolutionary conserved mechanisms aimed at combating against invading viral pathogens [69]. In general, innate immune responses to non-virally delivered siRNAs are mediated by members of the toll-like receptor (TLR) family or by the two different dsRNA-sensing proteins: retinoic acid-inducible gene-1 and dsRNA-binding protein kinase [70]. Certain siRNA sequence motifs invoked TLR7-dependent immune stimulation [71]. The particular sequence motif (5′-GUCCUUCAA-3′) seems to be recognized by TLR7 in plasmacytoid dendritic cells and activates immune responses. The GU-rich regions, so-called "danger motifs," stimulated innate immune responses and lead to secretion of inflammatory cytokines in a cell type and sequence-specific manner. As siRNA-mediated immune induction seems to rely on endosome-located TLR receptors (TLR7 and TLR8) [72], the delivery and compartmentalization of the siRNA significantly influence the cellular responses [3]. These interactions can occur during endosomal or lysosomal compartments' internalization or intracellular release of the siRNA molecule. It has a manner of dose and sequence dependence. Importantly, the chemically modified or nanoparticle-encased siRNA complexes avoid stimulation of immune response.

2.5.3. *Suppression of off targets*

Harmfulness of RNAi is "OTE." Genome-wide sequencing analyses have clearly demonstrated that siRNA-treated cells show off-target silencing of a large number of genes [73]. The research result suggests that siRNAs with a 2′-*O*-MOE modification at the second base can significantly reduce off target without compromising the degree of silencing target [74]. Experimentally, it has been verified that off targets have 6~7-nt long matching to the siRNA, and it is called "seed" region [75]. When the siRNA guide strand contains seed-sequence matching to mRNA 3′-UTR regions, the siRNA guide strand functions as a miRNA, which might lead to harmful OTEs by translational repression [76]. To avoid siRNA seed matching with mRNA 3′ UTRs, the use of online 3′-UTR search algorithms would potentially reduce the detrimental OTEs [75].

The OTEs can also derive from non-specific changes in gene expression due to the activation of the interferon response (IR) [77]. The OTEs can change another gene by binding either strand of the shRNA to partially complementary sequences rather than binding to the intended target gene [77]. In case of dsRNA, it can result in a signaling cascade that culminates with the activation of interferon responsive genes and global translational repression [78]. Nevertheless, IR activation was variable among the siRNAs used for each of these studies, and one recent report did not detect IR activation by siRNAs [79]. In mice, injection of naked siRNA did not show detectable induction of an IR in one study while another study showed sequence-dependent induction of innate immunity [79, 80].

3. Applications of RNAi

RNAi has been used to generate model systems to identify novel molecular targets [81], to study gene function [82], and to create a new niche for clinical therapeutics [83]. Many researchers reported that siRNAs have successfully been tested in various disease animal models. Recent reports reviewed the therapeutic potential of synthetic siRNAs in various human diseases and disorders [84].

3.1. Application for therapy with RNAi *in vivo*

Applications, such as gene function analysis, target identification and validation, and therapeutic agents, are the main spots of this new technology [26]. Although RNAi is an efficient technique for *in vitro* studies, there are some challenges for *in vivo* applications. siRNAs have undesired characteristics, such as non-specific silencing of non-targeted genes and dose-dependent immunogenic response [85]. In addition, it is extremely complicated to avoid the OTEs due to spatiotemporal gene expression pattern of these molecules [73]. Furthermore, age, sex, tissue, organ, tumor, and individual-specific specificity should be also considered as other variables [86]. Prediction of susceptible off-target domains that can influence silencing efficiency is the first step for applying *in vivo* therapy [73, 87]. Some studies recommend utilization of more sensitive alignment algorithms or siDirect instead of BLAST database [85, 88] to predict a target for siRNA matching without cross-reactivity [89].

The administration route for siRNA, such as oral or intravenous, is not feasible and not efficiently delivered the siRNA into target cells. A single injection of naked siRNA into the brain parenchyma failed to good efficacy [90]. A study reported that continuous infusion of siRNA into the ventricular CSF success with very high concentration [91]. To penetrate the blood–brain barrier (BBB) and reach the target cells in the interesting site, receptor-specific pegylated immunoliposome (PIG) is used. PIGs encapsulate the plasmid vector–encoding siRNA or shRNA and are administered with peripheral route to the brain. This tool has been tried in brain cancer animal model and successfully worked [92]. Another study showed effective and long-term knock down of endogenous tyrosine hydroxylase (TH) in rodent brain using shRNA-expressing adeno-associated virus (AAV) [93]. There have been many successful *in vivo* studies with using viral vector. They are included two models of autoimmune hepatitis

[94], hepatitis B virus [95], respiratory viruses such as influenza virus [96], respiratory syncytial virus [97], parainfluenza virus, and sexually transmitted disease such as herpes simplex virus-2 [98]. Both non-viral and viral shRNA delivery systems have been trailed.

3.2. Application for therapy with RNAi in brain diseases

Many works using RNAi to suppress dominant disease genes have occurred primarily in cell culture models [99, 100]. Allele-specific silencing aims to suppress the disease gene without affecting any other normal genes. The possible therapeutic applications of RNAi for neurological diseases are broad, ranging from acquired diseases, such as viral infections, to purely genetic disorders.

Particularly, one attractive group of candidate diseases for RNAi therapy is the dominantly inherited neurodegenerative diseases, including polyglutamine disorders such as Huntington's disease (HD) [101], amyotrophic lateral sclerosis (ALS) [102], familial Alzheimer's disease (AD) [103], and frontotemporal dementia caused by tau mutations [104]. HD has been approaching with animal model mimicking the human disease to provide some therapeutic clues with various ways. In the new preclinical study, single injection of a cholesterol conjugated-siRNA was targeting mutant Huntingtin (mhtt), and, subsequently, the pathologic symptoms containing behavioral dysfunction were improved [105].

The exciting recent works have taken place *in vivo* in mouse models of neurodegenerative brain disease. The best example of RNAi-mediated therapy to date is in spinocerebellar ataxia type-1 (SCA-1) [106]. As another case, RNAi-mediated therapy was tried on DYT1 dystonia with animal disease model. DYT1 dystonia is another inherited dystonia. DYT1 dystonia is caused by deletion of GAG that is coding TOR1A, which results in one of a pair of glutamic acid from the carboxyl terminal of the torsin A (TA) protein-coding region [107].

Prion disease is one of the brain diseases that is invariably fatal, and no therapy is available. Once serious damage to the brain has already occurred, clinical symptoms manifest after the untreatable brain damage. Causing this reason, prion disease treatments have aimed not to cure the disease but to slow disease progression [108]. Prion disease is caused by prions, in which a self-replicating, infectious protease resistant form of PrP (termed PrPSc), is the only essential component identified to date. PrPSc multiplies through conversion of the normal cellular PrP (PrPC) [109]. Some reviews are presenting that lentivector-mediated anti-PrPC shRNA expression effectively suppressed prion replication in a murine neuroblastoma cell line, and researchers created chimeric mice using embryonic stem cells, which were transfected with a lentiviral vector carrying an anti-PrPC shRNA. Results showed that the survival time after prion inoculation was markedly prolonged [110, 111].

4. Prospects of RNA therapeutics in CNS disease

The current phamaceuticals required more knowledge to decipher potentials of the RNAi in spite of flourishing future. It is crucial that each disease has not only a unique pattern but also the understanding for pathogenesis relating pathways and activating or inhibiting factors [112]. To introduce the DNA therapeutics into the CNS is much more complicated due to the BBB, which can be only permeable to lipophilic molecules of less than 400 Da [113]. Using human viruses, DNA delivery system has been extensively trailed for over three decades. However, the results have been not satisfactory. Therefore, a critical goal for clinical neuroscience is to develop the efficient RNAi therapy to prevent the neuronal damage [77]. We categorized the neurological disease containing cancers in below sections.

4.1. Genetic neuronal disease-familial neurological disease

The application of siRNA has been advanced in development of various incurable disease therapies, apart from the widespread usage of RNAi in fundamental biological application. Particularly, dominant inherited disorders are major application field. Among familial neurobiological diseases, HD has been tried to lots of therapies based on RNAi and may be beneficial effect from the therapy using siRNA. In the N171-82Q transgenic HD mouse model, a study using shRNA showed a 50–55% decrease in the N171-82Q mRNA when injected to striatum and a complete elimination of mHtt protein inclusions from the neuronal cells [114]. There was also a rescue of motor dysfunctions. siRNAs against the "R6/2 huntingtin (htt) mRNA" reduced brain atrophy and neuronal inclusions in the R6/2 transgenic mouse model [115]. With using a rAAV5 vector and administrating to the striatum, long-term expression of a mHtt-siRNA partially reduced in neuropathology condition [116].

Besides AAV, there is lentiviral vector that can be applied after onset of symptoms [117]. Using lentivirus vector decreased htt protein expression by up to 35% and altered htt-related pathways but did not reduce cellular viability for at least 9 months after treatment. To enhance cellular uptake of siRNA, cholesterol-conjugated duplexes (cc-siRNA) have been applied to target htt mRNA [118]. Allele-specific targeting of mhtt helped to overcome the side effects of RNAi where ASO or single nucleotide polymorphisms (SNPs) in the mHtt allele have been used to specifically target only the mutant gene product [119]. Intra-cellular antibody fragments bind to abnormal aggregations, and allele-specific siRNA disrupts mhtt gene [120, 121]. Targeting of just three SNPs with five siRNAs covered most of the HD patients in the population studied [122].

Tuberous sclerosis is a common, dominantly inherited disorder caused by mutations in the tumor suppressor complex-1 (TSC1) or tumor suppressor complex-2 (TSC2) genes [123]. The proteins hamartin (encoded by TSC1) and tuberin (encoded by TSC2) form a complex. This protein complex represses mTOR-S6K-4E-BP signaling pathway [123]. Mutated TSC1 and TSC2 lead to loss of activity resulting in unchecked cell growth and hamartoma formation in the CNS. Recent studies propose that the target may be the GTPase Rheb [124]. RNAi suppression of Rheb might respond the dysregulated cell proliferation in tuberous sclerosis.

Particularly, allele-specific silencing is apt for inherited neurological diseases. DYT1 is the most commonly inherited dystonia [125]. Although the pathogenesis of DYT1 is unclear, several facts make DYT1 a good candidate to explore the therapeutic potential of RNAi [77]. The three nucleotide difference between the wild type and the mutated gene has been enough to allow allele-specific silencing against mutant TA (the mutated protein in DYT1) in cultured cells using *in vitro* synthesized siRNA [107].

Allelic discrimination has also been demonstrated for superoxide dismutase (SOD) mutations responsible for familial ALS [100], and also a mutation in an acetylcholine receptor subunit causes congenital myasthenia [126]. In a tau mutation responsible for fronto-temporal dementia, siRNAs can act by discriminating between sequences differing by a single nucleotide [99].

An important role for RNAi in the brain is also presented for Fragile X syndrome (FXS) in human [127]. FXS is the one of the most common forms of inherited mental retardation caused by mutations in Fragile X Mental Retardation Protein (FMRP), a protein influencing synaptic plasticity [127]. FXS is stemmed from mutations in FMRP and is supported by the involvement of the RNAi process in human neurological disease [127]. Increasing evidences from different studies support the view that FMRP regulates protein translation by regulating RNAi in neurons [128, 129].

4.2. Sporadic neurodegenerative diseases

Neurodegenerative diseases are age dependent, and many of them are inherited. However, non-genetic neurological diseases, such as sporadic AD or migraine, are much more common than diseases due to single-gene mutations.

The most common sporadic neurodegenerative disease, AD, is also the best studied with siRNA therapy. Many studies of AD pathogenesis investigate an essential role for β-amyloid (Aβ) in familial and sporadic forms of AD [130]. Different RNAi strategies have been applied to regulate this pathogenic cascade. Researchers tried by directly silencing of amyloid precursor protein (APP) [131], by silencing of β-secretase (BACE1) that is one of two proteases required for Aβ production but not essential gene in mice [132], or by silencing of tau expression that is a component of the neurofibrillary tangles of AD neurons. Therapeutic use of RNAi is now being tested in animal models of AD targeting these proteins.

Migraine, one of the most common neurological disorders, is caused by diminished production of calcitonin gene-related peptide (CGPR) in the trigeminal system. CGPR can protect from migraine attacks [133]. The CGPR-limited animals are normal, but the paroxysmal nature of this disorder necessitates to use promoters for CGPR. From the beginning of the pathogenic cascade, expression of the shRNA targeting CGPR can terminate the growing pain of this disease. This pain alleviating therapy for migraine is limited because of high threshold dose needed for RNAi [133].

4.3. Motor dysfunction disease

A viral delivery of shRNA was used to achieve a long-term RNAi in the CNS. In some reports, the delivery of shRNA-expressing lentivirus showed a rescue of spinal motor neurons with behavioral and histopathological phenotypes in a mouse model having dominant familial ALS [134].

Parkinson's disease (PD) is the second most common neurodegenerative disease. Patient brain of PD is often littered with Lewy body, which is abnormal protein aggregate primarily of alpha-synuclein (α-syn) [135, 136]. parkinsonism is linked to hereditary to a single-point mutation in the α-syn as well as genetic duplication or triplication of the α-syn (SCNA) [104]. The studies targeting the α-syn expression revealed RNAi as a therapeutic approach to PD [30, 137]. To date, conflicting results were reported. Regarding the effectiveness and tolerability, there is a report that nigrostriatal degeneration was detected after depleting the α-syn level in the brain [138]. It can be inferred that RNAi approaches can be used to validate them in genetic and sporadic models of PD.

4.4. Neurovascular disease

RNAi can be applied to cardiovascular and cerebrovascular diseases. Cardiovascular disease results from the progressive occlusion of arteries, and it is most common in a process called atherosclerosis, which can ultimately culminate in a myocardial infarction or stroke [139]. It may be a trigger for the death of cardiac muscle cells or neurons [139]. Although some of the cells die rapidly by necrosis, many other cells die more slowly by apoptosis in such cardiac myocytes and brain neurons [140, 141]. RNAi technology may be used to intervene in atherosclerosis or to reduce the damage of heart tissue and brain cells following a myocardial infarction or stroke [142].

Another vascular disease is an ocular disease. Representatively, there were two RNAi clinical trials. The trials performed direct intra-vitreal injection of siRNAs that are targeting VEGF or the VEGFR to test for the safety and efficacy in ocular diseases [143]. siRNAs, targeting VEGF and VEGFR1, are currently in the early stages of clinical trials. The direct injection approach can also prove its usefulness for the other ocular diseases.

4.5. Cancer

A chemo-resistance or radio resistance is a major obstacle in cancer treatment. Targeted therapies that enhance cancer cell sensitivity have the potential to increase drug efficacy while reducing toxic effects on untargeted cells (144). Actually, oncogenes expressed at abnormally high levels are attractive targets for RNAi-based therapies against cancers [145], and such approaches have effectively inhibited tumor growth *in vivo* in mouse models.

In nasopharyngeal carcinoma, hyaluronan receptor (CD44) gene silencing resulted in profound reduction of malignant potential of the cells: tumorigenesis and metastasis of tumors in nude mice [105, 146]. It is also suggested a possible therapeutic effect of direct introduction of siRNA to CD44 into some human solid tumors with high expression of the CD44 gene [146]. Although the role of epidermal growth factor receptor (EGFR) in altering tumor chemosensitivity has not yet been fully elucidated, selectively targeting EGFR supplies the reversal possibility of chemoresistance in many tumor types [147]. Reduction of EGFR expression and increased chemosensitivity to docetaxel are emerging an effective strategy for the sensitization of cancer cells to taxane chemotherapy [147]. siRNA-PG-Amine polyplexes can be systemically delivered to tumors in mice [148], and siRNA-nanocarrier system can efficiently inhibit expression of a specific gene in tumor cells. Once the intact siRNA molecule moves to the target, the gene of interest gets silenced. The PG-amine-based delivery system actually combines both tumor passive targeting with the sequence selectivity of siRNA [148].

The limiting point of targeted therapy is alternative pathway compensation by gene amplification. The "synthetic lethality" is proposed idea to overcome the above problem [149]. This concept suggests that two genes may be considered to have a synthetically lethal relationship [150]. When a mutation is existed either of the two genes alone has no effect on cell survival, but when mutations in both genes cell death is triggered at the same time. By genome-wide RNAi library screening, some synthetic lethal molecules have been discovered. Anaphase-promoting complex/cyclosome (APC/C) and polo-like kinase (PLK) are synthetically lethal with the RAS oncogene in colorectal cancer [151]. The STK33 gene is also synthetic lethal interacting with a RAS mutation in multiple cancer cells from different tumor types [152]. Modified EGFR (amplification or truncation) and hyperactivation of AKT play a major role in the development of glioblastoma, one of the extreme malignancies [153]. There are approaches to develop the siRNA delivery efficiency such as the use of dsRNA-binding domain (DRBD) with a TAT peptide transduction domain (PTD) delivery peptide [154]. These facilities are stable and efficient delivery of siRNAs into cells [155].

5. Conclusions

Small RNAs and non-coding small RNAs were important discovery for molecular cell biology; these small RNAs have a vital role in gene regulation that can be controlled by RNA interfering technology. Presently, attempts to integrate gene expression profiling and protein interaction mapping are the main research objectives. The proof-of-principle studies *in vivo* have clearly demonstrated that both viral and non-viral delivery methods can provide selective and efficient target gene suppression without any clear toxic effects. Initial results have been very promising, and many pharmaceutical companies are already focusing on commercialization of various disease-specific RNAi drugs. Despite successful trials in a large number of animal model studies including brain diseases, to develop an efficient therapeutic application, there are numerous hurdles and concerns regarding targeted delivery of siRNAs into brain subregions that must be overcome before wide clinical application of RNAi as a new therapeutic solution. The OTEs, competition with endogenous cellular RNAi components, and effective delivery *in vivo* remain to be optimized. Although recent research has improved the safety and toxicity from the OTEs, it still remains a crucial issue and needs to be addressed before RNAi-based drugs are ready for clinical use. Translational research using RNAi has taken place with an unprecedented speed, and already there are several RNAi-based human clinical trials in progress that will provide breakthrough therapeutic tools for effective treatment human CNS-related disease.

Author details

Kyoung Joo Cho and Gyung Whan Kim*

*Address all correspondence to: gyungkim@yuhs.ac

Department of Neurology, Severance Hospital, Yonsei University College of Medicine, Seoul, South Korea

References

[1] Leung RK, Whittaker PA. RNA interference: from gene silencing to gene-specific therapeutics. Pharmacol Ther. 2005;107:222–239. DOI: 10.1016/j.pharmthera.2005.03.004

[2] Wilson RC, Doudna JA. Molecular mechanisms of RNA interference. Annual Review of Biophysics 2013;42:217–239. DOI: 10.1146/annurev-biophys-083012-130404

[3] Aagaard L, Rossi JJ. RNAi therapeutics: principles, prospects and challenges. Advanced Drug Delivery Reviews 2007;59:75–86. DOI: 10.1016/j.addr.2007.03.005

[4] Almeida R, Allshire RC. RNA silencing and genome regulation. Trends in Cell Biology 2005;15:251–258. DOI: 10.1016/j.tcb.2005.03.006

[5] Carthew RW, Sontheimer EJ. Origins and mechanisms of miRNAs and siRNAs. Cell 2009;136:642–655. DOI: 10.1016/j.cell.2009.01.035

[6] Hannon GJ. RNA interference. Nature 2002;418:244–251. DOI: 10.1038/418244a

[7] Shabalina SA, Koonin EV. Origins and evolution of eukaryotic RNA interference. Trends in Ecology & Evolution 2008;23:578–587. DOI: 10.1016/j.tree.2008.06.005

[8] Mittal V. Improving the efficiency of RNA interference in mammals. Nature Reviews Genetics 2004;5:355–365. DOI: 10.1038/nrg1323

[9] Tang G. siRNA and miRNA: an insight into RISCs. Trends in Biochemical Sciences 2005;30:106–114. DOI: 10.1016/j.tibs.2004.12.007

[10] Lee Y, Ahn C, Han J, Choi H, Kim J, Yim J, et al. The nuclear RNase III Drosha initiates microRNA processing. Nature 2003;425:415–419. DOI: 10.1038/nature01957

[11] Han J, Lee Y, Yeom KH, Kim YK, Jin H, Kim VN. The Drosha-DGCR8 complex in primary microRNA processing. Genes & Development 2004;18:3016–3027. DOI: 10.1101/gad.1262504

[12] Saini HK, Griffiths-Jones S, Enright AJ. Genomic analysis of human microRNA transcripts. Proceedings of the National Academy of Sciences of United States of America 2007;104:17719–17724. DOI: 10.1073/pnas.0703890104

[13] Bagga S, Bracht J, Hunter S, Massirer K, Holtz J, Eachus R, et al. Regulation by let-7 and lin-4 miRNAs results in target mRNA degradation. Cell 2005;122:553–563. DOI: 10.1016/j.cell.2005.07.031

[14] Yuan X, Naguib S, Wu Z. Recent advances of siRNA delivery by nanoparticles. Expert Opinion on Drug Delivery 2011;8:521–536. DOI: 10.1517/17425247.2011.559223

[15] Singha K, Namgung R, Kim WJ. Polymers in small-interfering RNA delivery. Nucleic Acid Therapeutics 2011;21:133–147. DOI: 10.1089/nat.2011.0293

[16] Bertrand JR, Pottier M, Vekris A, Opolon P, Maksimenko A, Malvy C. Comparison of antisense oligonucleotides and siRNAs in cell culture and in vivo. Biochemical and Biophysical Research Communications 2002;296:1000–1004. DOI: 10.1016/S0006-291X(02)02013-2

[17] Schwarz DS, Hutvagner G, Du T, Xu Z, Aronin N, Zamore PD. Asymmetry in the assembly of the RNAi enzyme complex. Cell 2003;115:199–208. DOI: 10.1016/S0092-8674(03)00759-1

[18] Heale BS, Soifer HS, Bowers C, Rossi JJ. siRNA target site secondary structure predictions using local stable substructures. Nucleic Acids Research 2005;33:e30. DOI: 10.1093/nar/gni026

[19] Khvorova A, Reynolds A, Jayasena SD. Functional siRNAs and miRNAs exhibit strand bias. Cell 2003;115:209–216. DOI: 10.1016/S0092-8674(03)00801-8

[20] Gary DJ, Puri N, Won YY. Polymer-based siRNA delivery: perspectives on the fundamental and phenomenological distinctions from polymer-based DNA delivery. Journal of Controlled Release 2007;121:64–73. DOI: 10.1016/j.jconrel.2007.05.021

[21] Lingor P, Michel U, Scholl U, Bahr M, Kugler S. Transfection of "naked" siRNA results in endosomal uptake and metabolic impairment in cultured neurons. Biochemical and Biophysical Research Communications 2004;315:1126–1133. DOI: 10.1016/j.bbrc.2004.01.170

[22] McManus MT, Sharp PA. Gene silencing in mammals by small interfering RNAs. Nature Reviews Genetics 2002;3:737–747. DOI: 10.1038/nrg908

[23] Brummelkamp TR, Bernards R, Agami R. A system for stable expression of short interfering RNAs in mammalian cells. Science 2002;296:550–553. DOI: 10.1126/science.1068999

[24] Whitehead KA, Langer R, Anderson DG. Knocking down barriers: advances in siRNA delivery. Nature Reviews Drug Discovery 2009;8:129–138. DOI: 10.1038/nrd2742

[25] Lee JB, Hong J, Bonner DK, Poon Z, Hammond PT. Self-assembled RNA interference microsponges for efficient siRNA delivery. Nature Materials 2012;11:316–322. DOI: 10.1038/nmat3253

[26] Borna H, Imani S, Iman M, Azimzadeh Jamalkandi S. Therapeutic face of RNAi: in vivo challenges. Expert Opinion on Biological Therapy 2015;15:269–285. DOI: 10.1517/14712598.2015.983070

[27] Park TG, Jeong JH, Kim SW. Current status of polymeric gene delivery systems. Advanced Drug Delivery Reviews 2006;58:467–486. DOI: 10.1016/j.addr.2006.03.007

[28] Ganta S, Devalapally H, Shahiwala A, Amiji M. A review of stimuli-responsive nanocarriers for drug and gene delivery. Journal of Controlled Release 2008;126:187–204. DOI: 10.1016/j.jconrel.2007.12.017

[29] Behlke MA. Chemical modification of siRNAs for in vivo use. Oligonucleotides 2008;18:305–319. DOI: 10.1089/oli.2008.0164

[30] Boudreau RL, Rodriguez-Lebron E, Davidson BL. RNAi medicine for the brain: progresses and challenges. Human Molecular Genetics 2011;20:R21–R27. DOI: 10.1093/hmg/ddr137

[31] Peacock H, Kannan A, Beal PA, Burrows CJ. Chemical modification of siRNA bases to probe and enhance RNA interference. Journal of Organic Chemistry 2011;76:7295–7300. DOI: 10.1021/jo2012225

[32] Kennedy S, Wang D, Ruvkun G. A conserved siRNA-degrading RNase negatively regulates RNA interference in *C. elegans*. Nature 2004;427:645–649.

[33] Chiu YL, Rana TM. siRNA function in RNAi: a chemical modification analysis. RNA 2003;9:1034–1048. DOI: 10.1261/rna.5103703

[34] Amarzguioui M, Holen T, Babaie E, Prydz H. Tolerance for mutations and chemical modifications in a siRNA. Nucleic Acids Research 2003;31:589–595. DOI: 10.1093/nar/gkg147

[35] Hall AH, Wan J, Shaughnessy EE, Ramsay Shaw B, Alexander KA. RNA interference using boranophosphate siRNAs: structure-activity relationships. Nucleic Acids Research 2004;32:5991–6000. DOI: 10.1093/nar/gkh936

[36] Sheehan D, Lunstad B, Yamada CM, Stell BG, Caruthers MH, Dellinger DJ. Biochemical properties of phosphonoacetate and thiophosphonoacetate oligodeoxyribonucleotides. Nucleic Acids Research 2003;31:4109–4018. DOI: 10.1093/nar/gkg439

[37] Yamada CM, Dellinger DJ, Caruthers MH. Synthesis and biological activity of phosphonocarboxylate DNA. Nucleosides, Nucleotides & Nucleic Acids 2007;26:539–546. DOI: 10.1080/15257770701489896

[38] Odadzic D, Bramsen JB, Smicius R, Bus C, Kjems J, Engels JW. Synthesis of 2′-O-modified adenosine building blocks and application for RNA interference. Bioorganic & Medicinal Chemistry 2008;16:518–529. DOI: 10.1016/j.bmc.2007.09.019

[39] Bramsen JB, Laursen MB, Nielsen AF, Hansen TB, Bus C, Langkjaer N, et al. A large-scale chemical modification screen identifies design rules to generate siRNAs with

high activity, high stability and low toxicity. Nucleic Acids Research 2009;37:2867–2881. DOI: 10.1093/nar/gkp106

[40] Wengel J, Petersen M, Nielsen KE, Jensen GA, Hakansson AE, Kumar R, et al. LNA (locked nucleic acid) and the diastereoisomeric alpha-L-LNA: conformational tuning and high-affinity recognition of DNA/RNA targets. Nucleosides, Nucleotides & Nucleic Acids 2001;20:389–396. DOI: 10.1081/NCN-100002312

[41] Trang P, Medina PP, Wiggins JF, Ruffino L, Kelnar K, Omotola M, et al. Regression of murine lung tumors by the let-7 microRNA. Oncogene 2010;29:1580–1587. DOI: 10.1038/onc.2009.445

[42] Glud SZ, Bramsen JB, Dagnaes-Hansen F, Wengel J, Howard KA, Nyengaard JR, et al. Naked siLNA-mediated gene silencing of lung bronchoepithelium EGFP expression after intravenous administration. Oligonucleotides 2009;19:163–168. DOI: 10.1089/oli.2008.0175

[43] Vaish N, Chen F, Seth S, Fosnaugh K, Liu Y, Adami R, et al. Improved specificity of gene silencing by siRNAs containing unlocked nucleobase analogs. Nucleic Acids Research 2011;39:1823–1832. DOI: 10.1093/nar/gkq961

[44] Nauwelaerts K, Fisher M, Froeyen M, Lescrinier E, Aerschot AV, Xu D, et al. Structural characterization and biological evaluation of small interfering RNAs containing cyclohexenyl nucleosides. Journal of the American Chemical Society 2007;129:9340–9348. DOI: 10.1021/ja067047q

[45] Fisher M, Abramov M, Van Aerschot A, Xu D, Juliano RL, Herdewijn P. Inhibition of MDR1 expression with altritol-modified siRNAs. Nucleic Acids Research 2007;35:1064–1074. DOI: 10.1093/nar/gkl1126

[46] Bonoiu AC, Mahajan SD, Ding H, Roy I, Yong KT, Kumar R, et al. Nanotechnology approach for drug addiction therapy: gene silencing using delivery of gold nanorod-siRNA nanoplex in dopaminergic neurons. Proceedings of the National Academy of Sciences of United States of America 2009;106:5546–5550. DOI: 10.1073/pnas.0901715106

[47] Lasic DD. Novel applications of liposomes. Trends in Biotechnology 1998;16:307–321. DOI: 10.1016/S0167-7799(98)01220-7

[48] Lavigne C, Slater K, Gajanayaka N, Duguay C, Arnau Peyrotte E, Fortier G, et al. Influence of lipoplex surface charge on siRNA delivery: application to the in vitro downregulation of CXCR4 HIV-1 co-receptor. Expert Opinion on Biological Therapy 2013;13:973–985. DOI: 10.1517/14712598.2013.743526

[49] Sakurai F, Nishioka T, Saito H, Baba T, Okuda A, Matsumoto O, et al. Interaction between DNA-cationic liposome complexes and erythrocytes is an important factor in systemic gene transfer via the intravenous route in mice: the role of the neutral helper lipid. Gene Therapy 2001;8:677–686. DOI: 10.1038/sj.gt.3301460

[50] Kawakami S, Sato A, Nishikawa M, Yamashita F, Hashida M. Mannose receptor-mediated gene transfer into macrophages using novel mannosylated cationic liposomes. Gene Therapy 2000;7:292–299. DOI: 10.1038/sj.gt.3301089

[51] Kang H, DeLong R, Fisher MH, Juliano RL. Tat-conjugated PAMAM dendrimers as delivery agents for antisense and siRNA oligonucleotides. Pharmaceutical Research 2005;22:2099–2106. DOI: 10.1007/s11095-005-8330-5

[52] Liu M, Frechet JM. Designing dendrimers for drug delivery. Pharmaceutical Science & Technology Today 1999;2:393–401.

[53] Tomalia DA, Reyna LA, Svenson S. Dendrimers as multi-purpose nanodevices for oncology drug delivery and diagnostic imaging. Biochemical Society Transactions 2007;35:61–67. DOI: 10.1042/BST0350061

[54] Kaminskas LM, Kelly BD, McLeod VM, Sberna G, Boyd BJ, Owen DJ, et al. Capping methotrexate alpha-carboxyl groups enhances systemic exposure and retains the cytotoxicity of drug conjugated PEGylated polylysine dendrimers. Molecular Pharmaceutics 2011;8:338–349. DOI: 10.1021/mp1001872

[55] Samal SK, Dash M, Van Vlierberghe S, Kaplan DL, Chiellini E, van Blitterswijk C, et al. Cationic polymers and their therapeutic potential. Chemical Society Reviews 2012;41:7147–7194. DOI: 10.1039/c2cs35094g

[56] Wadia JS, Dowdy SF. Transmembrane delivery of protein and peptide drugs by TAT-mediated transduction in the treatment of cancer. Advanced Drug Delivery Reviews 2005;57:579–596. DOI: 10.1016/j.addr.2004.10.005

[57] Elliott G, O'Hare P. Intercellular trafficking and protein delivery by a herpesvirus structural protein. Cell 1997;88:223–233. DOI: 10.1016/S0092-8674(00)81843-7

[58] Morris MC, Vidal P, Chaloin L, Heitz F, Divita G. A new peptide vector for efficient delivery of oligonucleotides into mammalian cells. Nucleic Acids Research 1997;25:2730–2736.

[59] Oehlke J, Scheller A, Wiesner B, Krause E, Beyermann M, Klauschenz E, et al. Cellular uptake of an alpha-helical amphipathic model peptide with the potential to deliver polar compounds into the cell interior non-endocytically. Biochimica et Biophysica Acta 1998;1414:127–139.

[60] Futaki S, Suzuki T, Ohashi W, Yagami T, Tanaka S, Ueda K, et al. Arginine-rich peptides. An abundant source of membrane-permeable peptides having potential as carriers for intracellular protein delivery. Journal of Biological Chemistry 2001;276:5836–5840. DOI: 10.1074/jbc.M007540200

[61] El-Aneed A. An overview of current delivery systems in cancer gene therapy. Journal of Controlled Release 2004;94:1–14. DOI: 10.1016/j.jconrel.2003.09.013

[62] Pack DW, Hoffman AS, Pun S, Stayton PS. Design and development of polymers for gene delivery. Nature Reviews Drug Discovery 2005;4:581–593. DOI: 10.1038/nrd1775

[63] Schiffelers RM, Ansari A, Xu J, Zhou Q, Tang Q, Storm G, et al. Cancer siRNA therapy by tumor selective delivery with ligand-targeted sterically stabilized nanoparticle. Nucleic Acids Research 2004;32:e149. DOI: 10.1093/nar/gnh140

[64] Feng Y, Hu J, Ma J, Feng K, Zhang X, Yang S, et al. RNAi-mediated silencing of VEGF-C inhibits non-small cell lung cancer progression by simultaneously down-regulating the CXCR4, CCR7, VEGFR-2 and VEGFR-3-dependent axes-induced ERK, p38 and AKT signalling pathways. European Journal of Cancer 2011;47:2353–2363. DOI: 10.1016/j.ejca.2011.05.006

[65] Suk JS, Lai SK, Boylan NJ, Dawson MR, Boyle MP, Hanes J. Rapid transport of muco-inert nanoparticles in cystic fibrosis sputum treated with N-acetyl cysteine. Nanomedicine 2011;6:365–375. DOI: 10.2217/nnm.10.123

[66] McNamara JO, 2nd, Andrechek ER, Wang Y, Viles KD, Rempel RE, Gilboa E, et al. Cell type-specific delivery of siRNAs with aptamer-siRNA chimeras. Nature Biotechnology 2006;24:1005–1015. DOI: 10.1038/nbt1223

[67] Grimm D, Streetz KL, Jopling CL, Storm TA, Pandey K, Davis CR, et al. Fatality in mice due to oversaturation of cellular microRNA/short hairpin RNA pathways. Nature 2006;441:537–541. DOI: 10.1038/nature04791

[68] Yi R, Doehle BP, Qin Y, Macara IG, Cullen BR. Overexpression of exportin 5 enhances RNA interference mediated by short hairpin RNAs and microRNAs. RNA 2005;11:220–226. DOI: 10.1261/rna.7233305

[69] Elbashir SM, Harborth J, Lendeckel W, Yalcin A, Weber K, Tuschl T. Duplexes of 21-nucleotide RNAs mediate RNA interference in cultured mammalian cells. Nature 2001;411:494–498. DOI: 10.1038/35078107

[70] Robbins M, Judge A, MacLachlan I. siRNA and innate immunity. Oligonucleotides 2009;19:89–102. DOI: 10.1089/oli.2009.0180

[71] Hornung V, Guenthner-Biller M, Bourquin C, Ablasser A, Schlee M, Uematsu S, et al. Sequence-specific potent induction of IFN-alpha by short interfering RNA in plasmacytoid dendritic cells through TLR7. Nature Medicine 2005;11:263–270. DOI: 10.1038/nm1191

[72] Marques JT, Williams BR. Activation of the mammalian immune system by siRNAs. Nature Biotechnology 2005;23:1399–1405. DOI: 10.1038/nbt1161

[73] Jackson AL, Bartz SR, Schelter J, Kobayashi SV, Burchard J, Mao M, et al. Expression profiling reveals off-target gene regulation by RNAi. Nature Biotechnology 2003;21:635–637. DOI: 10.1038/nbt831

[74] Jackson AL, Burchard J, Leake D, Reynolds A, Schelter J, Guo J, et al. Position-specific chemical modification of siRNAs reduces "off-target" transcript silencing. RNA 2006;12:1197–205. DOI: 10.1261/rna.30706

[75] Lim LP, Lau NC, Garrett-Engele P, Grimson A, Schelter JM, Castle J, et al. Microarray analysis shows that some microRNAs downregulate large numbers of target mRNAs. Nature 2005;433:769–773. DOI: 10.1038/nature03315

[76] Jackson AL, Burchard J, Schelter J, Chau BN, Cleary M, Lim L, et al. Widespread siRNA "off-target" transcript silencing mediated by seed region sequence complementarity. RNA 2006;12:1179–1187. DOI: 10.1261/rna.25706

[77] Miller VM, Paulson HL, Gonzalez-Alegre P. RNA interference in neuroscience: progress and challenges. Cellular and Molecular Neurobiology 2005;25:1195–1207. DOI: 10.1007/s10571-005-8447-4

[78] Stark GR, Kerr IM, Williams BR, Silverman RH, Schreiber RD. How cells respond to interferons. Annual Review of Biochemistry 1998;67:227–264. DOI: 10.1146/annurev.biochem.67.1.227

[79] Heidel JD, Hu S, Liu XF, Triche TJ, Davis ME. Lack of interferon response in animals to naked siRNAs. Nature Biotechnology 2004;22:1579–1582. DOI: 10.1038/nbt1038

[80] Judge AD, Sood V, Shaw JR, Fang D, McClintock K, MacLachlan I. Sequence-dependent stimulation of the mammalian innate immune response by synthetic siRNA. Nature Biotechnology 2005;23:457–462. DOI: 10.1038/nbt1081

[81] Lu PY, Xie F, Woodle MC. In vivo application of RNA interference: from functional genomics to therapeutics. Advances in Genetics 2005;54:117–142. DOI: 10.1016/S0065-2660(05)54006-9

[82] Xie FY, Woodle MC, Lu PY. Harnessing in vivo siRNA delivery for drug discovery and therapeutic development. Drug Discovery Today 2006;11:67–73. DOI: 10.1016/S1359-6446(05)03668-8

[83] Martin SE, Caplen NJ. Applications of RNA interference in mammalian systems. Annual Review of Genomics and Human Genetics 2007;8:81–108. DOI: 10.1146/annurev.genom.8.080706.092424

[84] Pushparaj PN, Melendez AJ. Short interfering RNA (siRNA) as a novel therapeutic. Clinical and Experimental Pharmacology & Physiology 2006;33:504–510. DOI: 10.1111/j.1440-1681.2006.04399.x

[85] Reynolds A, Leake D, Boese Q, Scaringe S, Marshall WS, Khvorova A. Rational siRNA design for RNA interference. Nature Biotechnology 2004;22:326–330. DOI: 10.1038/nbt936

[86] Nishikawa M, Huang L. Nonviral vectors in the new millennium: delivery barriers in gene transfer. Human Gene Therapy 2001;12:861–870. DOI: 10.1089/104303401750195836

[87] Du Q, Thonberg H, Wang J, Wahlestedt C, Liang Z. A systematic analysis of the silencing effects of an active siRNA at all single-nucleotide mismatched target sites. Nucleic Acids Research 2005;33:1671–1677. DOI: 10.1093/nar/gki312

[88] Naito Y, Yamada T, Ui-Tei K, Morishita S, Saigo K. siDirect: highly effective, target-specific siRNA design software for mammalian RNA interference. Nucleic Acids Research 2004;32(Web Server issue):W124–W129. DOI: 10.1093/nar/gkh442

[89] Zufferey R, Dull T, Mandel RJ, Bukovsky A, Quiroz D, Naldini L, et al. Self-inactivating lentivirus vector for safe and efficient in vivo gene delivery. Journal of Virology 1998;72:9873–9880.

[90] Isacson R, Kull B, Salmi P, Wahlestedt C. Lack of efficacy of 'naked' small interfering RNA applied directly to rat brain. Acta Physiologica Scandinavica 2003;179:173–177. DOI: 10.1046/j.1365-201X.2003.01188.x

[91] Thakker DR, Natt F, Husken D, Maier R, Muller M, van der Putten H, et al. Neurochemical and behavioral consequences of widespread gene knockdown in the adult mouse brain by using nonviral RNA interference. Proceedings of the National Academy of Sciences of United States of America 2004;101:17270–17275. DOI: 10.1073/pnas.0406214101

[92] Pardridge WM. Intravenous, non-viral RNAi gene therapy of brain cancer. Expert Opinion on Biological Therapy 2004;4:1103–1113. DOI: 10.1517/14712598.4.7.1103

[93] Hommel JD, Sears RM, Georgescu D, Simmons DL, DiLeone RJ. Local gene knockdown in the brain using viral-mediated RNA interference. Nature Medicine 2003;9:1539–1544. DOI: 10.1038/nm964

[94] Song E, Lee SK, Wang J, Ince N, Ouyang N, Min J, et al. RNA interference targeting Fas protects mice from fulminant hepatitis. Nature Medicine 2003;9:347–351. DOI: 10.1038/nm828

[95] McCaffrey AP, Meuse L, Pham TT, Conklin DS, Hannon GJ, Kay MA. RNA interference in adult mice. Nature 2002;418:38–39. DOI: 10.1038/418038a

[96] Ge Q, Filip L, Bai A, Nguyen T, Eisen HN, Chen J. Inhibition of influenza virus production in virus-infected mice by RNA interference. Proceedings of the National Academy of Sciences of United States of America 2004;101:8676–8681. DOI: 10.1073/pnas.0402486101

[97] Bitko V, Musiyenko A, Shulyayeva O, Barik S. Inhibition of respiratory viruses by nasally administered siRNA. Nature Medicine 2005;11:50–55. DOI: 10.1038/nm1164

[98] Palliser D, Chowdhury D, Wang QY, Lee SJ, Bronson RT, Knipe DM, et al. An siRNA-based microbicide protects mice from lethal herpes simplex virus 2 infection. Nature 2006;439:89–94. DOI: 10.1038/nature04263

[99] Miller VM, Xia H, Marrs GL, Gouvion CM, Lee G, Davidson BL, et al. Allele-specific silencing of dominant disease genes. Proceedings of the National Academy of Sciences of United States of America 2003;100:71957–72000. DOI: 10.1073/pnas.1231012100

[100] Maxwell MM, Pasinelli P, Kazantsev AG, Brown RH, Jr. RNA interference-mediated silencing of mutant superoxide dismutase rescues cyclosporin A-induced death in cultured neuroblastoma cells. Proceedings of the National Academy of Sciences of United States of America 2004;101:3178–3183. DOI: 10.1073/pnas.0308726100

[101] Xia H, Mao Q, Eliason SL, Harper SQ, Martins IH, Orr HT, et al. RNAi suppresses polyglutamine-induced neurodegeneration in a model of spinocerebellar ataxia. Nature Medicine 2004;10:816–820. DOI: 10.1038/nm1076

[102] Xia XG, Zhou H, Zhou S, Yu Y, Wu R, Xu Z. An RNAi strategy for treatment of amyotrophic lateral sclerosis caused by mutant Cu,Zn superoxide dismutase. Journal of Neurochemistry 2005;92:362–367. DOI: 10.1111/j.1471-4159.2004.02860.x

[103] Liu Z, Li S, Liang Z, Zhao Y, Zhang Y, Yang Y, et al. Targeting beta-secretase with RNAi in neural stem cells for Alzheimer's disease therapy. Neural Regeneration Research 2013;8:3095–3106. DOI: 10.3969/j.issn.1673-5374.2013.33.003

[104] Hardy J. Genetic analysis of pathways to Parkinson disease. Neuron 2010;68:201–206. DOI: 10.1016/j.neuron.2010.10.014

[105] Pushparaj PN, Aarthi JJ, Manikandan J, Kumar SD. siRNA, miRNA, and shRNA: in vivo applications. Journal of Dental Research 2008;87:992–1003. DOI: 10.1177/154405910808701109

[106] Keiser MS, Boudreau RL, Davidson BL. Broad therapeutic benefit after RNAi expression vector delivery to deep cerebellar nuclei: implications for spinocerebellar ataxia type 1 therapy. Molecular Therapy 2014;22:588–595. DOI: 10.1038/mt.2013.279

[107] Gonzalez-Alegre P, Miller VM, Davidson BL, Paulson HL. Toward therapy for DYT1 dystonia: allele-specific silencing of mutant TorsinA. Annals of Neurology 2003;53:781–787. DOI: 10.1002/ana.10548

[108] White MD, Mallucci GR. RNAi for the treatment of prion disease: a window for intervention in neurodegeneration? CNS & Neurological Disorders – Drug Targets 2009;8:342–352.

[109] Kong Q. RNAi: a novel strategy for the treatment of prion diseases. Journal of Clinical Investigation 2006;116:3101–3103. DOI: 10.1172/JCI30663

[110] White MD, Farmer M, Mirabile I, Brandner S, Collinge J, Mallucci GR. Single treatment with RNAi against prion protein rescues early neuronal dysfunction and prolongs survival in mice with prion disease. Proceedings of the National Academy of

Sciences of United States of America 2008;105:10238–10243. DOI: 10.1073/pnas.0802759105

[111] Caughey B, Caughey WS, Kocisko DA, Lee KS, Silveira JR, Morrey JD. Prions and transmissible spongiform encephalopathy (TSE) chemotherapeutics: a common mechanism for anti-TSE compounds? Accounts of Chemical Research 2006;39:646–653. DOI: 10.1021/ar050068p

[112] Rider TH, Zook CE, Boettcher TL, Wick ST, Pancoast JS, Zusman BD. Broad-spectrum antiviral therapeutics. PLoS One 2011;6:e22572. DOI: 10.1371/journal.pone.0022572

[113] Boado RJ. Blood-brain barrier transport of non-viral gene and RNAi therapeutics. Pharmaceutical Research 2007;24:1772–1787. DOI: 10.1007/s11095-007-9321-5

[114] Harper SQ, Staber PD, He X, Eliason SL, Martins IH, Mao Q, et al. RNA interference improves motor and neuropathological abnormalities in a Huntington's disease mouse model. Proceedings of the National Academy of Sciences of United States of America 2005;102:5820–5825. DOI: 10.1073/pnas.0501507102

[115] Wang YL, Liu W, Wada E, Murata M, Wada K, Kanazawa I. Clinico-pathological rescue of a model mouse of Huntington's disease by siRNA. Neuroscience Research 2005;53:241–249. DOI: 10.1016/j.neures.2005.06.021

[116] Rodriguez-Lebron E, Denovan-Wright EM, Nash K, Lewin AS, Mandel RJ. Intrastriatal rAAV-mediated delivery of anti-huntingtin shRNAs induces partial reversal of disease progression in R6/1 Huntington's disease transgenic mice. Molecular Therapy 2005;12:618–633. DOI: 10.1016/j.ymthe.2005.05.006

[117] Drouet V, Perrin V, Hassig R, Dufour N, Auregan G, Alves S, et al. Sustained effects of nonallele-specific Huntingtin silencing. Annals of Neurology 2009;65:276–285. DOI: 10.1002/ana.21569

[118] DiFiglia M, Sena-Esteves M, Chase K, Sapp E, Pfister E, Sass M, et al. Therapeutic silencing of mutant huntingtin with siRNA attenuates striatal and cortical neuropathology and behavioral deficits. Proceedings of the National Academy of Sciences of United States of America 2007;104:17204–17209. DOI: 10.1073/pnas.0708285104

[119] Bennett CF, Swayze EE. RNA targeting therapeutics: molecular mechanisms of antisense oligonucleotides as a therapeutic platform. Annual Review of Pharmacology and Toxicology 2010;50:259–293. DOI: 10.1146/annurev.pharmtox.010909.105654

[120] Southwell AL, Ko J, Patterson PH. Intrabody gene therapy ameliorates motor, cognitive, and neuropathological symptoms in multiple mouse models of Huntington's disease. Journal of Neuroscience: The Official Journal of the Society for Neuroscience 2009;29:13589–13602. DOI: 10.1523/JNEUROSCI.4286-09.2009

[121] Southwell AL, Khoshnan A, Dunn DE, Bugg CW, Lo DC, Patterson PH. Intrabodies binding the proline-rich domains of mutant huntingtin increase its turnover and re-

duce neurotoxicity. Journal of Neuroscience: The Official Journal of the Society for Neuroscience 2008;28:9013–9020. DOI: 10.1523/JNEUROSCI.2747-08.2008

[122] Pfister EL, Kennington L, Straubhaar J, Wagh S, Liu W, DiFiglia M, et al. Five siRNAs targeting three SNPs may provide therapy for three-quarters of Huntington's disease patients. Current Biology 2009;19:774–778. DOI: 10.1016/j.cub.2009.03.030

[123] Davidson BL, Paulson HL. Molecular medicine for the brain: silencing of disease genes with RNA interference. Lancet Neurology 2004;3:145–149. DOI: 10.1016/S1474-4422(04)00678-7

[124] Garami A, Zwartkruis FJ, Nobukuni T, Joaquin M, Roccio M, Stocker H, et al. Insulin activation of Rheb, a mediator of mTOR/S6K/4E-BP signaling, is inhibited by TSC1 and 2. Molecular Cell 2003;11:1457–1466. DOI: 10.1016/S1097-2765(03)00220-X

[125] Fahn S, Bressman SB, Marsden CD. Classification of dystonia. Advances in Neurology 1998;78:1–10.

[126] Abdelgany A, Wood M, Beeson D. Allele-specific silencing of a pathogenic mutant acetylcholine receptor subunit by RNA interference. Human Molecular Genetics 2003;12:2637–2644. DOI: 10.1093/hmg/ddg280

[127] Jin P, Zarnescu DC, Ceman S, Nakamoto M, Mowrey J, Jongens TA, et al. Biochemical and genetic interaction between the fragile X mental retardation protein and the microRNA pathway. Nature Neuroscience 2004;7:113–117. DOI: 10.1038/nn1174

[128] Jin P, Alisch RS, Warren ST. RNA and microRNAs in fragile X mental retardation. Nature Cell Biology 2004;6:1048–1053. DOI: 10.1038/ncb1104-1048

[129] Caudy AA, Myers M, Hannon GJ, Hammond SM. Fragile X-related protein and VIG associate with the RNA interference machinery. Genes & Development 2002;16:2491–2496. DOI: 10.1101/gad.1025202

[130] Hardy J, Selkoe DJ. The amyloid hypothesis of Alzheimer's disease: progress and problems on the road to therapeutics. Science 2002;297:353–356. DOI: 10.1126/science.1072994

[131] Miller VM, Gouvion CM, Davidson BL, Paulson HL. Targeting Alzheimer's disease genes with RNA interference: an efficient strategy for silencing mutant alleles. Nucleic Acids Research 2004;32:661–668. DOI: 10.1093/nar/gkh208

[132] Kao SC, Krichevsky AM, Kosik KS, Tsai LH. BACE1 suppression by RNA interference in primary cortical neurons. Journal of Biological Chemistry 2004;279:1942–1949. DOI: 10.1074/jbc.M309219200

[133] Lipton RB, Dodick DW. CGRP antagonists in the acute treatment of migraine. Lancet Neurology 2004;3:332. DOI: 10.1016/S1474-4422(04)00764-1

[134] Ralph GS, Radcliffe PA, Day DM, Carthy JM, Leroux MA, Lee DC, et al. Silencing mutant SOD1 using RNAi protects against neurodegeneration and extends survival in an ALS model. Nature Medicine 2005;11:429–433. DOI: 10.1038/nm1205

[135] Halliday GM, McCann H. The progression of pathology in Parkinson's disease. Annals of the New York Academy of Sciences 2010;1184:188–195. DOI: 10.1111/j.1749-6632.2009.05118.x

[136] Spillantini MG, Schmidt ML, Lee VM, Trojanowski JQ, Jakes R, Goedert M. Alpha-synuclein in Lewy bodies. Nature 1997;388:839–840. DOI: 10.1038/42166

[137] Sapru MK, Yates JW, Hogan S, Jiang L, Halter J, Bohn MC. Silencing of human alpha-synuclein in vitro and in rat brain using lentiviral-mediated RNAi. Experimental Neurology 2006;198:382–390. DOI: 10.1016/j.expneurol.2005.12.024

[138] Gorbatyuk OS, Li S, Nash K, Gorbatyuk M, Lewin AS, Sullivan LF, et al. In vivo RNAi-mediated alpha-synuclein silencing induces nigrostriatal degeneration. Molecular Therapy 2010;18(8):1450–1457. DOI: 10.1038/mt.2010.115

[139] Angaji SA, Hedayati SS, Poor RH, Madani S, Poor SS, Panahi S. Application of RNA interference in treating human diseases. Journal of Genetics 2010;89:527–537.

[140] Mattson MP. Apoptosis in neurodegenerative disorders. Nature Reviews Molecular Cell Biology 2000;1:120–129. DOI: 10.1038/35040009

[141] Zhao ZQ, Vinten-Johansen J. Myocardial apoptosis and ischemic preconditioning. Cardiovascular Research 2002;55:438–455. DOI: 10.1016/S0008-6363(02)00442-X

[142] Reddy KS. India wakes up to the threat of cardiovascular diseases. Journal of the American College of Cardiology 2007;50:1370–1372. DOI: 10.1016/j.jacc.2007.04.097

[143] Kim DH, Rossi JJ. Strategies for silencing human disease using RNA interference. Nature Reviews Genetics 2007;8:173–184. DOI: 10.1038/nrg2006

[144] Michiue H, Eguchi A, Scadeng M, Dowdy SF. Induction of in vivo synthetic lethal RNAi responses to treat glioblastoma. Cancer Biology & Therapy 2009;8:2306–2313.

[145] Pai SI, Lin YY, Macaes B, Meneshian A, Hung CF, Wu TC. Prospects of RNA interference therapy for cancer. Gene Therapy 2006;13:464–477. DOI: 10.1038/sj.gt.3302694

[146] Shi Y, Tian Y, Zhou YQ, Ju JY, Qu L, Chen SL, et al. Inhibition of malignant activities of nasopharyngeal carcinoma cells with high expression of CD44 by siRNA. Oncology Reports 2007;18:397–403.

[147] Dickerson EB, Blackburn WH, Smith MH, Kapa LB, Lyon LA, McDonald JF. Chemosensitization of cancer cells by siRNA using targeted nanogel delivery. BMC Cancer 2010;10:10. DOI: 10.1186/1471-2407-10-10

[148] Ofek P, Fischer W, Calderon M, Haag R, Satchi-Fainaro R. In vivo delivery of small interfering RNA to tumors and their vasculature by novel dendritic nanocarriers. FASEB Journal 2010;24:3122–3134. DOI: 10.1096/fj.09-149641

[149] Dai B, Fang B, Roth JA. RNAi-induced synthetic lethality in cancer therapy. Cancer Biology & Therapy 2009;8:2314–2316.

[150] Hartwell LH, Szankasi P, Roberts CJ, Murray AW, Friend SH. Integrating genetic approaches into the discovery of anticancer drugs. Science 1997;278:1064–1068. DOI: 10.1126/science.278.5340.1064

[151] Luo J, Emanuele MJ, Li D, Creighton CJ, Schlabach MR, Westbrook TF, et al. A genome-wide RNAi screen identifies multiple synthetic lethal interactions with the Ras oncogene. Cell 2009;137:835–848. DOI: 10.1016/j.cell.2009.02.024

[152] Scholl C, Frohling S, Dunn IF, Schinzel AC, Barbie DA, Kim SY, et al. Synthetic lethal interaction between oncogenic KRAS dependency and STK33 suppression in human cancer cells. Cell 2009;137:821–834. DOI: 10.1016/j.cell.2009.03.017

[153] Hulleman E, Helin K. Molecular mechanisms in gliomagenesis. Advances in Cancer Research 2005;94:1–27. DOI: 10.1016/S0065-230X(05)94001-3

[154] Gump JM, Dowdy SF. TAT transduction: the molecular mechanism and therapeutic prospects. Trends in Molecular Medicine 2007;13:443–438. DOI: 10.1016/j.molmed.2007.08.002

[155] Prochiantz A. Protein and peptide transduction, twenty years later a happy birthday. Advanced Drug Delivery Reviews 2008;60:448–451. DOI: 10.1016/j.addr.2007.08.040

Chapter 9

RNAi-based Gene Therapy for Blood Genetic Diseases

Mengyu Hu, Qiankun Ni, Yuxia Yang and Jianyuan Luo

Additional information is available at the end of the chapter

http://dx.doi.org/10.5772/61644

Abstract

Therapies for blood genetic diseases can be divided into different categories, including chemotherapy, radiotherapy, gene therapy, and hematopoietic stem cell transplantation. Among these treatments, gene targeting is progressively becoming a therapeutic alternative that offers the possibility of a permanent cure for certain blood genetic diseases. In recent years, gene therapy has played a more important role in curing genetic blood disorders. RNA interference (RNAi) is one of the directions for gene therapy, which was intensively studied in the past decades for its potentials in the treatment of diseases. In order to provide useful references and prospective directions for further studies concerning RNAi-based gene therapy for blood genetic diseases, current RNAi-based gene therapies for several typical blood genetic diseases have been summarized and discussed in this chapter.

Keywords: RNA interference, gene therapy, mechanism, therapeutic strategy, blood genetic diseases

1. Introduction

Conceived in the 1960s, gene therapy did not produce any meaningful results until recent reports of success appeared in clinical studies. Gene therapy attempts to treat inherited diseases using normal copies of the defective genes. Insertion and expression of specific exogenous genetic materials via the transfer of nucleic acids directly *in vivo*, or through modified cells *in vitro*, correct a cellular dysfunction or provide a new cellular function. It has the potential to cure any genetic disease with long-lasting therapeutic benefits [1, 2]. Gene therapy can be classified into (i) germ line and (ii) somatic line gene therapy types. In the former, genomes of germ cells (sperms or eggs) are integrated by exogenous functional genes, which can be carried onto the patient's offsprings. In the latter, therapeutic genes are introduced into somatic cells and the effects will only be limited to the individual patient [3].

According to the mechanisms, gene therapy may include three major categories: (a) direct modulation of the disease-causing gene, which can be applied to monogenic hereditary diseases; (b) indirect treatment through gene modulation, which can be applied to multifactorial diseases; and (c) immunotherapy by gene modulation (DNA vaccines), which leads to the synthesis of the relevant antigen or an adjuvant [1].

RNA interference (RNAi) can be used for gene therapy. It was intensively studied in the past few decades for its potential in the treatment of blood genetic diseases. RNAi-based gene therapy possesses several therapeutic advantages such as high efficiency, sequence specificity, and potentially less immunogenicity. Less immunogenicity is largely due to the use of non-protein-coding "gene products" to trigger RNAi, which makes gene therapy less likely to be potentially hampered by the host immune system [4, 5]. Compared to traditional small molecules and protein drugs, the target specificity and universal treatment spectrum make RNAi-based gene therapy an ideal treatment for blood genetic diseases. However, there are still obstacles that remain, such as barriers in the blood circulation system and the diseased tissues that block the actualization of the RNAi effects [6]. RNAi technology is a relatively new discovery, and it has already become a potent method for gene regulation. In order to provide useful references and prospective directions for further studies, current RNAi-based gene therapies for blood genetic diseases have been summarized and discussed in this chapter.

2. The mechanism of RNAi-based gene therapy

Being a well-described gene regulatory mechanism, RNAi not only suppresses transcription by transcriptional gene silencing (TGS) but also activates a homology-based mRNA degradation process by post-transcriptional gene silencing (PTGS). Both silencing pathways resulted in the decrease of the coding transcript level (mRNA) [7]. We will focus on PTGS due to its important role in RNAi-based gene therapy. Two distinct mechanisms regulate PTGS. The first one is the repression and degradation of mRNAs with imperfect complementarity. Endogenous microRNAs (miRNAs) belong to this category. They induce translational repression and mRNA degradation when the guide (antisense) strand has limited complementarity to the target mRNA. The second one is the sequence-specific cleavage of perfectly complementary mRNAs. Exogenous small interfering RNAs (siRNAs) or short hairpin RNAs (shRNAs) belong to this category. They have perfect or near-perfect base-pairings with the intended target mRNA. The miRNAs production and processing rely on host machinery that is guided by complementary miRNA strands to the target mRNA [8, 9]. During the process, double-stranded RNAs (dsRNA) of the target gene are produced and then processed into 21–24 non-coding small RNA duplexes with the help of RNaseIII enzyme dicer and its homologs. These siRNAs are then incorporated into a multi-subunit endonuclease silencing complex called RNA-induced silencing complex (RISC). siRNAs are associated with the defense against parasites, heterochromatin formation, transposon and transgene silencing, and PTGS. These siRNAs, loaded into the RISC, are used as the guide to recognize and degrade or suppress the complementary gene or mRNA utilizing the endonucleases activity of RISC. Gene silencing by RNAi can be used in different biological situations when sequence-specific knockdown of

http://dx.doi.org/10.5772/61644

gene expression is required, thus providing a convenient tool for analysis of gene function as well as gene therapy [10, 11, 12].

Recent reports have shown that off-targeting can commonly occur during RNAi, despite the belief that initial gene silencing through RNAi was thought to be specific. Because nonspecific hybridization of siRNAs with non-target transcripts can induce undesired effects, it should be guaranteed that the dsRNA and corresponding siRNA sequences do not exert off-target effects that negatively influence host physiology. Off-target silencing is determined by the similarity of sequences between siRNA and non-target genes, or mRNA sequences not selected for RNAi, as well as the size of siRNA and transitive RNAi. Thus, off-targeting effects can be avoided by using highly specific sequences in siRNA expressed under specific and inducible promoters. In addition, it is important to examine the off-targeting effects of RNAi at multiple levels, since undesired effects on the host may occur through the silencing of genes associated with regulatory functions and multiple metabolic pathways, such as transcription factors or signaling molecules [10].

3. RNAi-based gene therapy for blood genetic diseases

3.1. Blood diseases

Blood diseases refer to the disorders in the hematopoietic system or plasma components. The development of blood disorders is always thought to be related with inheritance, the environment, drugs, and biological factors where the changes in chromosome and/or genes play a critical role in some specific hemopathies. Therapeutic approaches for blood diseases can be divided into different categories, including chemotherapy, radiotherapy, RNAi-based gene therapy, and hematopoietic stem cell transplantation. Among these, RNAi-based gene therapy is progressively becoming a therapeutic alternative which offers the possibility of a permanent cure for some blood diseases [13].

3.2. Hemophilia

Hemophilia A and B are X-linked monogenic bleeding disorders resulting from deficiencies of factor VIII and IX, respectively. Gene therapy, utilizing both viral and non-viral delivery vectors *in vivo* and *ex vivo*, has been attempted for the treatment of both hemophilia A and B [14, 15]. Given its recent clinical success, adeno-associated vector (AAV)-mediated hepatic gene transfer could be primarily used for the treatment of hemophilia B. However, a number of problems, such as current immunosuppressive regimen and pre-existing neutralizing antibodies, limit the broad applicability of this approach. For hemophilia A, while AAV-mediated gene therapy has potential, a number of limitations reduce its desirability, such as packaging capacity and inefficient expression. While a number of transgene modifications have increased the expression levels, the vector doses require the corrective F.VIII expression to remain significantly higher than the F.IX. These expression limitations lead to further concerns about immune responses to both the capsid and, if expression levels are not sufficient, the transgene. As such, *ex vivo* gene transfer may be more effective for hemophilia A due to its ability to enhance expression through cellular division. While a number of promising gene therapies for hemophilia have been elucidated, there are clearly numerous problems that still need to be addressed to develop approved gene therapies, especially RNAi, for both hemophilia A and B in humans [16]. RNAi-based gene therapy for hemophilia is still in its early stages of development.

3.3. β-Thalassemia

The globin chains have an extremely precise structure, ensuring their function of loading, delivering, and unloading oxygen. The globin chains are coded by genes in the chromosome 16 (α-gene) and 11(β-gene). The normal structure of globin is based on the balanced match between α-chains and β-chains. When the condition is not met, there will be a complete or partial defect in one or both allelic globin genes, such as β-thalassemia [17]. β-Thalassemia is a worldwide-distributed inherited hemoglobin disorder resulting in severe, chronic anemia [18, 19]. It is a heterozygous condition in which only a single β-globin gene is affected and results in the absence or reduced β-globin chain synthesis. The defects of β-globin synthesis lead to an excess of unmatched α-globin, which release free iron, non-heme iron, or hemichrome. These iron species promote a severe red cell membrane oxidative stress and lead to abnormal β-thalassemic red cell features. The abnormal red cells are finally removed by the macrophage system and results in anemia [20, 21].

Blood transfusion is a primary way to treat the most severe forms of β-thalassemia. Appropriate goals and optimal safety of transfused blood are necessary for routine administration of red blood cells to patients. The problem is that the high frequency of blood transfusion can lead to iron overload. In its less severe form, chronic transfusions are not required, but iron overload may still develop due to the chronic suppression of the synthesis of the iron regulatory hormone hepcidin by ineffective erythropoiesis. Untreated iron overload can be fatal, resulting in cardiac complications [3, 22]. Therefore, handling iron overload is a key factor for the successful treatment of this disease. TMPRSS6, a serine protease expressed predominantly in the liver, can inhibit an iron-responsive bone morphogenetic protein-mother against the decapentaplegic (BMP-SMAD) signaling pathway, resulting in the downregulation of hepcidin transcription. Researchers found that therapeutics with the lipid nanoparticle (LNP)-formulated RNAi targeting of TMPRSS6, in conjunction with oral deferiprone therapy, is superior to monotherapy with dietary iron deficiency and iron chelate for reducing hepatic iron storage [22].

3.4. B-lineage lymphoid malignancies

B-precursor acute lymphoblastic leukemia (BPL) is the most common form of cancer in children and adolescents. A dysfunctional CD22 is expressed in BPL cells due to the deletion of Exon 12 (CD22ΔE12) resulting from a splicing defect related to homozygous intronic mutations. CD22 is a negative regulator of multiple signal transduction pathways critical for the proliferation and survival of B-lineage lymphoid cells, and CD22ΔE12 leads to uncontrolled proliferation and the survival of B cells. Recently, researchers have found that CD22ΔE12 is especially associated with therapy-refractory clones in pediatric BPL, thus implicating the impact of the CD22ΔE12 genetic defect on the aggressive biology of relapsed or therapy-refractory pediatric BPL. At the same time, forced expression of CD22ΔE12 in transgenic mice causes fatal BPL, demonstrating that CD22ΔE12 alone is sufficient as an oncogenic driver lesion for malignant transformation and clonal expansion of B-cell precursors [23].

Recent studies have demonstrated that B-lineage lymphoid malignancies in children and adults are characterized by a high incidence of the CD22ΔE12 genetic alterations. Moreover, the relationship between CD22ΔE12 and aggressive biology of BPL cells is also reported through the demonstration that siRNA-mediated knockdown of CD22ΔE12 in primary BPL cells is associated with a remarkable inhibition of their carcinogenicity. A unique polypeptide-based nanoparticle formulation of CD22ΔE12-siRNA is described as a first-in-class RNAi therapeutic candidate targeting of CD22ΔE12. This formulation is capable of delivering siRNA cargo into the cytoplasm of leukemia cells, leading to a remarkable inhibition of leukemic cell growth [24]. It is expected that further development of this nanoparticle may promote an effective therapeutic RNAi strategy of aggressive or chemotherapy-resistant B-lineage lymphoid malignancies [23].

3.5. Myeloid leukemia

Leukemia arising from genetic alterations in normal hematopoietic stem or progenitor cells results in the impaired regulation of proliferation, differentiation, and apoptosis, as well as the survival of malignant cells. Overall, the relative 5-year survival rate for various leukemias is only around 50% [25]. Leukemia is still a worldwide health problem, although various therapies have been explored to cure the disease. Among them, chemotherapy is always considered to be a frontline treatment, mainly containing a broad spectrum of cytotoxic agents and therapeutic molecules. Although leukemic cells respond well to chemotherapy at the onset of treatment, over a period of 6–12 months the drugs might lose effectiveness in a considerable fraction of patients. Moreover, significant side effects of traditional cytotoxic agents are inevitable at efficacious doses, which limit its function with the progression of the disease. For example, in chronic myeloid leukemia (CML), resistance to current frontline therapy of imatinib and failure to a complete cytogenetic response may occur in 24% of patients within 18 months. With a better understanding of molecular changes in leukemia, the treatment targeting tumor-specific changes, such as RNAi, is expected to make a difference in the therapeutic effectiveness of the disease [26].

Researchers have explored the suitability of RNAi in suppressing the growth and proliferation of myeloid leukemia cell lines including HL-60, U937, THP-1, and K562, which express c-raf and bcl-2 genes. The results were exciting, as the siRNA duplexes succeeded in significantly decreasing the level of target proteins by eliminating the expression of c-raf and bcl-2 genes. This led to the inhibition of the differentiation and programmed cell death suppression of myeloid leukemia cells. These results demonstrated the possibility of RNAi as a novel therapeutic approach to myeloid leukemia [27]. In recent years, based on the molecular alteration of CML, two clinical trials of RNAi therapy have been conducted to target the aberrantly expressed isoforms of the BCR-ABL fusion protein. In one case, there are no publishable outcomes. In the other case, silencing aberrant proteins with RNAi have been found to be less prone to drug resistance [28]. In another *in vivo* application of targeted and non-virally delivered synthetic bcr-abl siRNA, a remarkable apoptosis of CML cells was found in a female patient with a recurrent Philadelphia chromosome with positive CML. The patient was resistant to imatinib and chemotherapy after hematopoietic stem cell transplantation. There were no clinically adverse events, implying feasibility and safety of the application of RNAi-based gene therapy for CML [29].

Furthermore, RNAi-based gene therapy also proves to be effective in acute promyelocytic leukemia (APL). APL is the M3 type of acute myeloid leukemia characterized by a clonal proliferation of abnormal promyelocytes in bone marrow and has a severe bleeding tendency. In 98% of APL patients, a balanced translocation between chromosomes 15 and 17 [t(15;17)(q22;q21)] was found, which leads to the formation and fusion of promelocytic leukemia protein (PML) and retinoic acid receptor alpha (RARα) [30, 31]. A variety of chromosomal aberrations have been identified in APL including t(11;17)(q23;q21), t(5;17)(q35;q12-21), t(11;17)(q13;q21), and der(17), in which the RARα gene is fused to the PLZF, NPM, NuMA, and STAT5b genes, respectively [32]. The differentiation of leukemic cells and complete remission of APL may occur after treatment with ATRA (all-trans retinoic acid). However, the alternative strategies of specific targeting of APL are required because of the ATRA resistance in patients with PLZF-RARα fusion mutation and a treatment of relapse. It has been found that the siRNA targeted knockdown of fused PML-RARα mRNA can induce differentiation and apoptosis of human APL cells; moreover, an injection of pretreated APL cells with anti-PML-RARα siRNA greatly inhibits the progression of APL in mice. Therefore, a targeted RNAi for PML-RARα fusion might be a promising treatment strategy for ATRA-resistant APL patients [33].

At present, several technological requirements and mechanistic challenges (i.e., targeted delivery of siRNAs) for efficient clinical trials have to be explored and overcome to make RNAi-based gene therapy readily applicable for the treatment of myeloid leukemia [26].

3.6. Multiple myeloma

Multiple myeloma (MM) of clonal plasma cells in bone marrow can cause damage to multiple organs. MM is the second most common hematological malignancy. Chromosomal abnormalities, oncogene activation, and growth factor dysregulation contribute to the development of MM. Like leukemia, chemotherapy is the most common treatment for MM right now. However, it is remarkably resistant to chemotherapy [34]. Molecular therapy became an alternative treatment, and the introduction of bortezomib has contributed to the improved survival of patients with MM. Resistance to this therapy inevitably occurs, and the clinical efficacy of bortezomib is significantly diminished. At present, RNAi is found to be helpful in sensitizing tumor cells to chemotherapy and radiation. Bmi-1, an oncogene, has been implicated in the pathogenesis of MM and might influence the response to bortezomib in MM patients. Bmi-1 has been silenced in two MM cell lines using shRNA targeting Bmi-1 (shBmi-1). The cell cycle progression and apoptosis of MM cells are evaluated. The prolonged G1 phase and enhanced apoptosis were observed that suggest RNAi-derived knockdown of Bmi-1 reducing the resistance to bortezomib. Therefore, Bmi-1-specific RNAi may serve as an important treatment strategy for MM [35].

4. Conclusions and future perspectives

As a powerful and novel treatment of blood genetic diseases, RNAi-based gene therapy has propelled the clinical testing of siRNAs for a variety of diseases at early stages. It is still too early to determine whether the RNAi-based therapeutics will be an efficient tool for the treatment of blood genetic diseases. Therefore, understanding the basic mechanisms of a targeted gene RNAi and its interconnection with genetic, biochemical, and physiological pathways, as well as "off-targets" and "side effects," are the most important factor for developing an efficient therapeutic RNAi strategy. It is highly possible that the RNAi-based gene therapy can be readily and efficiently used for clinical treatment in conjunction with other therapies. The power of sequence-specific suppression of gene expression without "off-targets" and undesired side effects makes RNAi-based gene therapy very promising. Although progress has been made [36], major obstacles, such as the development of methods for efficient targeted delivery of siRNAs in patients, still remain a critical task. In addition, uncovering target domains of genes related to blood genetic diseases and the discovery of more blood genetic disease-causing genes are also key research areas for developing RNAi-based gene therapy for important blood genetic diseases.

Acknowledgements

This study was supported by the Natural Science Foundation of Beijing [5122022].

Author details

Mengyu Hu[1 #], Qiankun Ni[1 #], Yuxia Yang[1*] and Jianyuan Luo[1,2*]

*Address all correspondence to: JLuo@som.umaryland.edu; yangyx@bjmu.edu.cn

1 Department of Medical Genetics, Peking University Health Science Center, Beijing, China

2 Department of Medical & Research Technology, School of Medicine, University of Maryland, Baltimore, USA

[#] These authors contributed equally.

References

[1] Linden R, Matte U. A snapshot of gene therapy in Latin America. Genet Mol Biol. 2014; 37(1 Suppl): 294–98.

[2] Chodisetty S, Nelson EJ. Gene therapy in India: A focus. J Biosci. 2014; 39: 537–41.

[3] Razi Soofiyani S, Baradaran B, Lotfipour F, Kazemi T, Mohammadnejad L. Gene therapy, early promises, subsequent problems, and recent breakthroughs. Adv Pharm Bull. 2013; 3: 249–55. DOI: 10.5681/apb

[4] Liu J, Harper SQ. RNAi-based gene therapy for dominant limb girdle muscular dystrophies. Curr Gene Ther. 2012; 12: 307–14. DOI:

[5] Liu J, Wallace LM, Garwick-Coppens SE, Sloboda DD, Davis CS, Hakim CH, Hauser MA, Brooks SV, Mendell JR, Harper SQ. RNAi-mediated gene silencing of mutant myotilin improves myopathy in LGMD1A mice. Nucleic Acids. 2014; 3: e160. DOI: 10.1038/mtna

[6] Zhou Y, Zhang C, Liang W. Development of RNAi technology for targeted therapy — a track of siRNA based agents to RNAi therapeutics. J Controll Release. 2014; 193: 270–81. DOI: 10.1016/j.jconrel

[7] Castanotto D, Rossi JJ. The promises and pitfalls of RNA-interference-based therapeutics. Nature. 2009; 457: 426-33. DOI: 10.1038/nature07758

[8] Burnett JC, Rossi JJ. RNA-based therapeutics: current progress and future prospects. Chem Biol. 2012; 19: 60-71. DOI: 10.1016/j.chembiol

[9] Kim D, Rossi J. RNAi mechanisms and applications. Biotechniques. 2008; 44: 613-6. DOI: 10.2144/000112792

[10] Kola VS, Renuka P, Madhav MS, Mangrauthia SK. Key enzyme and protein of crop insects as candidate for RNAi based gene silencing. Front Physiol. 2015; 6: 119. DOI: 10.3389/fphys

[11] Presloid JB, Novella IS. RNA viruses and RNAi: quasispecies implications for viral escape. Viruses. 2015; 7: 3226–40. DOI: 10.3390/v7062768

[12] Makkonen KE, Airenne K, Ylä-Herttulala S. Baculovirus-mediated gene delivery and RNAi applications. Viruses. 2015; 7: 2099–25. DOI: 10.3390/v7042099

[13] Porada CD, Stem C, Almeida-Porada G. Gene therapy: the promise of a permanent cure. N C Med J. 2013; 74: 526–9.

[14] Kay MA, Manno CS, Ragni MV, Larson PJ, Couto LB, McClelland A, Glader B, Chew AJ, Tai SJ, Herzog RW, Arruda V, Johnson F, Scallan C, Skarsgard E, Flake AW, High KA. Evidence for gene transfer and expression of factor IX in haemophilia B patients treated with an AAV vector. Nat Genet. 2000; 24: 257–61.

[15] Manno CS, Pierce GF, Arruda VR, Glader B, Ragni M, Rasko JJ, Ozelo MC, Hoots K, Blatt P, Konkle B, Dake M, Kaye R, Razavi M, Zajko A, Zehnder J, Rustagi PK, Nakai H, Chew A, Leonard D, Wright JF, Lessard RR, Sommer JM, Tigges M, Sabatino D, Luk A, Jiang H, Mingozzi F, Couto L, Ertl HC, High KA, Kay MA. Successful trans-

duction of liver in hemophilia by AAV-factor IX and limitations imposed by the host immune response. Nat Genet. 2006; 12: 342–7.

[16] Rogers GL, Herzog RW. Gene therapy for hemophilia. Front Biosci (Landmark Ed). 2015; 20: 556–603.

[17] Meo A, Cassinerio E, Castelli R, Bignamini D, Perego L, Cappellini MD. Effect of hydroxyurea on extramedullary haematopoiesis in thalassaemia intermedia: case reports and literature review. Int J Lab Hematol. 2008; 30: 425–31. DOI: 10.1111/j. 1751-553

[18] Parthasarathy V. A search for beta thalassemia trait in India. Turk J Haematol. 2012; 29: 427–9. DOI: 10.5505/tjh.2012.21703

[19] Hagag AA, Elfrargy MS, Gazar RA, El-Lateef AE. Therapeutic value of combined therapy with deferasirox and silymarin on iron overload in children with Beta thalassemia. Mediterr J Hematol Infect Dis. 2013; 5: e2013065. DOI: 10.4084/MJHID

[20] Kalpravidh RW, Tangjaidee T, Hatairaktham S, Charoensakdi R, Panichkul N, Siritanaratkul N, Fucharoen S. Glutathione redox system in beta-thalassemia/Hb E patients. Sci World J. 2013; 7: 543973. DOI: 10.1155/2013/543973

[21] De Franceschi L, Bertoldi M, Matte A, Santos Franco S, Pantaleo A, Ferru E, Turrini F. Oxidative stress and beta-thalassemic erythroid cells behind the molecular defect. Oxid Med Cell Longev, 2013; 985210. DOI: 10.1155/2013/985210

[22] Schmidt PJ, Racie T, Westerman M, Fitzgerald K, Butler JS, Fleming MD. Combination therapy with a *Tmprss6* RNAi-therapeutic and the oral iron chelator deferiprone additively diminishes secondary iron overload in a mouse model of β-thalassemia intermedia. Exp Toxicol Pathol. 2015; 90: 310–3. DOI: 10.1002/ajh.23934

[23] Uckun FM, Qazi S, Ma H, Yin L, Cheng J. A rationally designed nanoparticle for RNA interference therapy in B-lineage lymphoid malignancies. EBioMedicine. 2014; 1: 141–55.

[24] Uckun FM, Ma H, Cheng J, Myers DE, Qazi S. CD22ΔE12 as a molecular target for RNAi therapy. Br J Haematol. 2015; 169: 401–14. DOI: 10.1111/bjh.13306

[25] National Cancer Institute Surveillance Research Program. Fast Stats: An interactive tool for access to SEER cancer statistics. 2013. Available from: http://seer.cancer.gov/faststats [Accessed: 2013-02-02]

[26] Landry B, Valencia-Serna J, Gul-Uludag H, Jiang X, Janowska-Wieczorek A, Brandwein J, Uludag H. Progress in RNAi-mediated molecular therapy of acute and chronic myeloid leukemia. Mol Ther Nucleic Acids. 2015; 12: 4:e240. DOI: 10.1038/mtna

[27] Cioca DP, Aoki Y, Kiyosawa K. RNA interference is a functional pathway with therapeutic potential in human myeloid leukemia cell lines. Cancer Gene Ther. 2003; 10: 125–33.

[28] Sawyers CL. Perspective: combined forces. Nature. 2013; 498:S7. DOI: 10.1038/498S7a

[29] Koldehoff M. Targeting bcr-abl transcripts with siRNAs in an imatinib-resistant chronic myeloid leukemia patient: challenges and future directions. Methods Mol Biol. 2015; 1218: 277–92. DOI: 10.1007/978-1-4939-1538-5_17

[30] Marchwicka A, Cebrat M, Sampath P, Snieżewski L, Marcinkowska E. Perspectives of differentiation therapies of acute myeloid leukemia: the search for the molecular basis of patients' variable responses to 1,25-dihydroxyvitamin D and vitamin D analogs. Front Oncol. 2014; 4: 125. DOI: 10.3389/fonc.2014.00125

[31] Zhou GB, Zhang J, Wang ZY, Chen SJ, Chen Z. Treatment of acute promyelocytic leukaemia with all-trans retinoic acid and arsenic trioxide: a paradigm of synergistic molecular targeting therapy. Philos Trans R Soc Lond B Biol Sci. 2007; 362: 959–71.

[32] Pagnano KB, Rego EM, Rohr S, Chauffaille Mde L, Jacomo RH, Bittencourt R, Firmato AB, Fagundes EM, Melo RA, Bernardo W. Guidelines on the diagnosis and treatment for acute promyelocytic leukemia: Associacao Brasileira de Hematologia, Hemoterapia e Terapia Celular Guidelines Project: Associacao Medica Brasileira-2013. Rev Bras Hematol Hemoter. 2014; 36: 71–92. DOI: 10.5581/1516-8484.20140018

[33] Guo J, Cahill MR, McKenna SL, O'Driscoll CM. Biomimetic nanoparticles for siRNA delivery in the treatment of leukaemia. Biotechnol Adv. 2014; 32: 1396–409. DOI: 10.1016/j.biotechadv

[34] Mutlu P, Kiraz Y, Gündüz U, Baran Y. An update on molecular biology and drug resistance mechanisms of multiple myeloma. Crit Rev Oncol Hematol. 2015; S1040-8428: 30003-2. DOI: 10.1016/j.critrevonc

[35] Wu SQ, Xu ZZ, Niu WY, Huang HB, Zhan R. ShRNA-mediated Bmi-1 silencing sensitizes multiple myeloma cells to bortezomib. Int J Mol Med. 2014; 34: 616–23. DOI: 10.3892/ijmm.2014.1798

[36] Tiemann K, Rossi JJ. RNAi-based therapeutics–current status, challenges and prospects. EMBO Mol Med. 2009; 1: 142–51. DOI: 10.1002/emmm.200900023

Chapter 10

Non-viral siRNA and shRNA Delivery Systems in Cancer Therapy

Emine Şalva, Ceyda Ekentok, Suna Özbaş Turan and Jülide Akbuğa

Additional information is available at the end of the chapter

http://dx.doi.org/10.5772/62826

Abstract

RNA interference represents a promising therapeutic strategy for the silencing of specific target genes in cancer therapy. Small interfering RNAs and DNA-based vectors encoding short hairpin RNAs provide sequence-specific post-transcriptional gene silencing by binding to its complementary RNA. For the therapeutic use of siRNA in cancer, efficient intracellular delivery is necessary. The efficient cancer therapy with RNAi is not still accomplished because of internalization and intracellular trafficking problems such as low transfection efficiency, enzyme degradation, inappropriate subcellular localization, and endosomal trapping of siRNAs in cells. Cancer is a complex disease including multiple genes and pathways. The most important benefits of siRNA therapy are high target specificity and non-toxicity compared with chemotherapy. The uptake of siRNA by cells without a carrier system is possible, but naked siRNA is mostly degraded with nucleases and activates the immune responses. Development of appropriate delivery systems is an important issue in the use of siRNA-based therapeutics. Non-viral delivery systems have great potential for safe and effective delivery of siRNA therapeutics to tumor cells. Nanocarriers such as nanoplexes, lipoplexes, nanoparticles, and liposomes have been commonly used for siRNA delivery. This chapter highlights the importance of non-viral delivery systems *in vitro* and *in vivo* cancer therapy.

Keywords: Cancer, non-viral vectors, RNAi, siRNA, shRNA

1. Introduction

RNA interference (RNAi) is a conserved endogenous cellular process for post-transcriptional regulation in sequence-specific gene silencing. The regulatory RNA molecules include small interfering RNAs (siRNAs), and short hairpin RNAs (shRNAs) provide the specific degradation of target mRNA in mammalian cells [1]. siRNAs are the products of long double-stranded

RNA (dsRNA) molecules in cells, which are expressed transgenically or delivered exogenously. Synthetic siRNAs can be transfected into cells that specifically silence the expression of target genes. In the RNAi pathway, dsRNA (over 100 nt) molecules are cleaved into 21- to 23-nucleotide duplexed RNAs, termed as siRNA duplex, by endoribonuclease Dicer or RNAse III-type enzyme. The cleaved siRNA duplexes contain 5′-phosphate and two-base 3′ overhangs. siRNAs are incorporated into the endogenous RNA-induced silencing complex (RISC). One of the two strands of siRNA duplex is guide (antisense) strand, and the other is passenger (sense) strand. siRNA duplex is unwinded by RNA helicase activity. While the guide strand binds to the RISC, the passenger strand is degraded. The activated RISC binds to mRNA with base-pairing for sequence-specific degradation of complementary mRNA. The mRNA fragments cleaved by Argonaute (Ago) proteins are released from RISC and degraded by other endogenous nucleases. After mRNA degradation, the active RISC is rebuilt and can participate in another RNAi pathway [2, 3]. In the event, RNAi process decreases specific mRNA levels, and thus decreases target gene expression.

Among the nucleic acid–based drugs, siRNAs as potential novel drug candidates are offered a highly promising strategy in cancer therapy. The knockdown of abnormal gene overexpression, occuring in cancer by using siRNA, has been used in therapeutic applications [2]. Targets of chemical drugs are limited to certain classes of receptors, ion channels, and enzymes. In the treatment with siRNA, known sequence of any gene of interest is sufficient and its target choice is unlimited [4].

The potential advantages of siRNA treatment compared with other treatment methods are that siRNAs [5–7] (i) provide sequence-specific gene therapy; (ii) can specifically target many undruggable genes or downregulate gene products; (iii) are considered the safe therapeutics; (iv) are potent and efficient molecules and possess high gene silencing activity; and (iv) can be easily designed for any disease.

RNAi might be a promising new pharmaceutical area for treatment of incurable and severe diseases such as cancers and infections. RNAi applications have been recently achieved by using synthetic siRNAs and vector-based siRNA expression systems or short hairpin RNAs (shRNAs) synthesized within the cells by vector-mediated production. The expressed shRNAs from plasmid and viral vectors in nucleus are cleaved by Dicer in cytoplasm and siRNAs are formed. There both strategies have advantages and disadvantages. Vector-based siRNA expression systems have several advantages for applying RNAi compared to synthetic siRNAs. Both permanent and transient transfection with vector-based systems can be achieved, and thus vector-based system increases the period of siRNA-mediated inhibition of gene expression [8]. In addition, shRNA constructs are more stable than siRNAs [9]. Low amount (nM) of siRNA and less than five copies of shRNA are sufficient for stable transfection and for acheiving gene silencing effect [10]. The synthetic siRNAs can be easily synthesized in large amounts and chemically modified to improve stability, permeability, efficacy, and transfection control; however, the modified siRNAs are highly expensive [11]. siRNAs are not integrated into host genome. The modification of vector-based shRNA systems is difficult, but shRNA expression systems can be regulated or induced by appropriate promoters and termination sequences. Choice of promoter, loop structure of shRNA, length and arrangement of sense and antisense strands, and orientation of restriction enzyme regions are important for shRNA expression cassette preparation. Similar to the various RNAi applications for targeted gene silencing, the chimeric expression cassettes of siRNA and shRNA in the same expression unit might also be made [12].

Design of optimal siRNA sequence plays a key role for successful siRNA therapy. The choice of potent and specific siRNA sequences is important for minimization of immune responses and off-target effects. siRNAs are 19–27 base pairs in length, but mostly preferred to be 21 nt of siRNAs with a structure of 19 nt duplex region and two nucleotide overhangs at the 3′ end, usually TT and UU, which are important for recognition by the RNAi machinery. Increasing the length of the dsRNA may enhance its potency, dsRNAs with 27 nucleotides are up to 100 times more potent than the siRNAs containing 21 nucleotides. The longer (25–30 nt) duplexes act as a substrate for Dicer (Dicer-subtrate siRNAs). This Dicer-substrate siRNAs are more efficiently loaded into the RISC over the siRNAs with 21 bp and newly produced siRNAs from the long dsRNAs directly incorporated into the RISC complex. Thus, gene silencing mechanism can be facilitated [13, 14]. On the other hand, dsRNAs longer than about 30 bp can lead to interferon response, which is the defense mechanism against viral infection. The activation of interferon pathway causes non-specific mRNA degradation and apoptosis [15, 16]. The long dsRNAs activates innate immune response by interaction with protein kinase receptor (PKR) and Toll-like receptors (TLR7 and 8 are activated by ssRNA; TLR9 activated by unmethylated CpG; and TLR3 activated by dsRNA). The activation of these receptors induces interferon (IFN) and proinflammatory cytokines [10, 17].

In addition to immune responses, another important problem for efficient RNAi therapy is off-target effects of these molecules. The cause of off-target effects are the suppression of undesired or unpredicted genes other than the desired target genes. The absence of homolog sequences between siRNA and its target mRNA can cause cleavage of non-targeted mRNA regions. Off-target effects of siRNA can lead to problems in the interpretation of gene silencing studies, serious and unwanted side effects such as potential toxicity and even cell death [18]. There are many factors and mechanisms leading to occurence of off-target effects. These factors are the length of dsRNA or siRNA, the length and position of siRNA-target sequence mismatch, and coding sequences and untranslated regions in genes [19]. The mechanisms leading to off-target effects of siRNAs are (i) the regulation of unwanted transcripts by seed sequence homology to the 3′ UTR of cellular mRNAs, (ii) the saturation of RISC by affecting cellular miRNA activity of siRNAs in large amounts, (iii) the function of miRNAs as siRNAs or shRNAs because of similarities in gene silencing pathway, (iv) non-specific distribution by non-targeting systemic delivery, and (v) immunostimulatory motifs in siRNA sequences [14, 17, 20].

Many preclinical studies with siRNA indicated that it is a hopeful molecule for clinical research of various diseases. Up to date, at least 22 RNAi-based drugs have been evaluated in clinical trials [21]. The first clinical trial with siRNA was made in 2004 by Opko Health. The clinical studies of Bevasiranib, that is, siRNA targeting vascular endothelial growth factor (VEGF) to suppress ocular neovascularization in patients with age-related macular degeneration (AMD), continued to the phase III trial, but the clinical trials was terminated in 2009 because of its poor efficacy and causing vision loss. Allergan company has terminated the phase II clinical trials of siRNA AGN-745, targeting VEGF because of its off-target effects [21]. The clinical translation of RNAi can be possible with development of safe and efficient RNAi delivery systems that lack of off-target effects [7, 21].

Although siRNAs are used as the potential therapeutic molecules in cancer and other diseases, the most important challenge in the development of RNAi-based drugs is efficient and safe delivery of appropriate doses to target cells and tissues. Therefore, the development of siRNA-based viral and non-viral delivery systems are required to have an enhanced efficacy, improved stability, and minimized non-specific gene silencing such as off-target effects and immune responses. This chapter focuses on recent improvements in the non-viral siRNA delivery systems in cancer therapy.

2. RNAi in cancer therapy

Cancer is a multistep genetic disease, which develops as a consequence of changes in the control of cell proliferation and differentiation. In the transformation of normal cells to tumor cells, the affected cells undergo mutations such as downregulation of tumor suppressor genes and overexpression of oncogenes. RNAi-based therapeutics have been extensively used for knockdown of cancer-associated genes. The *in vitro* and *in vivo* studies with siRNA and shRNA have shown that silencing of genes related to tumor cell growth, invasion, angiogenesis, metastasis, and chemoresistance in various types of cancer [17]. RNAi technology, as a new approach for cancer therapeutics, offers many advantages over conventional cancer treatment strategies. Advantages of gene silencing by siRNA and shRNA are the high degree of specificity to target tumor cells and tissues, a capacity to inhibit target gene expression, a simple and rapid design, and synthesis [22]. While non-specific chemotherapy leads to death of cancer cells, it significantly damages the surrounding healthy tissues and organs, causing extensive systemic toxicity. The side-effects of chemotherapeutic drugs can be minimized with siRNA treatment.

Cancer cells have the ability to develop a resistance to chemotherapeutic drugs. RNAi-based therapeutics can simultaneously target multiple genes in cancer signaling pathway. The simultaneous silencing of multiple genes in cancer therapy have importance in terms of minimizing the multiple drug resistance caused by small chemical molecules given in high dose [23, 24]. This therapy inhibits survival signals and pathways that take part in the development of multi-drug resistance in cancer cells.

Oncogenes, mutated tumor supressor genes, survival and apoptotic genes, causing tumor initiation and progression, are major targets for RNAi-based therapy. Simultaneous suppression of one target gene or multiple genes has provided a significant advantage in cancer therapy. siRNAs can be designed for effective gene knockdown by targeting any gene or multiple genes in cells [25]. siRNAs are likely to be more effective than other antisense approaches because of many properties such as a highly specific mRNA degradation, cell-to-cell spreading of gene silencing effect, long silencing activity, improved stability *in vivo*, and their efficiency in lower concentrations [26, 27]. A single therapeutic strategy is insufficient for the inhibition of cancer growth and progression; RNAi as a new therapeutic strategy may be used as well as with chemotherapy, immunotherapy, anti-hormone therapy, and radiotherapy for achieving synergistic therapeutic effect.

In clinical trials, the most of siRNAs have been given by local administration. When siRNAs are delivered to target tissue locally, lower siRNA doses can be used for pharmacologic effect (e.g., saline-based formulation, or excipiants such as 5% dextrose) and any drug delivery approaches (e.g., liposome, nanoparticle, and complexes) [28]. However, systemic drug administration by intravenous injection is required for cancer diseases [7]. In systemic effect, siRNAs must encounter several extra- and intra-cellular barriers until it reaches the target cell and tissue. siRNAs cannot freely cross physiological and cellular barriers because of their high molecular weight and negative charge. The significant challenges of using siRNA are their poor cellular uptake, degradation by serum nucleases, and rapid elimination. These factors and barriers reduce therapeutic effect of siRNA. Therefore, efficient *in vitro* and *in vivo* delivery of siRNA-based therapeutics in cancer is dependent on the development of appropriate delivery systems. siRNA delivery systems should (a) protect siRNAs against degradation enzymes and serum proteins, (b) prolong the circulation time of siRNA, (c) provide siRNA stability in blood serum, (d) avoid sequestration in the reticuloendothelial system (RES), (e) avoid aggregation in serum, (f) minimize non-specific tissue and cellular uptake, (g) achieve target-specific siRNA delivery, (h) allow for immune evasion, (i) resist rapid renal clearance, (j) enhance vascular permeability to reach cancer tissues, (k) promote trafficking to the cytoplasm and uptake into RISC, and (l) have low or non-toxicity [7, 29, 30].

3. Delivery strategies of RNAi-based therapeutics

siRNAs have large molecular weight (~13 kDa) and are polyanionic nature (~40 negative phosphate charge) and are easily degraded by enzymes in cells, tissues, and bloodstream. In addition, siRNAs cannot easily cross the cell membrane [29]. The naked siRNAs are readily degraded by serum endonucleases. The half-life of circulating naked siRNA is less than 10 minutes because of its rapid clearance by the kidneys, so that they cannot reach to target cell efficiently. The gene silencing activity of unmodified or uncomplexed siRNAs is little or absent [31]. To solve this problem, two strategies are used: chemical modifications and conjugation of siRNA molecules or use of gene delivery systems for increasing efficiency of RNAi-based therapeutics.

Chemical modification is the major approach to overcome *in vivo* siRNA delivery problems. Chemical modifications of naked siRNAs have been performed to (i) enhance siRNA stability, (ii) protect siRNA from degradation, (iii) avoid recognition by the innate immune system and minimize immunostimulatory responses, (iv) minimize off-target effects, (v) reduce required dose for gene silencing, (vi) improve pharmacodynamic properties, (vii) increase delivery to target cells, and (viii) allow the delivery by systemic administration. The sugar, backbone and nucleobase modifications of siRNA, can significantly protect siRNA in both serum and cytoplasm. The commonly used chemical siRNA modifications are the incorporation of locked nucleic acids (LNA), phosphorothioate linkages, and 2′-o-methyl, 2′-amine, 2′-fluoro groups [7, 32, 33]. Chemical modifications must increase the stability of siRNA without affecting its gene silencing activity [23]. However, these substitutions may lead to off-target effects, cytotoxicity, reduced RNAi activity, and impaired biological activity [17, 34].

Other chemical strategies for siRNA are cholesterol, folate, and aptamer conjugation and peptide modification. siRNAs can associate with aptamers, ligands, and antibodies by electrostatic interaction or direct conjugation. The conjugation of these functional groups provides cell- or tissue-specific targeting and efficient delivery. As a result, the efficacy of silencing can be increased [1].

Viral and non-viral vectors have been extensively used in the siRNA-based therapy. Viral vectors encoding shRNA have a high gene transduction and gene silencing effects. Adeno-associated viral vectors, lentiviral vectors, and adenoviral vectors have been extensively used in gene knockdown studies [35]. The transfering of shRNA-encoding vectors into the nucleus of cells have obtained high and long-term shRNA expression. In addition, viral vectors can integrate the host genome [14]. Although viral vectors have a high gene transfection efficiency, the challenges such as inflammatory reactions, strong immunogenicity, insertional mutagenesis, and oncogenic transformation of viral vectors can cause important safety concerns. In addition, some viral vectors have low capacity for transgene insertion. To overcome these problems, non-viral vectors have been developed and used in siRNA delivery. Compared to viral vectors, non-viral vectors have several advantages such as lack of immunogenicity, low or no integration into genome, large-scale production, and use of wide variety of nucleic acids size [36]. However, the transfection efficiency of non-viral vectors is not as high as the viral vectors.

3.1. Non-viral vectors

The non-viral delivery of siRNA and shRNA therapeutics to target tumor cells is a multi-step process. To achieve efficient delivery and therapeutic gene silencing, siRNAs should be stable in biological fluids and must have above mentioned properties [37, 38]. The circulating siRNAs after systemic administration must be evaded from the reticuloendothelial system (RES). Negatively charged siRNAs gain the positive charge after complexed with cationic charged polymers. This positive charge facilitates cellular internalization of siRNAs; however, the cationic charge increase non-specific interactions by non-target cells, negatively charged serum proteins, and extracellular matrix. As a consequence of these non-specific interactions, clot-like accumulations or aggregations are formed. Complexes are entrapped in the endothelial capillary bed or taken up by RES recognition. While RES organs such as spleen, liver, and bone marrow uptake the major part of injected dose, the minor part of this reaches to tumors [25, 37, 39].

Non-viral delivery vectors prolong the biological half-life and mean residence time of siRNA, and they enhance accumulation of siRNA molecules in tumor tissues. siRNA therapeutics can be accumulated into cancer tissue by enhanced permeability and retention (EPR) effect as a result of discontinuous vasculature (permeation) and poor lymphatic drainage (retention) in the abnormal tumor blood vessels compared to the normal blood vessels. Tumor endothelium allows penetration of macromolecules [37, 38].

The other challanges of RNAi-based therapeutics delivery to the tumor tissues after systemic circulation are crossing of cellular membrane, intracellular traffic into the cells with endosomal/lysosomal compartments, release of siRNA or shRNA from carriers, and nuclear transport for vector-based siRNA/shRNA therapeutics and entry to cytoplasm for siRNA-based therapeutics. The cell membrane is an important extracellular barrier for siRNA uptake. The average size of a single siRNA molecule is less than 10 nm. Despite their small size, polyanionic nature and hydrophilicity of siRNA make crossing of biological membranes difficult [18]. To overcome this problem, the complexation of negatively charged siRNA with cationic polymers or lipids are performed. The net positive charge of this formulations facilitates binding to negatively charged cell membranes, following internalization by adsorptive pinocytosis. For cell-type specific delivery, targeting ligands, antibodies, and aptamer-binding non-viral vectors pass through the cell membrane by receptor-mediated endocytosis [1]. After crossing from the cell membrane, siRNAs and vector-based siRNAs/shRNAs encounter several intracellular barriers that include the endosomal trafficking, unpackaging of siRNA, and nuclear traffic. The intracellular traffic of endosomal content is important for succesful siRNA delivery. When siRNA released from the carrier reaches cytosol, RNAi mechanism is induced inside the cells. However, for the onset of RNAi effect, transfer of vector-based siRNA/shRNA to the nucleus is required. In the delivery process, early release of siRNA from endosome is required. If siRNA remains inside the endosome for long time, it will be degraded. Therefore, different agents (fusogenic protein) conjugated with polymers disrupt the endosomal membrane. In addition, polymers possess proton-sponge effect (polyethyleneimine, PEI), which have been used to induce osmotic swelling and subsequent disruption of the endosome [15].

3.1.1. Polymer-based RNAi delivery system in cancer therapy

Negatively charged siRNAs or shRNAs can readily bind to cationic polymers or load to the nanocarriers by ionic interactions. Nanosized complexes or polyplexes by electrostatic interactions and nanoparticle formulations by encapsulation have been developed for efficient siRNA/shRNA delivery. Thus, siRNAs can be protected from nuclease attack and cellular uptake of siRNAs via endocytic pathway faciliated. Many natural and synthetic polymers are used for gene delivery, such as polyethyleneimine (PEI), poly-l-lysine (PLL), chitosan, protamine, gelatin, atelocollagen, cationic polypeptides, cyclodextran polymers, dendrimers, poly-lactide-co-glycolide (PLGA), and polydimethylaminoethylmethacrylate (PDMAEMA) [34]. In addition, polyethyleneglycol (PEG) is widely used as a linker between polymer and ligand or nucleic acid or for binding of siRNA onto nanocarrier surface [40].

3.1.1.1. Chitosan

Among the non-viral vectors, chitosan or its derivatives are attractive where chitosan has been shown to be biodegradable, biocompatible, non-toxic, mucoadhesive, and non-inflammatory and has low cost of production. Chitosan is a cationic polysaccharide, consisting of *N*-acetyl-d-glucosamine and d-glucosamine units. In addition, chitosan has been designated as "Generally Recognized As Safe (GRAS)" by the FDA [41]. It has been widely used in *in vivo* siRNA and shRNA delivery applications because of positively charged amines, allowing electrostatic interactions with negatively charged nucleic acids to form stable complexes. The protonated amine groups allow transportation to cellular membranes and subsequent endocytosis into cells. Moreover, the high amounts of chitosan in siRNA complexes may lead to increase cellular accumulation of siRNA molecules and facilitate release of siRNA from endosomes to cytosol under high osmotic pressure in the endosomes of cells [42].

Chitosan-based nanocarriers are prepared by three different methods. These include simple complexation, ionic gelation (siRNA entrapment), and adsorption of siRNA onto the surface of chitosan nanoparticles [42]. The molecular weight and degree of deacetylation of chitosan influence its solubility, hydrophobicity, charge density, and thus the interaction ability with nucleic acids. The N/P ratio (ratio between chitosan nitrogen per siRNA phosphate) of chitosan/siRNA nanoplexes is an important factor for optimization of complex properties (size and zeta potential), transfection, and gene silencing efficiency. Increasing the N/P ratio not only helps to obtain a high transfection efficiency but also enhances toxicity. The excess of free chitosan in the formulations can interact with cell membrane and cellular process, and thus, may reduce cell viability [41].

Chitosan has a great potential in siRNA-based cancer therapy studies, because it can be safely and efficiently delivered to cancer cells. It is reported that chitosan or modified chitosan nanoplexes and nanoparticles as delivery system exerted antitumoral effects in different cancers [43–48].

Studies with chitosan formulations in different cancers

Howard et al. [43] developed chitosan nanoparticles using polyelectrolyte complexation method. The size of nanoparticles was between 40 and 600 nm. The endogenous enhanced green fluorescent protein (EGFP) silencing efficiency with nanoparticles was found to be 77.9 and 89.3% in human lung carcinoma cells (H1299) and murine peritoneal macrophages. The siRNA/chitosan nanoparticles reduced EGFP expression (43%) compared to untreated control in transgenic EGFP mice. They suggested that this chitosan-based system can be used in the treatment of systemic and mucosal diseases.

Salva and Akbuga [44] studied silencing effect of chitosan/*VEGF* shRNA nanoplexes in breast cancer cell lines. A significant *VEGF* gene silencing (60%) was obtained after nanoplexes application in MCF-7 cells. Salva et al. [44, 45] demonstrated the successful application of chitosan/siRNA or shRNA *VEGF* nanoplexes in *in vivo* breast cancer models. After intratumoral and intraperitoneal injection, comparison was made and higher tumor inhibition was obtained with intratumoral injection. qRT-PCR and Western Blot analysis showed that *VEGF* mRNA and protein expression was significantly reduced by chitosan nanoplexes.

Salva et al. [46] also studied the IL-4 encoded plasmid (pIL-4) to improve the therapeutic efficacy of siRNA targeting *VEGF* because of the anti-angiogenic effect of IL-4 molecule. Researchers prepared chitosan nanoparticles containing shRNA *VEGF* and pIL-4, and they have reported that co-delivery of shRNA *VEGF* and pIL-4 into chitosan nanoparticles caused additive effect on breast tumor cell growth in rat model (97% inhibition) [46].

In another study, Salva et al. [47] obtained enhanced silencing effect by using siRNAs targeting to *VEGF* and *HIF-1α* in different breast cancer cell lines such as MCF-7, MDA-MB-231, and MDA-MB-435. Two siRNAs were encapsulated into liposome coated with chitosan, and the co-delivery of siRNA *VEGF* and *HIF-1α* into liposomal form have significantly inhibited *VEGF* (89%) and the *HIF-1α* (62%) [47].

Yang et al. [48] reported that chitosan/siRNA *VEGF* nanoparticles prepared by complex coacervation method showed spherical morphology with a mean diameter of 110–200 nm and positively charged surface (20 mV). Chitosan nanoparticles were effectively transfected to mouse melanoma cells (B16-F10), and they have investigated 40% of the *VEGF* gene silencing efficiency in cells without any cytotoxicity.

Wang et al. [49] prepared the chitosan-TPP (tripolyphosphate) nanoparticles by ionic gelation method for the delivery of shRNA expressing vector to the human rhabdomyosarcoma (RD) cell line and for the inhibition of *TGF-β1* expression. Suppression of *TGF-β1* gene by chitosan nanoparticles containing shRNA has resulted in decrease of RD cell growth *in vitro* and tumorigenicity in nude mice.

Huang et al. [50] studied the effect of chitosan/shRNA *VEGF* nanocomplexes on angiogenesis and tumor growth in hepatocellular carcinoma (HCC). The administration of low molecular weight chitosan/shRNA *VEGF* complexes by intratumoral or intravenous injection demonstrated more effective suppression of tumor angiogenesis and tumor growth in the different HCC models. They showed that LMWC could effectively deliver shRNA into tumor tissue. shRNA *VEGF* concentrations in tumor tissue dramatically increased after intravenous administration of chitosan/shRNA *VEGF* complexes.

Studies with chitosan derivatives and conjugation with other polymers and ligands in different cancers

In order to increase the transfection efficiency of chitosan, different modifications are made on the structure of chitosan. Modified forms of chitosan such as carboxymethyl or trimethyl chitosan, trisaccharide-substituted chitosan oligomers, and succinated or galactosylated chitosan are formed. Chitosan is also conjugated with folic acid or PEG [51].

Jere et al. [52] used chitosan-graft-polyethylenimine (CHI-g-PEI) copolymer for delivery of shRNA *Akt1* expressing plasmid in lung cancer cells. The formed complexes were silenced *Akt1* onco-protein and significantly reduced the survival, proliferation, and growth progression of lung cancer cell. *Akt1* silencing induced apoptosis in cancer cells. The suppression of *Akt1* oncoprotein decreased A549 cell malignancy and metastasis. The therapeutic efficiency of CHI-g-PEI-shRNA *Akt* was found higher than PEI25K-shRNA *Akt* compared to carrier.

Noh et al. [53] prepared a copolymer containing additional cationic moieties linked with chitosan to enhance the cationic charge of chitosan. Therefore, chitosan derivation with poly-l-arginine (PLR) and polyethyleneglycol (PEG) (PLR-grafted CS) polyplexes were used for *in vitro* and *in vivo* delivery of siRNA *RFP*. PLR alone can be cytotoxic, thus conjugation of PLR to chitosan both decreased cytotoxicity of PLR and enhanced siRNA delivery efficiency. The pegylation of cationic polymers reduces the charge of polymers and limits the interaction with cell membranes. PEG-CS-PLR did not significantly reduce the cellular delivery of siRNA. Three intratumoral injections of 120 μg of PEG-CS-PLR/siRNA *RFP* complexes to B16F10-RFP tumor-bearing mice had decreased *RFP* expression at 90% level in tumor tissues. It is indicated that PEG-CS-PLR can be a useful carrier for delivery of oncogene-specific siRNAs.

Fernandes et al. [54] investigated folate conjugation to improve gene transfection efficiency of chitosan. When chitosan was conjugated with folate, the folate-chitosan-siRNA complexes have increased gene silencing efficiency because of promoted uptake in HeLa and OV-3 cell lines, which are known to have high folate receptor expression. Higher transfection efficiency and lower toxicity of folate-chitosan complexes are reported in folate receptor–positive cells.

Cell penetrating peptide-based systems may improve cellular uptake and gene silencing efficiency of siRNAs without side effects. Protamine is a cationic, non-toxic polypeptide that has membrane translocation and nuclear localization activities because of its arginine-rich amino acid sequences. In addition to its stabilization enhancing properties, protamine is known to exhibit cell penetrating activity and is an important compound for several cancer targeting systems [55].

Salva et al. [46] have developed ternary nanoplexes of chitosan/protamine/siRNA targeting *VEGF* in breast cancer cell lines for efficient siRNA uptake and inhibition effect. Ternary nanoplexes showed the highest cellular uptake than binary nanoplexes.

Erdem-Cakmak et al. [56] reported that addition of protamine to chitosan complexes increased the silencing of *VEGF* genes after using chitosan/shRNA/protamine nanoplexes. In terms of the gene silencing and transfection, when the molecular weight of chitosans were compared at the different cell lines including HEK293, HeLa, and MCF-7, low molecular weight chitosan (70 kDa) proved more efficient than medium molecular weight chitosan. Gene inhibition values in cell lines after transfection of binary and ternary complexes followed the rank HEK293>HeLa>MCF-7. In addition, any cytotoxicity was not found after the complexes.

Song et al. [57] used protamine/antibody fusion protein to deliver siRNAs targeting *c-my*, *MDM2*, and *VEGF* specifically to HIV envelope-expressing B16 melanoma cells and envelope-expressing subcutaneous B16 tumors. The positively charged protamine served as binding partner for negatively charged siRNA and showed cell internalization and release of the siRNA cargo. The antibody-protamine delivery system can target siRNA specifically to cells.

Choi et al. [58] reported that complexes prepared with low molecular weight protamine (LMWP) inhibited cell growth by suppressing *VEGF* expression in hepatocarcinoma cancer cells. In tumor tissues, the expression of *VEGF* was inhibited through the systemic application of peptide complex, thereby suppressing tumor growth.

3.1.1.2. Polyethylenimine

Polyethylenimines (PEIs) are water-soluble cationic synthetic polymers. They can be synthesized in different lengths and different molecular weights such as branched (bPEI) or linear (lPEI) and low molecular weight (<1000 Da) or high molecular weight (>1000 kDa). PEI has a high cationic charge density because of the protonation of its primary, secondary, and tertiary amine groups positioned at every third nitrogen [59]. While in linear PEI all nitrogen atoms are protonable, in the branched form, two-thirds of nitrogens can be charged. PEI can lead to proton accumulation in endosome, which was brought in by endosomal ATPase with an influx of chloride anion. Proton accumulation in endolysosome counteracts pH decrease, inhibits nucleases and unbalances endosome osmolarity depend on CI concentration and results in osmotic swelling of endosome. This effect of PEI is named as "proton sponge effect". PEI may enhance intracellular delivery by facilitating endosomal escape and induce lysosomal distruption, endosomal release, and DNA/siRNA protection from lysosomal degradation by buffering endosomes [60].

The molecular weight of PEI is important in the development of gene delivery and level of cytotoxicity in cells. The high molecular weight PEI has higher transfection efficiency than low molecular weight PEIs. PEI has a high electrostatic capacity, which can provide strong electrostatic interactions with the siRNA and contribute to cell membrane binding and internalization. Especially, the 25 kDa bPEI is one of the most effective non-viral vectors in gene silencing because of efficient endosomal escape. However, the high positive charge of bPEI leads to severe cytotoxicity and non-specific interactions with serum proteins [61, 62]. The cytotoxicity of PEIs can be decreased with modification of free amine groups or conjugation of cell binding and targeting ligands. Therefore, graft copolymers have been usually preferred as a delivery system.

Schiffelers et al. [63] prepared PEGylated PEI nanoplexes with Arg-Gly-Asp (RGD) peptide ligand containing siRNA targeting *VEGFR-2* and investigated the effect of angiogenesis and tumor growth in tumor-bearing mice. This study indicated that nanoplexes containing siRNA *VEGFR-2* reached tumor tissues after systemic administration. This delivery system has sequence-specific inhibition effect and reduced the tumor growth.

Jiang et al. [64] studied anti-*VEGF* siRNA/PEI-HA complex prepared by PEI-hyaluronic acid (PEI-HA). Complexes at the dose of 4.5 μg of siRNA/mouse were applied intratumorally to C57BL/6 mice by daily injection for 3 days. At 24 hours post-injection, the siRNA *VEGF* formulations were distributed mainly in the tumor, spleen, lung, heart, liver, and kidney. This study suggested that siRNA *VEGF*/PEI-HA complexes can be used for the treatment of cancer in the tissues having HA receptors such as the liver and kidney.

Park et al. [61] synthesized siRNA/(PEI-SS)-b-HA complexes and, after characterization, applied to *in vitro* and *in vivo* gene silencing for target-specific tumor treatment. This delivery system demonstrated an excellent *in vitro* gene silencing efficiency (50–80%). siRNA *VEGF*/(PEI-SS)-b-HA complexes were administrated intratumorally to colorectal tumor bearing mice every 3 days. After the treatment of tumor, *VEGF* gene silencing and reduction in tumor growth were seen.

3.1.2. Other non-viral delivery systems

Among cationic polymers, poly (l-Lysine) (PLL) is one of the mostly studied polymers used for nucleic acid delivery. It formed complexes with DNA smaller than 100 nm. Its complexes can target different cells after binding suitable ligands. PLL can be easily produced in large scale and is physiologically stable and biosafe [65]. PLL may protect siRNA from degradation effect of nucleases. However, PLL has some hurdless that impade its clinical application. PLL does not have the proton buffering ability to enhance lysosomal release of transported siRNA. It can be modified also by addition of ligands [66].

The ternary copolymer mPEG-b-PLL-g(ss-IPEI) was used for siRNA delivery to SKOV-3 ovarian cancer treatment. Nanocomplexes were administered to SKOV-3-implated Balb/c mice and tumor growth inhibition was observed [67].

Dendrimers are highly branched spherical and synthetic multifunctional macromolecules. The surface functional groups of dendrimers can be modified to enhance biocompatibility and decrease toxicity. Polycationic dendrimers such as poly(amidoamine) (PAMAM) and poly(propyleneimine) (PPI) dendrimers, because of the high density of positive charges on the surface, are highly attractive for delivery of negatively charged pDNA, antisense oligonucleotide (AsODN), and siRNAs. PAMAM dendrimers have primary amine groups on their surface and tertiary amine groups inside. Their amine groups are complexed with siRNAs. Thus, compact structure promote cellular uptake of siRNA and tertiary amine groups initiate the proton sponge effect to enhance endosomal release of siRNA [68, 69].

Waite et al. [70] conjugated cationic PAMAM dendrimers with RGD targeting peptides to enhance the delivery efficiency of siRNA to glioma cells. They suggested a promising strategy of RGD-conjugated dendrimers for siRNA delivery to solid tumors.

Liu et al. [71] investigated *in vitro* characterization and anticancer effect of PAMAM dendrimer-mediated shRNA against human telomerase reverse transcriptase (*hTERT*) in oral cancer. Dendriplexes had 110 nm size and +30 mV zeta potential which were favorable parameters for escape from the vasculature and intracellular delivery. shRNA *hTERT* dendriplexes were applied by intratumoral administration to tumors. Dendrimer-mediated shRNA *TERT* resulted in cell growth inhibition and apoptosis *in vitro* and tumor growth inhibition *in vivo* in the xenograft model. In addition, expression of *HTERT* and *PCNA* proteins was reduced in tumors.

Atelocollagen, which is produced from bovine type I collagen, has biomaterial properties such as high biocompatibility, biodegredability, and low immunogenicity. Atelocollagen forms a helix of three polypeptide chains and has positive charge, which enable its binding to nucleic acid molecules [72]. At low temperature, atelocollagen exists in liquid form (2–10°C), therefore, it can be easily mixed with nucleic acid solutions [72, 73]. Thus, atelocollagen can increase cellular uptake, nuclease resistance, and prolong release of nucleic acids. The size, charge, and sustained release of atelocollagen/siRNA complexes can be altered by ratio of siRNA to atelocollagen [74, 75].

Takei et al. [76] first studied anti-tumoral effect of atelocollagen complexes containing siRNA *VEGF in vitro* and *in vivo*. They showed that siRNA *VEGF* with atelocollagen inhibited tumor angiogenesis and tumor growth in PC-3 cell lines *in vitro* and xenograft tumor *in vivo* model.

Koyanagi et al. [77] reported that siRNA targeting vasohibin-2 (*VASH-2*) using atelocollagen complexes siginificantly inhibited ovarian tumor growth and angiogenesis in ovarian cancer xenograft model. The knockdown of *VASH2* with atelocollagen/siRNA *VASH2* complexes exerted a significant antitumor effect and helped in tumor vascularization.

PLGA has been widely used as gene delivery system because of its biodegredability, biocompatibility, and non-toxic properties. FDA has approved PLGA as a pharmaceutical excipient. PLGA nanoparticles enter the cells efficiently by specific and non-specific endocytosis. Nanoparticles can release the encapsulated drug slowly leading to sustained drug effect [25].

Murata et al. [78] investigated anti-tumor effect of long-term sustained release of PLGA microspheres encapsulating anti-*VEGF* siRNA. The release of siRNA from microspheres was sustained for over one month. Intratumoral injection of PLGA microspheres containing siRNA *VEGF* inhibited tumor growth.

Su et al. [79] prepared PEI-coated PLGA nanoparticles loaded with paclitaxel and *Stat3* siRNA. PLGA-PEI nanoparticles more rapidly released *Stat3* siRNA than paclitaxel. Thus, decrease of *Stat3* expression by siRNA in human lung cancer cells (A549) and A549-derived paclitaxel-resistant A549/T12 cell lines reduced resistance of cell to paclitaxel. The released paclitaxel from nanoparticles killed the cancer cells that induce microtubule aggregation. In summary, inhibition of *Stat3* expression decreased cell viability, increased apoptosis, and reduced cellular resistance to paclitaxel.

3.1.3. Lipid-based siRNA delivery systems in cancer therapy

Cationic lipids are used as carrier for siRNA delivery. Liposomes and lipoplexes, as lipid-based delivery systems, have been widely used in local and systemic siRNA or shRNA delivery. Liposomes are microscopic vesicles that consist of single or multiple lipid bilayer, form in a sphere with an aqueous core. Nucleic acids can either be entrapped in the aqueous core of liposomes or attached to the lipid surface for delivery. The advantages of liposomes as delivery system include a high gene transfection efficiency, enhanced stabilization, easy penetration into cell membranes, efficient *in vivo* delivery, and flexible and versatile physicochemical properties. The disadvantages of liposomes are the short half-life in serum, lack of tissue specificity, rapid liver clearence, and cell toxicity [17]. Three different liposomes, such as neutral, anionic, and cationic liposomes, are used in the siRNA delivery studies [22]. Cationic liposomes for siRNA delivery can easily cross the cell membrane, promote escape from the endosomal compartment, and reach the target genes with good biocompatibility. However, cationic lipids can induce an interferon response and cause unwanted interactions with negatively charged serum proteins because of its high cationic charge density [32, 67]. Interferon responses can lead to not only change in gene expression but also show dose-dependent cytotoxicity and pulmonary inflammation [80, 81]. The toxicity and transfection efficiency of cationic lipids depend on length and structure of hydrocarbon chains of lipids [82].

Neutral lipids lead to less cellular toxicity and do not induce immune responses without the down-regulation of gene expression. However, neutral liposomes have shown low transfection efficiency because of their lack of surface charges [17]. The commonly used cationic lipids for siRNA delivery include 1,2-dioleoyloxy-3-trimethylammonium propane (DOTAP) and 1,2-di-o-octadecenyl-2-trimethylammonium propane (DOTMA) have combined with neutral lipids such as 1,2-dioleoyl-sn-glycero-3-phosphoethanolamine (DOPE). This combination can enhance transfection efficiency. Because neutral lipids facilitate fusion to the host cell's membrane, cationic lipids can facilitate electrostatically complexation with siRNA to obtain more stable formulation and entry to cells more easily [18]. Liposomes are usually more stable than lipoplex in biological fluids [5].

Lipid-based siRNA delivery strategies have shown as promising in cancer therapy. Tumor-targeting approaches have been used to enhance antitumor efficacy of these delivery systems. Specific delivery to target cells can be achieved by conjugation of ligands or molecules such as transferin or PEG on the surface of liposomes [20]. The targeting and prolonged circulation half-life of liposomes allow for the enhanced permeability of tumor vasculature, increased delivery to tumor tissue, and reduced side effects [34, 82]. Cationic liposomes containing siRNA targeting tumor-associated genes have been used to inhibit tumor growth and proliferation, induce apoptosis, and enhance the radiosensitivity of tumor cells [83–85].

Cationic lipids can interact with negatively charged siRNA by ionic interactions. Thus, self-assembly formed lipoplexes protect siRNA from enzymatic degradation, enhance cellular uptake of siRNA by endocytosis, enhance the release of siRNA from endosomal/lysosomal entrapment, and thus, promote siRNA accumulation in the cytosol [16]. Commercially available cationic lipid formulations such as Lipofectin®, Lipofectamine® (Invitrogen), Dharmafect® (Dharmacon), RNAifect® (Qiagen), and TransIT TKO® (Mirus) have been studied as tranfection reagents for siRNA delivery *in vitro* [86]. The ratio of lipid and siRNA (lipid/siRNA ratio) affects the colloidal properties of the lipoplexes (particle size and zeta potential). Lipid/siRNA or shRNA ratio is important to facilitate the cellular internalization of lipoplexes and to dissociate the nucleic acids in the cytosol. Lipid/siRNA ratio can be optimized in terms of biological activity [16]. Developing a lipid-based delivery system, choice of lipids, and appropriate formulations are essential to decrease cytotoxicity and increase the transfection efficiency of formulation.

To overcome the drawbacks of lipoplexes and liposomes, different nanostructures such as neutral lipid-based nanoliposomes, stable nucleic acid lipid particles (SNALP), and solid lipid nanoparticles (SLN) have been developed as siRNA delivery system. SNALPs are composed of cationic, neutral, and fusogenic lipid mixture. SNALPs increase cellular uptake and endosomal release of siRNA [4]. PEG-conjugated SNALPs represent exciting lipid-based systemic RNAi. The PEG-lipid conjugate improves the retention time to >10 hours [87]. Recently, Tekmira Pharmaceuticals [88] has developed siRNA-based drugs that are encapsulated in the SNALPs for delivery of siRNAs to target tissue by intravenous injection. SNALP-encapsulated siRNA targeting *PLK1* initiated phase I trial in December 2010. Alnylam Pharmaceuticals [89] has developed first dual-targeted siRNA drug, SNALP-encapsulated siRNAs targeting *VEGF,* and kinesin spindle protein (*KSP*) for the treatment of hepatocellular carinoma. Phase I trial was initiated in April 2009 [90].

Tekedereli et al. [91] indicated that knockdown of *Bcl-2* by intravenously administered nanoliposomal-siRNA *Bcl2* (150 μg siRNA/kg) twice a week lead to antitumoral activity in breast tumors of orthotopic xenograft models. In addition, nanoliposomal-siRNAs have enhanced the efficacy of chemotherapeutic agents in the breast cancer therapy.

http://dx.doi.org/10.5772/62826

Landen et al. [92] studied neutral nanoliposomes incorporating siRNA targeting *EphA2* in orthotopic mouse model of ovarian cancer. Three weeks of treatment with *EphA2*-targeting siRNA nanoliposomes (150 µg/kg twice weekly) reduced tumor growth. The combination therapy with paclitaxel reduced tumor growth.

Salva et al. [47] investigated the effect of co-delivery of siRNA *HIF1-α* and *VEGF* in liposomal form in the breast cancer cell lines. Chitosan-coated liposomal formulation for co-delivery of siRNA *VEGF* and *HIF1-α* were developed. The co-delivery of siRNA *VEGF* and *HIF1-α* was greatly enhanced *in vitro* gene silencing efficiency in the breast camcer cell lines (95%). In addition, chitosan-coated liposomes showed 96% cell viability. Salva et al. has suggested that siRNA-based therapies with chitosan-coated liposomes may have some promises in cancer therapy [47].

In conclusion, siRNA-based therapeutics are new and potential targets in cancer studies. In cancer, different mechanisms including angiogenesis, and cell growth were studied as target pathways. However, siRNAs have different hurdles in treatment because of their short biological life in blood, instability, and poor cellular internalization. In order to overcome these hurdles two solutions are present: one is modification of siRNA and the other is use of suitable siRNA delivery system. In cancer treatment, viral and non-viral delivery systems are evaluated as siRNA delivery. Although limited information is available related to *in vivo* delivery, more papers are present in literature. Viral delivery systems have serious problems. Therefore, non-viral systems are more attractable than viral systems for siRNAs. Cationic lipids, liposomes, and polymers such as chitosan, PEI, PLL, and PLGA are used as non-viral siRNA delivery system. However, more suitable carriers are needed for siRNA delivery systems.

Author details

Emine Şalva[1*], Ceyda Ekentok[2], Suna Özbaş Turan[2] and Jülide Akbuğa[2]

*Address all correspondence to: emine_salva@yahoo.com

1 Faculty of Pharmacy, Department of Pharmaceutical Biotechnology, İnönü University, Turkey

2 Faculty of Pharmacy, Department of Pharmaceutical Biotechnology, Marmara University, Turkey

References

[1] Dominska M, Dykxhoorn DM. Breaking down the barriers: siRNA delivery and endosome escape. J Cell Sci. 2010;123:1183-1189. DOI:10.1242/jcs.066399

[2] Aravin A, Tuschi T. Identification and characterization of small RNA involved in RNA silencing. FEBS Lett. 2005;579:5830-5840. DOI:10.1186/1471-2164-10-443

[3] Liu X, Rocchi P, Peng L. Dendrimers as non-viral vectors for siRNA delivery. New J Chem. 2012;36:256-263. DOI:10.1039/C1NJ20408D

[4] Lee JM, Yoon TJ, Cho YS. Recent developments in nanoparticle-based siRNA delivery for cancer therapy. Biomed Res Int. 2013;2013:1-10. DOI:10.1155/2013/782041

[5] Chen Y, Huang L. Tumor-targeted delivery of siRNA by non-viral vector: Safe and effective cancer therapy. Expert Opin Drug Del. 2008;5:1301-1311. DOI: 10.1517/17425240802568505

[6] Draz MS, Fang BA, Zhang P, Hu Z, Gu S, Weng KC et al. Nanoparticle-mediated systemic delivery of siRNA for treatment of cancers and viral infections. Theranostics. 2014;4:872-892. DOI:10.7150/thno.9404

[7] Xu CF, Wang J. Delivery systems for siRNA drug development in cancer therapy. Asian J Pharm Sci. 2015;10:1-12. DOI:10.1016/j.ajps.2014.08.011

[8] Jones SW, deSouza PM, Lindsay MA. siRNA for gene silencing: A route to drug target discovery. Curr Opin Pharmacol. 2004;4:522-527. DOI:10.1016/j.coph.2004.06.003

[9] Laufer SD, Detzer A, Sczakiel G, Restle T. Selected strategies for the delivery of siRNA in vitro an in vivo. In: Erdmann VA, Barciszewski J, editors. *RNA Technologies and Their Applications*. Berlin: Springer-Verlog; 2010. pp. 29-58.

[10] Rao DD, Vorhies JS, Senzer N, Nemunaitis J. siRNA vs shRNA: Similarities and differences. Adv Drug Deliver Rev. 2009;61:746-759. DOI:10.1016/j.addr.2009.04.004

[11] Latterich M, editor. *RNAi*. New York:Taylor & Francis Group; 2008, 23 p.

[12] Amarzguioui M, Rossi JJ, Kim D. Approaches for chemically synthesized siRNA and vector-mediated RNAi. FEBS Lett. 2005;579:5974-5981. DOI:10.1016/j.febslet.2005.08.070

[13] Aigner A. Delivery systems for the direct application of siRNAs to induce RNA interference (RNAi) in vivo. J Biomed Biotechnol. 2006;2006:1-15. DOI:10.1155/JBB/2006/71659

[14] Lam JKW, Chow MYT, Zhang Y, Leung SWS. siRNA versus miRNA as therapeutics for gene silencing. Mol Ther-Nuc Acids. 2005;4:e252. DOI:10.1038/mtna.2015.23

[15] Gary DJ, Puri N, Won YY. Polymer-based siRNA delivery: Perspectives on the fundamental and phenomenological distinctions from polymer-based DNA delivery. J Control Release. 2007;121:64-73. DOI:10.1016/j.jconrel.2007.05.021

[16] Wang J, Lu Z, Wientjes MG, Au JLS. Delivery of siRNA therapeutics: Barriers and carriers. AAPS J. 2010;12:492-503. DOI:10.1208/s12248-010-9210-4

[17] Deng Y, Wang CC, Choy KW, Du Q, Chen J, Wong Q et al. Therapeutic potentials of gene silencing by RNA interference: Principles, challenges and new strategies. Gene. 2014;538:217-227. DOI:10.1016/j.gene.2013.12.019

[18] Guo P, Coban O, Snead NM, Trebley J, Hoeprich S, Guo S et al. Engineering RNA for targeted siRNA delivery and medical application. Adv Drug Deliver Rev. 2010;62:650-666. DOI:10.1016/j.addr.2010.03.008

[19] Qiu S, Adema CM, Lane T. A computational study of off-target effects of RNA interference. Nuc Acids Res. 2005;33:1834-1847. DOI:10.1093/nar/gki324

[20] Kim SS, Garg H, Joshi A, Manjunath N. Strategies for targeted nonviral delivey of siRNA in vivo. Trends Mol Med. 2009;15:491-500. DOI:10.1016/j.molmed.2009.09.001

[21] Cheng K, Mahata RI, editors. *Advanced Delivery and Therapeutic Applications of RNAi*. Chichester: Wiley; 2013. 509 p.

[22] Zhang J, Li X, Huang L. Non-viral nanocarriers for sirNA delivery in breast cancer. J Control Release. 2014;190:440-450. DOI:10.1016/j.jconrel.2014.05.037

[23] Bora RS, Gupta D, Mukkur TKS, Saini KS. RNA interference therapeutics for cancer: Challenges and opportunities. Mol Med Rep. 2012;6:9-15. DOI:10.3892/mmr.2012.871

[24] Mansoori B, Shotorbani SS, Baradaran B. RNA interference and its role in cancer therapy. Adv Pharm Bull. 2014;4:313-321. DOI:10.5681/apb.2014.046

[25] Guo J, Bourre L, Soden DM, O'Sullivan GC, O'Driscoll C. Can non-viral technologies knockdown the barriers to siRNA delivery and achieve the next generation of cancer therapeutics?. Biotechnol Adv. 2011;29:402-417. DOI:10.1016/j.biotechadv.2011.03.003

[26] De Rosa G, La Rotonda MI. Nano and microtechnologies for the delivery of oligonucleotides with gene silencing properties. Molecules. 2009;14:2801-2823. DOI:10.3390/molecules14082801

[27] Fattal E, Brratt G. Nanotechnologies and controlled release systems for the delivery of antisense oligonucleotides and small interfering RNA. Brit J Pharmacol. 2009;157:179-194. DOI:10.1111/j.1476-5381.2009.00148.x

[28] De Fougerolles AR. Delivery vehicles for small interfering RNA in vivo. Hum Gene Ther. 2008;19:125-132. DOI:10.1089/hum.2008.928

[29] Akhtar S, Benter IF. Nonviral delivery of synthetic siRNAs in vivo. J Clin Invest. 2007;117:3623-3632. DOI:10.1172/JCI33494

[30] Gupta GJC, Pednekar PP, Jadhav KR, Chilajwar SV, Kadam VJ. Non viral synthetic siRNA delivery system an efficient tool for cancer treatment. World J Pharm Pharmaceutical Sci. 2014;3:351-387.

[31] Gad SC, editor. *Handbook of Pharmaceutical Biotechnology*. New Jersey: Wiley; 2007, 1072 p.

[32] Gao Y, Liu XL, Li XR. Research progress on siRNA delivery with nonviral carriers. Int J Nanomed. 2011;6:1017-1025. DOI:10.2147/IJN.S17040

[33] Juliano R, Bauman J, Kang H, Ming X. Biological barriers to therapy with antisense and siRNA oligonucleotides. Mol Pharm. 2009;6:686-695. DOI:10.1021/mp900093r

[34] Ozpolat B, Sood AK, Lopez-Berestein G. Nanomedicine based approaches for the delivery of siRNA in cancer. J Intern Med. 2010;267:44-53. DOI:10.1111/j. 1365-2796.2009.02191.x

[35] Amer MH. Gene therapy for cancer: Present status and future perspective. Mol Cell Ther. 2014;2:27. DOI:10.1186/2052-8426-2-27

[36] Oliveirea S, Storm G, Schiffelers RM. Targeted delivery of siRNA. J Biomed Biotechnol. 2006;2006:1-9. DOI:10.1155/JBB/2006/63675

[37] Zhang Y, Satteriee A, Huang L. In vivo gene delivery by nonviral vectors: Overcoming hurdles? Mol Ther. 2012;20:1298-1304. DOI:10.1038/mt.2012.79

[38] Scomparin A, Polyak D, Krivitsky A, Satchi-Falnaro R. Achieving successful delivery of oligonucleotides – From physico-chemical characterization to in vivo evaluation. Biotechnol Adv. DOI: http://dx.doi.org/10.1016/j.biotechadv.2015.04.008.

[39] Zhou Y, Zhang C, Liang W. Development of RNAi technology for targeted therapy – A track of siRNA based agents to RNAi therapeutics. J Control Release. 2014;193:270-281. DOI:10.1016/j.jconrel.2014.04.044

[40] Martimprey H, Vauthier C, Malvy C, Couvreur P. Polymer nanocarriers for the delivery of small fragments of nucleic acids: Oligonucleotides and siRNAs. Eur J Pharm Biopharm. 2009;71:490-504. DOI:10.1016/j.ejpb.2008.09.024

[41] Ragelle H, Vandermeulen G, Preat V. Chitosan-based siRNA delivery systems. J Control Release. 2013;172:207-218. DOI:10.1016/j.jconrel.2013.08.005

[42] Mao S, Sun W, Kissel T. Chitosan-based formulations for delivery of DNA and siRNA. Adv Drug Deliver Rev. 2010;62:12-27. DOI:10.1016/j.addr.2009.08.004

[43] Howard KA, Rahbek UL, Liu X, Damgaard CK, Glud SZ, Andersen MØ, et al. RNA interference in vitro and in vivo using a chitosan/siRNA nanoparticle system. Mol Ther. 2006;14:476-484. DOI:10.1016/j.ymthe.2006.04.010

[44] Salva E, Akbuga J. In vitro silencing effect of chitosan nanoplexes containing siRNA expressing vector targeting VEGF in breast cancer cell lines. Pharmazie. 2010;65:896-902. DOI:10.1691/ph.2010.0192

[45] Salva E, Kabasakal L, Eren F, Ozkan N, Cakalagaoglu F, Akbuga J. Local delivery of chitosan/VEGF siRNA nanoplexes reduces angiogenesis and growth of breast cancer in vivo. Nucleic Acid Ther. 2012;22:40-48. DOI:10.1089/nat.2011.0312

[46] Salva E, Turan SO, Kabasakal L, Alan S, Ozkan N, Eren F, et al. Investigation of the therapeutic efficacy of codelivery of psiRNA-vascular endothelial growth factor and

pIL-4 into chitosan nanoparticles in the breast tumor model. J Pharm Sci. 2014;103:785-795. DOI:10.1002/jps.23815

[47] Salva E, Turan SO, Eren F, Akbuga J. The enhancement of gene silencing efficiency with chitosan-coated liposome formulations of siRNAs targeting HIF-1α and VEGF. Int J Pharm. 2015;478:147-154. DOI:10.1016/j.ijpharm.2014.10.065

[48] Yang Y, Liu X, Zhang D, Yu W, Iv G, Xie H, et al. Chitosan/VEGF-siRNA nanoparticle for gene silencing. J Control Release. 2011;152:e160-e161. DOI:10.1016/j.jconrel.2011.08.062

[49] Wang SL, Yao HH, Guo LL, Dong L, Li AG, Gu YP, Qin ZH. Selection of optimal sites for TGFB1 gene silencing by chitosan-TPP nanoparticle-mediated delivery of shRNA. Cancer Genet Cytogenet. 2009;190:8-14. DOI:10.1016/j.cancergencyto.2008.10.013

[50] Huang Z, Dong L, Chen J, Gao F, Zhang Z, Chen J, et al. Low-molecular weight chitosan/vascular endothelial growth factor short hairpin RNA for the treatment of hepatocellular carcinoma. Life Sci. 2012;91:1207-1215. DOI:10.1016/j.lfs.2012.09.015

[51] Rudzinski WE, Aminabhavi TM. Chitosan as a carrier for targeted delivery of small interfering RNA. Int J Pharm. 2010;399:1–11. DOI:10.1016/j.ijpharm.2010.08.022

[52] Jere D, Jiang HL, Kim YK, Arote R, Choi YJ, Yun CH, et al. Chitosan-graft-polyethylenimine for Akt1 siRNA delivery to lung cancer cells. Int J Pharm. 2009;378:194-200. DOI:10.1016/j.ijpharm.2009.05.046

[53] Noh SM, Park MO, Shim G, Han SE, Lee HY, Huh JH, et al. Pegylated poly-L-arginine derivatives of chitosan for effective delivery of siRNA. J Control Release. 2010;145:159-164. DOI:10.1016/j.jconrel.2010.04.005

[54] Fernandes JC, Qiu X, Winnik FM, Benderdour M, Zhang X, Dai K, et al. Low molecular weight chitosan conjugated with folate for siRNA delivery in vitro: Optimization studies. Int J Nanomedicine. 2012;7:5833-5845. DOI:10.2147/IJN.S35567

[55] Chen J, Yu Z, Chen H, Gao J, Liang W. Transfection efficiency and intracellular fate of polycation liposomes combined with protamine. Biomaterials. 2011;32:1412-1418. DOI:10.1016/j.biomaterials.2010.09.074

[56] Erdem-Cakmak F, Ozbas-Turan S, Salva E, Akbuga J. Comparision of VEGF gene silencing efficiencies of chitosan and protamine complexes containing shRNA. Cell Biol Int. 2014;38:1260-1270. DOI:10.1002/cbin.10317

[57] Song E, Zhu P, Lee SK, Chowdhury D, Kusman S, Dykxhoorn DM, et al. Antibody mediated in vivo delivery of small interfering RNAs via cell-surface receptors. Nat Biotechnol. 2005;23:709-717. DOI:10.1038/nbt1101

[58] Choi YS, Lee JY, Sun JS, Kwon YM, Lee SJ, Chung JK, et al. The systemic delivery of siRNAs by a cell penetrating peptide, low molecular weight protamine. Biomaterials. 2010;31:1429-1443. DOI:10.1016/j.biomaterials.2009.11.001

[59] Morille M, Passirani C, Vonarbourg A, Clavreul A, Benoit JP. Progress in developing cationic vectors for non-viral systemic gene therapy against cancer. Biomaterials. 2008;29:3477-3496. DOI:10.1016/j.biomaterials.2008.04.036

[60] Templeton NS, editor. *Gene and Cell Therapy Therapeutic Mechanisms and Strategies*. 3rd ed. New York: Taylor & Francis Group; 2008, 330 p.

[61] Park K, Lee MY, Kim KS, Hahn SK. Target specific tumor treatment by VEGF siRNA complexed with reducible polyethylenimine-hyaluronic acid conjugate. Biomaterials. 2010;31:5258-5265. DOI:10.1016/j.biomaterials.2010.03.018

[62] Yang J, Liu H, Zhang X. Design, preparation and application of nucleic acid delivery carriers. Biotechnol Adv. 2014;32:804-817. DOI:10.1016/j.biotechadv.2013.11.004

[63] Schiffelers RM, Ansari A, Xu J, Zhou Q, Tang Q, Storm G, et al. Cancer siRNA therapy by tumor selective delivery with ligand-targeted sterically stabilized nanoparticle. Nucleic Acids Res. 2004;32:e149. DOI:10.1093/nar/gnh140

[64] Jiang G, Park K, Kim J, Kim KS, Hahn SK. Target specific intracellular delivery of siRNA/PEI-HA complex by receptor mediated endocytosis. Mol Pharm. 2009;6:727-737. DOI:10.1021/mp800176t

[65] Howard KA. Delivery of RNA inerference therapeutics using polycation-based nanoparticles. Adv Drug Deliver Rev. 2009;61:710-720. DOI:10.1016/j.addr.2009.04.001

[66] Scholz C, Wagner E. Therapeutic plasmid DNA versus siRNA delivery: Common and different tasks for synthetic carriers. J Control Release. 2012;161:554-565. DOI: 10.1016/j.jconrel.2011.11.014

[67] Li J, Cheng D, Yin T, Chen W, Lin Y, Chen J, et al. Copolymer of poly(ethylene glycol) and poly-(L-lysine) grafting polyrthylenimine through a reducible disulfide linkage for siRNA delivery. Nanoscale. 2014;6:1732-1740. DOI:10.1039/C3NR05024F

[68] Zhou J, Shum KT, Burneti JC Rossi JJ. Nanoparticle-based delivery of RNAi therapeutics: Progress and challenges. Pharmaceuticals. 2013;6:85-107. DOI:10.3390/ph6010085

[69] McCarroll J, Kavallaris M. Nanoparticle delivery of siRNA as a novel therapeutic for human disease. Australian Biochemist. 2012;43:9-13.

[70] Waite CL, Roth CM. PAMAM-RGD conjugates enhance siRNA delivery through a multicellular spheroşd model of malignant glioma. Bioconjug Chem. 2009;20:1908-1916. DOI:10.1021/bc900228m

[71] Liu X, Huang H, Wang J, Wang C, Wang M, Zhang B, et al. Dendrimers-delivered short hairpin RNA targeting HTERT inhibits oral cancer cells growth in vitro and in vivo. Biochem Pharmacol. 2011;82:17-23. DOI:10.1016/j.bcp.2011.03.017

[72] Ashihara E, Kawata E, Maekawa T. Future prospect of RNA interference for cancer therapies. Curr Drug Targets. 2010;11:345-360. DOI:10.2174/138945010790711897

[73] Ochiya T, Honma K, Takeshita E, Nagahara S. Atelocollagen-mediated drug discovery technology. Expert Opin Drug Dis. 2007;2:159-167. DOI:10.1517/17460441.2.2.159

[74] Mu P, Nagahara S, Makita N, Tarumi Y, Kadomatsu K, Takei Y. Systemic delivery of siRNA specific to tumor mediated by atelocollagen: Combined therapy using siRNA targeting Bcl-XL and cisplatin against prostate cancer. Int J Cancer. 2009;125:2978-2990. DOI:10.1002/ijc.24382

[75] Takei Y, Yoshifumi T. Atelocollagen-mediated siRNA delivery: future promise for therapeutic application. Ther Deliv. 2014;5:369-371. DOI:10.4155/tde.14.8

[76] Takei Y, Kadomatsu K, Yuzawa Y, Matsuo S, Muramatsu T. A small interfering RNA targeting vascular endothelial growth factor as cancer therapeutics. Cancer Res. 2004;64:3365-3370. DOI:10.1158/0008-5472.CAN-03-2682

[77] Koyanagi T, Suzuki Y, Saga Y, Machida S, Takei Y, Fujiwara H, et al. In vivo delivery of siRNA targeting vasohibin-2 decreases tumor angiogenesis and suppresses tumor growth in ovarian cancer. Cancer Sci. 2013;104:1705-1710. DOI:10.1111/cas.12297

[78] Murata N, Takashima Y, Toyoshima K, Yamamoto M, Okada H. Anti-tumor effects of anti-VEGF siRNA encapsulated with PLGA microspheres in mice. J Control Release. 2008;126:246-254. DOI:10.1016/j.jconrel.2007.11.017

[79] Su WP, Cheng FY, Shieh DB, Yeh CS, Su WC. PLGA nanoparticles codeliver paclitaxel and Stat3 siRNA to overcome cellular resistance in lung cancer cells. Int J Nanomedicine. 2012;7:4269-4283. DOI:10.2147/IJN.S33666

[80] Ma Z, Li J, He F, Wilson A, Pitt B, Li S. Cationic lipids enhance siRNA-mediated interferon response in mice. Biochem Biophys Res Commun. 2005;330:755-759. DOI: 10.1016/j.bbrc.2005.03.041

[81] Dokka S, Toledo D, Shi X, Catranova V, Rojanasakul Y. Oxygen radical-mediated pulmonary toxicity induced by some cationic liposomes. Pharm Res. 2000;17:521-525. DOI:10.1023/A:1007504613351

[82] Ozpolat B, Sood AK, Lopez-Berestein G. Liposomal siRNA nanocarriers for cancer therapy. Adv Drug Deliver Rev. 2014;66:110-116. DOI:10.1016/j.addr.2013.12.008

[83] Tagami T, Suzuki T, Matsunaga M, Nakamura K, Moriyoshi N, Ishida T, et al. Anti-angiogenic therapy via cationic liposome-mediated systemic siRNA delivery. Int J Pharm. 2012;422:280-289. DOI: 10.1016/j.ijpharm.2011.10.059

[84] Yang W, Sun T, Cao J, Liu F. Survivin downregulation by siRNA/cationic liposome complex radiosensitises human hepatoma cells in vitro and in vivo. Int J Radiat Biol. 2010;86:445-457. DOI: 10.3109/09553001003668006

[85] Yao Y, Su Z, Liang Y, Zhang N. pH-Sensitive carboxymethyl chitosan-modified cationic liposomes for sorafenib and siRNA co-delivery. Int J Nanomedicine. 2015;10:6185–6198. DOI: 10.2147/IJN.S90524

[86] Zhang S, Zhi D, Huang L. Lipid-based vectors for siRNA delivery. J Drug Target. 2012;20:724-735. DOI: 10.3109/1061186X.2012.719232

[87] Li W, Szoka FC. Lipid-based nanoparticles for nucleic acid delivery. Pharm Res. 2007;24:438-449. DOI:10.1007/s11095-006-9180-5

[88] Ozcan G, Ozpolat B, Coleman RL, Sood AK, Lopez-Berestein G. Preclinical and clinical development of siRNA-based therapeutics. Adv Drug Deliv Rev. 2015;87:108-119. DOI:org/10.1016/j.addr.2015.01.007

[89] Davidson BL, McCray PB Jr. Current prospects for RNA interference-based therapies. Nat Rev Genet. 2011;12:329-340. DOI:10.1038/nrg2968

[90] siRNA clinical trials [Internet]. Available from: https://www.clinicaltrials.gov/ct2/show/NCT00882180 [Accessed 2016-01-15]

[91] Tekedereli I, Alpay SN, Akar U, Yuca E, Ayugo-Rodriguez C, Han HD, et al. Therapeutic silencing of Bcl-2 by systemically administered siRNA nanotherapeutics inhibits tumor growth by autophagy and apoptosis and enhances the efficacy of therapy in orthotopic xenograft models of ER(-) and ER(+) breast cancer. Mol Ther-Nucleic Acids. 2013;2:e121. DOI:10.1038/mtna.2013.45

[92] Landen CN, Chavez-Reyes A, Bucana C, Schmandt R, Deavers M, Lopez-Berestein G, et al. Therapeutic EphA2 gene targeting in vivo using neutral liposomal small interfering RNA delivery. Cancer Res. 2005;65:6910-6918. DOI: 10.1158/0008-5472.CAN-05-0530

siRNA-Induced RNAi Therapy in Acute Kidney Injury

Cheng Yang and Bin Yang

Additional information is available at the end of the chapter

http://dx.doi.org/10.5772/61838

Abstract

siRNA therapy has great potential in humans, and its applications have been significantly improved. The kidney is a comparatively easy target organ of siRNA therapy due to its unique structural and functional characteristics. Here, we reviewed recent achievements in the design, delivery, and utilization of RNAi with a focus on kidney diseases, in particular acute kidney injury. In addition, the perspectives and challenges of siRNA therapy such as increasing its serum stability and immune tolerance, targeting single/double/multiple genes, cell/allele-specific delivery, time-controlled silencing, and siRNA-modified stem cell therapy were also discussed. Finally, selecting target genes and therapeutic time windows were addressed.

Keywords: Small interfering RNA, kidney diseases, delivery, off-target effects, compensative responses

1. Introduction

Acute kidney injury (AKI) is very common and critical in clinical practice. The incidence of hospital-acquired AKI is increasing, and many patients require renal replacement therapy [1]. AKI significantly increases the risk of chronic renal disease, end-stage renal disease (ESRD), and death, presenting a major burden to the patient and the health care system. Because of high metabolic activity in handling and transporting ions, amino acids, and other small molecules, the kidney is highly susceptible to acute injuries from lack of sufficient perfusion, exposure to, and accumulation of nephrotoxic substances. Despite numerous clinical trials, AKI remains a cause of significant morbidity and mortality for which there is no effective intervention [2].

RNA interference (RNAi) is a highly conserved biological phenomenon in all eukaryotes, including renal cells. Although RNAi naturally exists, synthetic artificial siRNA exerts similar effects as natural endogenous microRNA (miRNA). Both sense and antisense strands of siRNA can be synthesized separately and annealed to form double stranded siRNA duplexes *in vitro.* After the siRNA is delivered into the cytoplasm, the artificial siRNA silences the target gene using similar biological processes as endogenous miRNA. Since the introduction of 21-nucleotide artificial siRNAs that triggered gene silencing in mammalian cells [3], synthetic siRNA has generated much interest in biomedical research, in which the kidney is one of important key players. siRNA as a strategic molecule has been highly expected in the field of innovative therapy. Because siRNA is highly efficient at gene silencing, it is possible to develop specific siRNA-based drugs that could target any genes, including those that have unknown pharmacological antagonists or inhibitors. Different types of synthetic siRNA have been tested for their efficacy in various disease models, including cancer [4], autoimmune disorders [5], cardiovascular injuries [6], and organ transplantation [7], including native and transplanted kidney injuries [8].

As siRNA is a posttranscriptional regulator, it must first be absorbed into the target cells. Therefore, the kidney could be an excellent target organ for siRNA therapy because it benefits from rapid and vast blood flow physically, subsequent glomerular filtration, and tubular absorption. In fact, the systemic administration of siRNA leads to rapid uptake by the kidney, yielding a significant decrease of target protein expression [8]. Consequently, RNAi by siRNA has advantages for the treatment of renal diseases due to the unique urological system [9]. In addition, the preservation of donor kidneys before transplantation also provides a suitable time window for the intervention of siRNA.

In this chapter, we highlighted the design and delivery of siRNA and its therapeutic effects with a focus on kidney diseases. We also discussed future challenges of siRNA therapy, targeting single/double/multiple genes, cell/allele specific delivery, time-controlled silence, and siRNA-modified stem cell therapy.

2. Current principle of siRNA design

The design of potent siRNAs has been greatly improved over the past decade. The basic criteria for choosing siRNAs include the consideration of thermodynamic stability, internal repeats, immunostimulatory motifs, such as GC content, secondary structure, base preference at specific positions in the sense strand, and appropriate length [10].

Chemical modifications significantly enhance the stability and uptake of naked siRNAs. Importantly, siRNAs can be directly modified without crippling the silencing ability. Chemical modifications have been rigorously investigated for virtually every part of siRNA molecules, from the termini and backbone to the sugars and bases, with the goal of engineering siRNA to prolong half-life and increase cellular uptake. The most common chemical modification involves modifying the sugar moiety. For example, the incorporation of 2′-fluoro (2′-F), -O methyl, -halogen, -amine, or -deoxy can significantly increase the stability of siRNA in serum.

Locked nucleic acid (LNA) has been also applied to modify siRNA. The commonly used LNA contains a methylene bridge connecting the 2′-oxygen with the 4′-carbon of the ribose ring.

This bridge locks the ribose ring in the 3′-endo conformation characteristic of RNA [11]. Additionally, recent studies, including ours [12], have proven the efficacy of LNA-modified siRNA in terms of prolonged half-life in serum, but without detectable adverse effects, suggesting that the natural RNAi machinery could accommodate a certain degree of alterations in the chemical structure of siRNAs [13].

3. siRNA delivery

The biggest obstacle faced by siRNA therapies is the *in vivo* delivery of genetic materials. The systemic delivery of synthetic siRNA has the most medical and commercial potential. This type of delivery, however, remains a major challenge for translating siRNA from the research to the clinic. Overcoming the delivery challenge requires effective siRNA delivery vehicles. The virus-based delivery system, while efficient, may be fatally flawed due to raised safety concerns, such as inducing mutations and triggering immunogenic and inflammatory responses [14]. Therefore, extensive research had been performed to develop efficacious nonviral delivery systems, including direct chemical modification of siRNA (as described above) and/or optimization of delivery materials, such as liposome formulation, nanoparticle conjugation and antibodies that target cellular moieties [14].

To date, studies on synthetic siRNA therapy have been performed in a variety of cell culture and rodent models [15] that produced exciting results and were cost effective but failed to faithfully mimic human diseases. Therefore, large animal models, such as porcine models, are indispensable to compensate for the limitations of rodent models due to their greater similarity to human beings. The investigations on siRNA conducted in our laboratory have reflected this trend in the field [7, 12, 16].

3.1. Direct delivery of synthetic siRNA *in vitro/ex vivo*

The siRNA could be easily transduced into various cells for scientific research. For example, we transfected synthetic caspase-3 siRNA in porcine proximal tubular cells (LLC-PK1) using cationic lipid-based transfection reagent. The caspase-3 siRNA inhibited apoptosis and inflammation in LLC-PK1 cells that were subjected to hydrogen peroxide stimulation [17]. In addition to *in vitro* delivery of siRNA, *ex vivo/in vivo* siRNA delivery to target organs is an indispensable step before its clinical application. If it was directly delivered into the kidneys, siRNA could obtain higher local concentrations, which would result in improved gene silencing efficacy. During kidney transplantation, *ex vivo* local delivery of siRNA into the donor kidney is feasible because it could be facilitated by the unique structure of the kidney and the characteristics of kidney transplantation. We utilized an *ex vivo* isolated porcine kidney reperfusion system to assess the efficacy of naked caspase-3 siRNA. The caspase-3 siRNA was directly infused into the renal artery (locally) and autologous blood perfusate (mimic systemic delivery) before 24-h cold storage (CS), followed by a further reperfusion for 3 h. The results demonstrated that the caspase-3 siRNA improved ischemia reperfusion (IR) injury with reduced caspase-3 expression and apoptosis, better renal oxygenation, and acid–base homeostasis [16]. These promising proof-of-principle observations provide valuable guidance for further development before siRNA used in clinical practice.

3.2. Local or systemic delivery of siRNA *in vivo*

Delivery of siRNA via *ex vivo* route can be applied in donor kidneys, but most renal diseases need *in vivo* delivery. Based on the anatomical and physiological characteristics of the kidney, local delivery can be achieved through several routes: (1) renal artery, first targeting the glomeruli or tubules [18, 19]; (2) renal vein, predominately targeting tubulointerstitium [20]; (3) intraureteral, administered into the renal pelvis and interstitium [21]; and (4) subcapsular administration, achieves intraparenchymal silencing [22]. Due to the rich blood flow through the glomeruli, siRNA injection via the renal artery followed by electroporation could silence specific genes in the glomeruli, such as TGF-β1, which subsequently ameliorates matrix expansion in an experimental glomerulonephritis model [18].

We then used naked caspase-3 siRNA in a porcine kidney autotransplant model for the first time. The left kidney was retrieved from mini pigs and was infused with University of Wisconsin solution, with or without 0.3 mg of naked caspase-3 siRNA, via the renal artery, which was followed by renal artery and renal vein clamping for 24-h cold storage (CS, mimicking donor kidney preservation before transportation in clinic). After right nephrectomy, the left kidney was autotransplanted into the right nephridial pit for 48 h without systemic siRNA treatment (Figure 1). The expression of caspase-3 mRNA and active caspase-3 protein, as well as its precursor, was downregulated by siRNA in the post-CS kidney. In the siRNA preserved posttransplant kidney, however, caspase-3 precursor was further decreased while caspase-3 mRNA, and its activated subunits were upregulated, which resulted in increased apoptosis and inflammation. This study indicated that the naked caspase-3 siRNA was effective for cold preservation but was not effective at protecting posttransplant kidneys, which may be due to systemic compensative responses overcoming local effects. Therefore, to overcome the systemic response and to prolong the therapeutic time window, we subsequently utilized a novel, serum-stable caspase-3 siRNA, both locally as before and systemically via a pretransplantation intravenous injection, and observed the animals for up to 2 weeks post-transplantation. The effectiveness of the novel caspase-3 siRNA was confirmed by downregulated caspase-3 mRNA and protein in the post-CS and/or posttransplant kidneys, as well as reduced apoptosis and inflammation. More importantly, renal function, associated with active caspase-3, HMGB1, apoptosis, inflammation, and tubulointerstitial damage, was improved by this novel, serum-stable caspase-3 siRNA [12].

It has also been revealed that an injection of a single-dose Fas siRNA through the renal vein post ischemia provided a survival advantage in a murine IR model, which was due to the antiapoptosis and antiinflammation effects of the Fas siRNA [20]. Unilateral ureteral obstruction (UUO) is a well-established model for tubulointerstitial fibrosis. Xia et al. injected the siRNA of heat shock protein 47 once via the ureter at the time of UUO preparation, leading to significantly reduced fibrosis-related protein expression and a remarkable alleviation of the accompanying interstitial fibrosis [21]. Subcapsular administration is still used in some experiments due to its unique advantages, although it requires an invasive procedure and has

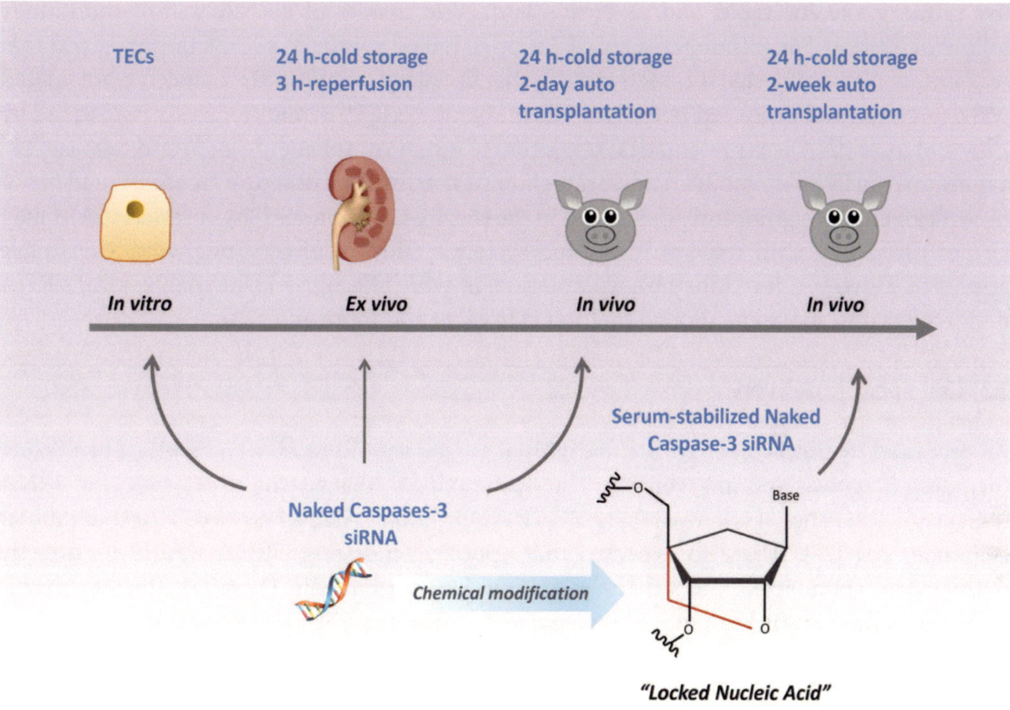

Figure 1. Schematic drawing showed a series of our studies using caspase-3 siRNA. The caspase-3 siRNA was first used to protect porcine renal tubular epithelia cells against hydrogen peroxide-induced injury [17]. The renoprotection of naked caspase-3 siRNA with the same sequences was further validated in a porcine *ex vivo* isolated reperfusion model and showed that the siRNA was effective for cold preservation [16], but not in autotransplanted kidneys without systematic siRNA treatment [7, 12, 16]. Finally, the chemically modified siRNA of caspase-3 via locked nucleic acid stabilized the siRNA in serum and significantly protected autotransplanted kidneys [7, 12, 16].

limitations in clinical practice. Cuevas et al. reported that an infusion of DJ-1 (an antioxidant)-specific siRNA into the subcapsule silenced DJ-1 expression in the renal cortex and increased ROS production [22].

Systemic delivery is a common and convenient clinical practice, although current clinical trials using siRNAs are almost directly administered to the target site, such as the nostril, eye, and lung, thereby avoiding the complexity of systemic delivery [23]. The most common method of systemic siRNA delivery is a hydrodynamic intravenous injection with hydraulic pressure to assist siRNA cell entry. However, the pharmacokinetic metabolism of siRNA is more complicated during systemic delivery because siRNAs can be rapidly degraded by nucleases in the serum and cleared by the kidney and liver. To enhance the *in vivo* efficacy of siRNA treatment, a variety of approaches have been attempted for both siRNA itself and delivery techniques [22–24], as mentioned above.

Due to its anatomical and physiological characteristics, the kidney is the most preferable target organ of systemic siRNA administration. siRNA access to the kidney is thought to be dependent on the filtration and reabsorption functions of the kidney. Proximal tubule cells (PTCs) are the primary site for rapid and extensive endocytic uptake of siRNA within the kidney following glomerular filtration. In an AKI model, naked synthetic siRNA targeting p53 that was intravenously injected 4 h after renal ischemic injury significantly reduced upregulated p53 expression and protected both the PTCs and kidneys [25]. In another study performed by Zheng et al., siRNA was systematically injected to target complement 3 (C3) and caspase-3 in a murine renal IR injury model. The results showed that the level of serum creatinine and blood urea nitrogen was significantly decreased in the siRNA-treated mice [26]. As most of AKI may be not associated with renal surgery, the systemic siRNA delivery might be a desirable approach. However, for kidney transplantation, in which IR injury is inevitable, local siRNA delivery via any above-mentioned method is feasible and more effective.

3.3. Cell-specific delivery

As proposed by precision medicine, individual person should receive customized healthcare including diagnosis and intervention. The dysfunctional cells are the true targets for siRNA delivery. For instance, it is known that p53 in PTCs promotes AKI, whereas p53 in other tubular cells does not [27]. It is also expected that apoptosis-inducing siRNA should be directly delivered into tumor cells rather than the surrounding normal cells. Therefore, the cell-specific delivery method is our key point in the next generation of siRNA development.

Recently, antibody conjugation technology has made tumor-targeting drug delivery systems available. The conjugate can be regarded as a "guided molecular missile" that specifically targets unique antigens [28]. Inspired by cancer therapy strategies, siRNAs have also been "packed" to be delivered to target organs, even cells. Recently, a type of asymmetric liposome particle (ALP) has been developed, which highly efficiently encapsulates siRNA without nonspecific cell penetration. The ALPs protected siRNA from ribonuclease degradation. ALPs without any surface modification elicited almost no uptake into cells, while the polyarginine peptide surface-modified ALPs induced nonspecific cell penetration [29]. Leus et al. delivered siRNA targeting vascular cell adhesion molecule-1 (VCAM-1) into inflammation-activated endothelium using anti-VCAM-1-SAINTPEGarg formulated with additional 2 mol% DOPE-PEG_{2000} *in vivo*. The antibody recognizes VACM-1, which can create specificity for inflammation activated endothelial cells. The siRNA homed to VCAM-1 protein expressing vasculature in TNF-α-treated mice without any kidney and liver toxicity [30]. These results represent great progress in siRNA delivery system development. Antibody-mediated specific recognition rather than virus-mediated recognition may be a mainstream in the future.

3.4. Allele-specific RNAi

RNAi, in addition, discriminates between two sequences only differing by one nucleotide conferring a high specificity of RNAi for its target mRNA. This property was used to develop a particular therapeutic strategy called "allele-specific RNAi" devoted to silence the mutated allele of genes causing dominant inherited diseases without affecting the normal allele. Therapeutic benefit was now demonstrated in cells from patients and animal models, and promising results of the first phase Ib clinical trial using siRNA-based allele-specific therapy were reported in pachyonychia congenita, an inherited skin disorder due to dominant mutations in the *keratin 6* gene [31]. The allele-specific siRNA silencing of the mutant *keratin 12* allele was also applied in corneal limbal epithelial cells grown from patients with Meesmann's epithelial corneal dystrophy [32, 33]. It has also been shown that modified siRNAs conferring allele-specific silencing against disease-causing ALK2 mutants found in fibrodysplasia ossificans progressiva, without affecting normal ALK2 allele [34].

3.5. Delivery of siRNA using a cargo system

Although lentivirus vectors as vehicles together with liposome reagents are widely applied in the transduction of siRNA, nanoparticle systems have emerged in last few years as an alternative carrier for advanced diagnostic and therapeutic applications. The nanotechnology offers many merits and overcomes the range of challenges/barriers summarized in the previous section, such as the bioavailability and biodistribution of therapeutic agents. Recent reports have demonstrated that the kidney, the glomerulus especially, is a readily accessible site for nanoparticles. Zuckerman at al. intravenously administered nanoparticles containing polycationic cyclodextrin and siRNA/CDP-NPs, most of which deposited in the glomerular mesangial areas. Furthermore, the cultured mouse and human mesangial cells could rapidly internalize siRNA/CDP-NPs. This process could be accelerated by attaching targeting ligand mannose or transferrin to the nanoparticle surface [35].

Complex nanoparticles, especially cationic polyplexes/lipoplexes and liposomes, dominated the scene in the early days of RNAi therapeutic development. Their main advantage lies in their endosomal release activity and their ability to concentrate multiple RNAi triggers in one particle [36]. Forbes and Peppas cross-linked polycationic nanoparticle formulations using ARGET ATRP or UV-initiated polymerization. The advantage of this method is the one-step, one-pot, and surfactant-stabilized monomer-in-water synthesis, which is simpler and faster compared with traditional complicated multistep techniques involving toxic organic solvents [37].

Regardless of how much each mechanism plays in the transport of the drug, cell entry remains a focus for drug design and discovery. An exciting and relatively new approach to transporting pharmaceutical agents into cells is making use of cell-penetrating peptides (CPPs). CPPs are relatively short peptides, typically less than 30 amino acids, and could be vectors for the delivery of genetic and biologic products. CPPs provide a safe, efficient, and noninvasive mode of transport for various cargos into cells [38]. Recently, van Asbeck et al. discovered that CPP/siRNA complexes with the most negative zeta-potentials in serum were the most resistant to siRNA release over a 20-h incubation period compared to less negatively charged complexes [39]. They also found that the zeta-potential of CPP/siRNA complexes in serum did not correlate with improved cellular association, which might demonstrate the importance of serum proteins or CPP conformation on the ability of CPP/siRNA complexes to associate with the cell membrane. Huang et al. designed a bifunctional peptide named RGD10-10R, by which siRNA was delivered *in vitro* and *in vivo*. Because of their electrostatic interactions with polyarginine (10R), negatively charged siRNAs were readily complexed with RGD10-10R peptides, forming spherical RGD10-10R/siRNA nanoparticles. This is also a novel siRNA delivery tool [40].

Gemini or dimeric lipids (GCLs) are a recent type of amphiphilic molecules that contain two polar headgroups linked by a rigid or flexible spacer that may be hydrophobic or hydrophilic. As each headgroup has a hydrophobic moiety, GCLs may be considered as two conventional monomeric surfactants connected by a spacer group [41]. GCLs have been proved as promising candidates to transfect nucleic acids in gene therapy. The molecular structure of the GCLs offers a high number of alternatives to develop and to improve their capability as transfecting agents.

4. siRNA therapy in AKI

To date, siRNA therapy has been successfully applied in a variety of acute kidney injuries. IR injury is the primary cause of AKI, particularly during kidney transplantation, in which the kidney is exposed to hypoxia and experiences a series of oxidative, inflammatory and apoptotic responses [42, 43]. Consequently, specific siRNAs targeting critical molecules that are involved in the processes of oxidation, inflammation, and apoptosis have been developed.

Caspase-3, which mediates apoptosis and inflammation, is upregulated by IR injury. Multiple pharmacological interventions against caspase-3, including enzyme inhibitors and genetic modification, have been investigated. In recent years, our group studied the delivery and efficacy of caspase-3 siRNA in *in vitro, ex vivo,* and *in vivo* kidney injury models. The synthetic caspase-3 siRNA was initially tested in porcine PTCs (LLC-PK1), with or without hydrogen peroxide (H_2O_2) stimulation. Apoptotic cells and activated IL-1β protein expression were significantly reduced by the caspase-3 siRNA, with improved cell viability [17]. This outcome led to siRNA application in an isolated organ perfusion system, as described above, and the efficacy of caspase-3 siRNA was further proven, in terms of silenced caspase-3 mRNA and protein expression, attenuated inflammation and apoptosis, and improved renal function and histology [16].

The porcine kidney preserved by caspase-3 siRNA was then autotransplanted in a 2-day model. However, the transplanted kidney was not protected without systemic treatment of the recipient. Moreover, new serum-stabilized caspase-3 siRNAs were applied locally in kidney preservation and intravenously in recipient in a 2-week autotransplant model. The transplanted kidneys were protected without significant off-target effects. These serials of step-by-step studies provided promising evidence to support siRNA treatment to be further applied in clinic.

p53, another pivotal protein in the apoptotic pathway, has been identified as a mediator of transcriptional responses to IR injury [44]. Molitoris et al. revealed that intravenously injected p53 siRNA attenuated ischemic and cisplatin-induced AKI [25]. Fujino et al. also tested the efficacy siRNA targeting p53 via transarterial administration siRNA injected into the left renal artery immediately after ischemia improved tubular injury and downregulated GSK-3β expression [45]. In a diabetic mouse model, p53 inhibition by siRNA also reduced ischemic AKI [46].

Silencing of other important transcription factors or immunity related receptors using siRNAs have also been studied. Renal IR injury and inflammation are related to postsurgical healing and both processes can be influenced by toll-like receptor (TLR) signals. Effective TLR9 silencing by siRNA decreases renal cell apoptosis, mitigates AKI severity, and increases the mice survival [47]. NF-κB, a pro-inflammatory transcription factor induced by TLR and other signals, plays a key role in AKI. NF-κB activation depends on the activation of the inhibitor of κB kinase β (IKKβ). Wan et al. demonstrated that silencing IKKβ using siRNA diminished inflammation and protected the kidneys against IR injury [19]. These studies clearly demonstrate the therapeutic potential of siRNA-induced silencing of key AKI mediators, which are activated and involved in the pathways of apoptosis, inflammation, immunity, etc.

5. Off-target side effects and toxicities of siRNA

The siRNA has been likened to a "magic bullet" due to this potency and specificity, but off-target side effects and toxicities create additional challenges for researchers. The induction of various side effects may be caused by unexpected perturbations between RNAi molecules and cellular components. The off-target effects of siRNA were first reported by Jackson and colleagues in 2003 [48]. Broadly speaking, off-target effects can be siRNA specific or nonspecific. The former are caused by limited siRNA complementarity to nontargeted mRNAs. The latter, resulting in immune- and toxicity-related responses, are due to the construction of the siRNA sequence, its modification, or the delivery vehicle.

The off-target effects associated with siRNA delivery fall into three broad categories: (1) miRNA-like off-target effects, referring to siRNA-induced sequence-dependent regulation of unintended transcripts through partial sequence complementarity to their 3′UTRs; (2) inflammatory responses through the activation of TLR triggered by siRNAs and/or delivery vehicles (such as cationic lipids and viruses), and (3) widespread effects on miRNA processing and function through the saturation of the endogenous RNAi machinery by exogenous siRNAs [49, 50].

5.1. miRNA-like off-target effects

The siRNAs and miRNAs share similar machinery downstream of their initial processing. Using several different siRNAs targeting the same gene, microarray profiling showed that each siRNA produced a unique, sequence-dependent signature. Sequence analysis of off-target transcripts revealed that the 3′ UTR regions of these transcripts were complementary to the 5′ end of the transfected siRNA guide strand [48]. It is now understood that for the off-targeting effects to occur, a perfect complementarity between the seed region of the antisense strand such as nucleotide positions 2–7 or 2–8 and the 3′ UTR of the transcript is necessary [49, 51]. Silencing the set of original off-target transcripts could be induced by base mismatches in the 5′ end of siRNA guide strands. However, a new set of off-target transcripts within 3′ UTRs that were complementary to the mismatched guide strand could be generated [49].

RNAi regulation by miRNAs involves partial complementarity between the targeting RNA and miRNA. Because miRNAs cause gene silencing through mRNA degradation and translation inhibition, the siRNA-mediated off-target effects may also be acting at two levels. For this reason, there should be greater emphasis on improving siRNA design as well as monitoring gene and protein levels following RNAi therapy to account for any off-target effects.

5.2. Recognition and stimulation of the innate immune system

The recognition and stimulation of the immune system arenonspecific off-target effects of siRNA therapy. The RNA-sensing pattern recognition receptors (PRRs), localized in endosomes, are the most important components of the innate immune system. The responses of PRRs to siRNAs are either TLR-mediated or non-TLR-mediated. The PRR responses are also associated with siRNA sequence-specific side effects and have recently attracted many attentions from researchers [52]. RNA-sensing TLRs (TLR3 and TLR7) are predominantly located intracellularly and recognize nucleic acids released from invading pathogens. The non-TLR-mediated innate immune responses triggered by siRNA binding are linked to RNA-regulated expression of protein kinase (PKR) and retinoic acid inducible gene 1 (RIG1), which further induce caspase-3 and NF-κB expression, respectively. The activation of PRRs generates excessive cytokine release and subsequent inflammation [53].

Based on this second type of off-target RNAi effects, our group further investigated the mechanism of how short-acting caspase-3 siRNA impaired posttransplanted kidneys. The results suggested that the amplified inflammatory responses in caspase-3 siRNA preserved autotransplant kidneys were associated with TLR3, TLR7, and PKR activation, which may be due to systemic compensative responses, although persistent actions initiated by short-acting caspase-3 siRNA cannot be completely excluded [54]. Other studies have also indicated that the horseshoe-like structure of TLR3 facilitates dsRNA recognition [55, 56]. Interactions between TLR3 and dsRNA were originally reported in 2001 when TLR3-deficient mice exhibited reduced immune responses to dsRNA viruses [57].

Several studies have demonstrated that the immune response to siRNAs is cell type-dependent due to the selective expression of TLRs. siRNAs stimulate monocytes and myeloid dendritic cells through TLR8 to produce proinflammatory cytokines, or activate plasmacytoid dendritic cells through TLR7 to produce type I interferons [58–60]. In addition, the volume of hydrodynamic naked siRNA delivery influences immune activation. Rácz et al. compared the immune responses induced by 50 μg siRNA dissolved in either low-volume (1 mL/mouse) or high-volume (10% of body weight, 2.5 mL/mouse in average) physiological salt solution delivered *in vivo*. Low-volume hydrodynamic injection induced slight alanine aminotransferase (ALT) elevation and mild hepatocyte injury, whereas high-volume hydrodynamic injection resulted in higher ALT levels and extensive hepatocyte necrosis. High-volume hydrodynamic injection also led to a time-dependent slight increase in IFN-related gene expression [61]. Collectively, these studies suggest that there is a need for improving siRNA design, establishing experimental controls and carefully interpreting results.

6. From bench to bedside: Clinical trials

The numbers of RNAi-based preclinical studies and clinical trials have grown over the past several years. To date, there have been 27 registered clinical trials using siRNA worldwide. These studies include retinal degeneration, dominantly inherited brain and skin diseases, viral infections, respiratory disorders, metabolic diseases, and of particular note, kidney diseases. In 2011, Quark Pharmaceuticals completed a phase I, randomized, double-blind, dose escalation, safety, and pharmacokinetic study (NCT00554359) on QPI-1002, also designated I5NP, which was a synthetic siRNA that temporarily inhibits p53 expression that is in early development for acute kidney failure therapy. I5NP is the first siRNA to be systemically administered in humans. Based on the preclinical data obtained from animal models, the siRNA was intravenously injected within 4 h to bypass surgery patients. Pharmacokinetic data were collected during the first 24 h, and safety and dose-limiting toxicities were monitored until hospital discharge and 6–12 months after surgery. Recently, Quark initiated a subsequent clinical trial to determine whether a single administration of I5NP can prevent delayed graft function in kidney transplant recipients. Data from this study will be used to identify I5NP doses for follow-on efficacy studies (NCT00802347). Another ongoing phase I trial investigating solid tumors, including Renal cell carcinoma (RCC), was conducted by Calando Pharmaceuticals. The investigators used CALAA-01, whose active ingredient is a type of siRNA, to inhibit tumor growth and/or reduce tumor size. This siRNA inhibits the expression of the M2 subunit of ribonucleotide reductase and resists nuclease degradation by using a stabilized nanoparticle that targets tumor cells (NCT00689065).Besides, there is an ongoing study, in which patients with melanoma, kidney cancer, pancreatic cancer, or other solid tumors that are metastatic or cannot be removed by surgeryare treated by APN401, siRNA-transfected autologousperipheral blood mononuclear cells.These cells were modified by siRNA targeting factors inhibiting the killing ability of immune cells in vitro and transfused back into the body, in order to kill more cancer cells (NCT02166255, the above clinical trials can be found at ClinicalTrials.gov, Table 1).

Study	Target/siRNA drug	Status	Disease
NCT00554359	I5NP	Phase I, completed	Kidney injury; acute renal failure
NCT00802347	I5NP	Completed	Delayed graft function in kidney transplantation
NCT00689065	CALAA-01	Phase I, terminated	Solid tumor cancers including RCC
NCT02166255	APN401	Phase I, recruiting	Melanoma, kidney cancer, pancreatic cancer, or other solid

Table 1. Clinical trials of siRNA therapy in kidney diseases.

7. Perspectives and challenges

Despite the enormous potential advantages of siRNA therapy, additional research must be performed before its large-scale clinical application.

7.1. Target gene selection

Genome-wide or pathway-specific siRNA libraries have become available using high-throughput screening approaches. Establishing *in vitro* prescreening leads to signaling pathway prediction and target validation in *in vivo* renal disease. However, choosing one or a set of reasonable target genes is the key for designing specific siRNA treatments. The pathophysiological changes during kidney disease, like any other disease, refer to a complex gene and protein regulation network. For example, the network that exists during kidney transplantation involves the original conditions of the donors and the interactions between the donor kidneys and the recipients, which could direct the progression, as well as the recovery, of the injury. Fortunately, transcriptome measurements of the transplanted kidney may provide a comprehensive understanding of gene regulation and would be beneficial for target gene selection.

Mueller et al. analyzed the transcriptome of postreperfusion implant biopsies in living donors (LD) and deceased donors (DD). Hundreds of mRNAs were identified that predicted delayed graft function [62]. In a recent prospective study using human posttransplant kidney biopsies, 20 mRNAs and two miRNAs were identified as molecular signatures of AKI. Elevated secretory leukocyte peptidase inhibitor in AKI allografts was validated and miR-182-5p was identified as a molecular regulator [63]. These genes could be used as potential targets of siRNA therapy. We recently identified 3 times more differentially expressed genes in renal allograft biopsies between living donors and cadaveric donors at 30 min than 3 months posttransplantation. The majority of these differentially expressed genes are responsible for acute responses at 30 min, but also involved in inflammation, nephrotoxicity, and proliferation at 3 months. These divergent transcriptome signatures between two types of donors might be linked with not only the initial injury of the donors, but also the immune responses of the recipients.

Another method for selecting target genes is by identifying their translation product proteins. To find a single or a set of crucial proteins involved in kidney allograft rejection, Wu et al. explored potential transcriptional factors and regulation networks in 352 kidney transplant recipients, of which 85 suffered from acute rejection (AR). The results demonstrated that the dominant processes and responses were associated with inflammation and complement activation in AR. A number of transcription factors were identified in AR patients, including NF-κB, signal transducer, and activator of transcription (STAT) 1 and STAT3 [64]. Their recent study further revealed inflammation-derived kidney allograft injury, such as AR, chronic rejection, and impaired renal function without rejection. Wu et al. 12 common proteins and 11 level-specific proteins from the phenotype-related protein–protein interaction networks [65]. These potential biomarkers also provide valuable targets for siRNA design relating to the treatment of transplant-related injury.

7.2. Timely application

Compared with shRNA, an advantage of siRNA for AKI therapy is time-controlled, transient treatment. Silencing the target gene for a short time or a long time should be assessed before RNAi application. The silenced genes may be multifunctional according to the surrounding milieu. For example, caspase-3, generally considered an executor in cellular apoptosis, should be inhibited in injured tissues. However, it is also a loyal scavenger in malignantly transformed cells, which could be an unavoidable side effect in any caspase-3-targeting siRNA therapy. For AKI, siRNA ineffectiveness is needed after the therapeutic time window. Additionally, siRNA application avoids intracellular traffic. In certain circumstances, shRNA delivery could be harmful to the organ or even fatal.

A study from Grimm et al. investigated the long-term effects of sustained high-level shRNA expression in the livers of adult mice. An evaluation of 49 distinct adeno-associated virus/ shRNA vectors, with unique lengths and sequences that were directed against six targets, showed that 36 vectors resulted in dose-dependent liver injury, with 23 ultimately causing death. The observed morbidity was associated with the downregulation of liver-derived miRNAs, indicating possible competition of the latter with shRNAs (through saturation of the endogenous RNAi machinery by the exogenous siRNAs) for the limited cellular factors required for the processing of various small RNAs [66]. Therefore, controlling intracellular shRNA expression levels will be imperative, but siRNA would not influence the endogenous process of RNA degradation mediated by miRNAs.

7.3. siRNA targeting single, double or multiple genes

The knockdown of two or more genes simultaneously using siRNA cocktail has been recently reported. Many applications of siRNA cocktail have demonstrated significant benefits compared with siRNA targeted to a single gene, particularly in anticancer and antiviral therapy [67, 68]. A high concentration of individual siRNAs may represent the key off-target effect in terms of competition for endogenous miRNA biogenesis machinery. Therefore, the other advantage of siRNA cocktail is the relatively low concentration of each siRNA, which may also reduce off-target signatures without sacrificing silencing potency [69].

7.4. Cell-specific siRNA targeting

We have showed that the apoptosis of different types of cells leads to different outcomes. For instance, the apoptosis of inflammatory cells is associated with inflammation clearance and tissue remodeling, whereas the apoptosis of renal parenchymal cells is link to tubular atrophy and renal fibrosis. Therefore, using the genetic material such as siRNA targeting specific cell at particular time frame is crucial to achieve high efficacy of treatment in AKI and also avoid site-effects [12, 54].

It is still challenging to administrate siRNA cell specifically, but it is feasible as there were a few studies showed delivering siRNA into liver cells and antigen-presenting cells [70–72] using carbon nanotubes and mannose-conjugated liposomes. In addition, surface pegylation and cell-specific targeting ligands incorporation in the carriers may improve the pharmacokinetics, biodistribution, and siRNA selectivity. Choosing appropriate siRNA carriers has to consider the safety, effectiveness, ease of manufacturing, off-target effects [12], and innate immune responses. Of course, the efficacy of siRNA is still a most important factor dominating the selection of its carriers [54].

7.5. siRNA-modified stem cell therapy

Mesenchymal stem cell (MSC) transplantation has attracted much attention in cell therapy in different organ systems such as myocardial infarction. One of the limitations is the poor survival of grafted cells in the ischemic microenvironment. To tackle this issue, a novel siRNA-mediated prolyl hydroxylase domain protein 2 (PHD2) silencing system has been developed based on arginine-terminated generation 4 poly (amidoamine) nanoparticles. This system, for the first time, exhibited effective and biocompatible siRNA delivery and PHD2 silencing in MSCs *in vitro*. After transplant PHD2 siRNA-modified MSC in myocardial infarction models, MSC survival and paracrine function of IGF-1 were enhanced significantly *in* vivo, with decreased cardiomyocyte apoptosis, scar size, and interstitial fibrosis, and increased angiogenesis in the diseased myocardium, which ultimately attenuated ventricular remodeling and improved heart function. This study demonstrated that a great potential of siRNA-modified stem cells in therapeutic applications, which, of course, might be used in AKI [73].

8. Conclusions

The kidney is a comparatively easy target organ for siRNA therapy due to its unique structural and functional characteristics. siRNA intervention is effective, feasible, and has great potential for fighting against kidney diseases. For the next-generation siRNA development, cell-specific precise delivery should be pursued. Although the safety of siRNA therapy has been proven by rapidly emerging clinical studies, off-target and compensative responses still need be overcome via various modification strategies. The time for realizing the therapeutic potential of RNAi has come because optimized siRNA therapy, in conjunction with advanced genetic screening technologies, could facilitate timely and specific treatment of kidney as well as other organ diseases in the near future.

Author details

Cheng Yang[1,2] and Bin Yang[3,4*]

*Address all correspondence to: by5@le.ac.uk

1 Department of Plastic Surgery, Zhongshan Hospital, Fudan University, Shanghai, China

2 Shanghai Key Laboratory of Organ Transplantation, Shanghai, China

3 Medical Research Centre, Medical School of Nantong University; Department of Nephrology, Affiliated Hospital of Nantong University, Nantong, China, United Kingdom

4 Renal Group, Department of Infection, Immunity and Inflammation, University of Leicester,University Hospitals of Leicester, United Kingdom

References

[1] Bellomo R, Kellum JA, Ronco C: Acute kidney injury. *Lancet* 2012; 380:756–766.DOI: 10.1016/S0140-6736(11)61454-2

[2] Palevsky PM, Molitoris BA, Okusa MD, Levin A, Waikar SS, Wald R, Chertow GM, Murray PT, Parikh CR, Shaw AD, et al: Design of clinical trials in acute kidney injury: report from an NIDDK workshop on trial methodology. *Clin J Am Soc Nephrol* 2012; 7:844–850. DOI:10.2215/CJN.12791211

[3] Elbashir SM, Harborth J, Lendeckel W, Yalcin A, Weber K, Tuschl T: Duplexes of 21-nucleotide RNAs mediate RNA interference in cultured mammalian cells. *Nature* 2001; 411:494–498. DOI:10.1038/35078107

[4] Petrocca F, Lieberman J: Promise and challenge of RNA interference-based therapy for cancer. *J Clin Oncol* 2011; 29:747–754. DOI:10.1200/JCO.2009.27.6287

[5] Jeker LT, Bluestone JA: Small RNA regulators of T cell-mediated autoimmunity. *J Clin Immunol* 2010; 30:347–357. DOI:10.1007/s10875-010-9392-7

[6] Latronico MV, Condorelli G: RNA silencing: small RNA-mediated posttranscriptional regulation of mRNA and the implications for heart electropathophysiology. *J Cardiovasc Electrophysiol* 2009; 20:230–237. DOI:10.1111/j.1540-8167.2008.01357.x

[7] Yang C, Jia Y, Zhao T, Xue Y, Zhao Z, Zhang J, Wang J, Wang X, Qiu Y, Lin M, et al: Naked caspase 3 small interfering RNA is effective in cold preservation but not in autotransplantation of porcine kidneys. *J Surg Res* 2013; 181:342–354. DOI:10.1016/j.jss.2012.07.015

[8] Racz Z, Hamar P: RNA interference in research and therapy of renal diseases. *Contrib Nephrol* 2008; 159:78–95. DOI:10.1159/000125587

[9] Yang C, Zhang C, Zhao Z, Zhu T, Yang B: Fighting against kidney diseases with small interfering RNA: opportunities and challenges. *J Transl Med* 2015; 13:39. DOI: 10.1186/s12967-015-0387-2

[10] Chaudhary A, Srivastava S, Garg S: Development of a software tool and criteria evaluation for efficient design of small interfering RNA. *Biochem Biophys Res Commun* 2011; 404:313–320. DOI:10.1016/j.bbrc.2010.11.114

[11] Elmen J, Thonberg H, Ljungberg K, Frieden M, Westergaard M, Xu Y, Wahren B, Liang Z, Orum H, Koch T, Wahlestedt C: Locked nucleic acid (LNA) mediated improvements in siRNA stability and functionality. *Nucleic Acids Res* 2005; 33:439–447. DOI:10.1093/nar/gki193

[12] Yang C, Zhao T, Zhao Z, Jia Y, Li L, Zhang Y, Song M, Rong R, Xu M, Nicholson ML, et al: Serum-stabilized naked caspase-3 siRNA protects autotransplant kidneys in a porcine model. *Mol Ther* 2014; 22:1817–1828. DOI:10.1038/mt.2014.111

[13] Mook OR, Baas F, de Wissel MB, Fluiter K: Evaluation of locked nucleic acid-modified small interfering RNA in vitro and in vivo. *Mol Cancer Ther* 2007; 6:833–843. DOI: 10.1158/1535-7163.MCT-06-0195

[14] Kanasty R, Dorkin JR, Vegas A, Anderson D: Delivery materials for siRNA therapeutics. *Nat Mater* 2013; 12:967–977. DOI:10.1038/nmat3765

[15] Deng Y, Wang CC, Choy KW, Du Q, Chen J, Wang Q, Li L, Chung TK, Tang T: Therapeutic potentials of gene silencing by RNA interference: principles, challenges, and new strategies. *Gene* 2014; 538:217–227. DOI:10.1016/j.gene.2013.12.019

[16] Yang B, Hosgood SA, Nicholson ML: Naked small interfering RNA of caspase-3 in preservation solution and autologous blood perfusate protects isolated ischemic porcine kidneys. *Transplantation* 2011; 91:501–507. DOI:10.1097/TP.0b013e318207949f

[17] Yang B, Elias JE, Bloxham M, Nicholson ML: Synthetic small interfering RNA down-regulates caspase-3 and affects apoptosis, IL-1 beta, and viability of porcine proximal tubular cells. *J Cell Biochem* 2011; 112:1337–1347. DOI:10.1002/jcb.23050

[18] Takabatake Y, Isaka Y, Mizui M, Kawachi H, Shimizu F, Ito T, Hori M, Imai E: Exploring RNA interference as a therapeutic strategy for renal disease. *Gene Ther* 2005; 12:965–973. DOI:10.1038/sj.gt.3302480

[19] Wan X, Fan L, Hu B, Yang J, Li X, Chen X, Cao C: Small interfering RNA targeting IKKbeta prevents renal ischemia-reperfusion injury in rats. *Am J Physiol Renal Physiol* 2011; 300:F857–F863. DOI:10.1152/ajprenal.00547.2010

[20] Hamar P, Song E, Kokeny G, Chen A, Ouyang N, Lieberman J: Small interfering RNA targeting Fas protects mice against renal ischemia-reperfusion injury. *Proc Natl Acad Sci U S A* 2004; 101:14883–14888. DOI:10.1073/pnas.0406421101

[21] Xia Z, Abe K, Furusu A, Miyazaki M, Obata Y, Tabata Y, Koji T, Kohno S: Suppression of renal tubulointerstitial fibrosis by small interfering RNA targeting heat shock protein 47. *Am J Nephrol* 2008; 28:34–46. DOI:10.1159/000108759

[22] Cuevas S, Zhang Y, Yang Y, Escano C, Asico L, Jones JE, Armando I, Jose PA: Role of renal DJ-1 in the pathogenesis of hypertension associated with increased reactive oxygen species production. *Hypertension* 2012; 59:446–452. DOI:10.1161/HYPERTENSIONAHA.111.185744

[23] Gooding M, Browne LP, Quinteiro FM, Selwood DL: siRNA delivery: from lipids to cell-penetrating peptides and their mimics. *Chem Biol Drug Des* 2012; 80:787–809. DOI:10.1111/cbdd.12052

[24] Braasch DA, Jensen S, Liu Y, Kaur K, Arar K, White MA, Corey DR: RNA interference in mammalian cells by chemically-modified RNA. *Biochemistry* 2003; 42:7967–7975. DOI:10.1021/bi0343774

[25] Molitoris BA, Dagher PC, Sandoval RM, Campos SB, Ashush H, Fridman E, Brafman A, Faerman A, Atkinson SJ, Thompson JD, et al: siRNA targeted to p53 attenuates is-

chemic and cisplatin-induced acute kidney injury. *J Am Soc Nephrol* 2009; 20:1754–1764. DOI:10.1681/ASN.2008111204

[26] Zheng X, Zhang X, Sun H, Feng B, Li M, Chen G, Vladau C, Chen D, Suzuki M, Min L, et al: Protection of renal ischemia injury using combination gene silencing of complement 3 and caspase 3 genes. *Transplantation* 2006; 82:1781–1786. DOI:10.1097/01.tp.0000250769.86623.a3

[27] Zhang D, Liu Y, Wei Q, Huo Y, Liu K, Liu F, Dong Z: Tubular p53 regulates multiple genes to mediate AKI. *J Am Soc Nephrol* 2014; 25:2278–2289. DOI:10.1681/ASN.2013080902

[28] Ojima I: Guided molecular missiles for tumor-targeting chemotherapy--case studies using the second-generation taxoids as warheads. *Acc Chem Res* 2008; 41:108–119. DOI:10.1021/ar700093f

[29] Mokhtarieh AA, Cheong S, Kim S, Chung BH, Lee MK: Asymmetric liposome particles with highly efficient encapsulation of siRNA and without nonspecific cell penetration suitable for target-specific delivery. *Biochim Biophys Acta* 2012; 1818:1633–1641. DOI:10.1016/j.bbamem.2012.03.016

[30] Leus NG, Morselt HW, Zwiers PJ, Kowalski PS, Ruiters MH, Molema G, Kamps JA: VCAM-1 specific PEGylated SAINT-based lipoplexes deliver siRNA to activated endothelium in vivo but do not attenuate target gene expression. *Int J Pharm* 2014; 469:121–131. DOI:10.1016/j.ijpharm.2014.04.041

[31] Trochet D, Prudhon B, Vassilopoulos S, Bitoun M: Therapy for dominant inherited diseases by allele-specific RNA interference: successes and pitfalls. *Curr Gene Ther* 2015; 15:503–510. DOI:10.2174/1566523215666150812115730

[32] Courtney DG, Atkinson SD, Allen EH, Moore JE, Walsh CP, Pedrioli DM, MacEwen CJ, Pellegrini G, Maurizi E, Serafini C, et al: siRNA silencing of the mutant keratin 12 allele in corneal limbal epithelial cells grown from patients with Meesmann's epithelial corneal dystrophy. *Invest Ophthalmol Vis Sci* 2014; 55:3352–3360. DOI:10.1167/iovs.13-12957

[33] Allen EH, Atkinson SD, Liao H, Moore JE, Leslie Pedrioli DM, Smith FJ, McLean WH, Moore CB: Allele-specific siRNA silencing for the common keratin 12 founder mutation in Meesmann epithelial corneal dystrophy. *Invest Ophthalmol Vis Sci* 2013; 54:494–502. DOI:10.1167/iovs.12-10528

[34] Takahashi M, Katagiri T, Furuya H, Hohjoh H: Disease-causing allele-specific silencing against the ALK2 mutants, R206H and G356D, in fibrodysplasia ossificans progressiva. *Gene Ther* 2012; 19:781–785. DOI:10.1038/gt.2011.193

[35] Zuckerman JE, Gale A, Wu P, Ma R, Davis ME: siRNA delivery to the glomerular mesangium using polycationic cyclodextrin nanoparticles containing siRNA. *Nucleic Acid Ther* 2015; 25:53–64. DOI:10.1089/nat.2014.0505

[36] Haussecker D: Current issues of RNAi therapeutics delivery and development. *J Control Release* 2014; 195:49–54. DOI:10.1016/j.jconrel.2014.07.056

[37] Forbes DC, Peppas NA: Polycationic nanoparticles for siRNA delivery: comparing ARGET ATRP and UV-initiated formulations. *ACS Nano* 2014; 8:2908–2917. DOI: 10.1021/nn500101c

[38] Li H, Tsui TY, Ma W: Intracellular delivery of molecular cargo using cell-penetrating peptides and the combination strategies. *Int J Mol Sci* 2015; 16:19518–19536. DOI: 10.3390/ijms160819518

[39] van Asbeck AH, Beyerle A, McNeill H, Bovee-Geurts PH, Lindberg S, Verdurmen WP, Hallbrink M, Langel U, Heidenreich O, Brock R: Molecular parameters of siRNA —cell penetrating peptide nanocomplexes for efficient cellular delivery. *ACS Nano* 2013; 7:3797–3807. DOI:10.1021/nn305754c

[40] Huang Y, Wang X, Huang W, Cheng Q, Zheng S, Guo S, Cao H, Liang XJ, Du Q, Liang Z: Systemic administration of siRNA via cRGD-containing peptide. *Sci Rep* 2015; 5:12458. DOI:10.1038/srep12458

[41] Junquera E, Aicart E: Recent progress in gene therapy to deliver nucleic acids with multivalent cationic vectors. *Adv Colloid Interface Sci* 2015. DOI:10.1016/j.cis.2015.07.003

[42] Kosieradzki M, Rowinski W: Ischemia/reperfusion injury in kidney transplantation: mechanisms and prevention. *Transplantation Proceedings* 2008; 40:3279–3288. DOI: 10.1016/j.transproceed.2008.10.004

[43] Eltzschig HK, Eckle T: Ischemia and reperfusion-from mechanism to translation. *Nature Medicine* 2011; 17:1391–1401. DOI:10.1038/nm.2507

[44] Vaseva AV, Moll UM: The mitochondrial p53 pathway. *Biochim Biophys Acta* 2009; 1787:414–420. DOI:10.1016/j.bbabio.2008.10.005

[45] Fujino T, Muhib S, Sato N, Hasebe N: Silencing of p53 RNA through transarterial delivery ameliorates renal tubular injury and downregulates GSK-3beta expression after ischemia-reperfusion injury. *Am J Physiol Renal Physiol* 2013; 305:F1617–F1627. DOI:10.1152/ajprenal.00279.2013

[46] Peng J, Li X, Zhang D, Chen JK, Su Y, Smith SB, Dong Z: Hyperglycemia, p53, and mitochondrial pathway of apoptosis are involved in the susceptibility of diabetic models to ischemic acute kidney injury. *Kidney Int* 2015; 87:137–150. DOI:10.1038/ki.2014.226

[47] Liu L, Li Y, Hu Z, Su J, Huo Y, Tan B, Wang X, Liu Y: Small interfering RNA targeting Toll-like receptor 9 protects mice against polymicrobial septic acute kidney injury. *Nephron Exp Nephrol* 2012; 122:51–61. DOI:10.1159/000346953

[48] Jackson AL, Bartz SR, Schelter J, Kobayashi SV, Burchard J, Mao M, Li B, Cavet G, Linsley PS: Expression profiling reveals off-target gene regulation by RNAi. *Nat Biotechnol* 2003; 21:635–637. DOI:10.1038/nbt831

[49] Jackson AL, Burchard J, Schelter J, Chau BN, Cleary M, Lim L, Linsley PS: Widespread siRNA "off-target" transcript silencing mediated by seed region sequence complementarity. *RNA* 2006; 12:1179–1187. DOI:10.1261/rna.25706

[50] Jackson AL, Linsley PS: Recognizing and avoiding siRNA off-target effects for target identification and therapeutic application. *Nat Rev Drug Discov* 2010; 9:57–67. DOI:10.1038/nrd3010

[51] Lin X, Ruan X, Anderson MG, McDowell JA, Kroeger PE, Fesik SW, Shen Y: siRNA-mediated off-target gene silencing triggered by a 7 nt complementation. *Nucleic Acids Res* 2005; 33:4527–4535. DOI:10.1093/nar/gki762

[52] Kabilova TO, Meschaninova MI, Venyaminova AG, Nikolin VP, Zenkova MA, Vlassov VV, Chernolovskaya EL: Short double-stranded RNA with immunostimulatory activity: sequence dependence. *Nucleic Acid Ther* 2012; 22:196–204. DOI:10.1089/nat.2011.0328

[53] Robbins M, Judge A, MacLachlan I: siRNA and innate immunity. *Oligonucleotides* 2009; 19:89–102. DOI:10.1089/oli.2009.0180

[54] Yang C, Li L, Xue Y, Zhao Z, Zhao T, Jia Y, Rong R, Xu M, Nicholson ML, Zhu T, Yang B: Innate immunity activation involved in unprotected porcine auto-transplant kidneys preserved by naked caspase-3 siRNA. *J Transl Med* 2013; 11:210. DOI:10.1186/1479-5876-11-210

[55] Bell JK, Askins J, Hall PR, Davies DR, Segal DM: The dsRNA binding site of human Toll-like receptor 3. *Proc Natl Acad Sci U S A* 2006; 103:8792–8797. DOI:10.1073/pnas.0603245103

[56] Choe J, Kelker MS, Wilson IA: Crystal structure of human toll-like receptor 3 (TLR3) ectodomain. *Science* 2005; 309:581–585. DOI:10.1126/science.1115253

[57] Alexopoulou L, Holt AC, Medzhitov R, Flavell RA: Recognition of double-stranded RNA and activation of NF-kappaB by Toll-like receptor 3. *Nature* 2001; 413:732–738. DOI:10.1038/35099560

[58] Hornung V, Guenthner-Biller M, Bourquin C, Ablasser A, Schlee M, Uematsu S, Noronha A, Manoharan M, Akira S, de Fougerolles A, et al: Sequence-specific potent induction of IFN-alpha by short interfering RNA in plasmacytoid dendritic cells through TLR7. *Nat Med* 2005; 11:263–270. DOI:10.1038/nm1191

[59] Judge AD, Sood V, Shaw JR, Fang D, McClintock K, MacLachlan I: Sequence-dependent stimulation of the mammalian innate immune response by synthetic siRNA. *Nat Biotechnol* 2005; 23:457–462. DOI:10.1038/nbt1081

[60] Sioud M: Induction of inflammatory cytokines and interferon responses by double-stranded and single-stranded siRNAs is sequence-dependent and requires endosomal localization. *J Mol Biol* 2005; 348:1079–1090. DOI:10.1016/j.jmb.2005.03.013

[61] Racz Z, Godo M, Revesz C, Hamar P: Immune activation and target organ damage are consequences of hydrodynamic treatment but not delivery of naked siRNAs in mice. *Nucleic Acid Ther* 2011; 21:215–224. DOI:10.1089/nat.2010.0248

[62] Mueller TF, Reeve J, Jhangri GS, Mengel M, Jacaj Z, Cairo L, Obeidat M, Todd G, Moore R, Famulski KS, et al: The transcriptome of the implant biopsy identifies donor kidneys at increased risk of delayed graft function. *Am J Transplant* 2008; 8:78–85. DOI:10.1111/j.1600-6143.2007.02032.x

[63] Wilflingseder J, Sunzenauer J, Toronyi E, Heinzel A, Kainz A, Mayer B, Perco P, Telkes G, Langer RM, Oberbauer R: Molecular pathogenesis of post-transplant acute kidney injury: assessment of whole-genome mRNA and MiRNA profiles. *PLoS One* 2014; 9:e104164. DOI:10.1371/journal.pone.0104164

[64] Wu D, Zhu D, Xu M, Rong R, Tang Q, Wang X, Zhu T: Analysis of transcriptional factors and regulation networks in patients with acute renal allograft rejection. *J Proteome Res* 2011; 10:175–181. DOI:10.1021/pr100473w

[65] Wu D, Liu X, Liu C, Liu Z, Xu M, Rong R, Qian M, Chen L, Zhu T: Network analysis reveals roles of inflammatory factors in different phenotypes of kidney transplant patients. *J Theor Biol* 2014; 362:62–68. DOI:10.1016/j.jtbi.2014.03.006

[66] Grimm D, Streetz KL, Jopling CL, Storm TA, Pandey K, Davis CR, Marion P, Salazar F, Kay MA: Fatality in mice due to oversaturation of cellular microRNA/short hairpin RNA pathways. *Nature* 2006; 441:537–541. DOI:10.1038/nature04791

[67] Liu K, Chen H, You Q, Shi H, Wang Z: The siRNA cocktail targeting VEGF and HER2 inhibition on the proliferation and induced apoptosis of gastric cancer cell. *Mol Cell Biochem* 2014; 386:117–124. DOI:10.1007/s11010-013-1850-0

[68] Zhou J, Neff CP, Liu X, Zhang J, Li H, Smith DD, Swiderski P, Aboellail T, Huang Y, Du Q, et al: Systemic administration of combinatorial dsiRNAs via nanoparticles efficiently suppresses HIV-1 infection in humanized mice. *Mol Ther* 2011; 19:2228–2238. DOI:10.1038/mt.2011.207

[69] Ge Q, Xu JJ, Evans DM, Mixson AJ, Yang HY, Lu PY: Leveraging therapeutic potential of multi-targeted siRNA inhibitors. *Future Med Chem* 2009; 1:1671–1681. DOI: 10.4155/fmc.09.131

[70] Jiang N, Zhang X, Zheng X, Chen D, Siu K, Wang H, Ichim TE, Quan D, McAlister V, Chen G, Min WP: A novel in vivo siRNA delivery system specifically targeting liver cells for protection of ConA-induced fulminant hepatitis. *PLoS One* 2012; 7:e44138. DOI:10.1371/journal.pone.0044138

[71] Siu KS, Chen D, Zheng X, Zhang X, Johnston N, Liu Y, Yuan K, Koropatnick J, Gillies ER, Min WP: Non-covalently functionalized single-walled carbon nanotube for topi-

cal siRNA delivery into melanoma. *Biomaterials* 2014; 35:3435–3442. DOI:10.1016/j.biomaterials.2013.12.079

[72] Chen D, Koropatnick J, Jiang N, Zheng X, Zhang X, Wang H, Yuan K, Siu KS, Shunnar A, Way C, Min WP: Targeted siRNA silencing of indoleamine 2, 3-dioxygenase in antigen-presenting cells using mannose-conjugated liposomes: a novel strategy for treatment of melanoma. *J Immunother* 2014; 37:123–134. DOI:10.1097/CJI.0000000000000022

[73] Zhu K, Lai H, Guo C, Li J, Wang Y, Wang L, Wang C: Nanovector-based prolyl hydroxylase domain 2 silencing system enhances the efficiency of stem cell transplantation for infarcted myocardium repair. *Int J Nanomedicine* 2014; 9:5203–5215. DOI:10.2147/IJN.S71586

Preclinical Development of RNAi-Inducing Oligonucleotide Therapeutics for Eye Diseases

Tamara Martínez, Maria Victoria González, Beatriz Vargas,
Ana Isabel Jiménez and Covadonga Pañeda

Additional information is available at the end of the chapter

http://dx.doi.org/10.5772/61803

Abstract

RNA interference (RNAi) is a posttranscriptional mechanism of gene regulation present in eukaryotic cells. Inducers of RNAi are small molecules of RNA that act in the cytoplasm where they are able to impair translation of a specific mRNA to protein, hence modifying gene expression. The discovery of this mechanism in mammals led to the development of a new class of therapeutics with the aim of exploiting this endogenous mechanism of action. In the last decade, great efforts have been put into understanding RNAi and translating this accumulated knowledge into the design of modern therapeutics. With several compounds in phase III clinical development, the field is getting closer to its first market authorization. Here we make a thorough overview of the field of RNAi therapeutics in ophthalmology, one of the fields in which RNAi has been most successful.

Keywords: RNAi, eye diseases, ophthalmology, drug development

1. Introduction

Short interference RNAs (siRNA) are small molecules of double-stranded RNA of around 21 base pair long that specifically downregulate the expression of a target gene [1]. This mechanism of endogenous gene expression regulation, present in most eukaryotic cells, has been thoroughly used to study gene function [2]. SiRNAs exert their function in the cytoplasm of the cell, where they assemble with a several proteins to yield the RNA-induced silencing complex (RISC), a multimeric RNA–protein complex that recognizes complementary messenger RNAs (mRNA) and promotes their degradation, thus blocking the synthesis of specific proteins. RNAi may be activated by endogenous siRNAs synthesized in the nucleus of the cell and generated by subsequent processing within the cell cytoplasm to yield siRNAs. Alternatively, siRNAs can be exogenously introduced to mimic the action of endogenous RNAi triggers [3]. Among the benefits of RNAi are the potential of transiently silencing any given gene at any stage of development and to affect gene expression in specific anatomical regions without affecting nontargeted regions. These benefits are being used as a basis to develop a new class of innovative drugs that may reach the market in the next five years; the present report highlights the advances made in RNAi therapeutics on the field of ophthalmology.

2. The special environment of the eye: advantages and disadvantages

The eye has traditionally been considered a good organ for proof-of-concept studies to assess the efficacy of innovative therapies. It has a very particular anatomy that allows the transformation of sensory information into electrical signals that can be thereafter interpreted by the brain. Transformation and partial processing of sensory information takes place in the retina, located at the back of the eye. The correct function of the eye requires light to travel through several anatomical structures in order to reach the photosensitive retina; hence, these structures have to be transparent or semi-transparent to allow passage of light. The environment of the eye is extremely specialized to ensure that transparency is maintained, and there are several mechanisms in place to ensure that this specialized environment is preserved. One of the anatomical characteristics of the eye to allow light to travel through its structures is restricting the blood flow to regions where transparency is not strictly required.

In addition, access to the innermost regions of the eye is controlled by several barriers; these barriers isolate the eye from external aggressions and pathogens to but also limit the access of therapeutics. The influence of the particular anatomical features of the eye on drug delivery is further explained in Section 4 of this review. The barriers of the eye do not only isolate this organ from external aggressions or substances but also limit the access of internal elements; as such, the immune system has only limited access to the eye making the eye a partially immune-privileged region. Finally, the aqueous humor, the clear liquid that fills the eye and maintains its shape and pressure, has a very low content in proteins compared to serum. Among the proteins that are significantly reduced compared to other tissues are RNases and elements of the complement cascade. The reduced concentration of RNases increases the half-life of RNAs used as therapeutics, and reduction in the elements of the complement cascade further decreases the likelihood of an unwanted immune reactions to drugs.

In order to preserve its integrity, the eye has efficacious barriers to block the entrance of pathogens and substances that could potentially affect its sensory function. The eye has developed specific features that ensure that light travels through its tissues; this specialization of tissues to preserve visual function is also observed by the immune system [4]. Immune responses change the local environment of tissues and are frequently associated to tissue inflammation. In order to avoid these potentially harmful changes, the eye has a relatively immune privileged status. This immune privilege status is maintained by several mechanisms. Absence of lymphatic and blood vessels in certain areas and abundance of immunosuppressive factors in the aqueous humor are among these mechanisms [5]. On the other hand, the eye needs to be able to respond to situations in which its integrity can be compromised such as viral or bacterial infections. The innate immune response is the first system activated in response to aggressions; it acts like a watchdog mechanism recognizing pathogen-associated molecular patterns (PAMP). Depending on the molecular characteristics and location of the PAMP, different effectors of the innate response are activated; these responses can be mediated by toll-like receptors (TLR) or independent of these receptors. Toll-like receptors discriminate self-motifs from non-self-motifs [6]. There are ten known TLRs, and they differ in their subcellular localization and in the type of non-self-pattern they recognize. TLR1, TLR2, TLR4, TLR5, and TLR6 recognize components of bacterial walls and are located in the cell surface, whereas TLR3, TLR7, TLR8, and TLR9 recognize oligonucleotides and are sequestered in intracellular compartment. TLR3 binds to single- and double-stranded RNA, TLR7 binds to single-stranded RNA, and TLR9 binds to unmethylated CpG motifs, usually found in bacterial DNA. In the eye, the expression pattern of each TLRs varies depending on the anatomical structure; all TLRs are present in the corneal and retinal pigment epithelia; TLR4 is the predominant TLR in the rest of the eye structures where it localizes in resident antigen presenting cells [7, 8]. TLR-independent response mechanisms to cytoplasmic oligonucleotides include dsRNA-binding protein kinase, the RNA helicase (RIG-I), and oligoadenylate synthase enzyme. These proteins are cytoplasmic dsRNA sensors belonging to the antiviral innate immune system, which plays an important role in antiviral defense in response to viral infection and replication [9].

The first proof-of-concept studies to demonstrate the viability of silencing genes in the eye showed that the injection of siRNAs into the subretinal space or vitreous cavity could indeed downregulate specific genes. In these experiments, the downregulation of genes of the vascular endothelial growth factor (VEGF) family with siRNAs correlated with the inhibition of ocular neovascularization [10, 11]. The first set of these experiments used an adenoviral vector that codified for an siRNA designed against VEGF1. The subretinal injection of this vector 36 h after the induction of coroidal neovascularization (CNV) by laser reduced the areas of neovascularization compared to areas of mice injected with vector codifying for a scrambled siRNA [10] In a subsequent study, Campochiaro and coworkers [10] demonstrated that the inhibition of ocular neovascularization could also be achieved by injecting a VEGFR1 siRNA directly, without an expression vector, into the vitreous cavity. The siRNA used in this study had the so-called canonical design, which comprises a 21-nucleotide guide strand and a complementary passenger strand annealed to form an siRNA duplex with a 19-bp dsRNA stem and 2 nucleotide 3′ overhangs at both ends [11].

In 2008, Kleinman and coworkers published a study in *Nature* demonstrating that the effect of siRNAs on CNV was mediated by activation of TLR3 rather than an effect on target [12]. The results of these studies showed that the effect of the siRNAs on CNV was dose-dependent but not dependent on sequence. In addition, the authors demonstrated that a minimum length of the siRNA was required in order for the molecules to have an effect on CNV; this length was show to be at least 21 nucleotides. The study also showed that the internalization of the siRNAs was not required for the inhibition of CNV as cells of the retinal pigment epithelium (RPE) abundantly express TLR3 on the cytoplasmic surface. The authors used several sequences to point out that the inhibition of CNV was mediated through an off-target effect. Using docking models, the authors showed that TLR3 and siRNAs were indeed able to interact with each other but the interaction was unstable when siRNAs were shorter than 21 nucleotides. A subsequent study by the same group showed that activation of TLR3 by IVT siRNAs led to caspase-3-mediated degeneration of the RPE questioning the safety these compounds as therapeutics for back of the eye diseases [13]. The findings of Kleinman and coworkers boosted research on alternative designs that could successfully block immune recognition; among the most commonly used strategies are incorporation of delivery systems and 2′-ribose modifications.

Finally, exogenous RNAs are quickly degraded by RNases present in tissues and body fluids [14]. These enzymes cut RNA into smaller components that are subsequently incorporated into the route of degradation of nucleotides. RNAses are present at high concentrations both in tissues, such as in spleen, liver, and pancreas, and in biological fluids, such as in serum [15]. In the eye, the tear fluid is rich in nucleases but the presence of these enzymes is considerably lower in most eye tissues, thus allowing for increased half-life of the siRNAs used for therapeutic purposes.

3. Efficacy studies: Animal models to study the eye

Proof-of-concept studies are required in order to demonstrate that a particular drug has the proposed activity. siRNAs are designed using bioinformatics tools to target specific regions of the human genome. Therefore, assessing the activity of these molecules in animal models requires that the siRNA has biological activity in the species chosen to perform the proof-of-concept study. With the sequencing of the genome of most animal models used in biomedical research, evaluating the homology of a given sequence between two species is nowadays common practice, but this does not warrant finding a fully homologous siRNA for all targeted genes. In cases where homologous sequences cannot be found, a surrogate compound can be used to perform animal efficacy studies; this entails designing a compound that targets the exact same region as the human version but with the sequence of the gene of the animal species to be used. Several animal models can be used to assess the activity of a compound. Here we highlighted the animal models used in the developmental programs of products included in the ophthalmic siRNA pipeline.

3.1. Ischemic optic neuropathy

Ischemic optic neuropathy is a sudden loss of vision caused by interruption or decreased blood flow in the optic nerve. There is a disagreement as to its pathogenesis, clinical features, and management because ischemic optic neuropathy is not a unique disease, but a spectrum of different types [16]. Ischemic optic neuropathy can be primarily of two types: anterior (AION) caused by the interruption of blood flow in the optic nerve head and posterior (PION) involving the posterior part the optic nerve. Both types can be further classified into different subtypes. AION comprises arteritic (A-AION) caused by giant cell arteritis and nonarteritic (NA-AION) caused by other than giant cell arteritis. NA-AION is by far the most common type and typically affects individuals between 55 and 67 years of age. The incidence of AION has only been thoroughly studied in the USA where there are 2.3–10.3 cases per 100,000 inhabitants; for the nonarteritic type, the numbers are lower: 0.36 per 100,000 inhabitants. NA-AION is characterized by visual loss, optic disc swelling, sometimes with flame hemorrhages on the swollen disc or nearby neuroretinal layer, and sometimes with nearby cotton wool exudates. Visual loss is usually sudden and may progress over several hours to days and even weeks [17].

Animal modes of this disease are used to assess efficacy of pharmaceuticals in development for these conditions and include the optic nerve crush model and the photoembolic stroke model. The optic nerve crush model is a general model in which surviving of the ganglionar cells can be studied in response to a physical damage to the optic nerve [18]. In the photoembolic stroke model, a photosensitive dye, such as rose bengal, is injected intravenously, and laser is specifically applied to the optic nerve head to activate the dye. The activation of the dye results in damage to the endothelial cells of the optic nerve vascular system that ultimately leads to thrombosis of vessels and edema of the optic nerve head [19].

3.2. Glaucoma

Glaucoma is a group of progressive optic neuropathies characterized by vision impairment and degeneration of retinal ganglion cells that if left untreated can lead to blindness. Glaucoma is the second leading cause of global irreversible blindness, and it has been estimated that 60.5 million people were affected by primary open-angle glaucoma (POAG) and primary angle–closure glaucoma (PACG) globally in 2010, a number expected to increase to nearly 80 million by 2020 [20]. The degeneration of the optic nerve is thought to be produced as a result of changes in intraocular pressure (IOP), but specific molecular mediators of these changes have yet to be identified. Because glaucoma may be asymptomatic until a relatively late stage where the nerve damage has already occurred, early diagnosis and treatment are crucial for halting the progression of the condition [21]. Reduction of IOP is the only proven strategy to treat the disease; thus, first-line treatments are aimed toward achieving this goal. There are several compounds currently used to lower IOP, and although most of them are efficacious in lowering IOP, they all come with their own set of side effects and tolerance to the drug is a frequent phenomenon. Tolerance or reduced response of the drug requires change of drug regimen, frequently increasing the dose or combining the prescribed pharmaceutical with another drug [22, 23].

Depending on the specific phase of the disease one wants to model, several animal models can be used [24]. If studying the degeneration of the retina is the main objective, the models mentioned in the previous section can be used. For assessing the IOP lowering efficacy of pharmaceuticals, models with increased IOP are generally used. The increased IOP model induced by oral water overloading in rabbits is a very easy and physiologic model to screen compounds. The basis behind this model is to give the animal an oral overload of water that will result in a transient increase in IOP [25]. Although the specific mechanism behind the increase in IOP following water overloading is uncertain, the model has been extensively used to perform rapid screens of IOP-lowering compounds. The main advantage of this model over other existing models of increased IOP is that the anatomical structure and physiology of eye structures are preserved allowing a normal response to hypotensive drugs. Other models of increased IOP include laser photocoagulation, intracameral injection of latex microspheres, topical application of prednisolone, light-induced reduced outflow facility, subconjunctival injection of betamethasone, or episcleral vein occlusion [24].

3.3. Dry eye disease

Dry eye disease (DED) is a multifactorial disease of the tear-fluid and ocular surface that results in symptoms of discomfort, visual disturbance, and tear film instability. It is accompanied by increased osmolarity of the tear film and inflammation of the ocular surface [26]. Common symptoms of this condition include blurry vision, tearing, and ocular pain. There are several factors that contribute to the etiology of the disease, among them are insufficient tear secretion, excessive evaporation, and alteration in the composition of the tear film [27]. Temporary changes of the composition of the tear film can cause an acute form of DED; if changes persist, the condition can turn into chronic DED. Damage to the ocular surface is usually more severe in the chronic forms than in the acute types. DED is frequently associated to other conditions such as Sjögren's disease or lachrymal gland dysfunction, but it can also be caused by vitamin deficiency, contact lens wear, and use of several prescription drugs. Acute DED is handled with lubricants and avoiding preservatives in concomitant eye drops. If DED persists, treatment options include procedures that favor tear retention such as punctal occlusion, moisture chamber spectacles, contact lenses, or pharmacologic agents that stimulate tear secretion. More severe forms may require the use of anti-inflammatory therapy [28]. Although some advances have been made toward alleviating some of the symptoms of DED, pain associated to this condition is not usually addressed. Pain in the eye results from stimulation of sensory axons of the trigeminal ganglion neurons innervating the cornea [29]. Animal models to assess the efficacy of ocular analgesics are extremely complex in terms of interpreting efficacy outcomes [30]. One of the commonly used models to study pain is the capsaicin-induced ocular pain model developed by Gertrudis and colleagues [31]. This model is based on the evaluation of animal behavior after topical ocular administration of capsaicin, a selective agonist of transient receptor protein vaniloid type 1 (TRPV1). Capsaicin applied locally to the eye activates TRPV1 inducing palpebral closure. Latency to open the eye and time required for complete palpebral opening can be used as measurements of the discomfort caused by capsaicin. Reference products used in this model include analgesics, in particular, capsazepine, the antagonist of TRPV1 channels.

3.4. Ocular allergy

Ocular allergies constitute a heterogenic group of diseases with a broad spectrum of clinical manifestations and include mild forms such as seasonal allergic conjunctivitis (SAC) and perennial allergic conjunctivitis (PAC), and more severe manifestations such as vernal keratoconjunctivitis (VKC), atopic keratoconjunctivitis (AKC), and giant papillary conjunctivitis (GPC). The severe forms can be associated to complications such as corneal damage and may cause vision loss. SAC and PAC are commonly IgE-mast cell-mediated hypersensitivity reaction to external allergens, whereas AKC and VKC are characterized by chronic inflammation involving several immune cell types. In SAC and PAC, allergens, with the help of antigen presenting cells, trigger a Th2-predominant immune response that induces B cells to release IgE. In SAC and PAC, allergen-induced local release of IgE prompts infiltration and degranulation of mast cells in Ca^{2+}-dependent mechanism. Mast cells liberate preformed inflammatory mediators such as histamine and leukotriene 4 that subsequently attract eosinophils amplify the allergic response [32]. The prevalence of ocular allergies in the general population is estimated to be around 40% in the United States [33] and up to 35% in Europe and the Middle East [34], but it is probably underestimated in most epidemiologic studies [35]. The primary treatment for ocular allergies includes avoidance of allergens, cold compresses, and lubrication. In persisting cases, symptoms can be treated using topical and oral decongestants, antihistamines, mast-cell stabilizers, or anti-inflammatory agents [36]. Allergic conjunctivitis can be modeled in animals by exposing them to allergens in the presence of an adjuvant [37]. The model developed by Magone and coworkers uses Female Balb/C mice that are sensitized with short ragweed and alum and several days later animals receive a topical dose of short ragweed pollen in the eye. A prescreening of mice can be performed in order to select only those animals that respond to allergens.

3.5. Age-related macular degeneration with choroidal neovascularization

Age-related macular degeneration (AMD) is the leading cause of severe vision loss in individuals over 50 years of age [38, 39]. AMD is caused by a combination of genetic and environmental factors. Risk factors include hypertension, cardiovascular disease, smoking, and high BMI. Among the genetic factors that confer susceptibility to developing AMD are variants in genes encoding complement pathway proteins [40, 41].

The underlying cause for AMD is accumulation of drusen or residual material produced by the renewal process of the external part of the photoreceptors of the retina in the retinal pigment epithelium (RPE). The accumulation of this material in the RPE leads to the production of inflammatory mediators that cause photoreceptor degeneration in the macula and severe vision loss [42]. In the early stages of the disease, accumulated drusen are small; the size and amount of this material increase as the disease progresses and central vision deteriorates.

There are two types of AMD: dry or wet. Dry AMD is characterized by the degeneration of the RPE and photoreceptors along with changes in pigmentation of the RPE. In the wet form, or choroidal neovascularization (CNV), fragile blood vessels of the choriocapillaris grow into the RPE and frequently leak blood and fluid that accumulate between RPE and choriocapillaris. As a result of these abnormal growths, dense scars are formed in the macula, and the RPE can detach. The wet form is more severe than the dry form and sometimes dry AMD can develop into wet AMD [43].

The characteristic invasion of leaky blood to the RPE in wet AMD is mediated by VEGF. The discovery of the relationship between VEGF and changes in vasculature in AMD led to the development of different approaches aimed to decrease the levels of this growth factor. Antibodies targeting VEGF are currently the first-line treatment for wet AMD [44]. The hallmark of wet AMD is CNV; thus, this is the lesion most extensively modeled in animals to assess efficacy of compounds targeting this disease. The laser-induced CNV model is by far the most used animal model. This model, initially developed for nonhuman primates (NHP), was later adapted into rodents. The basis for this model is to induce a break in Bruch's membrane using a high-energy laser. The experimental CNV can be analyzed in vivo using fluorescein angiography or optical coherence tomography or postmortem studying the retina explants. The model has been successfully transferred and validated to rat and mouse, and in both species, the chain of events taking place after lesion induction resembles the events that tale place in humans with the disease. Other models include the injection of subretinal materials such as Matrigel, angiogenic substances, macrophages, lipid peroxides, or polyethylene glycol. Although these models are promising, they have yet to be appropriately validated in order to be used as a proof of concept tools [45].

3.6. Diabetic retinopathy

Diabetic retinopathy (DR) is an ocular complication of diabetes mellitus characterized by microaneurysms in the retinal vasculature that eventually lead to ischemia and macular edema. Changes in the retina can cause rapid vision loss, and this complication is the main cause of visual loss in working-age individuals [46, 47].

The initial phase of DR, known as nonproliferative DR, is characterized by the thickening of the capillary basement membrane and apoptosis and migration of pericytes. These microchanges cause microaneurysms and small leakages in the vessels that irrigate the retina. As the disease progresses, interaction between endothelial cells and pericytes weakens and the capillaries become permeable; subsequent accumulation of fluids in the macula leads to edema. The microaneurysms in the retinal capillaries cause occlusions that compromise blood flow through the retina and cause ischemia. Local hypoxia upregulates angiogenic factors that cause capillaries to grow into the retina, preretinal space, and vitreous cavity; stage known as proliferative DR [48]. Among the upregulated angiogenic factors, one of the most critical is VEGF; the newly formed vessels are structurally deficient and very responsive to this growth factor. As such, antibodies used to treat AMD are also used for the treatment of diabetic retinopathy. DR is usually treated with laser photocoagulation, a procedure that does not cure the disease but mitigates the damage. IVT steroids can also be used to reduce accumulation of fluids within the retina. If accumulation of blood in the vitreous humor physically impedes laser photocoagulation, a vitrectomy has to be performed in order to remove the blood accumulated in the vitreous prior to laser photocoagulation.

There are several animal models of diabetic retinopathy, each of them comes with its own set of advantages and disadvantages. One of the most extensively used is the streptozotocin (STZ)-induced diabetes model. Intravenous or intraperitoneal injection of STZ causes a rapid and selective destruction of β-pancreatic cells leading to hyperglycemia and development of type I diabetes. The model has been used successfully in several animal species including rat, mouse, rabbit, dog, and monkey. Nonproliferative DR develops in this model, but microaneurysms and neovascularization are seldom observed; hence, this model can be complemented with the laser-induced CNV model explained in the AMD section. Larger animal models can be generated by surgically removing the pancreas, but this model is significantly more complicated to generate than the STZ model and has the same drawbacks. Alternatively, animals can be fed a high-galactose diet, but the induction of diabetes is considerably slower [50].

4. Biodistribution studies

Despite the extraordinary potential that RNAi technology displays in the treatment of ocular conditions, the transition of siRNAs programs to the clinical setting still presents challenges. The *in vivo* efficacy of therapies based on siRNAs depends on the ability of a given siRNA to reach the cytoplasm of its target cell in sufficient quantities to achieve its desired biological effect. The intrinsic characteristics of siRNAs such as their sensitivity to degradation by endogenous enzymes, their relative large size, and its negative charge limit their ability to cross biological barriers and reach the cytoplasm. Approaches used to overcome the hurdles associated to the use of siRNAs range from delivery strategies to chemical modifications aimed towards improving the pharmacological properties of the therapeutic siRNAs.

Drug delivery into the eye is challenging due to the presence of static and dynamics barriers that protect the internal tissues. The eye consists of two anatomically differentiated regions: the anterior and posterior segments. The anterior segment includes the cornea, conjunctiva, iris, ciliary body, lens, and anterior and posterior chambers; this segment occupies approximately the anterior third of the eyeball. The posterior segment is of greater size and comprises the sclera, choroid, retina, and vitreous cavity. There are significant anatomical, molecular, and immune differences between the two segments; thus, strategies to deliver molecules to the eye will be very different depending on the targeted segment [51]. The anterior region of the eye is protected from exterior aggressions by the cornea and tear film. The former is a specialized tissue composed of five layers that constitutes the main physical barrier to external molecules; the latter is an enzyme-rich fluid that degrades many biological molecules, lubricates the eye surface, and washes away materials from the cornea. In addition, many components of the tear film impede adhesion of molecules to the eye surface further restricting the access of external molecules to the inside of the eye.

Topical ocular administration of drugs is a patient-friendly administration route typically used for the treatment of pathologies affecting the anterior segment of the eye. However, molecules applied as eye drops are quickly cleared from the ocular surface being the bioavailability of a compound administered via this route less than 5% of the initially applied dose. The standard volume of a commercial eye drop is approximately 40 μL whereas the normal volume of the tear fluid in the ocular surface is 7-9 μl. Once an eye drop is instilled in the inferior conjunctival sac, there is a transient increase of volume that activates the blinking reflex and increases the turnover of the tear film. Most of the content of the eye drop is spilled out by the blinking process or drained via the nasolacrimal duct, drastically reducing the amount of compound available to the eye.

The cornea is a specialized tissue covering the anterior part of the eye whose main functions are protecting against harmful agents and provide the eye with a refractive surface that allows the entrance of light. The human cornea is approximately 0.5–0.8 mm thick, and it is comprised of three layers: the outer five cell layer-epithelium, a thick stroma rich in type I collagen fibrils and glycosaminoglycans, and the innermost endothelium consisting in a single layer of cuboidal cells. The corneal epithelium is separated from the stroma by the Bowman's membrane, while the stroma and the corneal endothelium are separated by the Descemet's membrane. There are no blood vessels irrigating the cornea; this provides the required transparency for the transmission and refraction of light. Drugs can take two paths to penetrate the corneal epithelium: the intracellular path crossing through the cells or the paracellular path bypassing between cells. The cells of the corneal epithelium are tightly attached to each other with gap and tight junctions that restrict the diffusion of large molecules between them [52–54]. The cross-cellular pathway requires molecules to be able to cross cell membranes; thus, lipophilic molecules have an easier access through this route. The stroma is an aqueous matrix composed mainly of hydrated collagen and proteoglycans with few keratinocytes interspersed [55]. The hydophilicity/lipophilicity index determines the diffusion of molecules through this layer [56]. The remaining layers of the cornea do not significantly hamper the diffusion of molecules.

Contrary to the cornea, the conjunctiva is a highly vasculated tissue that covers the sclera and lines the inner surface of the eyelids. Its main functions are producing mucus and tears to lubricate the eye surface and preventing the entrance of pathogens. The human conjunctiva is composed of three layers: the outer epithelium, the substantia propia, containing nerves and blood vessels, and the submucosa layer, which provides a lightweight attachment to the underlying sclera [57]. The histology of the stratified outer epithelium varies among the different regions of the conjunctiva, but it is always its apical portion that controls the permeability of the conjunctiva. The conjunctiva offers an attractive route for drug delivery when compared to the cornea as it presents an extended exchange surface as well as a superior rate of permeation to large hydrophilic molecules. The sclera is structurally continuous with the cornea and extends posteriorly from the limbus. The composition of the sclera is similar to that of the corneal stroma, mainly collagen and mucopolysaccharides leaving numerous channels through which drugs can freely diffuse [58]. The sclera is poorly vascularized and significantly more permeable than the cornea but less permeable than conjunctiva. There are contradictory reports on the ability of charged molecules to cross the sclera. Some authors suggest that this layer is more permeable to negatively charged molecules [59, 60], whereas other studies suggest that positively charged molecules cross the sclera more easily [61, 62]. Ranta and colleagues suggested that the negative charge of mucopolysaccharides in the sclera prevented the diffusion of negatively charged molecules as a consequence of charge repulsion. Other studies have shown that negatively charged molecules are indeed able to cross the sclera, pointing out that size is the limiting factor in drug diffusion through this layer [52]. It should be noted, however, that scleral drug binding does not necessarily impair drug delivery to inner structures of the eye; it can also act as a drug-depot if the molecules are subsequently released [63].

Ophthalmic drugs topically administered to de eye can thus be absorbed through two pathways: crossing the cornea to reach the aqueous humor or through the conjunctival-scleral pathway reaching the uvea. The relative quantity that enters through each of the above-mentioned routes varies significantly depending on the size and hydrophilic/lipophilic ratio of the molecule. Generally, the conjunctival route is favored for large hydrophilic molecules, whereas small lipophilic drugs are mainly absorbed through the cornea. The ability of siRNAs to penetrate the cornea has been thoroughly demonstrated as well as the ability of these compounds to enter the cytoplasm of cells within the cornea. However, the capacity of siRNAs to cross the cornea is limited, as shown by the limited amount of siRNAs detected in the aqueous humor following eye drop instillation [64].

Increasing the amount of compound in the anterior part may be of interest for treating specific conditions. For this purpose, several strategies can be used in order to improve delivery: (a) increasing the residence time of the compound within the eye surface, (b) directing the molecule to a specific region to increase the concentration locally, and (c) increasing absorption by using physical methods. Increasing the contact time of the molecule with the eye surface can be achieved by the use of formulations or depots. Formulations that increase viscosity and/or mucoadhesion of ophthalmic solutions are generally believed to increase absorption into the eye. Polymers such as methylcellulose or polyvinyl alcohol can be added to solutions to increase viscosity and consequently increase residence and reduce clearance time. Mucoadhesion may be increased by formulating the oligonucleotides in polymers such as chitosans. These polymers have been used to deliver DNA vectors into the eye [65]. Encapsulation in liposomes and in thermosensitive gels has also been attempted as a means to increase the absorption and residence time of oligonucleotides in the eye [53]. In these studies, a 16-mer was formulated in liposomes, a thermosensitve 27% poloxamer gel, and HEPES; the results of these studies showed that the amount of compound reaching external tissues such as the conjunctiva or the cornea was higher when the compound was prepared in HEPES. By contrast, access to deeper regions of the anterior chamber such as the sclera or the iris benefited from the increased viscosity of the gel formulation [53]. One of the main drawbacks of biodistribution studies to assess the fate of a given siRNA in a formulation is that most of these studies focus on the fate of nanocarrier rather than on that of the oligonucleotide and the relative distribution of the molecule among the tissues of the eye. Therefore, thorough biodistribution, studies are required to address the specific characteristics required for improving delivery for specific conditions. Targeting has scarcely been used to deliver oligonucleotides into the eye; there are a few reports using dendrimers with the goal of increasing the intracellular concentration of therapeutic oligonucleotides in specific regions of the eye, but advances toward this goal are as of today very limited [66]. Physical methods such as iontophoresis have also been studied aiming to increasing the amount of molecule that crosses the cornea and/or the sclera. Although iontophoresis certainly increases the amount of transcorneal and transcleral delivery of oligonucleotides mainly to the anterior chamber but also to some degree to the posterior chamber, the use of this method has not been extensively used most likely because the equipment required to apply the required current would entail in-office administration, which would significantly complicate repeated administrations [67].

Drugs administered systemically enter the eye from the bloodstream crossing the capillaries of the choroid. The choroid is a vascular layer composed of capillaries and supported by Bruch's membrane, a connective membrane of 2–4 μm thickness. Bruch's membrane separates the choroid from the retina, forming the main barrier to permeation across the choroid-Bruch's bilayer [68]. The permeability of Bruch's membrane is relatively high; charge and size do not generally affect drug diffusion through this membrane unless molecules are very big; in this particular case, size can reduce the rate of permeation [52]. The choroid is a thin and permeable membrane that is rich in melanin. Melanin has the ability to bind and retain many drugs hampering their entrance to the retina and inner tissues. Other drug-binding proteins, depending on the kinetic of binding/unbinding retention of drugs by melanin, can completely block the entrance or act as a reservoir for slow release [69]. Studies to assess the binding of oligonucleotides to melanin have yielded different results suggesting that at least some oligonucleotides bind to melanin reducing the rate of entrance to the retina; this is however not the case for all oligonucleotides [52, 70].

The main restriction to free permeation of molecules from systemic circulation to the eye is the blood–retinal barrier (BRB). The BRB is composed of the inner BRB and the outer BRB. The former includes the vessels of the retina, whereas the latter is constituted by the retinal pigment epithelium (RPE). Both barriers possess cells with well-developed intercellular junctions that control the permeation of substances through them. Larger molecules, such as proteins and nucleic acids, are mostly able to permeate through the choroid but have limited ability to cross the inner BRB; thus, drugs need to exit the choroid and penetrate the eye crossing the outer BRB. Crossing through the outer BRB usually requires high systemic doses increasing the likelihood of systemic side effects [71]. Delivery to the posterior segment of systemic or topically applied drugs requires thus crossing several biological barriers. Therefore, invasive administration procedures are frequently used to deliver drugs to the posterior segment. In addition, the outflow mechanisms of the eye rapidly remove drugs from the posterior chamber; thus, reaching clinically meaningful concentrations is challenging. Most of the programs developing siRNAs for eye conditions target the back of the eye; consequently, the route of administration is IVT injection. The concentration of siRNAs administered IVT is highest in the vitreous body, but they are also found in the RPE, choroid, and retina. Depending on the stability of the siRNAs, the compound can also be found in systemic circulation.

There are numerous reports describing strategies that can be of benefit for increasing the concentration of drugs in the back of the eye. Several nonbiodegradable (Retisert™, Illuvien™, and Vitrasert®) and one biodegradable (Ozurdex™) intravitreal ocular inserts are currently used in the clinical practice for delivering small molecules to the back of the eye. It is expected that these advances be soon incorporated into the pipelines of larger molecules such as proteins and oligonucleotides.

5. Toxicology

siRNAs are chemically synthesized oligonucleotides and are considered New Chemical Entities (NCEs) by the US and European Regulatory Authorities since 2009 when the European Commission excluded siRNAs from the definition of advanced medicinal products [72]. Toxicology assessment of RNAi-based drugs should be carried out following guidelines for NCEs, and the complete toxicology battery is usually performed following the recommendations of the ICH M3 (R2) guideline [73]. The guideline recommends the assessment of toxicology in two species, a rodent and a nonrodent, at three dose levels and for a duration that should be similar or superior to the clinical trial to be carried out. This assessment should include acute or maximum tolerated toxicology studies and repeated-dose toxicity studies. Additionally, pharmacokinetics, safety pharmacology, genotoxicity, carcinogenicity, and specific toxicology studies should be carried out depending of the nature, indication, and route of administration of the product. On the other hand, some aspects of RNAi-based products are closer to new biological entities (NBEs) rather than NCEs; therefore, some of the requirements of the ICH S6 guideline also apply to the design of their developmental programs [74]. As such, a tailored toxicology assessment program should be designed combining the recommendations outlined in the above-mentioned guidelines and the accumulated experience of numerous compounds tested in preclinical and clinical development.

Toxicology of ocular products depends on their biodistribution and on their biological activity. Moreover, the disease process, age, sex, or eye pigmentation are other potential factors affecting the toxicity profile of the ocular drug assessed. Additionally, the bioavailability of the RNAi compound will depend mainly on the route of ocular administration (topical versus injected) and on the physicochemical characteristics of the drug.

Toxicities arising from oligonucleotides, including siRNAs, can be classified into hybridization-dependent toxicities and hybridization-independent toxicities. Hybridization-dependent toxicities can be caused by (a) exaggerated pharmacology: excessive activity on the intended target or by (b) off-target effect: modulating gene expression of an unintended target by an RNAi-mediated mechanism. Hybridization-independent toxicities are often associated to the chemistry of the siRNA. Identified hybridization-independent toxicities include prolongation of activating partial thromboplastin time (aPTT), complement activation, and immunostimulation [75, 76, 77].

5.1. General toxicology

Up to date, numerous siRNAs indicated for different eye conditions have entered clinical trials (Table 1); the administration route of four of these compounds is by IVT injection, whereas the remaining two compounds are topically administered in eye drops. The toxicology assessment of these products follows the traditional schedule for NCEs; this schedule entails general toxicology studies in two species, a rodent and a nonrodent species of variable length. Most programs up to date have used NHP as the nonrodent species; this is because siRNAs are species specific, and it is likely that the assessment of toxicology was performed in the only species in which the compound was pharmacologically active. The rabbit is very frequently used to assess toxicology of compounds under development for eye conditions. Many sponsors of programs using NHP or dog as nonrodent species chose to use the rabbit as second species, although this animal is not a rodent per se. Reasons behind this choice include the similarity of the volume of the eye to that of humans and the difficulty of administering controlled doses to smaller animals. This is particularly relevant when the compound is administered by IVT injection. This rationale has also been followed for developing siRNAs for eye conditions; only in one case, PF-04523655, rats were used as the rodent species, and the rest of the programs developing siRNAs for eye indications used the rabbit (New Zealand White rabbits or Dutch Belted rabbit) as second species for toxicology assessment.

Most programs developing siRNAs for eye conditions include acute/maximum tolerated dose and repeat-dose toxicology studies. The length of these studies is determined by the indication, stage of development, and envisioned duration of treatment. In addition, most programs do not only perform toxicology studies using the envisaged route of administration but also include studies using intravenous route to challenge the systemic exposure to the drug and assess potential dose limitations and target organs.

5.2. Genotoxicity

As mentioned in the previous section, both the ICH M3 (R2) and the ICH S6 guidelines apply to programs developing siRNAs [73]. The ICH S6 states that the range and type of genotoxicity studies routinely conducted for NCEs are usually not applicable to NBEs; pointing out that performance of these studies is only required when there is a cause of concern. The European Medicines Agency (EMA) issued a reflection paper on the assessment of the genotoxic potential of antisense oligodeoxynucleotides in January 2005. This paper recommends addressing at least two issues in regards to oligonucleotides which may indicate a cause of genotoxic concern: (a) analyzing the potential of incorporation of phosphorothioated (PS) oligonucleotides into the DNA and (b) addressing the potential of triplex formation of oligonucleotides with the DNA fiber [78]. Several years of experience with siRNAs indicate that full-length molecules are very unlikely to interact with the DNA. Thus, the potential cause of concern may arise from the genotoxic potential of metabolites or chemical contaminants. The metabolism of nonmodified oligonucleotides yields naturally occurring nucleotides that are subsequently incorporated to the natural degradation pathways of endogenous nucleic acids; thus, toxicities derived from these degradation products are not expected. Modified oligonucleotides, on the other hand, incorporate very frequently backbone modifications to reduce nuclease activity and improve other pharmaceutical properties of the molecule. The most commonly used backbone modification is the replacement of a nonbridging oxygen on the backbone between two ribonucleotides with a sulfur to create a PS linkage [79]. Extensive genotoxicity studies performed with Vitravene, a PS antisense oligonucleotide administered by IVT injection, indicate that oligonucleotides with a PS backbone do not pose genotoxic potential [80, 81]. These results are in line with those obtained in the analysis of over 30 compounds studied in the standard battery, all of which have yielded negative results. Other modified nucleotides could potentially be incorporated into nucleotide pools and be thereafter used to synthesize DNA. The standard battery of tests would detect eventual damaging potential of theses degradation products.

The EMA reflection paper also recommends assessing the potential of triplex formation with the DNA fiber. For this to happen, siRNA molecules would have to enter the nucleus of the cell and their structure should include an uninterrupted homopurine stretch of at least 10–12 base pairs that should be homologous a given region of the DNA. In silico design of siRNAs usually addresses these issues and candidates with the ability of forming triplex are avoided prior to lead selection.

5.3. Carcinogenicity

Standard carcinogenicity studies are generally not required for NBEs, but these studies may be required for siRNAs depending on their chemical structure, clinical dosing, patient population, or biological activity. If the in vitro test genotoxic studies indicate that there is cause of concern for carcinogenic potential, further studies should be required in relevant models.

For RNAi products under development for eye conditions, the systemic bioavailability of these products is usually very low, and a waiver to perform these studies may be justified. Strategies should be discussed in a case-by-case base with the competent health authorities.

5.4. Reproductive and developmental toxicity

The assessment of reproductive and developmental toxicity is required to support the use of a given pharmaceutical in pregnant women, women of childbearing potential, or children. These studies are regulated by the ICH S5 guideline [82], which recommends assessing the effect of drugs on all phases of the reproductive cycle. These recommendations apply to siRNA-based products. Nevertheless, due to the unique features of these compounds, a case-by-case approach should be followed for each product, and the requirements for these studies should be discussed with the competent authorities. The target, indication, chemical modifications, and systemic bioavailability of the RNAi-based drugs are features that may influence in the nature of the required studies.

Because the toxicity of siRNAs can be caused by exaggerated pharmacology whenever reproductive toxicity studies are required, they should be performed in a pharmacologically active species. Standard reproductive toxicity species in rodents or rabbits can give information on toxicity related to chemical structure. However, if the compound is not active in these species or if the biological activity is not deemed to be equivalent to the foreseen activity in humans, the assessment of reproductive risk may be conducted using an active analog or in a nonrodent species in which the compound has biological activity. If the former strategy is chosen, the toxicity and toxicokinetic profile of the surrogate should be taken into account when interpreting the results. If the compound is only active in NHPs, studies should only be performed in cases where there is cause for concern. In these particular cases, the number of animals should be optimized, and a combined enhanced pre-and postnatal developmental study can be performed as recommended for NBEs. In NHP studies, the assessment of reproductive toxicology is usually studied by histopathologic examination of the reproductive organs as part of the general toxicology studies of at least three months. The timing of reproductive and developmental studies depends on when women of childbearing potential are to be included in clinical trials. If NHPs are required for the assessment, the timing is more flexible due to the length and complexity of the studies [83].

5.5. Local tolerance

Local tolerance studies are required for all topically administered drugs. In most cases, the potential adverse events caused by local tolerance issues are evaluated in the single or repeated-dose toxicology studies, reducing the number of animals required for the program.

5.6. Safety pharmacology

According to ICH S7A, safety pharmacology studies can be reduced or eliminated for locally applied products as well as for NBEs that achieve highly specific receptor targeting [84]. For siRNAs under development for ophthalmology indications, separate safety studies are not usually required; instead, functional safety end points are incorporated into the repeated-dose toxicity studies. If the results of the toxicology studies indicate that there is cause of concern, separate safety pharmacology studies should be performed.

6. Programs in development and future ahead

Table 1 summarizes the status of siRNA-based therapies under development for ocular conditions. As mentioned in Section 1, the eye offers multiple advantages for developing innovative therapies; therefore, studies in the eye pioneered the field of siRNA therapeutics. The first siRNA to enter clinical development for an ophthalmology indication was bevasiranib in 2004 shortly followed by sirna-027. Bevasiranib targeted VEGFA, whereas sirna-027 targeted VEGFR1. These compounds were being developed for the treatment of AMD as both showed a dose-dependent inhibition of experimental CNV in animal models that correlated with knockdown of their respective target genes [10, 85]. As mentioned in Section 1, in 2008 Kleinman and coworkers published a study demonstrating that the effect of siRNAs targeting VEGF and VEGFR on CNV was not mediated by an on-target effect but by activation of TLR3 [12]. The results of these studies indicated that the effect of the compounds on CNV was sequence-independent and mediated by siRNAs of 21 base pairs or longer. The study also showed that the internalization of the siRNAs was not required for the inhibition of CNV as cells of the RPE abundantly express TLR3 on the cytoplasmic surface. The authors used several sequences, including those of the siRNAs undergoing clinical trials at the time, to point out that the inhibition of CNV by both bevasiranib and sirna-027 was mediated through an off-target effect. A subsequent study by the same group showed that activation of TLR3 by IVT siRNAs led to caspase-3-mediated degeneration of the retinal pigment epithelium (RPE) questioning the safety of these compounds as therapeutics for back of the eye diseases [13].

The clinical development of bevasiranib was halted in 2007 and of sirna-027 in 2009 both as a result of not reaching or being unlikely to reach their respective efficacy end points in phase III trials.

The findings of Kleinman and coworkers boosted research on alternative designs that were not able to activate TLR3, and as result, a new generation of compounds is currently undergoing clinical trials. Currently, the most advanced siRNAs-based programs for ocular indications are Quark's QPI-007 and Sylentis' bamosiran (SYL040012). QPI-007 is a 19-nt modified siRNA-targeting caspase 2 currently in phase II/III for the treatment of nonarteritic anterior ischemic optic neuropathy (NAION) [86]. QPI-1007 has shown to be safe when IVT injected to animal models and humans. The ongoing phase II/III trial for this compound analyzes the potential of multiple IVT doses to improve visual acuity in patients suffering NAION [87, 88]. Bamosiran is a canonical-designed naked siRNA-targeting β2-adrenergic receptor (ADRB2) under development for the treatment of increased IOP associated to glaucoma [64, 89–91]. Glaucoma is a degenerative, chronic disease of the optic nerve that can lead to blindness if left untreated [92]. The mechanistic details of optic nerve degeneration observed in glaucoma are yet to be fully detailed, but it is well established that reduction of intraocular pressure avoids development of the disease. ADRB2 controls the production and release of aqueous humor. The aqueous humor is responsible for maintaining optimal IOP. Treatment with topic beta-blockers has shown to efficiently reduce intraocular pressure, but currently approved beta-blockers are small molecules and are thus able to reach systemic circulation and systemic organs were they cause unwanted effects. The rationale behind bamosiran is developing a locally active compound that efficiently knocks down ADRB2 in the eye but that is not able to reach systemic tissues reducing the likelihood of side effects. The compound is administered in eye drops and has been shown to be well tolerated in animal models and humans [64, 93]. Three different doses of bamosiran are currently being studied in an active controlled phase IIb trial. Previous clinical trials with this compound have shown promising results in healthy individuals and patients with ocular hypertension [91, 93].

SYL1001 is a naked 19-bp siRNA-targeting transient receptor potential vanilloid-1 (TRPV1) for the treatment of ocular pain. TRPV1 is a cation channel permeable to calcium activated by heat, low pH, and capsaicin among other signals. This receptor is present in several structures of the eye where it has been related, among other roles, to nociception [94]. SYL1001 has shown to be safe when administered in eye drops to animals and humans and to have analgesic effect in the capsaicin-induced eye pain model. The compound is currently undergoing a phase I/II for the treatment of ocular pain associated to dry eye disease, a condition for which no specific treatment currently exists [89].

PF-655 is a chemically stabilized siRNA-targeting RTP801, a stress-induced adaptor protein that inhibits mTOR function upstream to TSC1/TSC2 complex in response to a variety of stresses. Expression of RTP801 is upregulated in response to ischemia, hypoxia, and/or oxidative stress. Intravitreal injection of PF-655 in preclinical animal models of laser-induced CNV leads to silencing of RTP801 via a RNAi mechanism without TLR activation and reduction of CNV volume, vessel leakage, and infiltration of inflammatory cells into the choroid [95–97]. This compound has undergone phase II clinical trials for the treatment of diabetic macular edema and wet AMD. Treatment with PF-655 of patients with diabetic macular edema over a period of 12 months caused a dose-dependent improvement in visual acuity compared to the visual acuity observed in patients treated with laser photocoagulation [98]. A subsequent phase IIb trial was conducted with a new set of doses but terminated because the primary end point was not likely to be achieved. The compound was thereafter tested in combination with ranibizumab, a monoclonal antibody fragment that targets VEGF and is the current gold standards for treatment of the disease. The results of this study have not yet been disclosed. PF-655 has also been studied in patients suffering wet AMD. In this indication, the compound did not show improvement as a single agent or in combination with ranibizumab in mean visual acuity after 3 months of dosing.

Self-delivery rxRNAs (sd-rxRNAs) incorporate 2′-F and 2-′O-Me modifications and a sterol conjugate on the sense strand with the goal of improving stability and cellular uptake. These compounds have a 19-nt antisense strand and a sense strand usually shorter than 15 nt resulting in an asymmetric duplex with a phosphorothioated single-stranded tail on the antisense strand [99]. These compounds have been tested in vitro where they have shown to be able to induce target knockdown in different cell lines. In vivo analysis of their activity showed these compounds are readily taken-up by retinal cells and that the compound is evenly distributed throughout the mouse retina. Several of these compounds are under development for different eye conditions and are expected to enter clinical development shortly.

SYL116011 is a naked 19-bp siRNA targeting the calcium release-activated calcium modulator 1 (ORAI1). Store-operated Ca^{2+} entry (SOCE) is activated in response to depletion of endoplasmic reticulum Ca^{2+} pools. Activation of SOCE induces Ca^{2+} entry from extracellular compartments, and this is mediated by store-operated CRAC channels. CRAC channels are composed of calcium sensing proteins called STIM (stromal interaction molecule) and pore-forming subunits named ORAI [100]. Mammalian cells have three ORAI isoforms: ORAI1, ORAI 2, and ORAI3; although ORAI2 and 3 fulfill the same role as ORAI1, the Ca^{2+} currents generated by these proteins are around two- to threefold smaller than the ones generated by ORAI1 [101]. There is growing evidence that indicates that short-term and long-term activation of immune cells in allergic responses is mediated by influx of Ca^{2+} to immune cells from the extracellular compartment. Short-term responses include the degranulation of mast cells and the activation of effector cytolitic T cells. Indeed, mast cells lacking either STIM1 or ORAI1 show a considerable defect in degranulation [102, 103]. Long-term responses involve the modulation of gene expression that controls B and T cell proliferation and differentiation. SYL116011 is being developed for the treatment of ocular allergies and has shown to reduce immediate clinical signs in a mouse model of ragweed pollen-induced ocular allergy. The decrease in clinical signs was accompanied by a reduction in the number of infiltrating eosinophils in the conjunctiva and reduction of allergy biomarkers.

TT-211 is an AAV-encapsidated construct that expresses a single shRNA modeled into a miRNA backbone that inhibits the expression of VEGF-A for the treatment of wet AMD. VEGF-a protein is responsible initiating a signaling cascade that stimulates the growth of new blood vessels, a hallmark of wet AMD. TT-231 is a second-generation candidate designed to express three shRNAs, which target three different genes, VEGF receptor 2, PDGF-β, and human complement factor B, proteins that play a major role in the progression of wet AMD. Both these compounds are yet in a preclinical phase; IND filing is planned for 2017.

STP601 is a multitargeted siRNA cocktail nanoparticle formulation administered by IVT injection under development for treatment of wet AMD, proliferative diabetic retinopathy, and herpetic stromal keratitis. The cocktail includes three 25-mer siRNA duplexes targeting VEGF, VEGFR1, and VEGFR2. Inhibiting this clinically validated pathway at the endothelial cells lining the interior of the growing blood vessels is thought to halt the progression of AMD. This product is currently in preclinical stage.

AQA001 is a single-stranded long chain nonmodified ribonucleotide connected by a proline-derived linker that self-anneals to form a shot-hairpin structure within the molecule. The compound targeting periostin acts through an RNAi mechanism and is being developed for the treatment of diabetic retinopathy. The compound has shown positive result in a proof-of-concept study of CNV [104].

Name	Indication	Target	Route	Sponsor	Status
Bevasiranib	AMD with choroidal neovascularization	VEGFA	IVT	Opko Health	Halted in Phase III
Sirna-027	AMD with choroidal neovascularization	VEGFR1	IVT	Allergan	Halted in Phase III
QPI-1007	NAION	Caspase 2	IVT	Quark	Active, Phase II/III
	Primary Angle Closure Glaucoma				Active, Phase IIa
PF-655	AMD with choroidal neovascularization	RTP801	IVT	Quark/Pfizer	Completed, Phase II
	Diabetic macular oedema				Completed, Phase IIb
SYL040012	Glaucoma	β2 ADR	Eye Drop	Sylentis	Completed, Phase IIb
SYL1001	Ocular pain associated to dry eye disease	TRPV1	Eye Drop	Sylentis	Active, Phase IIa
Undisclosed	Retinal scaring	Undisclosed	Intraocular	RXi	Preclinical
Undisclosed	Corneal scaring	Undisclosed	Eye Drop	RXi	Preclinical
Undisclosed	Macular degeneration	Undisclosed	Intraocular	RXi	Preclinical
SYL116011	Ocular allergy	ORAI1	Eye Drop	Sylentis	Preclinical
TT-211	AMD	VEGF-A	IVT	Benitec	Preclinical
TT-231	AMD	VEGF-A, PDGFβ and CFB	IVT	Benitec	Preclinical
STP601	AMD and retinopathy	VEGF-VFGFR1-VEGF2	IVT	Sirnaomics	Preclinical
AQA001	Diabetic macular oedema	Periostin	IVT	Aqua Therapeutics	Preclinical

Table 1. siRNAs in development for ocular indication.

7. Conclusion

RNA interference is on the verge of becoming a new class of therapeutics [105]. The field of ophthalmology has played a major role in advancing siRNAs from laboratory tools to the clinic. In the last few years, significant advances have been made in the understanding of how these molecules enter and exert its action in the eye and in the identification of the main hurdles that still need to be addressed. The introduction of chemical modifications as well as the understanding of the immune activation in the eye has significantly improved the pharmaceutical properties of compounds for eye conditions. However, the following years will tell whether improvements on these molecules are enough to be of therapeutic value in the field of ophthalmology or not.

Author details

Tamara Martínez[#], Maria Victoria González[#], Beatriz Vargas, Ana Isabel Jiménez and Covadonga Pañeda[*]

*Address all correspondence to: cpaneda@sylentis.com

Sylentis SAU, Tres Cantos, Madrid, Spain

[#]These two authors contributed equally to the review.

References

[1] Zamore PD, Tuschl T, Sharp PA, Bartel DP. RNAi: double-stranded RNA directs the ATP-dependent cleavage of mRNA at 21 to 23 nucleotide intervals. Cell. 2000;101:25–33. DOI: 10.1016/S0092-8674(00)80620-0.

[2] Elbashir SM, Harborth J, Lendeckel W, Yalcin A, Weber K, Tuschl T. Duplexes of 21-nucleotide RNAs mediate RNA interference in cultured mammalian cells. Nature. 2001;411:494–8. DOI:10.1038/3507810735078107.

[3] Aagaard L, Rossi JJ. RNAi therapeutics: principles, prospects and challenges. Adv Drug Deliv Rev. 2007;59:75–86. DOI:10.1016/j.addr.2007.03.2005.

[4] Perez VL, Saeed AM, Tan Y, Urbieta M, Cruz-Guilloty F. The eye: a window to the soul of the immune system. J Autoimmun. 2013;45:7–14. DOI: 10.1016/j.jaut.2013.06.011.

[5] Stein-Streilein J. Immune regulation and the eye. Trends Immunol. 2008; 29:548–54. DOI: 10.1016/j.it.2008.08.002.

[6] Chang ZL. Important aspects of Toll-like receptors, ligands and their signaling pathways. Inflamm Res. 2010;59:791–808. DOI: 10.1007/s00011-010-0208-2

[7] Yu FS, Hazlett LD. Toll-like receptors and the eye. Invest Ophthalmol Vis Sci. 2006;47:1255–63. DOI: 10.1167/iovs.05-0956.

[8] Kumar MV, Nagineni CN, Chin MS, Hooks JJ, Detrick B. Innate immunity in the retina: Toll-like receptor (TLR) signaling in human retinal pigment epithelial cells. J Neuroimmunol. 2004;153:7–15. DOI: 10.1016/j.jneuroim.2004.04.018

[9] Sioud M. RNA interference and innate immunity. Adv Drug Deliv Rev. 2007 ;59:153–63. DOI: 10.1016/j.addr.2007.03.006.

[10] Reich SJ, Fosnot J, Kuroki A, Tang W, Yang X, Maguire AM, et al. Small interfering RNA (siRNA) targeting VEGF effectively inhibits ocular neovascularization in a mouse model. Mol Vis. 2003;9:210–6.

[11] Shen J, Samul R, Silva RL, Akiyama H, Liu H, Saishin Y, et al. Suppression of ocular neovascularization with siRNA targeting VEGF receptor 1. Gene Ther. 2006;13:225–34. DOI: 10.1038/sj.gt.3302641.

[12] Kleinman ME, Yamada K, Takeda A, Chandrasekaran V, Nozaki M, Baffi JZ, et al. Sequence- and target-independent angiogenesis suppression by siRNA via TLR3. Nature. 2008;452:591–7. DOI: 10.1038/nature06765.

[13] Kleinman ME, Kaneko H, Cho WG, Dridi S, Fowler BJ, Blandford AD, et al. Short-interfering RNAs induce retinal degeneration via TLR3 and IRF3. Mol Ther. 2011;20:101–8. DOI: 10.1038/mt.2011.212.

[14] Turner JJ, Jones SW, Moschos SA, Lindsay MA, Gait MJ. MALDI-TOF mass spectral analysis of siRNA degradation in serum confirms an RNAse A-like activity. Mol Biosyst. 2007;3:43–50. DOI: 10.1039/b611612d.

[15] Weickmann JL, Glitz DG. Human ribonucleases. Quantitation of pancreatic-like enzymes in serum, urine, and organ preparations. J Biol Chem. 1982 10;257:8705–10.

[16] Hayreh SS. Ischemic optic neuropathy. Prog Retin Eye Res. 2009;28:34–62. DOI: 10.1016/j.preteyeres.2008.11.002.

[17] Hayreh SS. Management of ischemic optic neuropathies. Indian J Ophthalmol. 2011;59:123–36. DOI: 10/4103/0301-4738.77024.

[18] Tang Z, Zhang S, Lee C, Kumar A, Arjunan P, Li Y, et al. An optic nerve crush injury murine model to study retinal ganglion cell survival. J Vis Exp. 2011;50:2685. DOI: 10.3791/2685.

[19] Bernstein SL, Guo Y, Kelman SE, Flower RW, Johnson MA. Functional and cellular responses in a novel rodent model of anterior ischemic optic neuropathy. Invest Ophthalmol Vis Sci. 2003;44:4153–62.

[20] Quigley HA, Broman AT. The number of people with glaucoma worldwide in 2010 and 2020. Br J Ophthalmol. 2006;90:262–7. DOI: 10.1136/bjo.2005.08-0875-7.

[21] Caprioli J, Varma R. Intraocular pressure: modulation as treatment for glaucoma. Am J Ophthalmol. 2011;152:340–4 e2. DOI: 10.1016/j.ajo.2011.05.029.

[22] Alward WL. Medical management of glaucoma. N Engl J Med. 1998;339:1298–307.

[23] Beckers HJ, Schouten JS, Webers CA, van der Valk R, Hendrikse F. Side effects of commonly used glaucoma medications: comparison of tolerability, chance of discon-

tinuation, and patient satisfaction. Graefes Arch Clin Exp Ophthalmol. 2008;246:1485–90. DOI: 10.1007/s00417-008-0875-7.

[24] Bouhenni RA, Dunmire J, Sewell A, Edward DP. Animal models of glaucoma. J Biomed Biotechnol. 2012;2012:692609. DOI: 10.1155/2012/692609.

[25] McDonald TO, Hodges JW, Borgmann AR, Leaders FE. The water-loading test in rabbits. A method to detect potential ocular hypotensive drugs. Arch Ophthalmol. 1969;82:381–4.

[26] The definition and classification of dry eye disease: report of the Definition and Classification Subcommittee of the International Dry Eye WorkShop (2007). Ocul Surf. 2007;5:75–92.

[27] Gayton JL. Etiology, prevalence, and treatment of dry eye disease. Clin Ophthalmol. 2009;3:405–12.

[28] Management and therapy of dry eye disease: report of the Management and Therapy Subcommittee of the International Dry Eye WorkShop (2007). Ocul Surf. 2007;5:163–78.

[29] Rosenthal P, Borsook D. The corneal pain system. Part I: the missing piece of the dry eye puzzle. Ocul Surf. 2012;10:2–14. DOI: 10.1016/j.jtos.2012.01.002.

[30] Johnson CB. New approaches to identifying and measuring pain. In: Scientific Assessment and Management of Animal Pain. OIE, OIE Technical Series; 2008. p. 131–44.

[31] Gonzalez GG, Garcia de la Rubia P, Gallar J, Belmonte C. Reduction of capsaicin-induced ocular pain and neurogenic inflammation by calcium antagonists. Invest Ophthalmol Vis Sci. 1993;34:3329–35.

[32] Bielory L. Allergic and immunologic disorders of the eye. Part II: ocular allergy. J Allergy Clin Immunol. 2000;106:1019–32. DOI: 10.1067/mai.2000.111238.

[33] Singh K, Axelrod S, Bielory L. The epidemiology of ocular and nasal allergy in the United States, 1988–1994. J Allergy Clin Immunol. 2010;126:778–83 e6. DOI: 10.1016/j.jaci.2010.06.050.

[34] Petricek I, Prost M, Popova A. The differential diagnosis of red eye: a survey of medical practitioners from Eastern Europe and the Middle East. Ophthalmologica. 2006;220:229–37. DOI: 10.1159/000093076.

[35] Leonardi A, Bogacka E, Fauquert JL, Kowalski ML, Groblewska A, Jedrzejczak-Czechowicz M, et al. Ocular allergy: recognizing and diagnosing hypersensitivity disorders of the ocular surface. Allergy. 2012;67:1327–37. DOI: 10.1111/all.12009.

[36] van Cauwenberge P, Bachert C, Passalacqua G, Bousquet J, Canonica GW, Durham SR, et al. Consensus statement on the treatment of allergic rhinitis. European Academy of Allergology and Clinical Immunology. Allergy. 2000;55:116–34.

[37] Magone MT, Chan CC, Rizzo LV, Kozhich AT, Whitcup SM. A novel murine model of allergic conjunctivitis. Clin Immunol Immunopathol. 1998;87:75–84.

[38] Rudnicka AR, Jarrar Z, Wormald R, Cook DG, Fletcher A, Owen CG. Age and gender variations in age-related macular degeneration prevalence in populations of European ancestry: a meta-analysis. Ophthalmology. 2011;119:571–80. DOI: 10.1016/j.ophtha.2011.09.027.

[39] Smith W, Assink J, Klein R, Mitchell P, Klaver CC, Klein BE, et al. Risk factors for age-related macular degeneration: pooled findings from three continents. Ophthalmology. 2001;108:697–704.

[40] Clemons TE, Milton RC, Klein R, Seddon JM, Ferris FL, 3rd. Risk factors for the incidence of advanced age-related macular degeneration in the Age-Related Eye Disease Study (AREDS) AREDS report no. 19. Ophthalmology. 2005;112:533–9. DOI:10.1016/j.ophtha.2004.10.047.

[41] Chen Y, Bedell M, Zhang K. Age-related macular degeneration: genetic and environmental factors of disease. Mol Interv. 2010;10:271–81. DOI: 10.1124/mi.10.5.4.

[42] Ding X, Patel M, Chan CC. Molecular pathology of age-related macular degeneration. Prog Retin Eye Res. 2009;28:1–18. DOI: 10.1016/j.preteyeres.2008.10.001.

[43] Sallo FB, Peto T, Leung I, Xing W, Bunce C, Bird AC. The international classification system and the progression of age-related macular degeneration. Curr Eye Res. 2009;34:238–40. DOI: 10.1080/02713680802714058.

[44] Keane PA, Tufail A, Patel PJ. Management of neovascular age-related macular degeneration in clinical practice: initiation, maintenance, and discontinuation of therapy. J Ophthalmol. 2011;2011:752543. DOI: 10.1155/2011/752543.

[45] Pennesi ME, Neuringer M, Courtney RJ. Animal models of age related macular degeneration. Mol Aspects Med. 2012;33:487–509. DOI: 10.1016/j.mam.2012.06.003.

[46] Scanlon PH, Aldington SJ, Stratton IM. Epidemiological issues in diabetic retinopathy. Middle East Afr J Ophthalmol. 2013;20:293–300. DOI: 10.4103/0974-9233.120007.

[47] Yau JW, Rogers SL, Kawasaki R, Lamoureux EL, Kowalski JW, Bek T, et al. Global prevalence and major risk factors of diabetic retinopathy. Diabetes Care. 2012;35:556–64. DOI: 10.2337/dc11-1909.

[48] Qian H, Ripps H. Neurovascular interaction and the pathophysiology of diabetic retinopathy. Exp Diabetes Res. 2011;2011:693426. DOI: 10.1155/2011/693426.

[49] Willard AL, Herman IM. Vascular complications and diabetes: current therapies and future challenges. J Ophthalmol. 2012;2012:209538. DOI: 10.1155/2012/209538.

[50] Mi XS, Yuan TF, Ding Y, Zhong JX, So KF. Choosing preclinical study models of diabetic retinopathy: key problems for consideration. Drug Des Devel Ther. 2014;8:2311–9. DOI: 10.2147/DDDT.S72797.

[51] Ghate D, Edelhauser HF. Ocular drug delivery. Expert Opin Drug Deliv. 2006;3:275–87. DOI: 10.1517/17425247.3.2.275.

[52] Pescina S, Govoni P, Antopolsky M, Murtomaki L, Padula C, Santi P, et al. Permeation of proteins, oligonucleotide and dextrans across ocular tissues: experimental studies and a literature update. J Pharm Sci. 2015;104:2190–202. DOI: 10.1002/jps.24465.

[53] Bochot A, Mashhour B, Puisieux F, Couvreur P, Fattal E. Comparison of the ocular distribution of a model oligonucleotide after topical instillation in rabbits of conventional and new dosage forms. J Drug Target. 1998;6:309–13. DOI: 10.3109/10611869808996838.

[54] Fattal E, Bochot A. Ocular delivery of nucleic acids: antisense oligonucleotides, aptamers and siRNA. Adv Drug Deliv Rev. 2006;58:1203–23. DOI: 10.1016/j.addr.2006.07.020.

[55] Barar J, Javadzadeh AR, Omidi Y. Ocular novel drug delivery: impacts of membranes and barriers. Expert Opin Drug Deliv. 2008;5:567–81. DOI: 10.1517/17425247.5.5.567.

[56] Prausnitz MR, Noonan JS. Permeability of cornea, sclera, and conjunctiva: a literature analysis for drug delivery to the eye. J Pharm Sci. 1998;87:1479–88.

[57] Ahmed I, Patton TF. Importance of the noncorneal absorption route in topical ophthalmic drug delivery. Invest Ophthalmol Vis Sci. 1985;26:584–7.

[58] Hamalainen KM, Kananen K, Auriola S, Kontturi K, Urtti A. Characterization of paracellular and aqueous penetration routes in cornea, conjunctiva, and sclera. Invest Ophthalmol Vis Sci. 1997;38:627–34.

[59] Cheruvu NP, Kompella UB. Bovine and porcine transscleral solute transport: influence of lipophilicity and the Choroid–Bruch's layer. Invest Ophthalmol Vis Sci. 2006;47:4513-22. DOI: 10.1167/iovs.06–0404.

[60] Maurice DM, Polgar J. Diffusion across the sclera. Exp Eye Res. 1977;25:577–82.

[61] Wen H, Hao J, Li SK. Influence of permeant lipophilicity on permeation across human sclera. Pharm Res. 2010;27:2446–56. DOI: 10.1007/s11095-010-0237-0.

[62] Lin CW, Wang Y, Challa P, Epstein DL, Yuan F. Transscleral diffusion of ethacrynic acid and sodium fluorescein. Mol Vis. 2007;13:243–51.

[63] Dubey S, Kalia YN. Understanding the poor iontophoretic transport of lysozyme across the skin: when high charge and high electrophoretic mobility are not enough. J Control Release. 2014;183:35–42. DOI: 10.1016/j.jconrel.2014.03.027.

[64] Martinez T, Gonzalez MV, Roehl I, Wright N, Paneda C, Jimenez AI. In vitro and in vivo efficacy of SYL040012, a novel siRNA compound for treatment of glaucoma. Mol Ther. 2014;22:81–91. DOI: 10.1038/mt.2013.216.

[65] de la Fuente M, Seijo B, Alonso MJ. Novel hyaluronic acid-chitosan nanoparticles for ocular gene therapy. Invest Ophthalmol Vis Sci. 2008;49:2016–24. DOI: 10.1167/iovs.07-1077.

[66] Marano RJ, Wimmer N, Kearns PS, Thomas BG, Toth I, Brankov M, et al. Inhibition of in vitro VEGF expression and choroidal neovascularization by synthetic dendrimer peptide mediated delivery of a sense oligonucleotide. Exp Eye Res. 2004;79:525–35. DOI: 10.1016/j.exer.2004.06.023.

[67] Berdugo M, Valamanesh F, Andrieu C, Klein C, Benezra D, Courtois Y, et al. Delivery of antisense oligonucleotide to the cornea by iontophoresis. Antisense Nucleic Acid Drug Dev. 2003;13:107–14. DOI: 10.1089/108729003321629647.

[68] Hussain AA, Starita C, Hodgetts A, Marshall J. Macromolecular diffusion characteristics of ageing human Bruch's membrane: implications for age-related macular degeneration (AMD). Exp Eye Res. 2010;90:703–10. DOI: 10.1016/j.exer.2010.02.013.

[69] Cheruvu NP, Amrite AC, Kompella UB. Effect of eye pigmentation on transscleral drug delivery. Invest Ophthalmol Vis Sci. 2008;49:333–41. DOI: 10.1167/iovs.07-0214.

[70] Pitkanen L, Ranta VP, Moilanen H, Urtti A. Binding of betaxolol, metoprolol and oligonucleotides to synthetic and bovine ocular melanin, and prediction of drug binding to melanin in human choroid-retinal pigment epithelium. Pharm Res. 2007;24:2063–70.DOI: 10.1007/s11095-007-9342-0.

[71] Rowe-Rendleman CL, Durazo SA, Kompella UB, Rittenhouse KD, Di Polo A, Weiner AL, et al. Drug and gene delivery to the back of the eye: from bench to bedside. Invest Ophthalmol Vis Sci. 2014;55:2714–30. DOI: 10.1167/iovs.13-13707.

[72] Srivatsa S. Regulatory challenges. Eur Biopharm Rev. 2012;Spring.

[73] ICH Harmonised Tripartite Guideline. Guidance on Nonclinical Safety Studies for the Conduct of Human Clinical Trials and Marketing Authorization for Pharmaceuticals M3(R2). 2009.

[74] Addendum to ICH Harmonised Tripartite Guideline preclinical safety evaluation of biotechnology-derived pharmaceuticals S6(R1). 2011.

[75] Kornbrust D, Cavagnaro J, Levin A, Foy J, Pavco P, Gamba-Vitalo C, et al. Oligo safety working group exaggerated pharmacology subcommittee consensus document. Nucleic Acid Ther. 2013;23:21–8. DOI: 10.1089/nat.2012.0399.

[76] Levin AA, Henry S. Toxicology of oligonucleotide therapeutics and understanding the relevance of the toxicities. In: Preclinical Safety Evaluation of Biopharmaceuticals: A Science-Based Approach to Facilitating Clinical Trials. John Wiley & Sons, Inc.; 2008. p. 537–75.

[77] Lindow M, Vornlocher HP, Riley D, Kornbrust DJ, Burchard J, Whiteley LO, et al. Assessing unintended hybridization-induced biological effects of oligonucleotides. Nat Biotechnol. 2012;30:920–3. DOI: 10.1038/nbt.2376.

[78] CHMP SWP reflection paper on the assessment of the genotoxic potential of antisense oligodeoxynucleotides, EMEA/CHMP/SWP/199726/2004. 2005.

[79] Eckstein F. Phosphorothioates, essential components of therapeutic oligonucleotides. Nucleic Acid Ther. 2014;24:374–87. DOI: 10.1089/nat.2014.0506.

[80] Henderson S. Preclinical safety evaluation of oligonucleotides. Developments in Life-Sciences 2008;9:4–8.

[81] Safety of intravitreous fomivirsen for treatment of cytomegalovirus retinitis in patients with AIDS. Am J Ophthalmol. 2002;133:484–98.

[82] ICH Harmonized Tripartite Guideline on detection of toxicity to reproduction for medicinal products & toxicity to male fertility S5(R2), CPMP/ICH136/95 modification. 2000.

[83] Cavagnaro J, Berman C, Kornbrust D, White T, Campion S, Henry S. Considerations for assessment of reproductive and developmental toxicity of oligonucleotide-based therapeutics. Nucleic Acid Ther. 2014;24:313–25. DOI: 10.1089/nat.2014.0490.

[84] ICH Harmonised Tripartite Guideline on the Safety Pharmacology Studies for Human Pharmaceuticals, CPMP/ICH/539/00-ICH S7A. 2000.

[85] Garba AO, Mousa SA. Bevasiranib for the treatment of wet, age-related macular degeneration. Ophthal Eye Dis. 2010;2:75–83. DOI: 10.4137/OED.S4878.

[86] Anderson J, Akkina R. CXCR4 and CCR5 shRNA transgenic CD34+ cell derived macrophages are functionally normal and resist HIV-1 infection. Retrovirology. 2005;2:53. DOI: 10.1186/1742-4690-2-53.

[87] Ahmed Z, Kalinski H, Berry M, Almasieh M, Ashush H, Slager N, et al. Ocular neuroprotection by siRNA targeting caspase-2. Cell Death Dis. 2011;2:e173. DOI: 10.1038/cddis.2011.54.

[88] Solano EC, Kornbrust DJ, Beaudry A, Foy JW, Schneider DJ, Thompson JD. Toxicological and pharmacokinetic properties of QPI-1007, a chemically modified synthetic siRNA targeting caspase 2 mRNA, following intravitreal injection. Nucleic Acid Ther. 2014;24:258–66. DOI: 10.1089/nat.2014.0489.

[89] Pañeda C, Martínez T, Wright N, Jimenez AI. Recent advances in ocular nucleic acid-based therapies: the silent era. In: Adio A, editor. Ocular Diseases. InTech; 2012. p. 157–86. DOI: 10.5772/48454

[90] Pañeda C. SYL040012, a siRNA for the treatment of glaucoma. Acta Ophthalmol. 2013;91:0–0. DOI: 10.1111/j.1755-3768.2013.4227.x.

[91] Pañeda C, Gonzalez V, Martínez T, Ruz V, Vargas B, Jiménez AI, editors. RNAi based therapies for ocular conditions. Proceedings of the 11th ISOPT 2014; 19–22 June 2014, Reykjavik. Medimond; 2014. p. 25–30.

[92] Weinreb RN, Khaw PT. Primary open-angle glaucoma. Lancet. 2004;363:1711–20. DOI: 10.1016/S0140-6736(04)16257-0.

[93] Moreno-Montanes J, Sadaba B, Ruz V, Gomez-Guiu A, Zarranz J, Gonzalez MV, et al. Phase I clinical trial of SYL040012, a small interfering RNA targeting beta-adrenergic receptor 2, for lowering intraocular pressure. Mol Ther. 2014;22:226–32. DOI: 10.1038/mt.2013.217.

[94] Martinez-Garcia MC, Martinez T, Paneda C, Gallego P, Jimenez AI, Merayo J. Differential expression and localization of transient receptor potential vanilloid 1 in rabbit and human eyes. Histol Histopathol. 2013;28:1507–16. 10.14670/HH-28.1507.

[95] Brafman A, Mett I, Shafir M, Gottlieb H, Damari G, Gozlan-Kelner S, et al. Inhibition of oxygen-induced retinopathy in RTP801-deficient mice. Invest Ophthalmol Vis Sci. 2004;45:3796–805. DOI: 10.1167/iovs.04-0052.

[96] Lee DU, Huang W, Rittenhouse KD, Jessen B. Retina expression and cross-species validation of gene silencing by PF-655, a small interfering RNA against RTP801 for the treatment of ocular disease. J Ocul Pharmacol Ther. 2012; 28:222–30. DOI: 10.1089/jop.2011.0116.

[97] Rittenhouse KD, Johnson TR, Vicini P, Hirakawa B, Kalabat D, Yang AH, et al. RTP801 gene expression is differentially upregulated in retinopathy and is silenced by PF-04523655, a 19-Mer siRNA directed against RTP801. Invest Ophthalmol Vis Sci. 2014;55:1232–40. DOI: 10.1167/iovs.13-13449.

[98] Nguyen QD, Schachar RA, Nduaka CI, Sperling M, Basile AS, Klamerus KJ, et al. Dose-ranging evaluation of intravitreal siRNA PF-04523655 for diabetic macular edema (the DEGAS study). Invest Ophthalmol Vis Sci. 2012;53:7666–74. DOI: 10.1167/iovs.12-9961.

[99] Byrne M, Tzekov R, Wang Y, Rodgers A, Cardia J, Ford G, et al. Novel hydrophobically modified asymmetric RNAi compounds (sd-rxRNA) demonstrate robust efficacy in the eye. J Ocul Pharmacol Ther. 2013;29:855–64. DOI: 10.1089/jop.2013.0148.

[100] Liao Y, Erxleben C, Abramowitz J, Flockerzi V, Zhu MX, Armstrong DL, et al. Functional interactions among Orai1, TRPCs, and STIM1 suggest a STIM-regulated heteromeric Orai/TRPC model for SOCE/Icrac channels. Proc Natl Acad Sci U S A. 2008;105:2895–900. DOI: 10.1073/pnas.0712288105.

[101] Prakriya M, Feske S, Gwack Y, Srikanth S, Rao A, Hogan PG. Orai1 is an essential pore subunit of the CRAC channel. Nature. 2006;443:230–3. DOI: 10.1038/nature05122.

[102] Holowka D, Calloway N, Cohen R, Gadi D, Lee J, Smith NL, et al. Roles for ca(2+) mobilization and its regulation in mast cell functions. Front Immunol. 2012;3:104. DOI: 10.3389/fimmu.2012.00104.

[103] Ma HT, Beaven MA. Regulators of Ca(2+) signaling in mast cells: potential targets for treatment of mast cell-related diseases? Adv Exp Med Biol. 2011;716:62–90. DOI: 10.1007/978-1-4419-9533-9_5.

[104] Nakama T, Yoshida S, Ishikawa K, Kobayashi Y, Zhou Y, Nakao S, et al. Inhibition of choroidal fibrovascular membrane formation by new class of RNA interference therapeutic agent targeting periostin. Gene Ther. 2014;22:127–37. DOI: 10.1038/gt.2014.112.

[105] Martinez T, Jiménez AI, Pañeda C. Short-interference RNAs: becoming medicines. EXCLI J. 2015;14:714–46. DOI: 10.17179/excli2015-297

Section 5

RNA Interference for Immune and Infectious Diseases

Chapter 13

RNAi-Induced Immunity

Wenyi Gu

Additional information is available at the end of the chapter

http://dx.doi.org/10.5772/61632

Abstract

RNA interference has a close relationship with the host defense system including adaptive immunity. It is not only involved in regulating immune cells at different stages of the immune response but also directly induces or enhances antigen presentation and subsequent immune responses. We have previously reported that a small hairpin RNA (shRNA) targeted the downstream site of a dominant cytotoxic T lymphocyte (CTL) epitope of human papillomavirus (HPV) type 16 oncogene E7 can stimulate an immune response against E7 expressing tumors in C57BL/6 mice. This results in the elimination of tumor growth *in vivo*, whereas an shRNA that targets the upstream site does not. Our recent data further confirm the long half-life of the 5'-mRNA fragment after shRNA degradation and its involvement in protein synthesis. This chapter summarizes these findings and provides some updated explanations for the findings.

Keywords: RNAi, shRNA, immune response, HPV E7, miRNA

1. Introduction

RNA interference (RNAi) is a conserved gene-regulation mechanism in all eukaryotic cells, where small RNAs including small interfering RNA (siRNA), small hairpin RNA (shRNA), and micro-RNA (miRNA, miR) interact with message RNAs (mRNAs) in a sequence-specific manner and cause the cleavage or translational blockage of a gene [1, 2]. Because of its specificity and efficiency, it has been widely utilized as a routine tool for gene functional studies in biology laboratories worldwide. In addition, since RNAi blockage is very specific and at the transcriptional level, RNAi-based gene therapy (RNAi therapy) is thought to hold a great potential for treating many diseases, especially viral infections and genetic disorders. Synthesized siRNA is thus regarded as a specialized drug for gene therapies. So far, promising results have been obtained with RNAi therapy in various diseases and many are being tested in clinical trials, including viral infections, cancers, and genetic or inflammatory disorders [3-7]. As cancers and other emerging diseases such as dementia and super-bug infections become major public health issues, RNAi therapy can offer a new solution and has the additional ability to overcome drug resistances.

Beside the fundamental gene-silencing and gene-regulating roles of RNAi, which will also regulate the gene functions of immune cells and thus the immune responses, RNAi pathway itself has an additional function and involvement in inducing adaptive immunity. This function has not been well-studied, and the mechanism is not clear. Its relationship with the immune system in terms of antigen reactivation and antigen presentation is still a new area to be investigated. Indeed, in plants and primitive species, RNAi is a part of the defense system against viral infections. However, in mammals, RNAi seems not directly involved in the immune system, probably due to the development of an advanced and sophisticated immune system. This chapter summarizes the evidence of RNAi-induced immunity against tumors and provides some updated possible explanations for the findings. The possible link between miRNA and its degraded products with the immune system has been also discussed. Exploring the relationship between RNAi and the immune system may lead to new discoveries in RNAi biology and approaches for more effective cancer immunotherapy or treatment for viral and intracellular pathogen infections.

2. The discovery of RNAi-induced adaptive immunity against tumors

In 2009, we reported a discovery about RNAi-induced immunity [7]. We investigated two shRNAs encoded by lentiviral vectors on their ability to suppress tumor cell growth and stimulate antitumor immunity *in vivo*. One shRNA targeted the downstream site of a dominant cytotoxic T lymphocyte (CTL) epitope of the oncogene E7 of human papillomavirus (HPV) type 16 (termed downstream shRNA), while another shRNA targeted the upstream site of this epitope (termed upstream shRNA). Both shRNAs were equally effective at silencing E7 gene expression (in mRNA and protein levels) and led to the inhibition of tumor cells growth *in vitro* and *in vivo* [7]. In spite of this, TC1 tumor cells (expressing HPV E6 and E7) treated with downstream shRNA stimulated an immune response against E7 in C57BL6 mice and resulted in elimination of tumor growth *in vivo*, whereas cells treated with the upstream shRNA did not. When untreated TC1 tumor cells were injected to the same mice (challenging tumors), the group of downstream shRNA exhibited a total inhibition of challenging tumor growth, whereas no inhibition was observed in the upstream shRNA group. This ability of downstream shRNA was absent in $Rag^{-/-}$ mice (lack of T- and B-cells), suggesting adaptive immune response or T-cell response was required. To prove that the immune response was antigen-specific, we carried out a same animal experiment by immunizing C57BL/6 mice with TC-1 cells treated with these shRNAs but challenged with another tumor cell line C2, which has the E7 expression and H-2b genetic background as C57BL/6 mice. Again, we observed that only mice immunized with downstream shRNA treated cells had a loss of tumor formation, indicating tumor clearance was specific to E7. Our data indicate that a more effective treatment can be developed for cervical cancer by combining RNAi

http://dx.doi.org/10.5772/61632

treatment with immunotherapy. Our results also reveal that RNAi may be widely used as an antitumor immunity stimulator or enhancer (Fig 1).

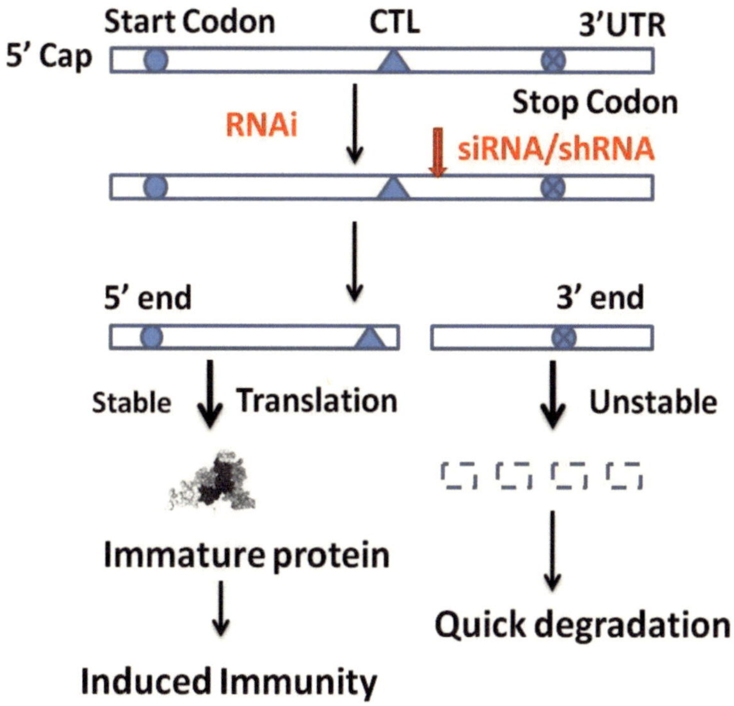

Figure 1. Schematic diagram shows RNAi targeting site and 5' mRNA fragment. It is known that in cervical cancer HPV E7 and mouse lymphoma EG7/OVA (ovalbumin) models, the shRNA targets the downstream site of the CTL epitope that produce the 5' fragment of mRNA. This makes immature proteins and further induces an immune response.

To prove the applicability of immune response to general tumor antigens, we tested a model antigen ovalbumin (OVA) expressed in EG7 cells that are a mouse thymoma cell line with C57BL6 genetic background. We chose the major CTL epitope of OVA, SIINFEKL, as the target site and designed two upstream shRNAs OVA-1 and -2 and a downstream shRNA OVA-3. The shRNA-treated EG7 cells were used to immunize the mice, which were subsequently challenged with untreated EG7 cells. We observed that only mice inoculated with OVA-3-shRNA treated cells had significantly reduced tumor formation but not with OVA-1 and -2 shRNAs.

3. Confirmation of mRNA fragments and truncated proteins in treated cells

To determine if the RNAi-induced immune response was actually from degraded products of RNAi, we designed a series of primers that would amplify RNA fragments inside and outside the targeting sites of upstream shRNA (E6-1) and downstream shRNA (E7-1, Fig 2A). If an inside fragment was present while the outside fragment was absent, it would indicate that the mRNA had been cleaved by shRNA at the target site. The cells were treated with E6-1 and E7-1 shRNAs and incubated for 2–4 days before real-time RT-PCR was carried out. As expected, the shortest PCR fragment, R3, was observed in all samples (Fig 2B). The full-length R1 PCR fragment was only observed in untreated TC1 cells or cells infected with the lentiviral vector control (PLL, Fig 2B). In cells treated with both E7-1 and E6-1, R1 was not found, indicating that shRNA-mediated cleavage was occurring. Of most interest was the R2 fragment which was found in all samples except cells treated with E6-1. These results suggest that R2 or R3 short fragments of E6-1 and E7-1 existed in the cells, at least temporarily at the time we isolated RNA. These short-form mRNAs may act as templates for short-form proteins (truncated proteins) and trigger antigen presentation to CD8+ T-cells and a CTL immune response to E7.

Apart from our data, a previous study reported that degradation of the 3' mRNA fragment resulting from siRNA-mediated cleavage was blocked for some mRNAs, leaving an mRNA fragment that could act as a template for cDNA synthesis. They suggested that this could give rise to false negative results and that this phenomenon may be avoided by the careful design of RT-qPCR primers for each individual siRNA experiment [8]. This report further confirms that mRNA fragments from RNAi do sometimes exist in the cells. In addition, it was noticed by researchers that un-degraded fragments of an siRNA-targeted mRNA may cause false positive effects of microarray analysis [9]. To avoid this, they developed a qRT-PCR protocol, which allowed for the determination of the optimal time point for mRNA analyses, indicating mRNA fragments after RNAi can be present in cell for a certain time.

What is the functional role of these mRNA fragments after RNAi? Our data demonstrated that they can be involved in translational machinery and produce truncated proteins. To experimentally prove this, we utilized the OVA-expressing EG7 cell model again. The cells were treated with downstream and upstream shRNAs and further treated with the protease inhibitor MG132 to reduce protein degradation before immunoblotting was performed. The blots were probed with an antibody against the N terminus of OVA protein. The predicted size of a truncated protein produced by the cleavage of OVA-2 shRNA was 14.7 kDa. We observed a protein band about 15-kDa in cells treated with the OVA-2 shRNA but not in untreated and OVA-1 or OVA-3 shRNA treated cells. It proves that truncated proteins can be produced in cells by the translation of mRNA fragment cleaved by shRNA. The predicted truncated product by shRNA-OVA3 was not observed due to cross-reacting proteins on the blot [7].

Our recent data (unpublished) showed that the cleaved 5′ and 3′ fragments of human papillomavirus type 16 (HPV-16) E6/7 mRNA after shRNA treatment were unevenly degraded. The 5′ mRNA fragment was more abundant and displayed a greater stability than the corresponding 3′ fragment in the treated cells. Further analysis revealed that the 5′ fragment was polysome-associated, indicating its active translation, and this was further confirmed by using tagged E7 protein to show that C-terminally truncated proteins were produced in treated cells (Singhania et al. submitted).

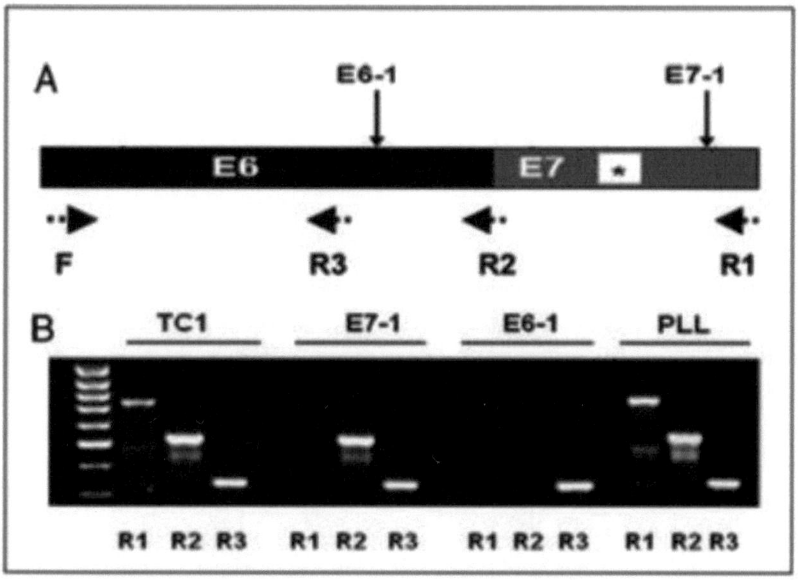

Figure 2. The shRNA targeting sites and primer design for HPV E6/E7 mRNA (Adapted from Gu et al 2009). (A) The shRNA and primer sites on E6/E7 mRNA. (B) The PCR products on an agarose gel. Notes: TC1, the untreated cell control. PLL, lentiviral vector control. *: indicates the site of CTL epitope. F: forward primer, R: reverse primer.

4. Possible models for explaining RNAi-induced immunity

It is well established that miRNAs play an important role in regulating innate and adaptive immune responses as a part of their gene-regulating roles. Evidence has accumulated that miRNAs are involved in the adaptive immune responses by regulating T-cells, B-cells, and antigen-presenting cells (APCs). For example, miR-214 was reported to target phosphatase and tensin homolog (PTEN) and increase proliferation and the activation of T-cells [10], while miR-150, -155, and let-7 have been shown to be involved in the development of T-cells into memory cells [11]. In addition, miR-184 was shown to inhibit nuclear factor of activated T-cells-1 (NFAT-1) in the activation of CD4 T-cell in the early stage of adaptive immune responses [12] and miR-181-a could promote CD4 and CD8 double positive T-cell development [13]. For B-cells, miR-155 is required for their normal function such as production of isotype-switched, high-affinity antibodies and for memory responses [14]. It has also been demonstrated that miR-155 is induced by B-cell receptor (BCR) [15]. However, overexpression of miR-155 can immortalize B-cells and lead to transformation, for instance, EBV was shown to have induced miR-155 expression and transformed B-cells [16, 17]. In addition, miR-150 is important in B-cell development [18] and so is miR-17 [19, 20].

For dendritic cells (DCs), a recent review summarized the need of miRNAs in their lineage commitment from bone marrow progenitors and for the development of subsets such as plasmacytoid DCs and conventional DCs [21]. Liu et al. (2010) used software to predict and then conducted experiments to confirm that three members of the miR-148 family, miR-148a, miR-148b, and miR-152 are negative regulators of the innate immune response and antigen-presenting capacity of DCs. They showed that miR-148/152 expression was upregulated in DCs on maturation and activation induced by TLR3, TLR4, and TLR9 agonists. These miRNAs in turn inhibited the production of cytokines including IL-12, IL-6, TNF-alpha, and IFN-beta and upregulation of MHC class II expression and DC-initiated antigen-specific T-cell proliferation by targeting Calcium/calmodulin-dependent protein kinase II alpha (CaMKIIα) [22]. In addition, miR-150 and miR-223 has been shown to play an important regulatory role in Langerhans cells (LCs) by cross-presenting a soluble antigen to antigen-specific CD8(+) T-cells [23, 24]. Beside APCs such as DC and LC, miRNA is shown to be directly involved in antigen presentation. For example, Bartoszewski et al. (2011) demonstrated that the mRNA of human endoplasmic reticulum (ER) antigen peptide transporter 1 (TAP1) is a direct target of miR-346. They showed that the 3'-UTR (un-translational region) of TAP1 contains a 6-mer seeding region for miR-346 and the ER stress-associated reduction of TAP1 mRNA and protein levels could be reversed by inhibitory miRNA of miR-346 [25]. As TAP plays an important role in MHC class I-associated antigen presentation, their data provide an insight for miRNA-regulating MHC class-I-associated antigen presentation during ER stress.

The above-highlighted results clearly indicate miRNA's regulatory role in many aspects of adaptive immunity. However, is it possible that miRNA also takes part in host immunity through mRNA fragments produced after RNAi just like shRNA described in section 2 and 3? Normally, miRNAs target the 3' UTR and lead to the translation block or degradation of the targeted mRNAs. So when they degrade mRNAs, it is supposed to produce long 5' mRNA fragments and may also produce truncated proteins. If this is true, the translated defective proteins could be treated as truncated protein and be processed by proteasome. If there is a CTL epitope in the defective structure, it could be coupled with the MHC class I molecule and presented to T-cells by DCs through antigen cross-presentation, as described above with shRNA. This could be a link between RNAi pathway and antigen presentation or adaptive immune response.

In the shRNA case discussed above, the target should be at the downstream of a CTL epitope to induce immunity. When miRNAs target 3' UTR, a site certainly at the downstream site of any possible CTL epitopes, it is assumed to have the ability to produce truncated proteins and so to induce immune responses. Therefore, an important question for miRNA biology is whether miRNAs can routinely induce immune responses by degrading mRNA at 3' UTR and generating 5' mRNA fragments or truncated proteins that contain CTL epitopes? So far, there is no answer for this question. Another critical question is: what is the difference between blocking and degrading mRNA by miRNAs at 3' UTR? Does this relate to antigen presentation of different proteins?

Because it has been shown that miRNA can act as siRNA and shRNA can be produced in the same pathway as miRNA [26], it is important and interesting to investigate if miRNA can induce the same immune response as shRNA. The systems of HPV 16 E7/TC1 and

http://dx.doi.org/10.5772/61632

OVA/EG7 can be used as good models to investigate this. As miRNAs are routinely transcribed and involved in interacting with mRNA, this mechanism can be considered as a routine way in cells to generate CTL containing truncated proteins. However, because most mRNAs in cells are for self-proteins, their CTL epitopes will not be presented to T-cells. This leaves the question of whether this is a mechanism just for cells that express viral genes (such as HPV E7 in TC1 and C2 as above) or for cells expressing foreign genes/antigens (such as OVA in EG7)? The next question is: can this be generalized to any tumor antigens including self-antigens? This is an interesting subject to investigate and will facilitate our understanding of how RNAi pathways interact with and are involved in adaptive immune responses (antigen presentation) to utilize them for cancer immunotherapy.

Although some miRNA are highly conserved between lower animals and higher animals, mammals have far more miRNAs compared to nonmammals. This suggests that during evolution, as gene regulation became so complex and important in higher animals, miRNA or RNAi pathway gradually specialized into gene regulation. At the same time, as the adaptive immune system became well developed and highly specialized, these two systems got separated, but as described above, they still have some links. Future investigations leading to insight into these links will provide answers to the above questions.

5. Conclusion

In summary, RNAi-induced immunity opens a new perspective in which to explore the relationship between RNAi pathways and the immune system, especially its involvement in antigen presentation in the adaptive immune response. For RNAi biology, it will provide an insight into the understanding of function roles of RNAi (including miRNA and siRNA) in host defense. In the field of gene therapy for cancers, RNAi can be used as an approach to silence oncogenes as well as a strategy to enhance immunity against cancer antigens (at least viral infection related cancers) and further explored as a novel cancer immunotherapy. Finally, for intracellar pathogens, it can be used as a strategy for developing new vaccine through RNAi reactivating their antigens to the immune system.

Author details

Wenyi Gu*

Address all correspondence to: w.gu@uq.edu.au

Australian Institute of Bioengineering and Nanotechnology, University of Queensland, QLD, Australia

References

[1] Sharp, P.A., *RNA interference--2001.* Genes Dev, 2001. 15(5): p. 485-90. doi:10.1101/gad.880001.

[2] Elbashir, S.M., et al., *Duplexes of 21-nucleotide RNAs mediate RNA interference in cultured mammalian cells.* Nature, 2001. 411(6836): p. 494-8. doi:10.1038/35078107.

[3] Jacque, J.M., K. Triques, and M. Stevenson, *Modulation of HIV-1 replication by RNA interference.* Nature, 2002. 418(6896): p. 435-8. doi:10.1038/nature00896.

[4] Harper, S.Q., et al., *RNA interference improves motor and neuropathological abnormalities in a Huntington's disease mouse model.* Proc Natl Acad Sci U S A, 2005. 102(16): p. 5820-5. doi:0501507102.

[5] Putral, L.N., et al., *RNA interference against human papillomavirus oncogenes in cervical cancer cells results in increased sensitivity to cisplatin.* Mol Pharmacol, 2005. 68(5): p. 1311-9. doi:10.1124/mol.105.014191.

[6] Bitko, V., et al., *Inhibition of respiratory viruses by nasally administered siRNA.* Nat Med, 2004. doi:10.1038/nm1164.

[7] Gu, W., et al., *Both treated and untreated tumors are eliminated by short hairpin RNA-based induction of target-specific immune responses.* Proc Natl Acad Sci U S A, 2009. 106(20): p. 8314-9. doi: 10.1073/pnas.0812085106.

[8] Holmes, K., et al., *Detection of siRNA induced mRNA silencing by RT-qPCR: considerations for experimental design.* BMC Res Notes, 2010. 3: p. 53. doi: 10.1186/1756-0500-3-53.

[9] Hahn, P., et al., *RNA interference: PCR strategies for the quantification of stable degradation-fragments derived from siRNA-targeted mRNAs.* Biomol Eng, 2004. 21(3-5): p. 113-7. doi:10.1016/j.bioeng.2004.09.001.

[10] Jindra, P.T., et al., *Costimulation-dependent expression of microRNA-214 increases the ability of T cells to proliferate by targeting Pten.* J Immunol, 2010. 185(2): p. 990-7. doi: 10.4049/jimmunol.1000793.

[11] Almanza, G., et al., *Selected microRNAs define cell fate determination of murine central memory CD8 T cells.* PLoS One, 2010. 5(6): p. e11243. doi: 10.1371/journal.pone.0011243.

[12] Weitzel, R.P., et al., *microRNA 184 regulates expression of NFAT1 in umbilical cord blood CD4+ T cells.* Blood, 2009. 113(26): p. 6648-57. doi: 10.1182/blood-2008-09-181156.

[13] Liu, G., et al., *Pre-miRNA loop nucleotides control the distinct activities of mir-181a-1 and mir-181c in early T cell development.* PLoS One, 2008. 3(10): p. e3592. doi: 10.1371/journal.pone.0003592.

[14] Calame, K., *MicroRNA-155 function in B Cells.* Immunity, 2007. 27(6): p. 825-7. doi: 10.1016/j.immuni.2007.11.010.

[15] Yin, Q., et al., *B-cell receptor activation induces BIC/miR-155 expression through a conserved AP-1 element.* J Biol Chem, 2008. 283(5): p. 2654-62. doi: 10.1074/jbc.M708218200.

[16] Rahadiani, N., et al., *Latent membrane protein-1 of Epstein-Barr virus induces the expression of B-cell integration cluster, a precursor form of microRNA-155, in B lymphoma cell lines.* Biochem Biophys Res Commun, 2008. 377(2): p. 579-83. doi:S0006-291X(08)01984-0.

[17] Linnstaedt, S.D., et al., *Virally induced cellular microRNA miR-155 plays a key role in B-cell immortalization by Epstein-Barr virus.* J Virol, 2010. 84(22): p. 11670-8. doi:JVI.01248-10.

[18] Xiao, C., et al., *MiR-150 controls B cell differentiation by targeting the transcription factor c-Myb.* Cell, 2007. 131(1): p. 146-59. doi:10.1016/j.cell.2007.07.021.

[19] Koralov, S.B., et al., *Dicer ablation affects antibody diversity and cell survival in the B lymphocyte lineage.* Cell, 2008. 132(5): p. 860-74. doi:S0092-8674(08)00268-7.

[20] Mendell, J.T., *miRiad roles for the miR-17-92 cluster in development and disease.* Cell, 2008. 133(2): p. 217-22. doi:S0092-8674(08)00449-2.

[21] Smyth, L.A., et al., *MicroRNAs affect dendritic cell function and phenotype.* Immunology, 2015. 144(2): p. 197-205. doi:10.1111/imm.12390.

[22] Liu, X., et al., *MicroRNA-148/152 impair innate response and antigen presentation of TLR-triggered dendritic cells by targeting CaMKIIalpha.* J Immunol, 2010. 185(12): p. 7244-51. doi:10.4049/jimmunol.1001573.

[23] Mi, Q.S., et al., *Lack of microRNA miR-150 reduces the capacity of epidermal Langerhans cell cross-presentation.* Exp Dermatol, 2012. 21(11): p. 876-7. doi:10.1111/exd.12008.

[24] Mi, Q.S., et al., *Deletion of microRNA miR-223 increases Langerhans cell cross-presentation.* Int J Biochem Cell Biol, 2013. 45(2): p. 395-400. doi:10.1016/j.biocel.2012.11.004.

[25] Bartoszewski, R., et al., *The unfolded protein response (UPR)-activated transcription factor X-box-binding protein 1 (XBP1) induces microRNA-346 expression that targets the human antigen peptide transporter 1 (TAP1) mRNA and governs immune regulatory genes.* J Biol Chem, 2011. 286(48): p. 41862-70. doi:10.1074/jbc.M111.304956.

[26] Zeng, Y., R. Yi, and B.R. Cullen, *MicroRNAs and small interfering RNAs can inhibit mRNA expression by similar mechanisms.* Proc Natl Acad Sci, 2003. 100(17): p. 9779-9784. doi: 10.1073/pnas.1630797100.

Chapter 14

Perspectives on RNA Interference in Immunopharmacology and Immunotherapy

Zhaohua Hou, Qiuju Han, Cai Zhang and Jian Zhang

Additional information is available at the end of the chapter

http://dx.doi.org/10.5772/61575

Abstract

RNA interference (RNAi), mediated by short interfering RNA (siRNA), vector-derived short hairpin RNA (shRNA) and microRNA (miRNA), brings about revolutionary features to basic biomedical research and clinical application. New drugs based on RNAi have been developed for therapeutic applications. The family of RNAi molecules are efficient agents to modulate mammalian immune system, and many studies reported that these molecules could manipulate immune defence, surveillance and homeostasis. Both perfect match of siRNA/shRNA and non-perfect match of miRNA could be beneficial for designing RNAi-based drugs for treatment of tumour and viral infection. This chapter provides a view to control or utilize the immune regulation of various small RNAs that should help researchers to understand the successful clinical application of RNAi.

Keywords: RNA interference, siRNA, miRNA, immunopharmacology, immunotherapy

1. Introduction

RNA interference (RNAi) is a conserved mechanism against exogenous nucleic acid and transposon transcripts in plants and lower animals. No matter of transfected siRNA, vector-delivered shRNA or pre-miRNA (transcribed mainly by Pol II) , Dicer (DCLs) and Agronaute (AGO) family proteins efficiently process small RNAs into short double-stranded RNA(dsRNA). Further, dsRNAs assemble into the RNAi-induced silencing (protein) complex (RISC) to guide and cleave target mRNA, promote mRNA degradation or inhibit mRNA translation. The great potential of RNAi is to specifically repress the expression of disease-causing genes while avoiding undesirable effects.

It is well accepted that siRNA can be recognized by endosomal pathways, Toll-like receptor 3 (TLR3), TLR7, TLR8 and cytoplasmic pathways, retinoic acid-inducible gene I (RIG-I), melanoma differentiation-associated antigen 5 (MDA-5) and RNA-activated protein kinase (PKR), resulting in immune activation [1–5]. For example, it has been demonstrated that siRNA can cause activation of at least three key transcription factors, including NF-κB, interferon regulatory factor 3 (IRF-3) and IRF-7, and stimulate interferon (IFN) secretion. This activates T cells and dendritic cells (DCs) in the spleen in a TLR7-dependent manner [2,6]. Furthermore, 5′-triphosphate siRNA was demonstrated to activate RIG-I signal pathway, and then natural killer (NK) cells and DCs were activated [7,8]. In most circumstances, immune system stimulation is regarded as an unwanted side effect; therefore, siRNA-induced immune response should be controlled by using proper delivery system or chemical modification, although immune stimulation has been proved to be essential in cancer treatment and viral infection.

miRNAs are critical in regulating the development, differentiation, function and destiny of immune cells, including DCs, granulocytes, monocytes/macrophages, NK and natural killer T (NKT) cells and B and T lymphocytes. miRNAs influence both innate and adaptive immune defence and individual miRNAs may contribute their implications to various immune-mediated diseases. Furthermore, pattern recognition receptors (PRRs), kinases, adaptors, inflammatory factors and IFN could all be targets of miRNAs. Extra effort has been made to develop miRNA-based oligos or vectors for anti-infection purpose by manipulating corresponding immune genes.

In addition to silencing of targeted genes in a sequence-specific manner, components of RNAi technology often induce immune response. Several strategies were reported to design RNAi molecules with gene silencing and immune regulatory properties. Bifunctional molecules rely on the activation of PRRs such as TLR7/8, TLR9 or RIG-I, or just rely on down-regulation of target gene. This chapter summarizes RNAi-involved immune responses in the past 10 years and discusses the anticipated therapeutic application.

2. Chemically synthesized siRNA and vector-derived shRNA

2.1. RNAi drugs based on targeting specific immune genes

Immune disorders, both autoimmune diseases and immune defective or deficiency, are always caused by high-level overexpression of certain immune genes. A variety of immune inhibitory genes can serve as targets for RNAi-mediated gene silencing. Targeting specific immune suppressor could re-balance immune network and subsets.

Elevated activity of signal transducer and activator of transcription 3 (STAT3) has been found in several kinds of human tumours. Use of RNAi to knockdown STAT3 expression and inhibit its activation would reduce the tumour cell growth such as pancreatic cancer, colorectal cancer, melanoma and hepatocarcinoma cells. STAT 3 knockdown could induce bystanders immune response in vitro and in vivo, where CD4+, CD8+ and NKT cells were activated as well as the secretion of interferon-γ (IFN-γ), interleukin-12 (IL-12) and tumour necrosis factor alpha (TNF-α) was increased significantly [9–11]. siRNA-STAT3, synthetically linked to CpG (agonist of TLR9), was demonstrated to silence immune suppressor STAT3 gene in TLR9+ myeloid cells and B cells. This strategy of therapy leads to activation of various populations of immune cells, including DCs and macrophages, that ultimately induce potent anti-tumour immune responses [10,12]. Hossain DM et al. recently reported that CpG-siRNA-STAT3 conjugates could efficiently silence the target expression, and abrogate inhibition of CD8+ T cells in patients who received myeloid-derived suppressor cells (MDSCs) [13]. Researchers proved that immune-stimulation-inducing CpG(A)-STAT3-siRNA was non-toxic for normal human leukocytes [14]. In another experiment, Luo Z et al. [15] generated a nano-vaccine loaded with poly I:C (a TLR3 agonist) and STAT3 siRNA. Researchers found this kind of siRNA could promote the maturation of DC and reverse immunosuppression in the tumour micro-environment; the function of inhibitory cells in tumour-draining lymph nodes were inhibited; thus, anti-tumour immune responses were potently induced; and the survival were prolonged [15]. Therefore, STAT3 siRNAs are expected to be a promising immunomodulatory drugs to improve the treatment efficacy of cancer vaccines by abrogating tumour immunosuppression.

Suppressor of cytokine signalling 1 (SOCS1) is a negative regulator of antigen-presenting cell (APC)-based immune response. Silencing of SOCS1 gene expression by RNAi is essential for DCs to enhance Ag-specific anti-tumour immunity [16]. SOCS1-silenced bone marrow dendritic cells (BMDCs) were more potent in suppressing tumour growth [17]. When SOCS1 was silenced, maturation of DCs (i.e. expressions of CD80, CD40, CD86 and major histocompatibility complex II [MHC II]) was significantly accelerated. As a result, SOCS1 inhibition up-regulated the expression of IFN-γ and IL-12, and decreased IL-4 secretions, which induced Th1 cell differentiation and thereby affected the development of Th2 cell. The combined nanoparticle (NP) delivery, which can render both tumour antigen and siRNA-SOCS1 to BMDCs, simultaneously could enhance immunotherapeutic effects in BMDC-based cancer therapy [16,18]. DC-targeted delivery of SOCS1 siRNA has been shown to enhance antifungal immunity in response to *Candida albicans* in vitro and HIV-specific cytotoxic T cell in mice [16, 19]. This evidence suggests the use of SOCS1–siRNA, as a potent adjuvant to improve immune response.

A20 is usually regarded as an attractive target for siRNA-mediated gene knockdown in DCs because it is a negative feedback regulator of multiple pro-inflammatory signal transduction. Several reports demonstrated that RNAi-mediated A20 silencing in DCs enhanced expression of co-stimulatory molecules (CD80, CD86, CD40 and MHC class II) and pro-inflammatory cytokines (IL-6 and TNF-α). Tumour-infiltrating cytotoxic T lymphocytes (CTLs), T helper cells that produced IL-6 and TNF-α were also activated by siA20-DC. A20 silencing in DCs can enhance the immune response against self-tumour-associated antigens [20,21]. Furthermore, A20-silenced DCs were proved to overcome CD4+CD25+regulatory T (Treg) cell suppression [21,22]. A20-silenced DCs could skew naive CD4+ T cells towards Th1 cell, but not Treg, Th2 or Th17 cells. Because a high amount of IL-10 was produced in A20-silenced DCs, simultaneous down-regulation of IL-10 and A20 resulted in enhanced T cell stimulatory capacity in DCs. A20 down-regulation resulted in enhanced CTLs immune response by the NF-κB and AP-1 pathways [20,23]. RNAi of A20 has enabled DCs to gain a potent ability to activate CTLs and Th cells, and inhibit Treg, providing a novel strategy to promote a tumour immune response.

Programmed death ligand (PD-L) is another exciting target on the surface of antigen-presenting cells (APCs); PD-L/PD-1 interactions were related to functional impairment and exhaustion of tumour antigen-specific CD8+ T cells. Although PD-L antibody exerts a potent anti-tumour effect, previous reports [24] have demonstrated that PD-L1-siRNA-PEI were preferentially and avidly engulfed by tumour-associated CD11c+PD-L1+ tolerogenic DCs at ovarian cancer locations. This kind of nanoparticle uptake stimulated multiple TLRs signalling, mainly via myeloid differentiation factor 88 (MyD88). Then, regulatory DCs activated into potent stimulators of CTLs that led to significant anti-tumour immunity in mouse models of ovarian cancer. Most importantly, PD-L knockdown DCs showed superior potential to expand minor histocompatibility antigen (MiHA)-specific CD8+ effector and memory T cells from leukaemia patients early after donor lymphocyte infusion and later during relapse. Combined PD-L1 and PD-L2 knockdown resulted in improved proliferation of CD4+ T cells and enhanced cytokine production [25,26]. In addition, another report demonstrated the improved effector functions of tumour-specific CD4+ and CD8+ human T cells by siRNA-mediated silencing of PD-1 ligands, PD-L1 or PD-L2 [27]. These results suggest that siRNA-mediated knockdown of PD-L is a fascinating strategy to inhibit a negative regulatory mechanism of tumour-specific T cells.

siRNA-CD40, delivered by a novel delivery system with a poly-dA extension at the 5'-end of the siRNA sense strand that was stably incorporated into 1,3-β-glucan, was captured and incorporated into DCs through its receptor, Dectin [28]. This strategy could induce antigen-specific Tregs, resulting in the permanent acceptance of mouse cardiac allografts. CD40 knockdown significantly suppressed Th1-type cytokines and induced Th2-type cytokines in rats with myocarditis. Knockdown of CD40 in experimental autoimmune myocarditis (EAM) rats promoted Foxp3 gene expression and increased Treg cells [29].

In addition, when silencing of CD40 or CD80/CD86, DCs exhibited suppressed allostimulatory activity with impaired APC function. In the well-established collagen-induced arthritis (CIA) model, multigene-silenced DCs were capable of delaying onset of joint pathology. Therapeutic effects of gene-silenced DCs were mediated by the inhibition of collagen II-specific Ab production and suppression of T cell recall responses. Also, multigene-silenced DCs inhibited Th1 and Th17 response, demonstrating IFN-γ and IL-2 inhibition [30]. Thus, inhibition of specific co-stimulatory molecules of DCs reveals a promising approach of suppressing immune responses in autoimmunity. These findings highlight the potential of immunomodulation of siRNA-CD40, and have important implications for developing RNAi-based clinical therapy in the transplantation field.

It is well documented that tumours could secrete immunosuppressive molecules, including the cytokines transforming growth factor β (TGF-β) and IL-10. This creates an immunosuppressive environment, which inhibits anti-tumour immunity. The suppression of Treg cell, induced by targeting TGF-β1 using siRNA, can enhance the efficacy of a DC vaccine against a poorly immunogenic tumour in mice [31]. Nanoparticle-delivered TGF-β siRNA enhances vaccination against advanced melanoma, and the tumour micro-environment was modified with increased levels of tumour-infiltrating CD8+ T cells and decreased level of regulatory T cells [32]. siRNA targeting IL-10 receptor α (siIL-10RA) initiated the significant antigen-specific CD8+ T cell immune responses. Concordantly, the combination of knockdown of IL-10RA and TGF-βR in DCs showed significant up-regulation of MHC I, enhancing co-stimulatory molecules CD40, CD80, CD86 and chemokine CCR7 after lipopolysaccharide (LPS) stimulation. It induced the strongest anti-tumour effects in the TC-1 P0 (a cervical cancer model expressing the human papillomavirus [HPV]-16 E7 antigen) tumour model, and even in the immune-resistant TC-1 (P3) ones [33]. These data revealed that siRNA co-targeting immunosuppressive molecules enhance the potency of DC-based immunotherapeutics.

High-mobility group box 1 (HMGB1) is highly expressed in tumour cells and increased levels of HMGB1 in tumour cells are usually associated with a greater tumour angiogenesis, growth, invasion and metastasis. Knockdown of tumour cell-derived HMGB1 by shRNA did not affect tumour cell growth, while naturally acquired long-lasting tumour-specific IFN-γ- or TNF-α-producing CD8+ T cell responses were induced, and ability to induce Treg was attenuated. This led to naturally acquired CD8 T cell-dependent anti-tumour immunity [34].

Foxp3, a master gene that controls the development and function of Treg cells, contributes to pathogenesis of several different tumours. Owing to the intracellular localization of Foxp3, RNAi technology was employed to knockdown its activation to suppress Treg activity in vivo. Tsai et al. [35] performed a study targeting silencing Foxp3 gene expression by shRNAs-mediated RNAi using a lentivirus vector in a murine model of leukaemia. The lentiviral vector was used to overcome poor transfection efficiency. Lentiviral-mediated Foxp3 RNAi showed suppressive effects on tumour growth and prolonged the survival of tumour-transplanted mice. Furthermore, Foxp3 knockdown mediated by siRNA increased the ratio of Th1/Th2 in chronic hepatitis B patients; transcription factors T-bet and GATA-3 may be partly involved in this progress [36]. This strategy provides a novel view about how to decrease the number of Treg cells and weaken its function.

Selective knockdown of CCL22 and CCL17 expression in monocyte-derived DC (MoDC) by siRNA decreased the ratios of CD4+ to CD8+ as well as lowered the frequency of Tregs recruited by MoDC. Furthermore, intratumoural injection of MoDC, which was transfected with siCCL22 and siCCL17, significantly reduced the number of Tregs while inducing CD8+ T cells infiltration in thymic nude mice with human tumour xenografts [37]. Using siRNA to selectively silence chemokines may lead to a new strategy for DC vaccine development to improve cancer biotherapy.

High expression of indoleamine 2, 3-dioxygenase (IDO) in DCs leads to the suppression of T cell responses. Gene silencing by siRNA or shRNA of IDO in DC would up-regulate IL-12 and IFN-γ and inhibit apoptosis in CD8 and CD4 T cells as well as Treg cells; IL-10 expression was significantly down-regulated, thus finally restraining tumour growth. DC-based vaccine with IDO silence was demonstrated to augment and enhance the anti-tumour response against breast cancer, melanoma, bladder tumour and liver cancer [38–40]. A novel APC-targeted siRNA delivery system using mannosed liposomes (Man-lipo) with encapsulated siRNA-IDO

(Man-lipo-siIDO) was demonstrated to preferentially silence IDO in APCs and efficiently enhance anti-tumour immune response [41–43].

It was reported that natural killer group 2, member D (NKG2D) activation was involved in NK cell and CD8+ cell-mediated liver inflammation, and blockade of NKG2D by silencing of multiple NKG2D ligands on hepatocytes was considered efficient in liver disease intervention. Huang et al. [44] constructed a plasmid containing the three shRNA sequences (shRae1-shMult1-shH60). After hydrodynamic injection into mice, they found that the expression of all three NKG2D ligands on hepatocytes was down-regulated, and fulminant hepatitis mediated through NKG2D in NK cell was attenuated. Furthermore, simultaneous knockdown of multiple human NKG2D ligands (MHC class I polypeptide-related sequence B/A(MICA/B), UL16-binding protein 2 [ULBP2] and ULBP3) also significantly attenuated NK cell cytolysis. Simultaneous knockdown of multiple ligands of NKG2D is a potential therapeutic approach to treat liver diseases induced by NKG2D-expressing NK cells and CD8+ cells. Furthermore, inhibition of human leukocyte antigen-G (HLA-G) by siRNA boosted NK cell lytic function [45,46].

Among several molecules involved in immune response, the choice of targets should be carefully reviewed and validated comprehensively according to the emerging knowledge about their function.

2.2. Advantage of non-target immune effect of siRNA/shRNA drugs

siRNA/shRNA have the potential to recruit immune receptors specialized in RNA sensor, such as TLR3, TLR7/8 [2,3]. 5′-triphosphate siRNA (3p-siRNA) was demonstrated to be detected by RNA sensors RIG-I. These immunostimulatory siRNA or shRNA can non-specifically induce innate immune response, the so-called 'off-target' effects that have considerable implications for clinical application to cure cancer and infection disease.

IFN response is a common side effect of siRNAs and siRNAs with GU-rich sequences, which are very potent in inducing IFN-α response. A newly published report demonstrated that siRNA could induce IFN-α responses, and then induced the analgesic effects in the spinal cord. This off-target analgesia is dose- and sequence-dependent while non-GU-rich sequences also produced off-target analgesia at high doses, where pain relief by a designed siRNA may not be attributable to target gene knockdown but IFN response [47].

Early in 2004, Karikó et al. [48] demonstrated that siRNAs and shRNAs induce immune activation by signalling through TLR3 and activate sequence-independent inhibition of gene expression. Kleinman et al. [4] showed that non-targeted (against non-mammalian genes) and targeted (against vascular endothelial growth factor [VEGF] or VEGFR1) siRNAs suppressed choroidal neovascularization (CNV) via cell-surface TLR3 and its adaptor TIR-domain-containing adaptor-inducing interferon-β (TRIF), leading to the induction of IFN-α and IL-12. The effect of non-targeted siRNA to suppress dermal neovascularization in mice was as effective as vascular endothelial growth factor (VEGF) siRNA. This finding showed that two investigational siRNAs in clinical trials owe their anti-angiogenic effect in mice, which was not due to target knockdown but due to TLR3 activation. The efficiency of RNAi by siRNA is believed to be comparable with anti-VEGF antibodies. Kleinman's group then concluded that a 21-nucleotide (nt) non-targeted siRNA suppresses both hemangiogenesis and lymphangiogenesis in mouse models of neovascularization, induced by corneal sutures or hindlimb ischemia, as efficiently as a 21-nt siRNA targeting VEGF-A [1].

Among 15 siRNAs, Khairuddin et al. [49] identified an extremely immunostimulatory siRNAs, targeting the HPV, which exerted potent anti-tumoural function. This bifunctional siRNA could reduce growth of established TC-1 tumours in C57BL/6 mice, and its effect was TLR7 dependent, where ablation of TLR7 recruitment via 2'O-methyl modification of the oligo backbone reduced these anti-tumour effects. Flatekval et al. [40] designed either monofunctional siRNAs devoid of immunostimulation or bifunctional siRNAs with IDO silencing and immunostimulatory activities. They showed that bifunctional siRNAs were able to knockdown IDO expression and induce cytokine production through either endosomal TLR7/8 or RIG-I.

In the past 10 years, several studies reported that bifunctional 3p-siRNA (Exp:targeting Bcl2/TGF-β/Survivin/Glutaminase/IDO) with target silencing and an innate immunity stimulation via RIG-I activation could confer potent anti-tumour efficacy. This is illustrated for the first time by the work of Poeck et al. [8], who reported that bifunctional siRNAs, with 5′-triphosphate targeting Bcl2 (3p-siRNA), led to better melanoma tumour reduction than OH-siRNA or 5′-triphosphate siRNAs containing target mismatches. Poeck and his colleagues revealed that siRNA with 5′-triphosphate ends could be recognized by RIG-I and activate an innate immune cells such as DC; then, expression of IFNs was directly induced, leading to apoptosis in tumour cells. These bifunctional 3p-siRNAs with RIG-I activation and RNAi-mediated Bcl2 silencing could provoke massive apoptosis of tumour cells in lung metastases in vivo. This was the first report demonstrating that 3p-siRNA represents a single molecule-based approach in which RIG-I function activates immune cell and gene silencing, leading to a key molecular event. Researchers subsequently found that 3p-TGFβ1-siRNA combining RIG-I activation with gene silencing of TGF-β1 induced profound tumour cell apoptosis and revealed potent anti-tumour efficacy in pancreatic cancer. This kind of 3p-siRNA induces a Th1 cytokine profile, demonstrating IFN-γ induction and IL-4 inhibition. High level of IFN and CXCL10 recruited more activated CD8+ T cells to the tumour. Frequency of immunosuppressive CD11b+ Gr-1+ myeloid cells was reduced after 3p-TGFβ1-siRNA treatment [50].

In addition, 3p-siRNA against survivin gene was designed and generated. This finding demonstrated that 3p-survivin-siRNA inhibited lung cancer cell proliferation and induced a RIG-I-dependent type-I interferon response [7]. Recently, 5′-triphosphate siRNA combining glutaminase (GLS) silencing with RIG-I activation was demonstrated to induce more prominent anti-tumour responses than RIG-I ligand or GLS silencing capability alone. 3p-siRNA-GLS effectively induced intrinsic proapoptotic signalling, and GLS silence sensitized malignant cells to apoptosis induced by RIG-I activation. Moreover, cytotoxicity was enhanced, resulting from disturbed glutaminolysis induced by GLS silencing. Finally, RIG-I activation by 3p-siRNA-GLS blocked autophagic degradation, leading to dysfunction of mitochondria, whereas GLS silencing severely impaired reactive oxygen species (ROS) scavenging systems, leading to a vicious circle of ROS-mediated cytotoxicity [51]. Immature monocyte-derived DCs had been transfected with siRNA-bearing 5′-triphosphate-activated T cells [40].

In addition, 3p-siRNA can inhibit hepatitis B virus (HBV), Influenza A Virus and Coxsackie-virus, by gene silencing and RIG-I activation. RNAi provides a promising approach for the specific treatment of HBV infection. Our laboratory has previously demonstrated that 3p-HBx-siRNA and shRNA-HBx not only directly inhibit HBV replication but also stimulate innate immunity against HBV, which are both beneficial for the inversion of HBV-induced immune tolerance [52]. In HBV-positive hepatoma HepG2.2.15 cells, 3p-HBx-siRNA combining RIG-I activation with HBx gene silencing induce stronger type I IFN response than non-target 3p-scramble-siRNA, indicating that a potent immunostimulatory effect may partly contribute to the reversal of immune tolerance through decreasing HBV load; 3p-HBx-siRNA more strongly inhibited HBV replication and promoted IFN production than HBx-siRNA in primary HBV(+) hepatocytes, and this effect was mediated by RIG-I activation [52]. This was consistent of the other two reports [53,54]. Our dually functional vector containing both an immunostimulatory single-stranded RNA (ssRNA) and an HBx-silencing shRNA could reverse HBV-induced hepatocyte-intrinsic immune tolerance; TLR7 signalling pathway was attributed to this progress [55].

Lin et al. [56] designed and tested a 3p-mNP1496-siRNA against influenza virus. They found that 3p-mNP1496-siRNA could activate the RIG-I-mediated IFN-β pathway and significantly reduce virus load and virus-induced pathogenesis. The inhibition effect was in an siRNA- and RIG-I-dependent manner, demonstrating siRNA playing dual antiviral roles: viral gene-specific silencing and non-gene-specific RIG-I activation. This strategy was also proved to elicit potent antiviral effects in coxsackievirus myocarditis, and virus-specific 3p-siRNA was superior to both conventional virus-specific siRNA and non-target 3p-siRNA in inhibiting viral replication and subsequent cytotoxicity [57].

In the attempt to inhibit the expression of woodchuck hepatitis virus (WHV), Meng et al. [58] found that innate immune responses could be enhanced by RNAi through the PKR- and TLR-dependent signalling pathways in primary hepatocytes. The immunostimulation by RNAi may contribute to the antiviral activity of siRNAs in vivo.

Furthermore, siRNA can also synergistically enhance DNA-mediated type III IFN (a newly characterized antiviral interferon) response in non-immune or primary immune cells. This enhancement is mediated by crosstalk signalling pathway between RIG-I (RNA sensor) and IFI16 (DNA sensor) [59].

Designing with GU sequences, addition of triphosphate motifs to siRNA, co-treatment with CpG oligos are believed to activate innate immunity when siRNA was applied in vitro and in vivo. Accumulating evidence suggests these bifunctional siRNAs could activate NK cells and CD8+ T cells in different models. Thus, specific clinical applications of RNAi can benefit from a concurrent activation of the immune system.

3. miRNA

It has been well discussed how miRNAs regulate signalling pathways, and the dynamics of the immune response, tolerance and homeostasis. Here we summarize and explore updated achievements of special miRNAs in immunopharmacology.

3.1. miRNAs as intrinsic targets in antiviral immunity

In addition to the conventional innate and adaptive immune responses, even in the earlier phase after virus invasion, the host cell suppresses viral replication by evolving the profile of special and constitutively expressed genes. These cell-intrinsic antiviral approaches based on host restriction factors may be no less important than in considerations of conventional immunity. At the same time, viruses also gain some countermeasures or adapt the unique phenotype of their hosts substantially to survive. Moreover, miRNAs may also be involved in the inextricably intertwined relationship between viruses and their hosts.

In 2005, a liver-specific miRNA, miR122, which is involved in cholesterol and lipid metabolism [60], was illustrated to be necessary for hepatitis C virus (HCV) accumulation in cultured liver cells [61]. Researchers found that miR122 directly binds to two close sites in the 5′ non-coding region of the HCV genome and promote HCV translation [62–64]. This miRNA kept conserved among all HCV subtypes [65,66]. Even in non-hepatic cell, miR122 could boost HCV replication [67]. Moreover, miR122 was further proved to be significantly reduced after IFN-β treatment, and miR122 mimics neutralized IFN-induced anti-HCV effect [68]. Epidemiological and genomic researches further suggested that the level of miR122 in individuals with HCV might be an 'indicator' for IFN therapy, and only those patients with high levels of miR122 responded well to IFN therapy [69,70]. Therefore, miR122 antagonist would also be called as IFN 'sensitizer' in HCV immune treatment.

Santaris Pharma designed and synthesized an LNA-based miR122 inhibitor, named Miravirsen (or SPC3649), to eradicate HCV. The product was first evaluated in preclinical studies in mice [71], cynomolgus monkeys [72], green African monkeys and chimpanzees [73,74]. Here the key concern is that whether miR122 inhibitor can effectively lower the level of free miR122 and inhibit HCV replication without disturbing normal cholesterol and lipid metabolism or without any potential chemical toxicity. Interestingly, although there was a reduction of cholesterol levels in plasma by nearly 40%, Miravirsen caused a dose-dependent reduction of miR122 and maintained ~5-week-long half-life in the liver of monkeys and chimpanzees [73, 74]. Moreover, in the high-dose treatment group, Miravirsen decreased HCV subtype 1a or 1b more than 2 orders of magnitude compared to control group. In all animal species, Miravirsen was reported to be safe, without serious adverse effects or dose-related toxicities in rats, monkeys and human [75,76].

In May 2008, Miravirsen was put into human clinical trials as the first miRNA-based drug (https://clinicaltrials.gov/ct2/show/NCT00979927). There was a significant, dose-dependent reduction and sustained decrease of HCV viremia after drug administration in human subjects, and several patients became even HCV undetectable during the study. At the same time, only infrequent and moderately adverse effects were caused to some volunteers and did not influence the trial process [77]. Because miR122 is only liver enriched in physiological conditions and there is high amount of miR122 in adult human liver, it may be an ideal target to design highly specific anti-HCV drugs with good resistance to HCV infected person, particularly to those who have no tolerance to traditional treatments. In the following years, miR196 [78], let-7b family [79] and some other miRNAs were then proved to influence HCV life cycle, providing new target to restrict hepatitis C infection and avoid chronic infection.

Besides HCV, some other kind of viruses also encode miRNAs or regulate the miRNAs expression in host cells to disturb the expression of many immune-associated genes directly and/or indirectly, so that they can be critical regulators for viral life cycle. For example, in HEK293T cell, prototype foamy virus I (PFV-1) encodes Tas protein to counteract cell-encoded miR32, which could inhibit PFV-1 gene expression and accumulation [80]. Kaposi's sarcoma-associated herpesvirus (KSHV)-induced miR132 could silence p300 expression, which is critical for the transcription initialization of many antiviral genes, to help themselves maintain long-time latency [81]. The hematopoietic-cell-specific miR142-3p potently restricts the replication of eastern equine encephalitis virus in myeloid-lineage cells by binding to the 3'-untranslated region (UTR) of viral genome [82]. Even Drosha, the enzyme that processes miRNA biogenesis and maturation, was an independent factor for limiting RNA virus replication along with canonical type I IFN system in particular cell type [83]. Above of all, it is much likely that miRNA mimics (for viral inhibitory miRNAs) or antagonists (for viral beneficial miRNAs) can be effective antiviral strategies as intrinsic immune drugs.

3.2. miRNA regulation antimicrobial and anti-tumour immunity

3.2.1. miRNA in antimicrobial innate immunity

Of the known PRRs, TLRs and RIG-like receptors (RLRs) have been well studied in mediating antimicrobial and inflammatory responses during infections, which may be targets of pathogens or host-encoded miRNAs.

The first PRR targeting miRNA let7i was reported in 2007 [84], which targeted TLR4 mRNA in a MyD88/NF-κB-dependent way during *Cryptosporidium parvum* infection, controlling the production of inflammatory factors. During *Bacillus Calmette-Guérin* (BCG) infection, miR124 exerts its function by targeting multiple components of the TLR signalling pathway, including TLR6, MyD88, TNF receptor-associated factor 6 (TRAF6) and TNF-α in mouse lung cell [85]. After HCV infection, miR373 was induced and negatively regulated the type I IFN signalling pathway by suppressing Janus kinase 1(JAK1) and IRF9 in hepatocytes [86]. Experimental evaluation using miR124 inhibitors or miR373 knockout up-regulated BCG-induced pro-inflammatory factors or type I IFN and so as to inhibit BCG or HCV more efficiently. Besides using host miRNAs, human cytomegalovirus (HCMV) targeted TLR2 by encoding its own miRNA, miR-UL112-3p, and reduced the expression of IL-1β, IL-6 and IL-8 upon stimulation with a TLR2 agonist [87]. Neutralizing this miRNA might recover normal cytokines production.

Besides immune inhibitory miRNAs, dengue virus (DENV)-induced miR30e* up-regulated IFN-β and the downstream IFN-stimulated genes (ISGs) by suppressing IkBα and promoting NF-κB-dependent IFN production [88]. The transfection of miR30e* would increase the expression of 2′-5′-oligoadenylate synthetase 1(OAS-1), myxovirus resistance A (MxA) and interferon-induced transmembrane protein (IFITM). In 2014, miR526 [89] was proved to enhance RIG-I-induced viral replication by suppression of the expression of cylindromatosis (CYLD), which suppresses RIG-I K-63-linked polyubiquitin. Moreover, Enterovirus 71(EV71) inhibited miR526 transcription in an IRF-dependent way and so as to attenuate virus-triggered type I interferon production. These studies suggested that recruitment or increase of miR30e* or miR526 would stimulate type I IFN expression and inhibit virus more quickly.

3.2.2. *'Immune miRs' as immunopharmaceutic agents*

With the general knowledge of immunologically relevant miRNAs established in the past 10 years, many miRNAs have been intensively investigated using gain- and loss-of-function methods, showing how this novel class of small non-coding RNA participates in mammalian immunity. And individual immune miRNA might contribute its implications to various immune-mediated diseases.

The role of miR125b in immune signalling may be paradoxical. After stimulation with LPS, miR125b was down-regulated and TNF-α, one of miR125b targets, was overexpressed in RAW264.7, which is essential for antimicrobial activity. Moreover, during *M. tuberculosis* infection, the overexpression of miR125a significantly attenuated the antimicrobial effects in macrophages through targeting UV radiation resistance–associated gene (UVRAG) [90]. Nevertheless, in diffuse large B cell lymphoma (DLBCL), miR125a and miR125b directly target a negative NF-κB regulator tumour necrosis factor alpha-induced protein 3(TNFAIP3) and present a positive self-regulatory property to maintain prolonged NF-κB activity. Taken together, whether overexpression or inhibition of miR125b in an anti-infection therapeutic study depends on concrete circumstances.

miR146a also acts as a negative regulator in immune sensing. Both in mouse and human, miR146a was always exploited by virus to attenuate innate and adaptive antiviral immunity mainly in DC [91], lymphocyte [92] and hepatocytes by inhibiting interleukin-1 receptor-associated kinase 1(IRAK1), TRAF6 [93], son of sevenless homolog 1 (SOS1) [94] and STAT1 [95]. Silencing of miR146a via the delivery of sponge or antagomiR could restore the expression of inflammatory factors, augment type I IFN production and promote clearance of vesicular stomatitis virus (VSV) [96], dengue virus [97], enterovirus 71 (EV71) [94,98] and HBV [95]. Because miR146a was also abnormally expressed in hepatocellular carcinoma (HCC) and exerted negative anti-tumour effects by up-regulation of immunoinhibitory cytokines such as TGF-β, IL-17, VEGF, miR146a may also be a novel immunotherapeutic target for HCC [99].

Unlike miR146a, miR155 always promotes immune signal transduction, enhances immune function or speeds lymphocyte proliferation. Mice lacking miR155 have impaired CTL cell responses to infections with lymphocytic choriomeningitis virus and the intracellular bacteria *Listeria monocytogenes* because of insufficient activation of Akt pathway after TCR cross-linking [100]. miR155 knockout mice died soon after Erdman (a variant from severe acute respiratory syndrome [SARS]) infection and held higher level of colony-forming units (CFU) in lungs than wild-type mice [101]. During HIV infection, miR155 inhibited the HIV-activating effects of tripartite motif-containing protein 32 (TRIM32), and therefore, it might promote a return to latency in CD4+ reservoir cells [102]. In addition, in NK cells, miR155 might regulate T cell immunoglobulin-3 (Tim-3)/T-bet/STAT-5-signalling axis, and following cytokine expression that balanced antiviral response and immune injury during chronic HCV infection [103]. A remarkably ectopic up-expression of miR155 can be observed by delivering hepatotropic adeno-associated virus 8 (AAV8) vectors to the liver of mice, and then high level of miR155-enhanced GAP's protective capacity against parasite [104]. These studies imply miR155 as an immune-augmenting adjuvant in improving the antigenicity of vaccination.

miR223 was already proved to be of importance in myeloid progenitor cells proliferation and responsiveness to pathogenic stimuli in neutrophils by targeting myocyte-specific enhancer factor 2C (MEF2C), acting as a fine-tune regulator both in normal granulocytes generation and in preventing aberrant expansion and over-activated inflammatory responses. In recent years, miR223 was involved in inflammasome response by targeting NLR family pyrin domain containing 3 (NLRP3) in human [105]. Moreover, Epstein–Barr virus (EBV) encoded a mimic of hsa-miR223, called miR-BART15, targeting the same site within the NLRP3 3′-UTR to repress inflammasome activation. Furthermore, this miRNA can be secreted from EBV-infected B cells into exosomes to rheostat NLRP3 inflammasome activity in non-infected cells [106]. miR223 sponge would balance the amount of NLRP3 and 'absorb' EBV-miR-BART15 in macrophages and DCs.

It is noteworthy that two groups of miRNAs, which shaped NK-mediated cytotoxicity, have potent value for developing antiviral and anti-tumour biodrugs. First, NKG2D–NKG2D-L interaction plays a predominant role in 'NK cell–abnormal cell' recognition. MICB/A, ULBPs targeting miRNAs, are not only encoded by human genome as stress regulators but also synthesized by some virus (e.g. HCMV-miR-UL112 [107], EBV-miRBART2 [108], KSHV-miR-K12-7 [108] and BK virus (BKV)-miR-B1-3p, JC virus (JCV)-miR-J1-3p[109]), to escape from NK cell killing. Meanwhile, viral infected cell and tumour cell always express low MICA/B because of up-regulated MICB/MICA, targeting miRNAs such as miR20a, 93, 103, 106b [110] to maintain a compromised micro-environment. Furthermore, non-classical human leukocyte antigen G (HLA-G) is known as an inhibitory ligand, which suppresses the cytotoxic activity of T and NK cells. Studies demonstrated a strong post-transcriptional gene regulation of the HLA-G by miR148a, miR148b and miR152, and lower expression of these miRNAs in renal carcinoma [111] and placental choriocarcinoma cells [112]. Stable manipulation of these activating and inhibitory miRNAs may enhance NK and LAK cell-mediated cytotoxicity against infected and tumour cells. Therefore, it could be concluded that modulating the expression or inhibition of specific miRNAs could boost immune response during viral infections or against cancers.

3.3. miRNA in maintaining immune homeostasis

Because several miRNAs participate in immune cell development and differentiation, abnormal expression of miRNA may cause a disturbance of homeostasis by changing the ratio of helper and regulatory cell subsets, or perturb the functionality and survival of effect-

memory cells that lead to lymphoproliferative disease. Utilization of miRNA interference techniques may recover regular immune balance.

3.3.1. *miR17-92, miR146a and miR155 in Systemic Lupus Erythematosus (SLE)*

In 2007, a unique mouse strain, 'sanroque', presented a pattern of lupus pathology, revealing the core role of T follicular helper (Tfh) in systemic autoimmunity [113]. miR17-92 was found to regulate Tfh cell differentiation, which is essential for maintenance of the germinal centre formation and sustained antibody responses. Overexpression of this miRNA in T cells would enhance Tfh cell proliferation and survive an autoantibody production [112]. Similarly, miR155 increased IL-21-mediated STAT3 signalling in T cell [114], which might accelerate Tfh differentiation and maturation as well. Moreover, miR155 deficiency ameliorates autoimmune inflammation of SLE by targeting s1pr1 in mice [115]. Therefore, miR17-92 and miR155 might be a new target to restrain aggressive autoimmune response in SLE.

3.3.2. *miR29 and miR146 in type 1 diabetes*

Type 1 diabetes (T1D) is a chronic autoimmune disease that results from the persisting destruction of pancreatic β-cells by autoreactive CD8+ T cell and Th1 cytokines. Dicer 1 deletion in β-cell would disrupt normal β-cell development and survival, lead to impairment of insulin secretion and diabetes development [116], apparently suggesting that miRNAs network is necessary for normal glycometabolism. Recently, endogenous miR29b released from pancreatic β-cells within exosomes stimulated TNF-α secretion in spleen cells isolated from diabetes-prone non-obese diabetic (NOD) mice. Delivery of miR29b to mice activated myeloid cell and pDCs to induce IFN-α, TNF-α and IL-6 production [117]. Abnormal expression of miR146 is associated with high serum titers of glutamic acid decarboxylase antibody in T1D patients, indicating the involvement of miR146 in the sustained immune imbalance during T1D progress [118]. These findings raised the possibility of developing a new clue for T1D immunotherapy using miRNA-based agents.

3.3.3. *miR146a and miR155 in rheumatoid arthritis*

The role of miR146a in controlling Treg-mediated decrease of Th1 responses has been demonstrated [119]. In contrast, miR155 promoted Th1 and Th17 differentiation and cell formation and lowered T cell sensitivity to IFN-γ-driven proliferation by targeting C-MAF and IFNγRα [120]. Therefore, imbalance of miR146a and miR155 may be an epigenetic phenotype for autoimmune response. In rheumatoid arthritis (RA), decreased expression of miR146a contributes to an abnormal Treg phenotype and allows Th1/Th17 skewing while low level of miR155 failed to support effective Th2 immunity [121]. Systemic administration of miR146a has potential therapeutic intervention for preventing bone destruction by inhibited Th1 and Th17 cells, as well as IL-1β, IL-6 and TNF-α [122].

3.3.4. *miR15 and miR326 in multiple sclerosis*

Multiple sclerosis (MS) is manifested by chronic and progressive inflammatory demyelination of the central nervous system and is one of the main causes of regressive neurological diseases.

Study on MS animal model illustrated that mice with fewer Th17 cells were less susceptible to experimental autoimmune encephalomyelitis (EAE) [123]. Therefore, Th17-targeting biotherapeutic approaches may be a promising way to cure multiple sclerosis. Gang Pei' s laboratory [124] found that miR326 promoted Th17 differentiation by targeting Ets-1 (a negative regulator of Th17 polarization) and antagonizing miR326 by sponge vector that resulted in fewer Th17 cells and Th17 cytokines and remitting EAE symptom. Inversely, increased miR155 in primary human microglia up-regulated pro-inflammatory cytokine secretion and co-stimulatory surface marker expression suggested that miR155 inhibition in myeloid cell might be useful to suppress allogeneic T cell responses [125]. In conclusion, reverse pathological expressed miRNAs and re-balance dysregulated immune genes are of consideration to treat multiple sclerosis.

4. Conclusion

RNAi technology holds promise for treating various human diseases. It is becoming apparent that clinical outcome of cancer immunotherapy and infectious diseases can be improved by targeted strategies to abrogate tumour-induced immunosuppression. Anti-tumour strategies using siRNA/shRNA/miRNA for both silencing of oncogenes and recruiting of innate receptors were designed. The present researches highlighted the potential therapeutic applications of this new generation of siRNAs in immunotherapy.

Additionally, but importantly, siRNA/shRNA or miRNA drugs with regard to pharmacodynamic difficulties and unwanted side effects are even more complicated compared to low molecular weight drugs and hard to be delivered into immune cells. This requires more extensive procedure than any other traditional drugs. Considering clinical challenges for RNA-based nucleic acid drugs, including barriers and RNases, the advanced tissue-directed delivery systems with safety, high efficiency and specificity, long-term function and controllability are required. Although the exploration of such tiny regulators causally bring pharmacists a considerable effort to draw up individualized and tailor-made strategies, we believe that immunoregulation triggered by siRNA/shRNA/miRNA can be used to regulate the host immunity against cancers or viruses. The development of multifunctional RNAi molecules will greatly contribute to the future arsenal of tools to combat not only microbial pathogens but also hard-to-treat cancer.

Acknowledgements

This work was supported by the Natural Science Foundation of China (81172789, 81373222, 31200651), National Basic Research Program of China (No. 2013CB531503) and National Mega Project on Major Infectious Diseases Prevention and Treatment (2012ZX10002006), The Special Foundation of Taishan Overseas Distinguished Experts and Scholars, The Priority Research Program of Shandong Academy of Sciences, Natural Science Foundation of Shandong

Province (No.BS2015YY023), Natural Science Foundation of Shandong Academy of Sciences (No. 2014QN004) and Science and Technology Development Foundation of Shandong Analysis and Test Center.

Author details

Zhaohua Hou[1], Qiuju Han[2*], Cai Zhang[2] and Jian Zhang[2]

*Address all correspondence to: hanqiuju@sdu.edu.cn

1 Laboratory of Immunology for Environment and Health, Shandong Analysis and Test Center, Shandong Academy of Sciences, Jinan, China

2 Institute of Immunopharmaceutical Sciences, School of Pharmaceutical Sciences, Shandong University, Jinan, China

References

[1] Cho WG, Albuquerque RJ, Kleinman ME: Small interfering RNA-induced TLR3 activation inhibits blood and lymphatic vessel growth. Proc Natl Acad Sci U S A. 2009; 106: 7137–7142. DOI: 10.1073/pnas.08123171060812317106

[2] Forsbach A, Nemorin JG, Volp K: Characterization of conserved viral leader RNA sequences that stimulate innate immunity through TLRs. Oligonucleotides. 2007; 17: 405–417. DOI: 10.1089/oli.2007.0098

[3] Judge AD, Sood V, Shaw JR: Sequence-dependent stimulation of the mammalian innate immune response by synthetic siRNA. Nat Biotechnol. 2005; 23: 457–462. DOI: 10.1038/nbt1081

[4] Kleinman ME, Yamada K, Takeda A: Sequence- and target-independent angiogenesis suppression by siRNA via TLR3. Nature. 2008; 452: 591–597. DOI: 10.1038/nature06765

[5] Melchjorsen J, Jensen SB, Malmgaard L: Activation of innate defense against a paramyxovirus is mediated by RIG-I and TLR7 and TLR8 in a cell-type-specific manner. J Virol. 2005; 79: 12944–12951. DOI: 10.1128/JVI.79.20.12944-12951.2005

[6] Hornung V, Guenthner-Biller M, Bourquin C: Sequence-specific potent induction of IFN-alpha by short interfering RNA in plasmacytoid dendritic cells through TLR7. Nat Med. 2005; 11: 263-270. DOI: 10.1038/nm1191

[7] Wang K, Chen X, Yan F: 5'-triphosphate-siRNA against survivin gene induces interferon production and inhibits proliferation of lung cancer cells in vitro. J Immunother. 2013; 36: 294–304. DOI: 10.1097/CJI.0b013e318294183b

[8] Poeck H, Besch R, Maihoefer C: 5'-Triphosphate-siRNA: turning gene silencing and Rig-I activation against melanoma. Nat Med. 2008; 14: 1256–1263. DOI: 10.1038/nm.1887

[9] Alshamsan A, Hamdy S, Haddadi A: STAT3 knockdown in B16 melanoma by siRNA lipopolyplexes induces bystander immune response in vitro and in vivo. DOI: Transl Oncol. 2011; 4: 178–188. DOI: 10.1593/tlo.11100

[10] Herrmann A, Kortylewski M, Kujawski M: Targeting Stat3 in the myeloid compartment drastically improves the in vivo antitumor functions of adoptively transferred T cells. Cancer Res. 2010; 70: 7455–7464. DOI: 10.1158/0008-5472.CAN-10-0736

[11] Alshamsan A, Haddadi A, Hamdy S: STAT3 silencing in dendritic cells by siRNA polyplexes encapsulated in PLGA nanoparticles for the modulation of anticancer immune response. Mol Pharm. 2010; 7: 1643–1654. DOI: 10.1021/mp100067u

[12] Kortylewski M, Swiderski P, Herrmann A: In vivo delivery of siRNA to immune cells by conjugation to a TLR9 agonist enhances antitumor immune responses. Nat Biotechnol. 2009; 27: 925–932. DOI: 10.1038/nbt.1564

[13] Hossain DM, Pal SK, Moreira D: TLR9-targeted STAT3 silencing abrogates immunosuppressive activity of myeloid-derived suppressor cells from prostate cancer patients. Clin Cancer Res. 2015; 21: 3771–3782. DOI: 10.1158/1078-0432.CCR-14-3145

[14] Zhang Q, Hossain DM, Nechaev S: TLR9-mediated siRNA delivery for targeting of normal and malignant human hematopoietic cells in vivo. Blood. 2013; 121: 1304–1315. DOI: 10.1182/blood-2012-07-442590b

[15] Luo Z, Wang C, Yi H: Nanovaccine loaded with poly I:C and STAT3 siRNA robustly elicits anti-tumor immune responses through modulating tumor-associated dendritic cells in vivo. Biomaterials. 2015; 38: 50–60. DOI: 10.1016/j.biomaterials.2014.10.050

[16] Shi D, Li D, Yin Q: Silenced suppressor of cytokine signaling 1 (SOCS1) enhances the maturation and antifungal immunity of dendritic cells in response to Candida albicans in vitro. Immunol Res. 2015; 61: 206-218. DOI: 10.1007/s12026-014-8562-8

[17] Akita H, Kogure K, Moriguchi R: Nanoparticles for ex vivo siRNA delivery to dendritic cells for cancer vaccines: programmed endosomal escape and dissociation. J Control Release. 2010; 143: 311–317. DOI: 10.1016/j.jconrel.2010.01.012

[18] Heo MB, Cho MY, Lim YT: Polymer nanoparticles for enhanced immune response: combined delivery of tumor antigen and small interference RNA for immunosuppressive gene to dendritic cells. Acta Biomater. 2014; 10: 2169–2176. DOI: 10.1016/j.actbio.2013.12.050

[19] Subramanya S, Armant M, Salkowitz JR: Enhanced induction of HIV-specific cytotoxic T lymphocytes by dendritic cell-targeted delivery of SOCS-1 siRNA. Mol Ther. 2010; 18: 2028–2037. DOI: 10.1038/mt.2010.148

[20] Zhang X, Su Y, Song H: Attenuated A20 expression of acute myeloid leukemia-derived dendritic cells increased the anti-leukemia immune response of autologous cytolytic T cells. Leuk Res. 2014; 38: 673–681. DOI: 10.1016/j.leukres.2014.03.011

[21] Warashina S, Nakamura T, Harashima H: A20 silencing by lipid envelope-type nanoparticles enhances the efficiency of lipopolysaccharide-activated dendritic cells. Biol Pharm Bull. 2011; 34: 1348–1351. DOI: 10.1248/bpb.34.1348

[22] Song XT, Evel-Kabler K, Shen L: A20 is an antigen presentation attenuator, and its inhibition overcomes regulatory T cell-mediated suppression. Nat Med. 2008; 14: 258–265. DOI: 10.1038/nm1721

[23] Breckpot K, Aerts-Toegaert C, Heirman C: Attenuated expression of A20 markedly increases the efficacy of double-stranded RNA-activated dendritic cells as an anticancer vaccine. J Immunol. 2009; 182: 860–870. DOI: 10.4049/jimmunol.182.2.860

[24] Cubillos-Ruiz JR, Engle X, Scarlett UK: Polyethylenimine-based siRNA nanocomplexes reprogram tumor-associated dendritic cells via TLR5 to elicit therapeutic antitumor immunity. J Clin Invest. 2009; 119: 2231–2244. DOI: 10.1172/JCI3771637716 [pii]

[25] Hobo W, Maas F, Adisty N: siRNA silencing of PD-L1 and PD-L2 on dendritic cells augments expansion and function of minor histocompatibility antigen-specific CD8+ T cells. Blood. 2010; 116: 4501–4511. DOI: 10.1182/blood-2010-04-278739

[26] van der Waart AB, Fredrix H, van der Voort R: siRNA silencing of PD-1 ligands on dendritic cell vaccines boosts the expansion of minor histocompatibility antigen-specific CD8(+) T cells in NOD/SCID/IL2Rg(null) mice. Cancer Immunol Immunother. 2015; 64: 645–654. DOI: 10.1007/s00262-015-1668-6

[27] Iwamura K, Kato T, Miyahara Y: siRNA-mediated silencing of PD-1 ligands enhances tumor-specific human T-cell effector functions. Gene Ther. 2012; 19: 959–966. DOI: 10.1038/gt.2011.185

[28] Zhang Q, Ichimaru N, Higuchi S: Permanent acceptance of mouse cardiac allografts with CD40 siRNA to induce regulatory myeloid cells by use of a novel polysaccharide siRNA delivery system. Gene Ther. 2015; 22: 1–10. DOI: 10.1038/gt.2014.119

[29] Gong X, Han B, Zou Y: Attenuation of experimental autoimmune myocarditis by siRNA mediated CD40 silencing. Int Heart J. 2014; 55: 539–545. DOI: 10.1536/ihj.14-125

[30] Zheng X, Suzuki M, Ichim TE: Treatment of autoimmune arthritis using RNA interference-modulated dendritic cells. J Immunol. 2010; 184: 6457–6464. DOI: 10.4049/jimmunol.0901717

[31] Conroy H, Galvin KC, Higgins SC: Gene silencing of TGF-beta1 enhances antitumor immunity induced with a dendritic cell vaccine by reducing tumor-associated regulatory T cells. Cancer Immunol Immunother. 2012; 61: 425–431. DOI: 10.1007/s00262-011-1188-y

[32] Xu Z, Wang Y, Zhang L: Nanoparticle-delivered transforming growth factor-beta siRNA enhances vaccination against advanced melanoma by modifying tumor microenvironment. ACS Nano. 2014; 8: 3636–3645. DOI: 10.1021/nn500216y

[33] Ahn YH, Hong SO, Kim JH: The siRNA cocktail targeting interleukin 10 receptor and transforming growth factor-beta receptor on dendritic cells potentiates tumour antigen-specific CD8(+) T cell immunity. Clin Exp Immunol. 2015; 181: 164–178. DOI: 10.1111/cei.12620

[34] Liu Z, Falo LD, Jr., You Z: Knockdown of HMGB1 in tumor cells attenuates their ability to induce regulatory T cells and uncovers naturally acquired CD8 T cell-dependent antitumor immunity. J Immunol. 2011; 187: 118–125. DOI: 10.4049/jimmunol.1003378

[35] Tsai BY, Suen JL, Chiang BL: Lentiviral-mediated Foxp3 RNAi suppresses tumor growth of regulatory T cell-like leukemia in a murine tumor model. Gene Ther. 2010; 17: 972–979. DOI: 10.1038/gt.2010.38

[36] Yongsheng Y, Xiaoliang L, Zhenghao T: siRNA-mediated knockdown of FoxP3 promotes the ratio of T-helper 1 (Th1) to Th2 in chronic hepatitis B patients. Turk J Gastroenterol. 2011; 22: 587–593. DOI: 10.4318/tjg.2011.0251

[37] Kang S, Xie J, Ma S: Targeted knock down of CCL22 and CCL17 by siRNA during DC differentiation and maturation affects the recruitment of T subsets. Immunobiology. 2010; 215: 153–162. DOI: 10.1016/j.imbio.2009.03.001

[38] Zheng X, Koropatnick J, Chen D: Silencing IDO in dendritic cells: a novel approach to enhance cancer immunotherapy in a murine breast cancer model. Int J Cancer. 2013; 132: 967–977. DOI: 10.1002/ijc.27710

[39] Zheng X, Koropatnick J, Li M: Reinstalling antitumor immunity by inhibiting tumor-derived immunosuppressive molecule IDO through RNA interference. J Immunol. 2006; 177: 5639–5646. DOI: 10.4049/jimmunol.177.8.5639

[40] Flatekval GF, Sioud M: Modulation of dendritic cell maturation and function with mono- and bifunctional small interfering RNAs targeting indoleamine 2,3-dioxygenase. Immunology. 2009; 128: e837–848. DOI: 10.1111/j.1365-2567.2009.03093.x

[41] Chen D, Koropatnick J, Jiang N: Targeted siRNA silencing of indoleamine 2, 3-dioxygenase in antigen-presenting cells using mannose-conjugated liposomes: a novel strategy for treatment of melanoma. J Immunother. 2014; 37: 123–134. DOI: 10.1097/CJI.0000000000000022

[42] Yen MC, Lin CC, Chen YL: A novel cancer therapy by skin delivery of indoleamine 2,3-dioxygenase siRNA. Clin Cancer Res. 2009; 15: 641–649. DOI: 10.1158/1078-0432.CCR-08-1988

[43] Huang TT, Yen MC, Lin CC: Skin delivery of short hairpin RNA of indoleamine 2,3 dioxygenase induces antitumor immunity against orthotopic and metastatic liver cancer. Cancer Sci. 2011; 102: 2214–2220. DOI: 10.1111/j.1349-7006.2011.02094.x

[44] Huang M, Sun R, Wei H: Simultaneous knockdown of multiple ligands of innate receptor NKG2D prevents natural killer cell-mediated fulminant hepatitis in mice. Hepatology. 2013; 57: 277–288. DOI: 10.1002/hep.25959

[45] Zeng XC, Zhang T, Huang DH: RNA interfering targeting human leukocyte antigen-G enhanced immune surveillance mediated by the natural killer cells on hepatocellular carcinoma. Ann Clin Lab Sci. 2013; 43: 135–144.

[46] Chen LJ, Han ZQ, Zhou H: Inhibition of HLA-G expression via RNAi abolishes resistance of extravillous trophoblast cell line TEV-1 to NK lysis. Placenta. 2010; 31: 519–527. DOI: 10.1016/j.placenta.2010.03.008

[47] Tan PH, Gao YJ, Berta T: Short small-interfering RNAs produce interferon-alpha-mediated analgesia. Br J Anaesth. 2012; 108: 662–669. DOI: 10.1093/bja/aer492

[48] Kariko K, Bhuyan P, Capodici J: Small interfering RNAs mediate sequence-independent gene suppression and induce immune activation by signaling through toll-like receptor 3. J Immunol. 2004; 172: 6545–6549. DOI: 10.4049/jimmunol.172.11.6545

[49] Khairuddin N, Gantier MP, Blake SJ: siRNA-induced immunostimulation through TLR7 promotes antitumoral activity against HPV-driven tumors in vivo. Immunol Cell Biol. 2012; 90: 187–196. DOI: 10.1038/icb.2011.19

[50] Ellermeier J, Wei J, Duewell P: Therapeutic efficacy of bifunctional siRNA combining TGF-beta1 silencing with RIG-I activation in pancreatic cancer. Cancer Res. 2013; 73: 1709–1720. DOI: 10.1158/0008-5472.CAN-11-3850

[51] Meng G, Xia M, Xu C: Multifunctional antitumor molecule 5'-triphosphate siRNA combining glutaminase silencing and RIG-I activation. Int J Cancer. 2014; 134: 1958–1971. DOI: 10.1002/ijc.28416

[52] Han Q, Zhang C, Zhang J: Reversal of hepatitis B virus-induced immune tolerance by an immunostimulatory 3p-HBx-siRNAs in a retinoic acid inducible gene I-dependent manner. Hepatology. 2011; 54: 1179–1189. DOI: 10.1002/hep.24505

[53] Chen X, Qian Y, Yan F: 5'-triphosphate-siRNA activates RIG-I-dependent type I interferon production and enhances inhibition of hepatitis B virus replication in HepG2.2.15 cells. Eur J Pharmacol. 2013; 721: 86–95. DOI: 10.1016/j.ejphar.2013.09.050

[54] Ebert G, Poeck H, Lucifora J: 5' Triphosphorylated small interfering RNAs control replication of hepatitis B virus and induce an interferon response in human liver cells

and mice. Gastroenterology. 2011; 141: 696–706, 706 e691-693. DOI: 10.1053/j.gastro.2011.05.001

[55] Lan P, Zhang C, Han Q: Therapeutic recovery of hepatitis B virus (HBV)-induced hepatocyte-intrinsic immune defect reverses systemic adaptive immune tolerance. Hepatology. 2013; 58: 73–85. DOI: 10.1002/hep.26339

[56] Lin L, Liu Q, Berube N: 5'-Triphosphate-short interfering RNA: potent inhibition of influenza A virus infection by gene silencing and RIG-I activation. J Virol. 2012; 86: 10359–10369. DOI: 10.1128/JVI.00665-12

[57] Ahn J, Ko A, Jun EJ: Antiviral effects of small interfering RNA simultaneously inducing RNA interference and type 1 interferon in coxsackievirus myocarditis. Antimicrob Agents Chemother. 2012; 56: 3516–3523. DOI: 10.1128/AAC.06050-12

[58] Meng Z, Zhang X, Wu J: RNAi induces innate immunity through multiple cellular signaling pathways. PLoS One. 2013; 8: e64708. DOI: 10.1371/journal.pone.0064708

[59] Sui H, Zhou M, Chen Q: siRNA enhances DNA-mediated interferon lambda-1 response through crosstalk between RIG-I and IFI16 signalling pathway. Nucleic Acids Res. 2014; 42: 583–598. DOI: 10.1093/nar/gkt844

[60] Esau C, Davis S, Murray SF: miR-122 regulation of lipid metabolism revealed by in vivo antisense targeting. Cell Metab. 2006; 3: 87–98. DOI: 10.1016/j.cmet.2006.01.005

[61] Jopling CL, Yi M, Lancaster AM: Modulation of hepatitis C virus RNA abundance by a liver-specific MicroRNA. Science. 2005; 309: 1577–1581. DOI: 10.1126/science.1113329

[62] Jopling CL, Schutz S, Sarnow P: Position-dependent function for a tandem microRNA miR-122-binding site located in the hepatitis C virus RNA genome. Cell Host Microbe. 2008; 4: 77–85. DOI: 10.1016/j.chom.2008.05.013

[63] Henke JI, Goergen D, Zheng J: microRNA-122 stimulates translation of hepatitis C virus RNA. EMBO J. 2008; 27: 3300–3310. DOI: 10.1038/emboj.2008.244

[64] Randall G, Panis M, Cooper JD: Cellular cofactors affecting hepatitis C virus infection and replication. Proc Natl Acad Sci U S A. 2007; 104: 12884–12889. DOI: 10.1073/pnas.0704894104

[65] Machlin ES, Sarnow P, Sagan SM: Masking the 5' terminal nucleotides of the hepatitis C virus genome by an unconventional microRNA-target RNA complex. Proc Natl Acad Sci U S A. 2011; 108: 3193–3198. DOI: 10.1073/pnas.1012464108

[66] Li YP, Gottwein JM, Scheel TK: MicroRNA-122 antagonism against hepatitis C virus genotypes 1-6 and reduced efficacy by host RNA insertion or mutations in the HCV 5' UTR. Proc Natl Acad Sci U S A. 2011; 108: 4991–4996. DOI: 10.1073/pnas.1016606108

[67] Chang J, Guo JT, Jiang D: Liver-specific microRNA miR-122 enhances the replication of hepatitis C virus in nonhepatic cells. J Virol. 2008; 82: 8215–8223. DOI: 10.1128/JVI.02575-07

[68] Pedersen IM, Cheng G, Wieland S: Interferon modulation of cellular microRNAs as an antiviral mechanism. Nature. 2007; 449: 919–922. DOI: 10.1038/nature06205

[69] Sarasin-Filipowicz M, Krol J, Markiewicz I: Decreased levels of microRNA miR-122 in individuals with hepatitis C responding poorly to interferon therapy. Nat Med. 2009; 15: 31–33. DOI: 10.1038/nm.1902

[70] Murakami Y, Tanaka M, Toyoda H: Hepatic microRNA expression is associated with the response to interferon treatment of chronic hepatitis C. BMC Med Genomics. 2010; 3: 48. DOI: 10.1186/1755-8794-3-48

[71] Elmen J, Lindow M, Silahtaroglu A: Antagonism of microRNA-122 in mice by systemically administered LNA-antimiR leads to up-regulation of a large set of predicted target mRNAs in the liver. Nucleic Acids Res. 2008; 36: 1153–1162. DOI: 10.1093/nar/gkm1113

[72] Hildebrandt-Eriksen ES, Aarup V, Persson R: A locked nucleic acid oligonucleotide targeting microRNA 122 is well-tolerated in cynomolgus monkeys. Nucleic Acid Ther. 2012; 22: 152–161. DOI: 10.1089/nat.2011.0332

[73] Lanford RE, Hildebrandt-Eriksen ES, Petri A: Therapeutic silencing of microRNA-122 in primates with chronic hepatitis C virus infection. Science. 2010; 327: 198–201. DOI: 10.1126/science.1178178

[74] Elmen J, Lindow M, Schutz S: LNA-mediated microRNA silencing in non-human primates. Nature. 2008; 452: 896–899. DOI: 10.1038/nature06783

[75] van der Ree MH, van der Meer AJ, de Bruijne J: Long-term safety and efficacy of microRNA-targeted therapy in chronic hepatitis C patients. Antiviral Res. 2014; 111: 53–59. DOI: 10.1016/j.antiviral.2014.08.015

[76] Masaki T, Arend KC, Li Y: miR-122 stimulates hepatitis C virus RNA synthesis by altering the balance of viral RNAs engaged in replication versus translation. Cell Host Microbe. 2015; 17: 217–228. DOI: 10.1016/j.chom.2014.12.014

[77] Janssen HL, Kauppinen S, Hodges MR: HCV infection and miravirsen. N Engl J Med. 2013; 369: 878. DOI: 10.1056/NEJMc1307787

[78] Hou W, Tian Q, Zheng J: MicroRNA-196 represses Bach1 protein and hepatitis C virus gene expression in human hepatoma cells expressing hepatitis C viral proteins. Hepatology. 2010; 51: 1494–1504. DOI: 10.1002/hep.23401

[79] Cheng JC, Yeh YJ, Tseng CP: Let-7b is a novel regulator of hepatitis C virus replication. Cell Mol Life Sci. 2012; 69: 2621–2633. DOI: 10.1007/s00018-012-0940-6

[80] Lecellier CH, Dunoyer P, Arar K: A cellular microRNA mediates antiviral defense in human cells. Science. 2005; 308: 557–560. DOI: 10.1126/science.1108784

[81] Lagos D, Pollara G, Henderson S: miR-132 regulates antiviral innate immunity through suppression of the p300 transcriptional co-activator. Nat Cell Biol. 2010; 12: 513–519. DOI: 10.1038/ncb2054

[82] Trobaugh DW, Gardner CL, Sun C: RNA viruses can hijack vertebrate microRNAs to suppress innate immunity. Nature. 2014; 506: 245–248. DOI: 10.1038/nature12869

[83] Shapiro JS, Schmid S, Aguado LC: Drosha as an interferon-independent antiviral factor. Proc Natl Acad Sci U S A. 2014; 111: 7108–7113. DOI: 10.1073/pnas.1319635111

[84] Chen XM, Splinter PL, O'Hara SP: A cellular micro-RNA, let-7i, regulates toll-like receptor 4 expression and contributes to cholangiocyte immune responses against Cryptosporidium parvum infection. J Biol Chem. 2007; 282: 28929–28938. DOI: 10.1074/jbc.M702633200

[85] Ma C, Li Y, Zeng J: Mycobacterium bovis BCG triggered MyD88 induces miR-124 feedback negatively regulates immune response in alveolar epithelial cells. PLoS One. 2014; 9: e92419. DOI: 10.1371/journal.pone.0092419

[86] Mukherjee A, Di Bisceglie AM, Ray RB: Hepatitis C virus-mediated enhancement of microRNA miR-373 impairs the JAK/STAT signaling pathway. J Virol. 2015; 89: 3356–3365. DOI: 10.1128/JVI.03085-14

[87] Landais I, Pelton C, Streblow D: Human cytomegalovirus miR-UL112-3p targets TLR2 and modulates the TLR2/IRAK1/NFkappaB signaling pathway. PLoS Pathog. 2015; 11: e1004881. DOI: 10.1371/journal.ppat.1004881

[88] Michael SF, Zhu X, He Z: MicroRNA-30e* suppresses dengue virus replication by promoting NF-κB–dependent IFN production. PLoS Neglected Tropical Diseases. 2014; 8: e3088. DOI: 10.1371/journal.pntd.0003088

[89] Xu C, He X, Zheng Z: Downregulation of microRNA miR-526a by enterovirus inhibits RIG-I-dependent innate immune response. J Virol. 2014; 88: 11356–11368. DOI: 10.1128/JVI.01400-14

[90] Kim JK, Yuk JM, Kim SY: MicroRNA-125a inhibits autophagy activation and antimicrobial responses during mycobacterial infection. J Immunol. 2015; 194: 5355–5365. DOI: 10.4049/jimmunol.1402557

[91] Park H, Huang X, Lu C: MicroRNA-146a and microRNA-146b regulate human dendritic cell apoptosis and cytokine production by targeting TRAF6 and IRAK1 proteins. J Biol Chem. 2015; 290: 2831–2841. DOI: 10.1074/jbc.M114.591420

[92] Wang S, Zhang X, Ju Y: MicroRNA-146a feedback suppresses T cell immune function by targeting Stat1 in patients with chronic hepatitis B. J Immunol. 2013; 191: 293–301. DOI: 10.4049/jimmunol.1202100

[93] Taganov KD, Boldin MP, Chang KJ: NF-kappaB-dependent induction of microRNA miR-146, an inhibitor targeted to signaling proteins of innate immune responses. Proc Natl Acad Sci U S A. 2006; 103: 12481–12486. DOI: 10.1073/pnas.0605298103

[94] Chang YL, Ho BC, Sher S: miR-146a and miR-370 coordinate enterovirus 71-induced cell apoptosis through targeting SOS1 and GADD45beta. Cell Microbiol. 2015; 17: 802–818. DOI: 10.1111/cmi.12401

[95] Hou ZH, Han QJ, Zhang C: miR146a impairs the IFN-induced anti-HBV immune response by downregulating STAT1 in hepatocytes. Liver Int. 2014; 34: 58–68. DOI: 10.1111/liv.12244

[96] Hou J, Wang P, Lin L: MicroRNA-146a feedback inhibits RIG-I-dependent Type I IFN production in macrophages by targeting TRAF6, IRAK1, and IRAK2. J Immunol. 2009; 183: 2150–2158. DOI: 10.4049/jimmunol.0900707

[97] Wu S, He L, Li Y: miR-146a facilitates replication of dengue virus by dampening interferon induction by targeting TRAF6. J Infect. 2013; 67: 329–341. DOI: 10.1016/j.jinf.2013.05.003

[98] Ho BC, Yu IS, Lu LF: Inhibition of miR-146a prevents enterovirus-induced death by restoring the production of type I interferon. Nat Commun. 2014; 5: 3344. DOI: 10.1038/ncomms4344

[99] Sun X, Zhang J, Hou Z: miR-146a is directly regulated by STAT3 in human hepatocellular carcinoma cells and involved in anti-tumor immune suppression. Cell Cycle. 2015; 14: 243–252. DOI: 10.4161/15384101.2014.977112

[100] Lind EF, Elford AR, Ohashi PS: Micro-RNA 155 is required for optimal CD8+ T cell responses to acute viral and intracellular bacterial challenges. J Immunol. 2013; 190: 1210–1216. DOI: 10.4049/jimmunol.1202700

[101] Iwai H, Funatogawa K, Matsumura K: MicroRNA-155 knockout mice are susceptible to mycobacterium tuberculosis infection. Tuberculosis (Edinb). 2015; 95: 246–250. DOI: 10.1016/j.tube.2015.03.006

[102] Ruelas DS, Chan JK, Oh E: MicroRNA-155 Reinforces HIV Latency. J Biol Chem. 2015; 290: 13736–13748. DOI: 10.1074/jbc.M115.641837

[103] Cheng YQ, Ren JP, Zhao J: MicroRNA-155 regulates interferon-gamma production in natural killer cells via Tim-3 signalling in chronic hepatitis C virus infection. Immunology. 2015; 145: 485–497. DOI: 10.1111/imm.12463

[104] Hentzschel F, Hammerschmidt-Kamper C, Borner K: AAV8-mediated in vivo overexpression of miR-155 enhances the protective capacity of genetically attenuated malarial parasites. Mol Ther. 2014; 22: 2130–2141. DOI: 10.1038/mt.2014.172

[105] Bauernfeind F, Rieger A, Schildberg FA: NLRP3 inflammasome activity is negatively controlled by miR-223. J Immunol. 2012; 189: 4175–4181. DOI: 10.4049/jimmunol.1201516

[106] Haneklaus M, Gerlic M, Kurowska-Stolarska M: Cutting edge: miR-223 and EBV miR-BART15 regulate the NLRP3 inflammasome and IL-1beta production. J Immunol. 2012; 189: 3795-3799. DOI: 10.4049/jimmunol.1200312

[107] Stern-Ginossar N, Elefant N, Zimmermann A: Host immune system gene targeting by a viral miRNA. Science. 2007; 317: 376–381. DOI: 10.1126/science.1140956

[108] Nachmani D, Stern-Ginossar N, Sarid R: Diverse herpesvirus microRNAs target the stress-induced immune ligand MICB to escape recognition by natural killer cells. Cell Host Microbe. 2009; 5: 376–385. DOI: 10.1016/j.chom.2009.03.003

[109] Bauman Y, Nachmani D, Vitenshtein A: An identical miRNA of the human JC and BK polyoma viruses targets the stress-induced ligand ULBP3 to escape immune elimination. Cell Host Microbe. 2011; 9: 93–102. DOI: 10.1016/j.chom.2011.01.008

[110] Nachmani D, Lankry D, Wolf DG: The human cytomegalovirus microRNA miR-UL112 acts synergistically with a cellular microRNA to escape immune elimination. Nat Immunol. 2010; 11: 806–813. DOI: 10.1038/ni.1916

[111] Jasinski-Bergner S, Stoehr C, Bukur J: Clinical relevance of miR-mediated HLA-G regulation and the associated immune cell infiltration in renal cell carcinoma. Oncoimmunology. 2015; 4: e1008805. DOI: 10.1080/2162402X.2015.1008805

[112] Zhu XM, Han T, Wang XH: Overexpression of miR-152 leads to reduced expression of human leukocyte antigen-G and increased natural killer cell mediated cytolysis in JEG-3 cells. Am J Obstet Gynecol. 2010; 202: 592 e591–597. DOI: 10.1016/j.ajog.2010.03.002

[113] Vinuesa CG, Cook MC, Angelucci C: A RING-type ubiquitin ligase family member required to repress follicular helper T cells and autoimmunity. Nature. 2005; 435: 452–458. DOI: 10.1038/nature03555

[114] Rasmussen TK, Andersen T, Bak RO: Overexpression of microRNA-155 increases IL-21 mediated STAT3 signaling and IL-21 production in systemic lupus erythematosus. Arthritis Res Ther. 2015; 17: 154. DOI: 10.1186/s13075-015-0660-z

[115] Xin Q, Li J, Dang J: miR-155 Deficiency Ameliorates Autoimmune Inflammation of Systemic Lupus Erythematosus by Targeting S1pr1 in Faslpr/lpr Mice. J Immunol. 2015; 194: 5437–5445. DOI: 10.4049/jimmunol.1403028

[116] Kalis M, Bolmeson C, Esguerra JL: Beta-cell specific deletion of Dicer1 leads to defective insulin secretion and diabetes mellitus. PLoS One. 2011; 6: e29166. DOI: 10.1371/journal.pone.0029166

[117] Salama A, Fichou N, Allard M: MicroRNA-29b modulates innate and antigen-specific immune responses in mouse models of autoimmunity. PLoS One. 2014; 9: e106153. DOI: 10.1371/journal.pone.0106153

[118] Yang M, Ye L, Wang B: Decreased miR-146 expression in peripheral blood mononuclear cells is correlated with ongoing islet autoimmunity in type 1 diabetes patients 1miR-146. J Diabetes. 2015; 7: 158–165. DOI: 10.1111/1753-0407.12163

[119] Lu LF, Boldin MP, Chaudhry A: Function of miR-146a in controlling Treg cell-mediated regulation of Th1 responses. Cell. 2010; 142: 914–929. DOI: 10.1016/j.cell.2010.08.012

[120] Banerjee A, Schambach F, DeJong CS: Micro-RNA-155 inhibits IFN-gamma signaling in CD4+ T cells. Eur J Immunol. 2010; 40: 225–231. DOI: 10.1002/eji.200939381

[121] Okoye IS, Czieso S, Ktistaki E: Transcriptomics identified a critical role for Th2 cell-intrinsic miR-155 in mediating allergy and antihelminth immunity. Proc Natl Acad Sci U S A. 2014; 111: E3081–3090. DOI: 10.1073/pnas.1406322111

[122] Zhou Q, Haupt S, Kreuzer JT: Decreased expression of miR-146a and miR-155 contributes to an abnormal Treg phenotype in patients with rheumatoid arthritis. Ann Rheum Dis. 2015; 74: 1265–1274. DOI: 10.1136/annrheumdis-2013-204377

[123] Ivanov II, McKenzie BS, Zhou L: The orphan nuclear receptor RORgammat directs the differentiation program of proinflammatory IL-17+ T helper cells. Cell. 2006; 126: 1121–1133. DOI: 10.1016/j.cell.2006.07.035

[124] Du C, Liu C, Kang J: MicroRNA miR-326 regulates TH-17 differentiation and is associated with the pathogenesis of multiple sclerosis. Nat Immunol. 2009; 10: 1252–1259. DOI: 10.1038/ni.1798

[125] Moore CS, Rao VT, Durafourt BA: miR-155 as a multiple sclerosis-relevant regulator of myeloid cell polarization. Ann Neurol. 2013; 74: 709–720. DOI: 10.1002/ana.23967

RNA Interference as a Tool to Reduce the Risk of Rejection in Cell-Based Therapies

Constanca Figueiredo and Rainer Blasczyk

Additional information is available at the end of the chapter

http://dx.doi.org/10.5772/61829

Abstract

Remarkable progress in the experimental and clinical applications of cell-based therapies has identified stem cells and their derived products as potential candidates for regenerative therapies for many disorders. The use of autologous stem cells as source for regenerative therapeutic products is strongly limited by their low availability. Therefore, the future applications of *in vitro* pharmed therapeutic cell products will most likely occur in an allogeneic manner. However, the high variability of the human leukocyte antigen (HLA) represents a major obstacle to the application of off-the-shelf products. We have developed a strategy to decrease the immunogenicity of *in vitro* generated cell products by silencing HLA expression using RNAi. HLA expression was permanently silenced in CD34+ hematopoietic stem and progenitor cells and induced the pluripotent stem cells to generate HLA-universal cells sources, which were then used for the differentiation of low immunogenic cell products. In this chapter, we will provide an overview about an RNAi-based strategy to reduce the immunogenicity of cell-based therapies, and in particular in the generation of HLA-universal platelets and tissues.

Keywords: HLA, immunogenicity, transplant rejection, blood pharming

1. Introduction

The high variability of the human leukocyte antigen (HLA) constitutes a major hurdle in allogeneic transplantation and to the application of off-the-shelf cell products in regenerative medicine. Recently, remarkable progresses in the field of stem cell biology, cell pharming, and tissue engineering have made feasible the differentiation of cells and tissues that might serve as a bridging strategy or even an alternative to the very scarce donated tissues and organs. However, HLA incompatibility may pose a threat to the applicability of such *in vitro* generated cell products by increasing the risk of immune rejection after the transplantation.[1] To overcome this major hurdle in the fields of transplantation, cell and tissue engineering, we have developed an RNA interference (RNAi)-based approach to reduce the immunogenicity of cells and tissues, allowing their application in an universal manner. A lentiviral vector encoding for specific short hairpins RNA (shRNA), targeting HLA transcripts were used to achieve a permanent silencing of HLA expression. As HLA residual expression is crucial to prevent the natural killer (NK) cell activity, RNAi appears as a superior tool in comparison to gene editing technologies that cause a complete gene deletion such as the transcription activator-like effector nuclease (TALEN) or clustered regularly interspaced short palindromic repeats (CRISPR)/Cas9 systems.[2-4] By decreasing the immunogenicity of cells and tissues, the need for immunosuppressive regimens might be reduced after HLA-mismatched transplantation. Furthermore, as HLA plays a pivotal role in the recognition of virus-infected cells and cancer cells, the combination of conditional promoter systems allows the re-expression of HLA and constitutes a safety mechanism. The generation of low immunogenic cells and tissues would bring enormous benefits to the patients and open novel horizons in the field of transplantation and regenerative medicine.

2. The HLA system

Evolution conferred highly refined mechanisms to all animals from sponges to mammals to distinguish self from non-self, and thereby allowing an immune response against potential pathogens. In humans, a tight interplay between adaptive and innate immune systems allows their defense against virtually all pathogens and cancer cells.[5, 6] Nevertheless, those sophisticated surveillance mechanisms pose a major hurdle to allogeneic transplantation. The alloimmune responses are mainly based on the recognition of mismatched major histocompatibility complex (MHC) antigens by antibodies and T-cells. In humans, the MHC is known as HLA and it comprises a group of linked genes. MHC class I and II regulate the immune response through the presentation of peptides to T-cells. Allogeneic MHC in the graft's antigen-presenting cells (APCs) is recognized after transplantation through a direct pathway. Afterwards, own patient APCs process and present the allogeneic antigens to T-cells by an indirect alloantigen recognition pathway.[7, 8] HLA loci are encoded on the short arm of human chromosome 6. Based on their structure, HLA molecules are grouped into class I and class II (Figure 1). HLA class I classical genes comprise the A, B, and C loci, and are expressed in the majority of cells. HLA class II genes include DR, DQ, and DP and are constitutively expressed only in professional APCs.[9] The non-self recognition mediated by the engagement of the T-cell receptor with the donor HLA is the basis for the allogeneic immune response.

2.1. HLA incompatibility increases the risk of rejection

Despite the progresses in the field of transplantation, graft rejection remains the major concern regarding the application of off-the-shelf products. HLA comprises the most polymorphic loci of the entire human genome. The probability to find a complete HLA-matched donor for a specific patient is very low and, therefore, in most of the cases, patients will be treated with partially HLA-mismatched tissues and organs. In addition, even in fully HLA donor/recipient

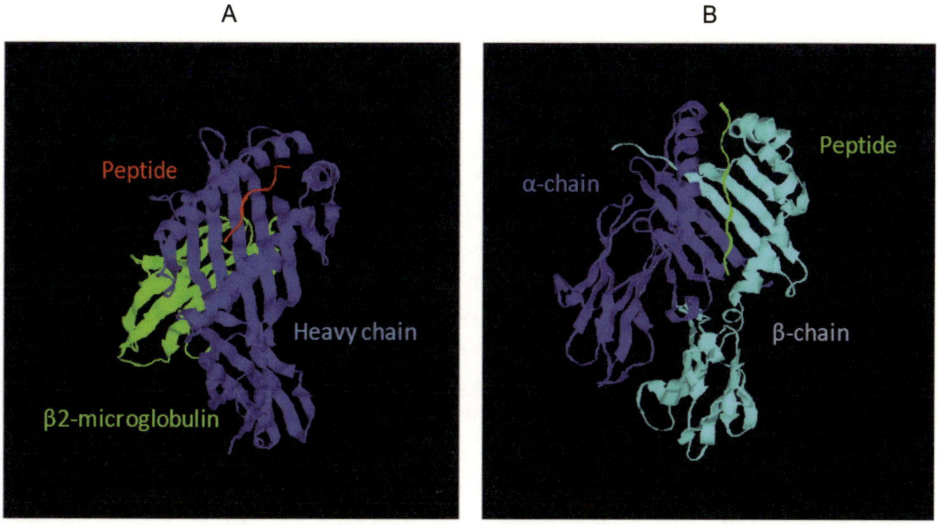

Figure 1. Structure representation of (A) HLA class I (HLA-B) and (B) HLA class II (HLA-DQ) molecules. The structures were designed using the software http://www.mh-hannover.de/institute/transfusion/histocheck/.

pairs, disparities at the minor histocompatibility antigens (mHAg) derived from other polymorphic proteins and presented at the HLA complexes are capable of triggering antigen-specific immune responses that cause graft rejection. Improved use of post-transplant immunosuppression to prevent acute and chronic rejection allowed allogeneic transplantation as a widespread, successful therapy.[10-13] However, graft rejection remains a major concern in the field of transplantation. The registry of the International Society for Heart and Lung Transplantation (ISHLT) reported that within the first year after lung transplantation, up to 55% patients need to be treated for acute rejection and only 50% are alive after five years.[14] Also, the number of HLA mismatches between a donor/recipient pair is associated with stronger immunosuppressive regimens. In particular, the number of HLA-DR mismatches and the number of HLA-A and -B mismatches as well as rejection treatment showed significant associations with the dose of maintenance steroids. Although immunosuppression allows the acceptance of the allogeneic graft, it has severe side effects that may contribute to death even with a functioning graft.[15] The occurrence of post-transplant complications related to the immunosuppressive therapy such as cancer, opportunistic infection, toxicity, and hip fractures have indicated the necessity to develop alternative strategies to allow the therapeutical use of off-the-shelf HLA and mHAg-mismatched cell-based products.[16] Furthermore, due to the shortage of organs and tissues for transplantation, there is a high demand regarding the development of *in vitro* pharmed cell products, and engineered tissues or organs. Progresses in the fields of stem cell biology and tissue engineering have demonstrated the feasibility to generate *in vitro* potential alternative cell-based products that might serve as an alternative or overcome the need for using donated tissues. Nevertheless, the future use of such products will occur in an allogeneic manner, and therefore, it will be required that those products will be able to escape an allogeneic immune response.

2.2. RNAi-mediated HLA targeting as a strategy to decrease the cell immunogenicity

Rejection of allogeneic grafts is based on the recognition of the HLA complexes by the specific pre-formed complement-binding anti-HLA antibodies or by the engagement of the T-cell receptor, which leads to T-cell activation and the initiation of the immune response.[17, 18] RNA interference is an invaluable technique in cell biology and regenerative strategies to silence the target gene expression. Our studies have focused on the downregulation of HLA class I and class II expression on the graft cells. So far, several strategies have been developed to induce the acceptance of the allogeneic graft. Similar to the immunosuppression, those strategies involve the modulation of immune responses and aim the induction of tolerance to the graft. In our studies, we genetically modify the graft to silence its HLA expression to prevent the recognition of the allogeneic graft as non-self by the recipient's immune system. In this approach, we do not induce tolerance toward the allogeneic graft, but we generate a condition of immunological blindness in which the recipient's immune system is not able to recognize the allogeneic cells (due to the missing HLA) but is fully capable of defending the patient against common clinical conditions associated with the use of immunosuppressive drugs such as opportunistic infections and leukemia. To prevent the recognition of the grafted cells as off the shelf, we have downregulated the expression of HLA class I and class II antigens using RNAi. We have constructed lentiviral vectors encoding for short-hairpin RNA sequences targeting β2-microglobulin (shβ2m) or the alpha-chain of HLA-DR (shDRA) to silence the expression of HLA class I and class II antigens, respectively. Our studies demonstrated the feasibility to stably downregulate HLA class I and II expression in several cell lines (e.g., B-LCL, MonoMac-6, HeLa) as well as in primary cells (e.g., endothelial cells, CD34+ progenitor, induced pluripotent stem cells). Cell transduction for the delivery of shRNAs targeting specific HLA transcripts resulted in a decrease by up to 90% of β2m or HLA-DRA transcript levels and HLA class I expression. *In vitro* assays have shown that HLA class I-silenced cells were protected against the antibody-mediated complement-dependent cytotoxicity. Furthermore, in T-cell cytotoxicity assays, significantly lower cell lysis rates were observed when HLA-silenced cells were used as targets in comparison to fully HLA-expressing cells. In addition, HLA-silenced cells demonstrated to induce significantly lower T-cell proliferation, pro-inflammatory cytokine secretion, and degranulation. The residual HLA class I expression showed to be sufficient to prevent NK cell cytotoxicity. Altogether, HLA-silenced cells showed a protective effect against the humoral and cellular allogeneic immune response.[2, 3, 19]

2.3. MHC-silenced cells survive after fully HLA-incompatible transplantation

Despite the widespread use of immunosuppressive regimens to prevent graft rejection, their therapeutic window is very narrow. Immunosuppressive drugs frequently cause adverse effects including thrombocytopenia, leukopenia, hypercholesterolemia, stomatitis, nephrotoxicity, and diarrhea, and they lead to an increased risk for infections and cancer.[20, 21] Silencing HLA expression using RNAi may represent an alternative to immunosuppression; hence it has the potential to offer many benefits for the patients. In addition, silencing HLA expression may allow the future application of HLA-mismatched off-the-shelf products in a universal manner independently of the genetic background of the donor and recipient. In an

http://dx.doi.org/10.5772/61829

allogeneic transplantation rat model, we have confirmed the improved capacity of MHC-silenced cells to survive in allogeneic environment upon transplantation and even in the absence of immunosuppression. A lentiviral vector encoding for a shRNA sequence targeting rat MHC class I (RT1-A) and the sequence for firefly luciferase as a reporter gene was used to silence MHC class I Lewis rat-derived fibroblasts. In contrast to nonmodified fibroblasts, MHC class I-silenced fibroblasts were able to survive after subcutaneous transplantation in a complete MHC-mismatched setting. MHC class I-silenced fibroblasts were able to engraft and were detectable during the entire monitoring period (8 weeks). Nonmodified cells were rejected in all animals.[22] This study showed the superior performance of MHC-silenced cells after MHC-incompatible transplantation.

2.4. Generation of HLA-silenced platelets

Since the 1950s, blood transfusion therapy has become routine clinical practice; however, the concept of blood pharming – ex vivo production of mature blood cells – is quite new. In humans, platelet production is sustained by a well-regulated process known as thrombopoiesis. In the bone marrow, CD34+ progenitor cells differentiate into polyploid megakaryocytes (the precursor of platelets). Megakaryocytes lack the expression of CD34, but express several glycoproteins essential for the platelet function.[23, 24] In general, platelet numbers in blood range from 150×10^9 to 400×10^9 per liter, and an estimated 1×10^{11} platelets are produced each day in the adult human. Thrombocytopenia and severe thrombocytopenia characterized as platelet counts less than 50×10^9 and 10×10^9 per liter, respectively, increase the risk of spontaneous bleeding and represent a threat for the patient's life.[25] Platelet transfusion has been widely used to prevent and treat life-threatening thrombocytopenia; however, preparation of a unit of concentrated platelets for transfusion requires at least 4–6 units of whole blood, thereby significantly increasing the risk of blood-borne infections and adverse immunologic reactions. Furthermore, platelet transfusion refractoriness – lack of adequate post-transfusion platelet counts remains a major complication often observed in patients receiving multiple transfusions. This condition is frequently caused by the development of antibodies specific to HLA. Currently, platelet transfusion relies on volunteer blood donation; however, the demand for blood products in particular of platelets often exceeds their availability.[25]

The potential of multipotent progenitor and stem cells in regenerative medicine has been recognized.[26, 27] Platelet transfusion refractoriness due to the presence of anti-HLA antibodies constitutes a life-threatening risk for many patients suffering from hematological disorders, and hence require multiple platelet transfusions. Thus, it would be highly desirable to produce HLA-deficient platelets to facilitate the management of severe alloimmunized thrombocytopenic patients. In our studies, we have combined the concept of blood pharming with RNAi as a strategy to downregulate HLA gene expression. The ultimate goal of this approach is the large-scale production of platelets *in vitro* that may be used as an alternative to the conventional donated blood platelets. In addition, we aim for the production of genetically modified platelets with the capacity to survive even under platelet transfusion refractoriness.

In our studies, CD34+ hematopoietic progenitor cells and induced pluripotent stem cells (iPSCs) were used to produce HLA-silenced platelets *in vitro*. CD34+ cells or iPSCs were transduced with a lentiviral vector encoding for the shRNA sequence targeting β2m which induces HLA class I silencing. We have demonstrated the feasibility to generate HLA-universal CD34+ cells and iPSCs which might be used for the differentiation of HLA-silenced cell-products. In our studies, we have differentiated HLA-silenced megakaryocytes and platelets from both cell sources. In our previous studies, we have demonstrated the possibility to generate HLA-silenced platelets with comparable function to blood-derived platelets. However, in contrast to blood-derived platelets, *in vitro* generated HLA-silenced platelets were able to escape antibody-mediated complement-dependent cytotoxicity as well as cellular-dependent cytotoxicity. Also, in a platelet transfusion refractoriness mouse model, HLA-silenced platelets showed the capacity to survive and were even detectable 10 days after transfusion.[28] The limited availability of CD34+ cells derived from G-CSF mobilized donors is a major obstacle to the large-scale production of *in vitro* pharmed platelets. The breakthrough Nobel Prize–winning research by Yamanaka and colleagues to induce pluripotency in somatic cells has reshaped the field of stem cell research. Human iPSCs can be used for studying embryogenesis, disease modeling, drug testing, and regenerative medicine.[29] In contrast to CD34+ cells, iPSCs represent an unlimited cell source for the *in vitro* production of a variety of cell-based products including platelets. Therefore, we have recently established an efficient protocol for the differentiation of megakaryocytes and platelets from iPSCs (Figure 2). First, we have generated an HLA-universal iPSC line. Then, the lentiviral vector containing the shRNA targeting β2-microglobulin was used to silence HLA expression on iPSCs. A significant and durable reduction of HLA expression was observed even after passaging. Nevertheless, the HLA-silenced iPSC line showed comparable expression of pluripotency markers (such as SSEA-4 and Tra-1-60) as the original HLA class I-expressing iPSC line (Figure 3). The data indicate that silencing HLA expression does not affect the pluripotency potential of iPSCs.

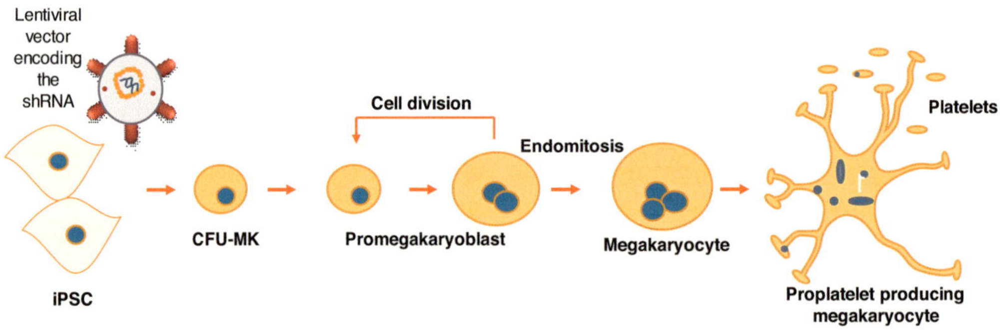

Figure 2. Schematic representation of the differentiation of HLA-silenced platelets from iPSCs. A lentiviral vector encoding for an HLA-specific shRNA is used to transduce the iPSCs. Afterward, HLA-silenced iPSCs will be differentiated using a cytokine cocktail containing thrombopoietin (TPO) until the release of platelets.

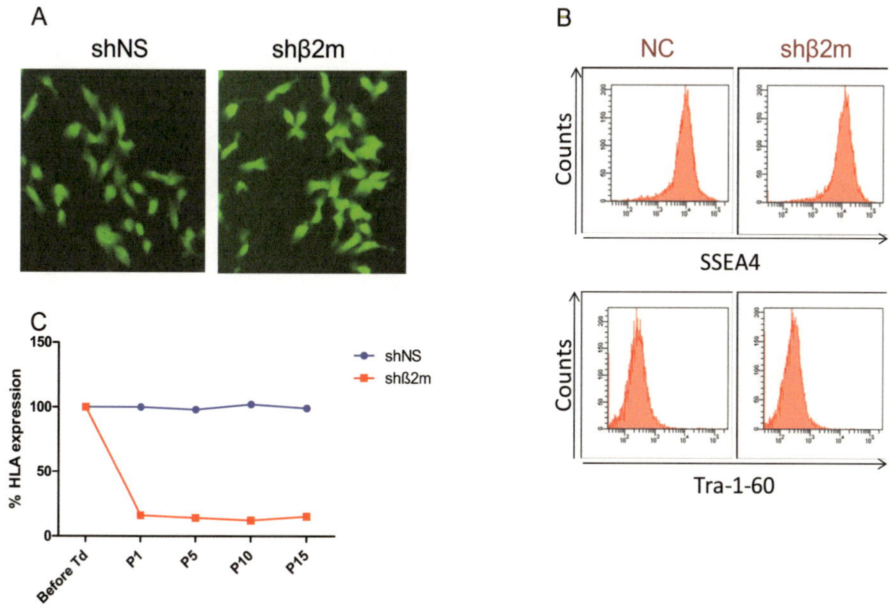

Figure 3. Generation of an HLA-universal iPSC line. (A) iPSCs were adapted to monolayer culture conditions and transduced with a lentiviral vector encoding for a nonspecific shRNA (shNS) or a β2-microglobulin-specific shRNA to silence the expression of HLA class I; (B) expression of SSEA4 and Tra-1-60 on nonmodified and shβ2m-expressing iPSCs; (C) expression of HLA class I of a HLA-silenced shNS-expressing iPSC lines. Cells were stained with an HLA class I antibody (W6/32) and the expression of HLA was measured by flow cytometry after different number of passages. Mean fluorescence intensities (MFI) detected on HLA-silenced iPSCs were normalized to the MFI measured on shNS-expressing iPSCs at the same passage.

In addition, the future application of iPSCs will occur most likely in an allogeneic manner to facilitate their availability during the time of need and standardization of the protocols. Hence, the use of HLA-silenced iPSCs may facilitate the application of HLA-mismatched iPSC-derived cell products. For megakaryocyte differentiation, HLA-silenced iPSCs were cultured in monolayer in the presence of vascular endothelial growth factor (VEGF) and BMP-4 for mesoderm induction and afterward in the presence of TPO. During ontogeny, definitive hematopoietic cells are generated de novo from a specialized subset of endothelium, known as hemogenic endothelium. Endothelial-to-hematopoietic transition during embryogenesis provides the first long-term hematopoietic stem and progenitor cells in the embryo.[30] In our differentiation cultures of iPSCs into megakaryocytes, structures resembling the hemogenic endothelium were observed (Figure 4). In suspension, megakaryocytes could be detected by an increase in DNA content higher than 4n and the expression of typical megakaryocytic markers such as CD41 and CD42a. In addition, the megakaryocytes showed the capability to build pro-platelets. Moreover, the shRNA-mediated silencing effect was maintained during the entire differentiation. Importantly, iPSC-derived megakaryocytes and pro-platelets showed a significant reduction of β2-microglobulin and HLA class I antigens in comparison to those differentiated from iPSC expressing a nonspecific shRNA (control) (Figure 5). Differentiation rates of iPSC into megakaryocytes by up to 82% were observed (Figure 6).

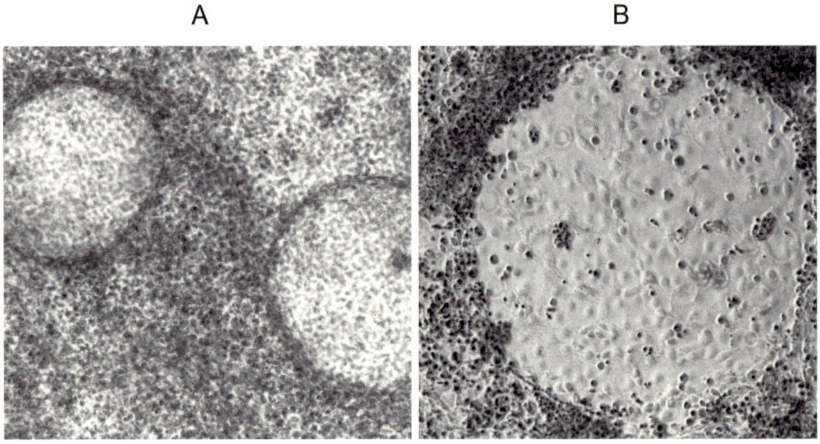

Figure 4. Formation of hemogenic-like endothelium during the differentiation of iPSCs into megakaryocytes. The photos display an island of hemogenic-like endothelium at a magnification of (A) 10x; (B) 20x.

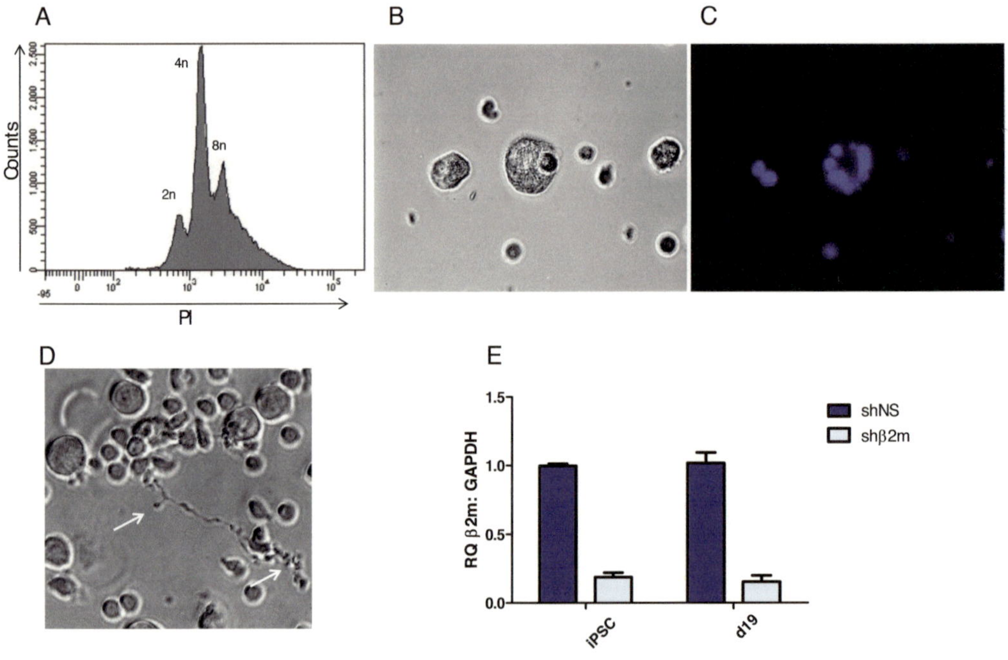

Figure 5. Differentiation of HLA-universal megakaryocytes from HLA-silenced iPSC. (A) The histogram represents the flow cytometric analysis of HLA-silenced iPSC-derived megakaryocytes after staining with propidium iodide; (B) light microscopic and (C) fluorescence microscopic analysis of an iPSC-derived megakaryocyte after staining with 4′,6-Diamidin-2-phenylindol (DAPI, blue); (D) light microscopic analysis of pro-platelets indicated with white arrows; (E) real-time PCR analysis of β2-microglobulin levels in megakaryocytes derived from iPSCs transduced with a lentiviral vector encoding the shRNA targeting β2-microglobulin (shβ2m) or a nonspecific shRNA (shNS) as a control.

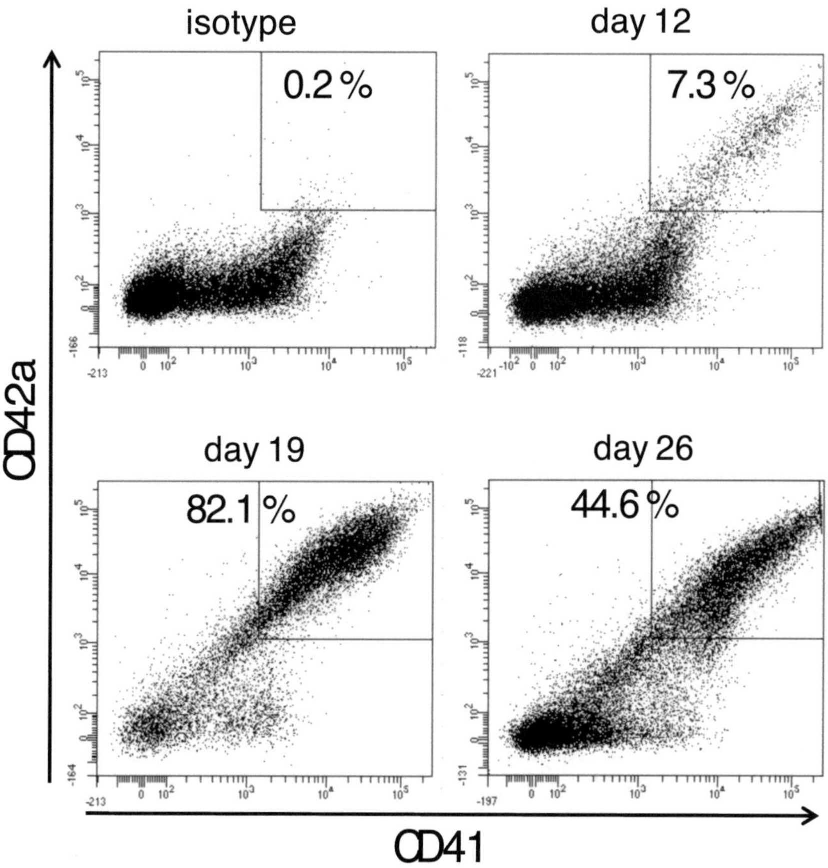

Figure 6. Phenotypic analysis of HLA-universal megakaryocytes derived from iPSCs. The expression of the megakaryocyte markers CD41 and CD42a was measured by flow cytometry in the cells harvested from the iPSC differentiation cultures at different time points. The gates in the dotplots indicate megakaryocytes characterized by the double expression of CD41 and CD42a.

The complement-dependent cytotoxic (CDC) crossmatch is an informative assay that detects alloantibodies in pre- and post-transplant patients, which may guide the most appropriate clinical management of transplant patients.[31] The capacity of *in vitro* generated HLA-silenced megakaryocytes and platelets to escape antibody-mediated complement-dependent cytotoxicity was evaluated in CDC tests. HLA-silenced megakaryocytes incubated with specific HLA antibodies and complement showed comparable cell lyses rates to the megakaryocytes incubated with nonspecific HLA antibodies. In contrast, significantly higher cell lysis rates were observed when HLA-expressing megakaryocytes were incubated with specific anti-HLA antibodies (Figure 7). These data suggest that HLA-universal iPSC-derived megakaryocytes are protected from anti-HLA antibody-mediated complement-dependent cytotoxicity and have the potential to survive under refractoriness conditions.

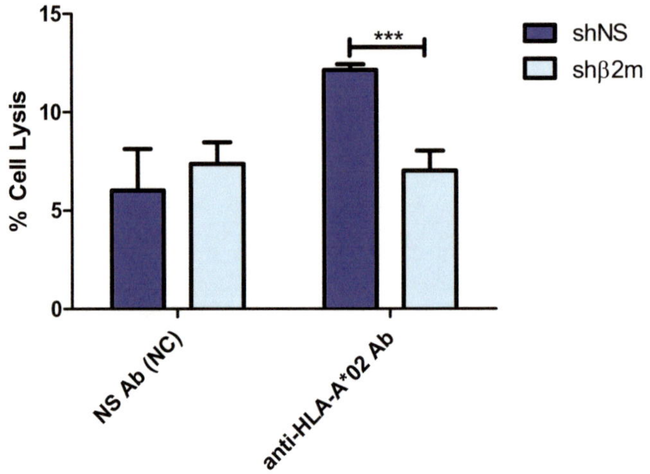

Figure 7. HLA-silenced megakaryocytes are protected from antibody-mediated complement-dependent cytotoxicity. HLA-expressing (shNS) or HLA-silenced (shβ2m) iPSC-derived megakaryocytes were incubated with a nonspecific antibody (NC) or an HLA-specific antibody and complement. Cell lysis was detected by flow cytometric analysis upon staining with propidium iodide. The bar graph represents means and standard deviations of three independent experiments. Statistical significance was calculated using Student's *t*-test (*$p < 0.05$, **$p < 0.01$; ***$p < 0.001$).

2.5. Generation of HLA-silenced tissues

Due to the high variability of the HLA loci and the shortage of organs and tissues for transplantation, it is very difficult to find a complete HLA-matched graft for a given recipient. The number of HLA mismatches between the graft and the recipient are associated with a higher risk for graft rejection and even morbidity and mortality due to immunosuppression-related side effects. Thus, it would be desirable to engineer the grafts in order to decrease their immunogenicity by silencing HLA expression. Worldwide, the demand for organs and tissues for transplantation is very high and it is not possible to satisfy all needs. This discrepancy is even accentuated in the Middle East and countries in the East such as India and China. According to the World Health Organization (WHO), there are over 10 million people in the world who are blind in one or both eyes due to corneal injury or disease and up to 45 million people could benefit from corneal transplants. However, according to data from eye banks and health agencies, less than 150,000 corneal transplants are done annually worldwide due to the shortage of human cadaver corneas. Furthermore, during the first five years after penetrating keratoplasty, rejection is responsible for 28–35% of total corneal graft loss. High risk-corneal recipients even showed increased rejection rates (30–56%).[32, 33]

The cornea presents a simple anatomical structure, in which the endothelium is easily accessible to the shRNA-encoding viral vector containing supernatant (Figure 8). The integrity of the endothelial cell layer is crucial for the transparency of the cornea and it is the major target for rejection. Therefore, silencing HLA expression on the corneal endothelium may improve cornea survival in high-risk patients after allogeneic keratoplasty.

http://dx.doi.org/10.5772/61829

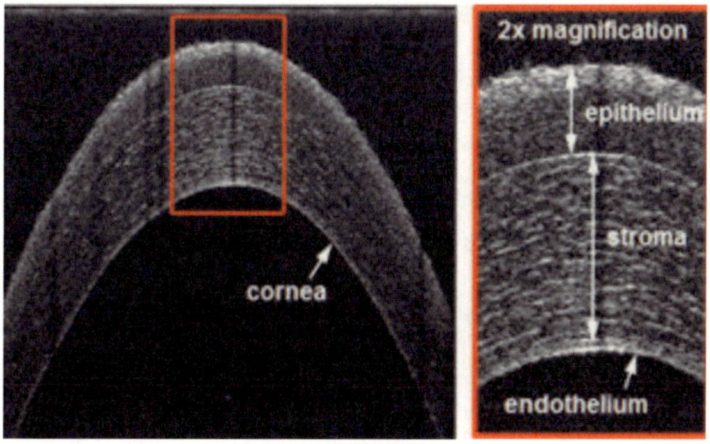

Figure 8. Anatomy of the cornea. Optical coherence tomography of a mouse cornea showing the three main layers.

We have silenced HLA expression in human and mice corneas. The tissue was transduced for 8 h with the lentiviral vector encoding for the MHC-specific shRNAs as described above. We were able to silence the MHC expression on the cornea endothelium, which is the major target during graft rejection. In this study, we demonstrated the feasibility to generate HLA universal tissues in their original 3D structure (Figure 9). Silencing HLA expression on tissues is expected to significantly improve graft survival rates in high-risk keratoplasty patients.

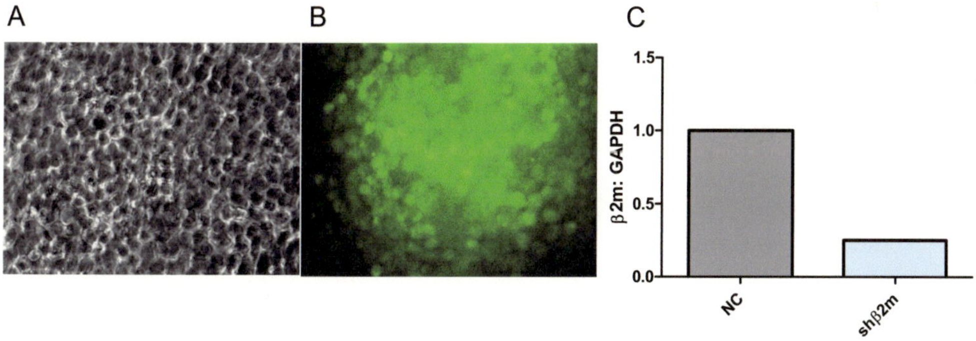

Figure 9. Generation of MHC-silenced corneas. A mouse cornea was explanted and transduced with a lentiviral vector encoding the shβ2m to cause a downregulation of MHC class I antigens and the expression of green fluorescence protein (GFP) sequences. (A) Light microscopic and (B) fluorescence microscopic analyses of a transduced mouse cornea.

2.6. Conclusion

Recently, gene regulation or editing strategies have emerged as powerful tools to improve the design and efficacy of personalized cell-based therapies. In the field of histocompatibility and transplantation, RNAi seems to be a favorite approach to reduce the immunogenicity of allogeneic and *in vitro* generated cells and tissues. The lentiviral vector-mediated delivery of shRNAs targeting HLA transcripts prevents the activation of cellular and humoral allogeneic immune responses that cause the rejection of the foreign cells. However, this RNAi-based strategy permits the residual expression of HLA class I antigens which are crucial to inhibit NK cell cytotoxicity. With the establishment of iPSCs, the concept of cell pharming came one step closer to reality as iPSCs may serve as unlimited cell sources for different cell products such as platelets. The combination of RNAi-mediated HLA silencing and the capacity to generate platelets *in vitro* may represent a novel therapeutic approach for the management of alloimmunized thrombocytopenic patients with an increased risk to develop refractoriness to platelet transfusion. Furthermore, our results also indicate the feasibility to reduce MHC expression in the 3D original structure of tissues. Abrogating the histocompatibility barrier between donors and recipients may improve therapeutic efficacy, reduce the adverse events associated with strong immunosuppressive regimens, and improve transplant patient life's quality. In conclusion, RNAi-mediated silencing of HLA expression may open new avenues in tissue engineering and transplantation.

Author details

Constanca Figueiredo* and Rainer Blasczyk

*Address all correspondence to: figueiredo.constanca@mh-hannover.de

Institute for Transfusion Medicine, Hannover Medical School, Hannover, Germany

References

[1] Barry J, Hyllner J, Stacey G, Taylor CJ, Turner M. Setting up a Haplobank: issues and solutions. *Curr Stem Cell Rep*. 2015;1(2):110–117.

[2] Figueiredo C, Seltsam A, Blasczyk R. Class-, gene-, and group-specific HLA silencing by lentiviral shRNA delivery. *J Mol Med (Berl)*. 2006;84(5):425–437.

[3] Jaimes Y, Seltsam A, Eiz-Vesper B, Blasczyk R, Figueiredo C. Regulation of HLA class II expression prevents allogeneic T-cell responses. *Tissue Antigens*. 2011;77(1): 36–44.

[4] Wiegmann B, Figueiredo C, Gras C, et al. Prevention of rejection of allogeneic endothelial cells in a biohybrid lung by silencing HLA-class I expression. *Biomaterials*. 2014;35(28):8123–8133.

[5] Hirano M, Das S, Guo P, Cooper MD. The evolution of adaptive immunity in vertebrates. *Adv Immunol*. 2011;109:125–157.

[6] Buchmann K. Evolution of innate immunity: clues from Invertebrates via fish to mammals. *Front Immunol.* 2014;5:459.

[7] Ali JM, Bolton EM, Bradley JA, Pettigrew GJ. Allorecognition pathways in transplant rejection and tolerance. *Transplantation.* 2013;96(8):681–688.

[8] Sagoo P, Lombardi G, Lechler RI. Relevance of regulatory T cell promotion of donor-specific tolerance in solid organ transplantation. *Front Immunol.* 2012;3:184.

[9] Shiina T, Hosomichi K, Inoko H, Kulski JK. The HLA genomic loci map: expression, interaction, diversity, and disease. *J Hum Genet.* 2009;54(1):15–39.

[10] Almoguera B, Shaked A, Keating BJ. Transplantation genetics: current status and prospects. *Am J Transplant.* 2014;14(4):764–778.

[11] de Rham C, Villard J. Potential and limitation of HLA-based banking of human pluripotent stem cells for cell therapy. *J Immunol Res.* 2014;2014:518135.

[12] Hess SM, Young EF, Miller KR, et al. Deletion of naive T cells recognizing the minor histocompatibility antigen HY with toxin-coupled peptide-MHC class I tetramers inhibits cognate CTL responses and alters immunodominance. *Transpl Immunol.* 2013;29(14):138–145.

[13] Kwun J, Malarkannan S, Burlingham WJ, Knechtle SJ. Primary vascularization of the graft determines the immunodominance of murine minor H antigens during organ transplantation. *J Immunol.* 2011;187(8):3997–4006.

[14] Trulock EP, Christie JD, Edwards LB, et al. Registry of the International Society for Heart and Lung Transplantation: twenty-fourth official adult lung and heart-lung transplantation report-2007. *J Heart Lung Transplant.* 2007;26(8):782–795.

[15] Opelz G, Dohler B. Association between steroid dosage and death with a functioning graft after kidney transplantation. *Am J Transplant.* 2013;13(8):2096–2105.

[16] Robson R, Cecka JM, Opelz G, Budde M, Sacks S. Prospective registry-based observational cohort study of the long-term risk of malignancies in renal transplant patients treated with mycophenolate mofetil. *Am J Transplant.* 2005;5(12):2954–2960.

[17] Wood S, Feng J, Chung J, et al. Transient blockade of delta-like Notch ligands prevents allograft rejection mediated by cellular and humoral mechanisms in a mouse model of heart transplantation. *J Immunol.* 2015;194(6):2899–2908.

[18] Wedel J, Bruneau S, Kochupurakkal N, Boneschansker L, Briscoe DM. Chronic allograft rejection: a fresh look. *Curr Opin Organ Transplant.* 2015;20(1):13–20.

[19] Figueiredo C, Horn PA, Blasczyk R, Seltsam A. Regulating MHC expression for cellular therapeutics. *Transfusion.* 2007;47(1):18–27.

[20] Moes DJ, Guchelaar HJ, de Fijter JW. Sirolimus and everolimus in kidney transplantation. *Drug Discov Today.* 2015;20(10):1243-9

[21] Khan S, Khan S, Baboota S, Ali J. Immunosuppressive drug therapy - biopharmaceutical challenges and remedies. *Expert Opin Drug Deliv*. 2015;12(8):1333–1349.

[22] Figueiredo C, Wedekind D, Muller T, et al. MHC universal cells survive in an allogeneic environment after incompatible transplantation. *Biomed Res Int*. 2013;2013:796046.

[23] Thon JN, Italiano JE. Platelet formation. *Semin Hematol*. 2010;47(3):220–226.

[24] Patel-Hett S, Wang H, Begonja AJ, et al. The spectrin-based membrane skeleton stabilizes mouse megakaryocyte membrane systems and is essential for proplatelet and platelet formation. *Blood*. 2011;118(6):1641–1652.

[25] Stanworth SJ, Navarrete C, Estcourt L, Marsh J. Platelet refractoriness - practical approaches and ongoing dilemmas in patient management. *Br J Haematol*. 2015;171(3): 297-305

[26] Crane AM, Kramer P, Bui JH, et al. Targeted correction and restored function of the CFTR gene in cystic fibrosis induced pluripotent stem cells. *Stem Cell Reports*. 2015;4(4):569–577.

[27] Tong Z, Solanki A, Hamilos A, et al. Application of biomaterials to advance induced pluripotent stem cell research and therapy. *EMBO J*. 2015;34(8):987–1008.

[28] Gras C, Schulze K, Goudeva L, Guzman CA, Blasczyk R, Figueiredo C. HLA-universal platelet transfusions prevent platelet refractoriness in a mouse model. *Hum Gene Ther*. 2013;24(12):1018–1028.

[29] Takahashi K, Yamanaka S. Induction of pluripotent stem cells from mouse embryonic and adult fibroblast cultures by defined factors. *Cell*. 2006;126(4):663–676.

[30] Zape JP, Zovein AC. Hemogenic endothelium: origins, regulation, and implications for vascular biology. *Semin Cell Dev Biol*. 2011;22(9):1036–1047.

[31] Lawrence C, Willicombe M, Brookes PA, et al. Preformed complement-activating low-level donor-specific antibody predicts early antibody-mediated rejection in renal allografts. *Transplantation*. 2013;95(2):341–346.

[32] Stuart PM, Yin X, Plambeck S, Pan F, Ferguson TA. The role of Fas ligand as an effector molecule in corneal graft rejection. *Eur J Immunol*. 2005;35(9):2591–2597.

[33] Yin XT, Zobell S, Jarosz JG, Stuart PM. Anti-IL-17 therapy restricts and reverses late-term corneal allorejection. *J Immunol*. 2015;194(8):4029–4038.

Chapter 16

Utility of Potent Anti-viral MicroRNAs in Emerging Infectious Diseases

Zhabiz Golkar, Donald G. Pace and Omar Bagasra

Additional information is available at the end of the chapter

http://dx.doi.org/10.5772/61687

Abstract

MicroRNAs (miRNAs) are small, noncoding RNA molecules that have emerged as important posttranscriptional regulators of gene expression. miRNA provides intracellular immune defense when the body is faced with challenges from transgenes, viruses, transposons, and aberrant mRNAs. miRNA molecules trigger gene silencing in eukaryotic cells. To date, more than 3,000 different human miRNAs (*hsa-miRs*) have been identified, and it is generally agreed that cellular gene regulation is significantly impacted by the presence of miRNAs. A single miRNA has the complex capacity to target multiple genes simultaneously. In a viral infection context, miRNAs have been connected with the interplay between host and pathogen, and occupy a major role in the host–parasite interaction and pathogenesis. While numerous viral miRNAs from DNA viruses have been identified, characterization of functional RNA virus-encoded miRNAs and their potential targets is still ongoing. Here, we describe an in silico approach to analyze the most recent Ebola virus (EBOV) genome sequences causing West African epidemics. We identified numerous "candidate" miRNAs that can be utilized to quell the Ebola virus. Future approaches will focus on experimental validation of these miRNAs during quelling the Ebola target transcripts for further elucidating their biological functions in primates and other animal models.

Keywords: Ebola virus, gene alignment, miRNA, prevention, vaccine

1. Introduction

1.1. Inhibition of Ebola virus by anti-Ebola miRNAs In silico

Since the HIV-1 pandemic of the 1980s and more recent outbreaks of bird flu, severe acute respiratory syndrome (SARS), and Middle East respiratory syndrome-Corona Virus (MER-CoV), it has been widely believed that there would be new pandemics of highly pathogenic viruses [1]. Fortunately, until recently, many of the new emerging pathogenic agents, such as Ebola virus (EBOV) and Marburg virus (MARV), have failed to demonstrate the transmissibility or animal reservoirs required to become true pandemic threats [2, 3]. Few, if any, antivirals can claim to be specific enough to halt the epidemic. Recently, a whole EBOV replication-defective vaccine—EBOVdVP30—has been found to be very effective in nonhuman primates, while two others are in Phase II trials [4].

The testing of the recently developed replication-defective recombinant chimpanzee adenovirus type 3–vectored ebolavirus (cAd3-EBO) vaccine is based on a demonstration of efficacy in a nonhuman primate model [5]. However, a curious finding has puzzled the investigators —preexisting neutralizing antibodies against cAd6 and cAd68 in human serum samples were found in ~40% of Ugandans and in 15% of the US and European volunteers. The increased prevalence of neutralizing antibodies against chimpanzee adenoviruses in sub-Saharan Africa may indicate cross-species transmission of these viruses from chimpanzees to humans. The possibility of fairly high levels of neutralizing antibodies against cAd3 may complicate the evaluation of the effectiveness of Ebola vaccines currently underway.

1.2. Virology of Ebola virus

Filoviruses are taxonomically classified within the order *Mononegavirales*, a large group of enveloped viruses whose genomes are composed of a nonsegmented, single-stranded minus [2, 3] RNA molecule. Following their discovery, filoviruses were originally grouped with rhabdoviruses, as the appearance of these virus particles appeared similar [3]. However, subsequent filamentous morphology and extensive genetic, physiochemical, and virologic studies of Marburg virus (MARV) and Ebola virus (EBOV) revealed distinctive characteristics, and these viruses were placed into a separate family, the *Filoviridae* [3]. Further characterization of these agents demonstrated that EBOV and MARV represent divergent lineages of filoviruses, and that their variances were significant enough to warrant the formation of the two genera, MARV and EBOV [4]. Subsequent to the International Committee on Taxonomy of Viruses recommendation, the MARV genus contains a single species, the Lake Victoria Marburg virus, as this strain exhibits only limited genetic variation.

EBOV is the causative agent of Ebola virus disease (EVD) [6]. The mortality rate can vary from 40% to 93% depending on the strains [6]. The viral life cycle begins with host cell entry through a mechanism that is still poorly understood. The incubation period for EVD is 2–21 days, and typical early symptoms include fever, chills, malaise, and myalgia (all of which could be misdiagnosed as malaria, which is highly prevalent in West African nations), followed by the onset of symptoms indicative of multi-organ stress and subsequent failure, sometimes followed by hemorrhagic episodes that can easily be misdiagnosed as Lassa fever.

EBOV is a negative, single-stranded RNA virus with an unusual, variable-length, filamentous, branched morphology whose helical capsid is enclosed inside a membrane. The mechanism of attachment and entry into the cell is still not completely defined (see discussion below). Once inside, the viral RNA polymerase (L protein) begins to copy the negative strand (–ve) RNA to make the positive strand (+ve) transcripts that mimic the structure of mRNA and are translated by host ribosomes. Replication is thought to occur in the cytoplasm. An unusual feature of the transcription and translation of the Ebola genes is the fact that the glycoproteins (GP) are only expressed through transcriptional editing. The genome of the Zaire Ebola virus (EBOV), the most pathogenic among all species of EBOV, is 18,959 nucleotides (nts) in length and contains seven transcriptional units that guide synthesis of at least nine distinct primary translation products: the nucleoprotein (NP), virion protein (VP) 35, VP40, glycoprotein (GP), soluble glycoprotein (sGP), small soluble glycoprotein (ssGP), VP30, VP24, and the large (L) protein. L is the catalytic subunit of the viral polymerase complex (Figure 1). Similar to other nonsegmented negative-sense (NNS) RNA viruses, EBOVs encode a multiprotein complex to carry out replication and transcription. In the case of EBOV, viral RNA synthesis requires the viral NP, VP35, VP30, and L proteins. Transcription of filovirus mRNAs is presumed to occur as in other NNS viruses, where there is a gradient of viral mRNAs with the abundance of each mRNA transcript decreasing as the polymerase transcribes toward the 5′ end of the template [7]. Each EBOV mRNA is presumed to be efficiently modified with a 5′–7′-methylguanosine (m^7G) cap and a 3′p (A) tail [8].

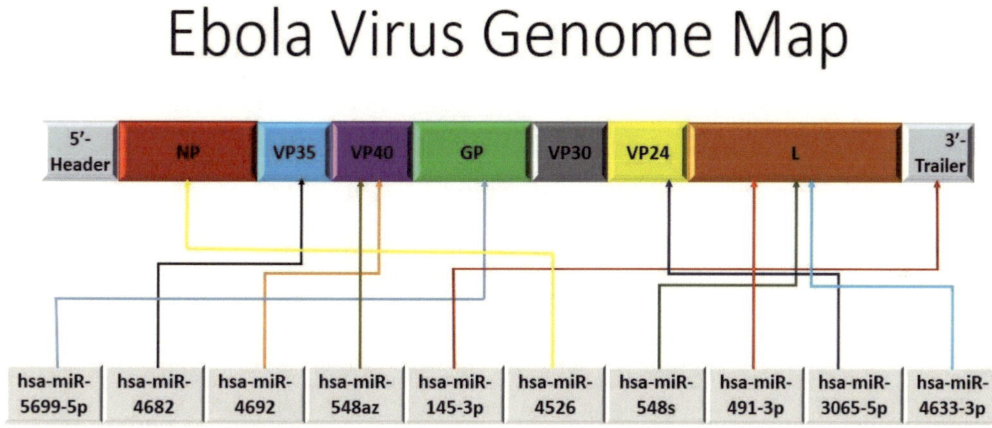

Figure 1. The genome of EBOV, 18 9 kb in length, has the following gene order: 3′ leader nucleoprotein (NP), virion proteins (VP) VP35-VP40, membrane glycoprotein (GP), viral polymerase (VP) VP30-VP24, viral polymerase L protein, and 5′ trailer.

The Ebola virus genus possesses greater diversity, and four viral species have been recognized: Zaire Ebola, Sudan Ebola, Reston Ebola, and Ivory Coast Ebola (EBOV-Z, EBOV-S, EBOV-R, and EBOV-IC, respectively). Each of the EBOV species has a different degree of pathogenicity and mortality rate [9]. Therefore, EBOV-S and EBOV-Z, which are the predominant EBOVs associated with known outbreaks, are more pathogenic than EBOV-R and EBOV-IC [10]. EBOV-IC has only caused a single nonfatal human infection, but EBOV-R has caused fatal infection in nonhuman primates [8]. However, EBOV-S, EBOV-Z, and EBOV-B often cause severe hemorrhagic diseases with markedly high case fatality rates (40–90%) [10]. The EBOV genome is 18.9 kb in length with the following gene order: 3′ leader nucleoprotein (NP), virion protein (VP) 35-VP40, glycoprotein (GP), VP30, VP24, polymerase (L), and 5′ trailer. The GP differences between any two species range from 37% to 41% at the nucleotide level and from

34% to 43% at the amino acid level [40]. However, variations within EBOV-Z species are very low (~2–3%) [11]. Thus, GP nucleotides are usually used in the phylogenetic analysis of EBOV (Figure 2).

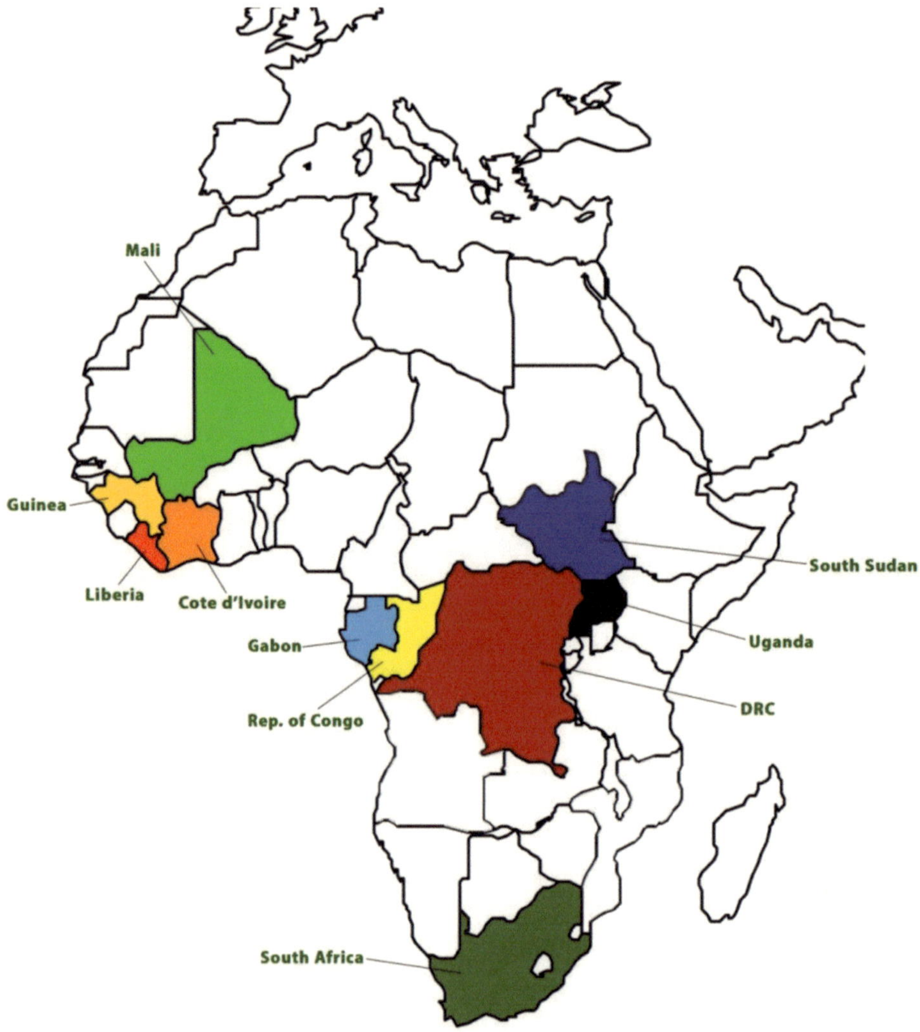

Figure 2. The Ebola Pandemic Map depicts the history of Ebola in Africa. The sporadic cases of Ebola were common in the central African countries such as the DRC (988 cases with 767 fatalities), Uganda (606 cases with 283 fatalities), South Sudan (335 cases with 180 fatalities), Gabon (214 cases with 150 fatalities), the Republic of the Congo (248 cases with 210 fatalities), and South Africa (2 cases with 1 fatality).

Because of their high mortality rate, which can vary from 40% to 93%, and their potential for person-to-person transmission and lack of an approved vaccine or antiviral therapy, MARV and EBOV are classified as biosafety level 4 (BSL-4) viruses by World Health Organization [12, 13]

http://dx.doi.org/10.5772/61687

1.3. History of MARV and EBOV

Viruses are obligate intracellular parasites and essentially rely on host cells for raw materials, replication, transcription, and translations of their genetic codes. Until a few years ago, we assumed that the major intracellular defenses against viral pathogens were interferons [13]. Since the discovery of RNA interference (RNAi) and miRNAs, we know that one of the fundamental functions of miRNAs is to prevent replication of foreign viruses by pre- and posttranscriptions and suppressions of viral expression [12]. Therefore, besides endogenous gene regulation, miRNAs are the primary intracellular immune defense system [13]. Viruses have also evolved to counter the antiviral effects of miRNAs by viral miRNAs (vmiRNAs).

Recently, Li and Chen [14] have conducted molecular epidemiologic analyses of presently extant Ebola viral genomes to ascertain their evolutionary viral history. Of considerable potential importance are interpretations derived from a dataset that is between 1,000 and 2,100 years old and includes four Ebola species (EBOV-Z, EBOV-S, EBOV-TF, EBOV-R) [15]. Logically, one could assume that over the past 2,000 years, humans have evolved countermeasures to the Ebola virus via innate, adaptive, and miRNA-based immunity. The identification in a human database of 71 miRNAs capable of potentially quelling EBOV strongly suggests that *Homo sapiens* already have developed primary intracellular defenses to quell EBOV infection [16]. This raises a question: Why have EBOVs been circulating for about 2,000 years, and yet they seem to have emerged only recently? The earliest known cases of Ebola date to the 1970s. One theory proposes that EBOV-Z experienced a recent genetic bottleneck [17]. Before Ebola viral strains were introduced to primates, they had already been circulating among small mammals, including bats, rodents, marsupials, shrews, and so on [16]. Although these bats and other animals were infected [15, 16], no evidence demonstrated that such infections were fatal to them [18]. This indicates that a natural balance had been achieved between the viruses' pathogenicity and the host's immune system, especially at the intracellular levels where miRNAs provide immunological protection [19]. This homeostasis, this balance, apparently was broken in 1900, when EBOV genetic diversity experienced a dramatic drop [16]. Accordingly, most lineages of the various EBOV species became extinct because of such influences as threatening human activities, climate change, and a steep decline in the number of animals to serve as a reservoir for viral replication. Probably due to altered patterns of positive selection in the glycoprotein (GP), which diversified substantially and was found to be part of fusion and receptor binding within cellular membranes, infection patterns through direct exposure were changing. Therefore, by about 1970, few lineages that possessed broader tropism and enhanced fitness had the capacity to infect primates via direct exposure [16]. Similar examples can be seen in the emergence of HIV-1, which appeared to have surfaced in the 1950s through a zoonotic event that involved common infections among chimpanzees (i.e., SIV) and then accidentally jumped to humans [16–18]. Due to the paucity of significant differences in EBOV genetic diversity since 1970, the decreased number of surviving viruses may have become the only circulating lineages in primates and viral reservoirs. EBOV-Z has the ability to traverse a long distance through bats, which serve as a migratory reservoir. Outbreaks with their epicenter in Congo have been caused by the EBOV-Z species [20–23].

Through analysis of miRNA numbers that demonstrate high homologies in seed sequences and that show high identity to EBOV species, we have deduced that the genetic variations at the GP may serve as a type of Achilles' heel. After all, only one miRNA showed identity to GP, while eight proved capable of blocking polymerase steps. This indicates that minor variations within the GP amino acid sequence could allow for viral entrance into host target cells in humans. The subsequent transcription of negative-stranded RNA viruses into positive RNA strands occurs amid a struggle to overcome the miRNAs with quelling potential that can halt this process. It is possible that at the time of exposure to EBOV, all of the protective miRNAs may not be present in the target cells, or may be present, but not in sufficient quantities to block early EBOV replication [24].

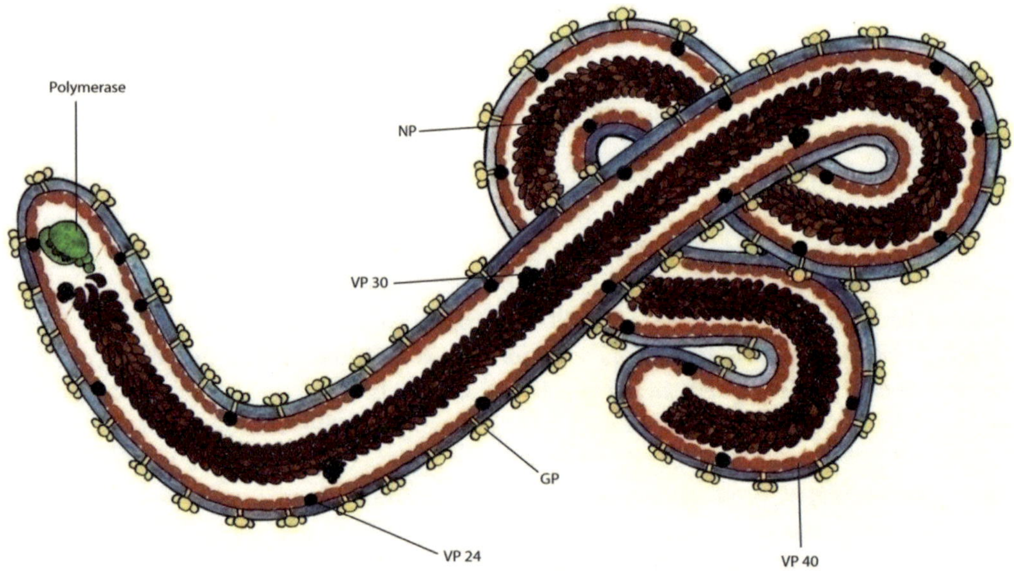

Figure 3. The illustration depicts a simplified structure of Ebola virus. The functions of various viral proteins are described in the text. GP, glycoprotein; NP, nucleoprotein; VP40, matrix protein; VP30, transcription factor; and polymerase enzyme.

Figure 3 shows the VP24, VP30, VP35, VP40, and L nucleoproteins that constitute the nucleocapsid, which is crucial in both the transcription and viral replication processes [25, 26]. The glycoprotein is located in the lipid membrane of the Ebola virus; this is also the place in the host target cells where receptors that facilitate viral entry are embedded [27]. Viral matrix proteins VP40 and VP24 are essential to viral budding, stability, and structure. VP40 is the primary matrix protein, and is the viral protein that is expressed most abundantly. It plays a central role in the process of Ebola budding from the plasma membrane. For example, in mammalian cells, the mere expression of VP40 is sufficient to create virus-like particles (VLPs) with morphological characteristics that are similar to those of the actual Ebola virus [28, 29]. Given VP40's absence, studies have found that the nucleocapsid was not transported effectively into the plasma membrane, and as this membrane is the site of assembly, budding, and incorporation into the virions, considerable attention should be given to the role of this matrix protein [30]. The utilization of miRNAs that specifically target VP40 mRNA degradation is important to our understanding of just how VP40 functions and what potential roles it might play in the regulation of VLP assembly in both in vitro and live cell settings. *hsa-miR-4692* and *hsa-miR-548-az* effectively target VP40; therefore, the overexpression of these particular miRNAs within host cells could totally disrupt the viral life cycle and may have a decisive impact in the categorization of therapeutic targets (data unpublished). The tendency of Ebola VP40 to assemble virus-like particles (VLPs) presents an appealing model for analysis of the Ebola viral assembly at biosafety level 2 made possible by the noninfectious nature of genetically engineered VLPs [31].

VP40's association with the plasma membrane is of fundamental importance [30]; it is here that assembly is initiated as well as oligomerization [31], and nucleoprotein recruitment. Besides membrane association, VP40 also associates or otherwise interacts with host cell factors, including the endosomal sorting complex that supports transport (ESCRT) machinery [27, 29], the vesicle coat II proteins (COPII) [24], as well as the protein actin [25, 30]; these host cell factors, respectively, have been shown to enable VP40 budding, transport, and movement. Moreover, host cell protein kinases could contribute to Ebola infectivity as c-Abl1 can phosphorylate Tyr^{13} in VP40 [32, 33]. Still we have an inadequate understanding of how VP40 actually assembles on the plasma membrane before virion release occurs. Localization of VP40 in the plasma membrane is believed to be important as studies give evidence that hydrophobic residues located within the C-terminal domain, including Leu^{213}, are essential in the localization and budding processes [32]. Detection of VP40 oligomers in VLPs and UV-inactivated virions has occurred [34, 35]; they have been detected mainly in filamentous structures stemming from the plasma membrane [36]. Therefore, VP40 oligomerization apparently occurs on the same plasma membrane in which oligomers selectively have found to reside [37]. In terms of structure, VP40 has predominantly been found to oligomerize into either hexamers or octamers [38, 39]. These share a comparable monomer–monomer (or intradimeric) antiparallel interface. However, the detection of oligomeric structures in live cells suggests that these structures, too, could exert a critical influence on both viral assembly and egress [40]. We discovered that *hsa-miR-4692* and *hsa-miR-548-az* both target VP40 (data unpublished).

The formation of virus-like particles (VLPs) requires VP40 oligomers; these are associated with membranes that are resistant to detergent [41], which underscores the active part that the plasma membrane may play in VP40 oligomerization. Moreover, on the plasma membrane, matrix protein oligomerization may function as a scaffold in host protein recruitment, and also supply the force needed to effect the formation of virus particles and the deformation of membranes. A comprehension of VP40 plasma membrane association thus becomes crucial to our understanding of how the formation of protein buds occurs on the plasma membrane. Gupta K [42] recently investigated the role that the VP40 C-terminal domain plays in membrane association as well as in membrane penetration. These investigators utilized the monolayer penetration methodology to conduct in vitro research into the molecular basis of the penetration of the VP40 membrane. To study VP40 assembly and its associated egress in cells, they employed a multipronged methodology that blended cellular imaging, number and brightness (N&B) analysis, analysis of the egress of virus-like particles, site-directed mutagenesis, and total internal reflection (TIRF) microscopy. N&B analysis permitted them to ascertain the average number of molecules and also the brightness within each pixel within a fluorescence microscopy image. This permitted them to detect the oligomeric status of proteins that are labeled fluorescently. They concluded that within the VP40 C-terminal domain, a hydrophobic interface actually penetrates the plasma membrane, which plays a key role in the oligomerization of VP40. The knocking out of plasma membrane penetration by hydrophobic mutants also substantially reduces the egress of VLPs [38, 39]. Therefore, degradation of VP40 mRNA by a two-pronged attack from *hsa-miR-4692* and *hsa-miR-548-az* can stop Ebola.

A distinguishing characteristic of filovirus genomes is their 3′- and 5′-UTRs that are long related to other RNA viruses of the nonsegmented negative-strand (NNS) variety [40]. Of particular note, Kochetov AV [41] concentrated on the 5′-UTRs in the mRNA of seven EBOV viruses, due to the critical importance of the 5′-UTRs in translation initiation. In four of these seven mRNAs, small alternate upstream open reading frames (uORFs) were identified, but their significance is yet to be fully characterized. In cellular mRNAs, uORFs are known to be a common feature; they are critical in modulating translation of primary ORFs (pORFs), which was accomplish by reducing the efficiency and quantity of the scanning ribosomes associated with the reinitiation that occurs at the start codon of pORFs [42]. At a uAUG, rather than a pAUG, translation initiation frequency is affected by a variety of factors, including the strength of the Kozak consensus sequence that surrounds the uAUG. Moreover, between the pAUG and the upstream open reading frame (uORF) is an intercistronic space that, combined with the phosphorylation status of and the eIF-2α [43, 44], controls whether translation takes place at the principal protein initiation site (pAUG) or at the termination codon (uAUG).

When eIF-2α~P is absent, cap-dependent translation has been found to be efficient, which permits higher ribosome initiation rates at the uORF [45]. When eIF2α~P is enhanced, impairment of translation initiation occurs, which causes a ribosome to continue scanning beyond the uAUG; in this case, initiation occurs at the pAUG. In short, when cell stress occurs, eIF2α~P facilitates translation initiation of select mRNAs that possess uORFs at the primary open ready frame (pORF) [46].

They characterized how the EBOV 5′-UTRs modulate translation. Mutating any of the four uAUGs present in the EBOV genome enhances translation at the corresponding pORF. The most dramatic effect was with the L gene where the L uAUG can potently suppress pORF translation; however, in response to eIF2α~P, the L uAUG maintains L translation. Modulating viral polymerase levels is biologically significant as ablating the L uORF in a recombinant EBOV reduces viral titers 10- to 100-fold in cell culture, severely impairs viral RNA synthesis, and functions to maintain virus titers in cells treated with stress-inducing agents. These data suggest that a uORF in the EBOV L mRNA regulates polymerase expression in response to the status of the cellular innate immune response and is required for optimal virus replication.

It would be relatively easy to incorporate a combination of relevant miRNAs in a miRNA-expression vector to test the utility of these miRNAs in genetically engineered VLP cell models in vitro that can be performed in a BSL-2 facility, and then to extend these studies in animal models utilizing safe vectors in a BSL-4 environment.

Currently, there are several genetically engineered vaccines containing genes for surface proteins (GP) that are in clinical trial. The first among these is a vaccine that Ebola GP genes stitched into a weakened chimpanzee adenovirus that serves as a vector. The second vaccine contains the Ebola surface protein gene inside a weakened version of vesicular stomatitis virus (VSV), which commonly infects farm animals. The potential dangers of employing of VSV are obvious: it can save men but potentially harm livestock in West Africa. The chimpanzee adenovirus will be a zoonotic event itself, and its potential danger cannot be underestimated [47, 48].

The third vaccine uses a vector known as MVA, a modified version of the smallpox vaccine virus, and involves protection from an Ebola virus "challenge" 10 months after the last vaccination.

We noted that none of these three approaches mentioned a simple and well-tested method of human and animal vaccination. What happened to the simple, whole formalin-killed or UV-killed, less pathogenic EBOV vaccines that have been tried in so many viral vaccinations [49, 50]?

With viruses like the major Ebola strands, where the mortality rate is over 50%, it will be difficult to find a reasonable and ethical way to carry out an unbiased clinical trial. However, if one can prepare a "dead Ebola virus" with antigenicity intact, it would be easy to immunize "high risk groups" without utilizing unusual vectors as exemplified by "harmless" chimpanzee adenovirus, VSV or MVA (modified smallpox virus), each with unknown long-term risk factors and accompanied by immediate concerns of viral vector-induced antigenic competition that may potentially quell proper immune responses to the Ebola antigens [51]. We believe that a dead vaccine may induce the protective miRNAs and quell the pandemic. Increasingly, miRNA-induced intracellular immunity is being better understood, and several clinical trials are under way to treat viral diseases and cancers [52–55]. The cost of each of these vaccines would run into millions of dollars and would be prohibitively expensive to any of the individuals who are predicted to be infected with the virus in West African nations. In contrast to the proposed recombinant vaccines, each of the more traditional "killed vaccines" has been very inexpensive to produce and has benefited billions of humans [56].

2. Conclusions

The current ongoing Ebola outbreaks in West Africa that began almost three years ago in March 2013 have already claimed 11,000 lives and over 27,000 cases. The rapid spread of the infection demands the need for rapid prevention methods. Currently, there are several vaccines that are in different phases of clinical trials. In this report, we highlight an alternative to the standard vaccine for Ebola prevention. We show that a preventive method based on miRNAs could be utilized and tested in nonhuman primates. Some of the lessons that we have learned from the recent West Africa Ebola outbreaks is to test the vaccine and other preventive methods that are currently available against Ebola before the major outbreaks occur. Therefore, we recommend that vaccines and preventive methods must be developed to the point that the measures correlate for human protection (Phase I level), so when the outbreaks occur, the vaccine and other measures can be rolled out quickly to prevent the spread of the disease.

Acknowledgements

We would like to thank Dr. Donald Gene Pace for his editorial assistance.

Author details

Zhabiz Golkar[1], Donald G. Pace[2] and Omar Bagasra[3*]

*Address all correspondence to: obagasra@claflin.edu

1 Department of Biology, School of Health and Natural Science, Voorhees College, Denmark, SC, USA

2 School of Humanities & Social Science, Claflin University, Orangeburg, SC, USA

3 School of Natural Science, Claflin University, Orangeburg, SC, USA

References

[1] Na W, Park N, Yeom M, Song D. Ebola outbreak in Western Africa 2014: what is going on with Ebola virus? ClinExp Vaccine Res. 2015; 4:1:17-22. DOI:10.7774/cevr.2015.4.1.17

[2] Zhou Y, Simmons G. Development of novel entry inhibitors targeting emerging viruses Expert Rev Anti Infect Ther. 2012; 10: 1129–1138 t. DOI:10.1586/eri.12.104

[3] Misasi J, Chandran K, Yang JY. Filoviruses require endosomal cysteine proteases for entry but exhibit distinct protease preferences. J. Virol. 2012; 86:6:3284–3292. DOI: 10.1128/JVI.06346-11

[4] Sarwar UN, Costner P, Enama ME, Berkowitz N, Hu Z, Hendel CS, Sitar S, Plummer S, Mulangu S, Bailer RT, Koup RA, Mascola JR, Nabel GJ, Sullivan NJ, Graham BS, Ledgerwood JE. Safety and immunogenicity of DNA vaccines encoding Ebola virus and Marburg virus wild-type glycoproteins in a phase I clinical trial. J Infect Dis. 2015; 211:4:549–557. DOI:10.1093/infdis/jiu511

[5] Zhang Q, Seto DChimpanzee Adenovirus Vector Ebola Vaccine--Preliminary Report. N Engl J Med. 2015 Aug 20; 373(8):775–6. DOI:10.1056/NEJMc1505499#SA1

[6] Gao J, Yin L. Drug development for controlling Ebola epidemic – a race against time.Drug DiscovTher. 2014; 85:229–31.

[7] Drake JW, Holland JJ. "Mutation rates among RNA viruses". Proc. Natl. Acad. Sci. 1999; 96:24:13910–13913. DOI:10.1073/pnas.96.24.13910

[8] Adu-Gyamfi E, Soni SP, Xue Y, Digman MA, Gratton E, Stahelin RV. The Ebola virus matrix protein penetrates into the plasma membrane: a key step in viral protein 40 (VP40) oligomerization and viral egress. J Biol Chem. 2013; 288:8:5779–5789. DOI: 10.1074/jbc.M112.443960

[9] Shabman RS, Hoenen T, Groseth A, Jabado O, Binning JM. An Upstream Open Reading Frame Modulates Ebola Virus Polymerase Translation and Virus Replication. 2013. PLoSPathog 9(1): e1003147. DOI:10.1371/journal.ppat.1003147

[10] Harty RN. No exit: Targeting the budding process to inhibit filovirus replication. Antiviral 2009; 81:189–197. DOI:10.1016/j.antiviral. 2008.12.003.

[11] Feldmann HME, Randolf A, Will C, Kiley MP, Sanchez A. Marburg virus, a Filovirus: messenger RNAs, gene order, and regulatory elements of the replication cycle. 1992; 24:1–19.

[12] Adu-Gyamfi E, Soni SP, Xue Y, Digman MA, Gratton E, Stahelin RV. The Ebola virus matrix protein penetrates into the plasma membrane: a key step in viral protein 40 (VP40) oligomerization and viral egress. J Biol Chem. 2013; 288:8:5779–5789. DOI: 10.1074/jbc.M112.443960

[13] Sanchez AKM. Identification and analysis of Ebola virus messenger RNA. Virology. 1987; 157:414–420.

[14] Weik M, Modrof J, Klenk HD, Becker S, Muhlberger E. Ebola Virus VP30-Mediated Transcription Is Regulated by RNA Secondary Structure Formation. J Virol. 2012; 76:8532–8539. DOI:10.1128/JVI.76.17.8532-8539.2002

[15] Bryan R. Cullen. The role of RNAi and microRNAs in animal virus replication and antiviral immunity. Genes & Dev. 2009; 23:1151–1164. DOI:10.1101/gad.1793309.

[16] Haasnoot J, Vries WD, Geutjes EJ, Prins M, Haan PD, Berkhout B.The Ebola virus VP35 protein is a suppressor of RNA silencing. PLoSPathog. 2007; 3:e86, DOI: 10.1371/journal.ppat.0030086

[17] Li YH, Chen SP. Evolutionary history of Ebola virus. Epidemiol Infect. 2014;142(6): 1138–1145. DOI: 10.1017/S0950268813002215.

[18] Biek R. Recent common ancestry of Ebola Zaire virus found in a bat reservoir. PLoS Pathogens. 2006; 2:e90. DOI: 10.1371/journal.ppat.0020090.

[19] Ramanan P, Shabman RS, Brown CS, Amarasinghe GK, Basler CF, Leung DW. Filoviral immune evasion mechanisms. Viruses. 2011; 3:9:1634-1649. DOI:10.3390/v3091634

[20] Taylor DJ, Leach RW, Bruenn J. Filoviruses are ancient and integrated into mammalian genomes. BMC evolutionary biology. 2010; 22:10:193. DOI: 10.1186/1471-2148-10-193

[21] Hunt CL, Kondratowicz AS, Bowman J, Sinn PL, McCray PB Jr, Quinn K, Weller ML, Chiorini JA, Maury W. Tyrosine kinase receptor Axl enhances entry of Zaire ebolavirus without direct interactions with the viral glycoprotein.Virology. 2011; 5:415:2: 83-94. DOI:10.1016/j.virol.2011.04.002

[22] Soni SP, Adu-Gyamfi E, Yong SS, Jee CS, Stahelin RV. The Ebola Virus Matrix Protein Deeply Penetrates the Plasma Membrane: An Important Step in Viral Egress. Biophysical Journal. 2013; 104:9:1940-1949. DOI:10.1016/j.bpj.2013.03.021

[23] Warfield KL, Warren TK, Lovejoy C, Hassinger JN, Ruthel G, Blouch RE, Moulton HM, Weller DD, Iversen PL, Bavari S. Chemical modifications of antisense morpholino oligomers enhance their efficacy against Ebola virus infection. Antimicrob Agents Chemother. 2009; 53:5:2089–2099. DOI:10.1128/AAC.00936-08

[24] Reynard O, Nemirov K, Volchkov VE. Conserved proline-rich region of Ebola virus matrix protein VP40 is essential for plasma membrane targeting and virus-like particle release. J. Infect. Dis. 2011; 204:3: 884–891. DOI:10.1093/infdis/jir305

[25] Makino A, Yamayoshi S, Kawaoka Y. Identification of amino acids in Marburg virus VP40 that are important for virus-like particle budding. J. Infect. Dis. 2011; 204: 3:871–877. DOI:10.1093/infdis/jir309.

[26] Harty RN, Brown ME, Hayes FP. A PPxY motif within the VP40 protein of Ebola virus interacts physically and functionally with a ubiquitin ligase: implications for filovirus budding. Proc. Natl. Acad. Sci. 2000; 97:13871–13876.

[27] Licata JM, Simpson-H M, Harty RN. Overlapping motifs (PTAP and PPEY) within the Ebola virus VP40 protein function independently as late budding domains: involvement of host proteins TSG101 and VPS-4.J. Virol. 2003; 77:1812–1819.

[28] Hoenen T, Volchkov V, Weissenhorn W. VP40 octamers are essential for Ebola virus replication. J. Virol. 2005; 79:1898–1905. DOI: 10.1128/JVI.00737-10

[29] Dessen A, Volchkov V, Weissenhorn W. Crystal structure of the matrix protein VP40 from Ebola virus. EMBO J. 2000; 19:4228–4236. DOI:10.1093/emboj/19.16.4228

[30] Adu-Gyamfi E, Soni SP, Stahelin RV. The Ebola virus matrix protein penetrates into the plasma membrane: a key step in viral protein 40 (VP40) oligomerization and viral egress. J. Biol. Chem. 2013; 288:5779–5789. DOI:10.3390/v6103837

[31] Adu-Gyamfi E, Digman MA, Stahelin RV. Investigation of Ebola VP40 assembly and oligomerization in live cells using number and brightness analysis. Biophys. J. 2012; 102:2517–2525. DOI:10.1016/j.bpj.2012.04.022

[32] Licata JM, Simpson-HM, Wright N T, Han Z, Paragas J, Harty RN. Overlapping motifs (PTAP and PPEY) within the Ebola virus VP40 protein function independently as

late budding domains: involvement of host proteins TSG101 and VPS-4. J. Virol. 2003; 77: 1812–1819.

[33] Neumann G, Ebihara H, Takada A, Noda T, Kobasa D, Jasenosky LD, Watanabe S, Kim J H, FeldmannH, Kawaoka Y. Ebola virus VP40 late domains are not essential for viral replication in cell culture. J. Virol. 2005; 79:10300–10307. DOI: 10.1128/JVI.79.16.10300-10307.2005

[34] Yamayoshi S, Noda T, Ebihara H, Goto H, Morikawa Y, Lukashevich IS, Neumann G, Feldmann H, Kawaoka Y. Ebola virus matrix protein VP40 uses the COPII transport system for its intracellular transport. Cell Host Microbe. 2008; 3:168–177. DOI: 10.1016/j.chom.2008.02.001

[35] García M, Cooper A, Shi W, Bornmann W, Carrion R, Kalman D, Nabel GJ. Produtive replication of Ebola virus is regulated by the c-Abl1 tyrosine kinase. Sci. Transl. Med. 2012; 4: 123ra24. DOI: 10.1126/scitranslmed.3003500

[36] McCarthy SE, Johnson RF, Zhang YA, Sunyer JO, Harty RN. Role for amino acids 212KLR214 of Ebola virus VP40 in assembly and budding. J. Virol. 2007; 81:11452–11460. DOI:10.1128/JVI.00853-07

[37] Hoenen T, Volchkov V, Kolesnikova L, Mittler E, Timmins J, Ottmann M, Reynard O, Becker S, Weissenhorn W. VP40 octamers are essential for Ebola virus replication. J. Virol. 2005; 79: 1898–1905. DOI:10.1128/JVI.79.3.1898-1905.2005

[38] Morris DR, Geballe AP. Upstream Open Reading Frames as Regulators of mRNA Translation. Molecular and Cellular Biology. 2000; 20: 8635–8642. DOI: 10.1128/MCB.20.23.8635-8642.2000

[39] Kozak M. Initiation of translation in prokaryotes and eukaryotes. Gene. 1999; 234:187–208.

[40] Meijer HA, Thomas AAM. Control of eukaryotic protein synthesis by upstream open reading frames in the 5′-untranslated region of an mRNA. BiochemJ. 2002; 367:1–11. DOI:10.1042/BJ20011706

[41] Kochetov AV, Ahmad S, Ivanisenko V, Volkova OA, Kolchanov NA, et al. uORFs, re-initiation and alternative translation start sites in human mRNAs. FEBS Letters 2008; 582:1293–1297. DOI:10.1016/j.febslet.2008.03.014

[42] Gupta KA. Regulation and Deregulation of mRNA translation during myeloid maturation. Experimental hematology. 2011; 39(2):133–141. DOI:10.1016/j.exphem.2010.10.011

[43] Wek RC, Jiang HY, Anthony TG. Coping with stress: eIF2 kinases and translational control. BiochemSoc Trans. 2006; 34: 7–11.

[44] Bukreyev AA, DiNapoli JM, Yang L, Murphy BR, Collins PL. Mucosal parainfluenza virus-vectored vaccine against Ebola virus replicates in the respiratory tract of vec-

tor-immune monkeys and is immunogenic. Virology. 2010; 399:2:290-298. DOI: 10.1016/j.virol.2010.01.015

[45] Passi D, Sharma S, Dutta SR, Dudeja P, Sharma V.Ebola Virus Disease (The Killer Virus): Another Threat to Humans and Bioterrorism: Brief Review and Recent Updates. J ClinDiagn Res. 2015; 9:6:LE01–8. DOI:10.7860/JCDR/2015/13062.6100

[46] Isere EE, Fatiregun AA, Ajayi IO.An overview of disease surveillance and notification system in Nigeria and the roles of clinicians in disease outbreak prevention and control. Niger Med J. 2015; 56:3:161–8. DOI: 10.4103/0300-1652.160347

[47] Sesmero E, Thorpe IF.Using the Hepatitis C Virus RNA-Dependent RNA Polymerase as a Model to Understand Viral Polymerase Structure, Function and Dynamics.Viruses. 2015 ; 7:7:3974–94. DOI: 10.3390/v7072808.

[48] Alexander KA, Sanderson CE, Marathe M, Lewis BL, Rivers CM, Shaman J, Drake JM, Lofgren E, DatoVM,Eisenberg MC, Eubank S.What factors might have led to the emergence of Ebola in West Africa?PLoSNegl Trop Dis. 2015; 9:6:e0003652. DOI: 10.1371/journal.pntd.0003652

[49] Falasca L, Agrati C, Petrosillo N, Di Caro A, Capobianchi MR, Ippolito G, Piacentini M.Molecular mechanisms of Ebola virus pathogenesis: focus on cell death.Cell Death Differ. 2015; 22:8:1250–9. DOI:10.1038/cdd.2015.67

[50] Rewar S, Mirdha D. Transmission of ebola virus disease: an overview. Ann Glob Health. 2014; 80:6:444–51. DOI: 10.1016/j.aogh.2015.02.005

[51] Cenciarelli O, Pietropaoli S, Malizia A, Carestia M, D'Amico F, Sassolini A, Di Giovanni D, Rea S, GabbariniV,Tamburrini A, Palombi L, Bellecci C, Gaudio P. Ebola virus disease 2013-2014 outbreak in west Africa: an analysis of the epidemic spread and response. Int J Microbiol. 2015; 2015:769121. DOI:10.1155/2015/769121

[52] Roca A, Afolabi MO, Saidu Y, Kampmann B.Ebola: a holistic approach is required to achieve effective management and control. J Allergy ClinImmunol. 2015; 135:4:856-67. DOI: 10.1016/j.jaci.2015.02.015

[53] Ibrahim F, Thio TH, Faisal T, Neuman M. The application of biomedical engineering techniques to the diagnosis and management of tropical diseases: a review. Sensors (Basel). 2015; 15:3:6947–95. DOI:10.3390/s150306947

[54] Shurtleff AC, Whitehouse CA, Ward MD, Cazares LH, Bavari S. Pre-symptomatic diagnosis and treatment of filovirus diseases. Front Microbiol. 2015; 20:6:108. DOI: 10.3389/fmicb.2015.00108

[55] Litterman N, Lipinski C, Ekins S. Small molecules with antiviral activity against the Ebola virus.F1000Res. 2015; 9:4:38. DOI:10.12688/f1000research.6120.1

[56] Bociaga-Jasik M, Piatek A, Garlicki A. Ebola virus disease – pathogenesis, clinical presentation and management. Folia Med Cracov. 2014; 54 :3:49–55.

Section 6

RNA Interference in Pest and Pathogen Control

Chapter 17

RNAi — Implications in Entomological Research and Pest Control

Nidhi Thakur, Jaspreet Kaur Mundey and Santosh Kumar Upadhyay

Additional information is available at the end of the chapter

http://dx.doi.org/10.5772/61814

Abstract

RNA interference (RNAi) has progressed swiftly in the past decade to become a convenient and dominant genetic tool that has immense utility in diverse fields. The entomological research, ranging from functional genomics to agriculture, has gained enormous momentum due to this technology. RNAi tool helped to discover the functions of new genes and study the complicated genetic networks, thus providing an evolutionary insight into various processes. RNAi is also becoming a method of choice for controlling insect pest populations. It is envisaged as tailor-made insecticide, which is highly species specific. However, the efficiency of this mechanism is limited by various factors such as the stability of the trigger molecule, the candidate gene selection, delivery system adopted and, most importantly, the choice of the target species. Apart from the successful implication in diverse areas, there are certain drawbacks of this technology such as 'off-target' effects, lack of sensitivity of various species, etc. Further research would relieve these limitations and support the manifestation of this genetic tool with much more reliability.

Keywords: RNAi, insects, pest management, efficiency of RNAi

1. Introduction

RNA interference (RNAi) is a highly conserved, sequence-specific mechanism of gene silencing which is triggered by the presence of double-stranded RNA (dsRNA). Since its discovery in 1998, RNAi has attained the status of a powerful genetic tool [1]. This reverse genetics technique is now immensely used in biomedical research, functional genetics and many other areas of biological research. Broadly, all the reactions that take place for RNA silencing are initiated when a long dsRNA is processed into small dsRNAs of about 21 to 24 bp by the RNaseIII enzyme, called Dicer. These small dsRNAs are called small interfering RNA (siRNA), which when unwound using ATP-dependent activity are incorporated into the multi-subunit RNA-induced silencing complex (RISC). Here, the siRNA guides the RISC complex to degrade cellular RNA molecules that are complementary to its sequence [2]. Earlier this process was described in the experimental RNAi studies, and now it is the most accepted tool for gene knockdown studies.

The advent of RNAi also revolutionised the entomological research, as novel gene functions were efficiently discovered. In 1998, Kennerdell and Carthew were the first to use RNAi *in vivo* to study the genes *Frizzled* and *Frizzled-2* in *Drosophila melanogaster* [3]. The tremendous success of RNAi in model organisms has prompted its use for research in other insect species as well. In genomics and post-genomics era with the availability of a large amount of sequence information, RNAi further provides an opportunity to investigate the vital functions and crucial interactions that are of importance in both biomedical research and agriculture [4–6]. RNAi studies on insects of economic importance would provide new insights into unravelling the molecular interactions between various disease vectors and ultimately helping in the discovery of novel vaccine and drug targets. Disease vectors such as mosquito, ticks, mites, lice and others were studied extensively using RNAi [7]. These insects cause many serious diseases in humans and animals.

Among other applications, this genetic tool is also gaining popularity as a promising technology in controlling a wide array of agricultural pests. There is a substantial amount of literature available which documents the success of RNAi as a feasible and sustainable strategy in managing the agricultural pests [8–11]. The core RNAi machinery being present in all the insects makes it possible to silence a wide variety of target genes to produce diverse physiological, developmental and reproductive restrains. The sequence specificity of endogenous RNAi pathway allows the targeted suppression of genes essential for insect survival and thus offers the development of a specific, logical and sustainable strategy to combat against insect pests.

Agricultural pests are notorious and they cannot be efficiently managed by employing a single control agent or technique. Most commonly, the integrated pest management (IPM) strategies are utilised for combating the diversity of insect pests in the agro-ecosystem [12]. Along with mechanical, cultural, biological and chemical methods, the transgenic technology should also be embraced in the IPM regime. In this regard, RNAi can play an important role along with the available insecticidal molecules. Among various transgenic approaches to manage insect pests, *Bacillus thuringiensis* (Bt) toxin has shown spectacular success [13]; however, many important insect pests (primarily sap-sucking pests) are not amenable to Bt protection [14]. RNAi can be harnessed to defend crops against insect pests. Successful application of RNAi technology in agricultural pest management requires (i) suitable candidate gene where its silencing can cause mortality of the insect and (ii) an effective method of dsRNA delivery. Nevertheless, prior to field application, many aspects of this multi-faceted technology including safety and possible risks to environment need to be evaluated in detail.

In this chapter, we discussed the potential of this technology in gene silencing experiments to study the gene function as well as on opportunity to combat against agricultural pests and other disease vectors. Further, the factors responsible for a successful RNAi experiment, the link with immune response and viral infections have been discussed, highlighting the possible shortcomings of this strategy.

2. RNAi in insects

RNAi offers species-specific molecules that can be flexibly manipulated and used in understanding various complicated biochemical pathways. The research application of RNAi in entomology has elucidated the functions of several genes. Decrease in the mRNA levels of a candidate gene due to introduction of a complementary dsRNA fragment, and the study of the corresponding phenotype, illuminates a gene function. RNAi has been used to study various mechanisms related to insect development (embryonic and post-embryonic), reproduction, behaviour and other complicated biosynthetic pathways [15].

Various insect orders have demonstrated amenability to RNAi-mediated silencing. Species of orders Coleoptera, Lepidoptera, Diptera, Hemiptera, Orthoptera, Blattodea and Hymenoptera have been studied for various aspects using RNAi technique [15]. The silencing efficiency ranges from 0% to 100% in different insects. A large majority of the target genes were gut-specific genes; however, genes from salivary glands, brain and antennae have also been targeted [16]. RNAi-based studies can be carried out by either *in vivo* or *in vitro* studies. The former method is much easier and involves incubating the cells with the dsRNA added to the medium. However, the *in vivo* approach is more useful in the field of functional genomics, especially in case of non-model organisms. Here, the dsRNA dosage and developmental stage of insect can be specified. In addition, RNAi can be very helpful in identifying the mutant genes that are fatal to the organism,. The significance and compilation of various categories of RNAi experiments in entomology are summarised in Table 1 [17–45].

Experiments	Insect	Gene and function
RNAi in developmental biology		
Parental RNAi	*Tribolium castaneum*	Zygotic genes [16]
Parental RNAi is an important method for analysing early embryogenesis. It is crucial for many insects whose eggs are not accessible or do not survive after microinjection.	*Oncopeltus fasciatus*	Determination of the role of the gap genes, *hunchback* and *Krüppel* [17,18]
	Gryllus bimaculatus	Antenna and appendages [19], *hedgehog*, *wingless* and *dpp* in the initiation of proximodistal axis formation during the regeneration of insect legs [20]
	Nasonia vitripennis	Various genes in demonstration of parental RNAi [21]
	Tetranychus urticae	*Distal-less* was used, resulting in phenotypes with canonical limb truncation as well as the fusion of leg segments [22]
Embryonic RNAi	*T. castaneum*	Role of *wingless* (*wg*) in leg development [23]

Experiments	Insect	Gene and function
	N. vitripennis	Role of *bicoid* gene in the structural pattern of the anterior body region. Also in the absence of *bicoid* gene, *orthodenticle, hunchback* and *giant* genes are responsible for proper head and thorax formation [24]
	Oplegnathus. fasciatus	*Hox* genes and genes involved in segmentation and segment specification [25]
Larval/nymphal/pupal RNAi	*T. castaneum* (larval RNAi)	To study the molecular basis of adult morphological diversity in various organs [26]
	T. castaneum (larval RNAi)	*Ubx/Utx* during hindwing/elytron development [27]
	T. castaneum (larval RNAi)	*Laccase* 2 [28]
	Bombyx mori (pupal RNAi)	Fatty acid transport protein (Bm'FATP) [29]
	Schistocerca Americana (Nymphal RNAi)	The eye colour gene of first-instar nymphs triggered a suppression of ommochrome formation in the eye [30]
	S. Americana	Importance of early retinal genes *eyes absent (eya)* or *sine oculis (so)* in eye development [31]
	Blattella germanica (nymphal RNAi)	RXR/USP, along with EcR, of the heterodimeric nuclear receptor of 20-hydroxyecdysone (20E) [32]
	G. bimaculatus	Mechanisms of leg regeneration [33]
	G. bimaculatus	*period* (*per*)gene for circadian-dependent locomotor activity rhythm [34]
	G. bimaculatus	Genes responsible for certain human disorders: *fragile X mental retardation 1* (*fmr1*) and *Dopamine receptor* (*DopR*) [35]
Regeneration-dependent RNAi	*G. bimaculatus*	Insect leg regeneration [36]
	G. bimaculatus	Orthologs of *Drosophila hedgehog* (*Gb'hh*), *wingless* (*Gb'wg*) and *decapentaplegic* (*Gb'dpp*) are expressed during leg regeneration and play essential roles in the establishment of the proximal–distal axis [37]
RNAi in behavioural biology	*Rhodnius prolixus*	Nitrophorin 2 a decrease of anticoagulant activity and less efficient feeding behaviour [38]
	Anopheles gambiae	Apyrase AgApy in the salivary glands shows important role in host probing behaviour [39]
	D. melanogaster	3-Hydroxy-3-methylglutaryl CoA reductase has been identified for the control of

Experiments	Insect	Gene and function
		sexual dimorphism of locomotor activity in [40]]
	B. germanica	Neuropeptide pigment dispersing factor in the regulation of locomotor circadian rhythms [41]
Mechanism of insecticidal action	Mosquitoes	NADPH cytochrome P450 reductase led to increased sensitivity of mosquitoes to pyrethroids [42]
	Spodoptera litura and *Helicoverpa armigera*	Aminopeptidase M led to decreased sensitivity to BT toxin [43]
Understanding the biosynthetic pathway	*T. castaneum*	Chitin synthases *CHS1* and *CHS2* are crucialexoskeleton and the midgut peritrophic matrix [28]
	Bombyx mori	*Bombykol* is the main component of sexual pheromone, as well as pheromone-binding proteins and the receptor of the pheromone biosynthesis activator neuropeptide [44]
	Epiphyas postvittana	Silencing of pheromone-binding protein of the antennae [45]

Table 1. RNAi in the study of gene function in insects.

Apart from deciphering the function of genes involved in various metabolic pathways, RNAi also finds relevance in other aspects of insect science. It is quite beneficial in maintaining the beneficial insects and saving them from various parasites and pathogens. Certainly, this is useful in case of those parasites and pathogens, which have operative RNAi machinery. A successful study in this regard shows the control of honey bee parasite *Nosema ceranae.* When the gene related to energy metabolism was silenced, it was observed that the honey bee population had reduced infestation of *Nosema,* and lower mortality [46]. In another study, multiple genes of an ectoparasite of honey bee *Varroa destructor* were targeted [47]. It poses a great threat to the health of bees, and its control is of utmost importance for the rearing industry. It is a blood-sucking parasite, so the bees were fed on a meal containing dsRNA against the genes of *Varroa.* The RNAi-mediated control decreased the mite population by 50%, causing no evident damage to the bees. RNAi has also been useful in elucidating the importance of various immunological pathways in *D. melanogaster* [48]. Host–parasite relationships such as that of *Anopheles–Plasmodium* have also been studied by using RNAi. Early research was conducted on *defensin* and it was shown to be important for protecting mosquitoes against infections of Gram-positive bacteria [49]. Later, the same group demonstrated how the development of Plasmodium is affected by *Anopheles gambiae* immune genes [50]. Similarly, in *Manduca sexta* haemocytes, knockdown of haemolin (a bacterial recognition protein) decreased the ability of insects to clear *Escherichia coli* from the haemolymph. This eventually reduced their ability to engulf bacteria and highlighted the role of haemolin in the *M. sexta* immune response [51].

3. RNAi in pest control

Plants are damaged by a plethora of insect pests. The losses due to these pests and expenditure on the chemical pesticides amount to billions of dollars. In an attempt to reduce these losses, many reports have been published which demonstrate the successful application of RNAi technique in crop protection. Huvenne and Smagghe [52] have summarised the reports on insects in which RNAi has been applied through feeding, and they discussed several factors that influence the success of RNAi on target insects, such as the concentration of dsRNA, the nucleotide sequence, the length of the dsRNA fragment and the life stage of the target insects. The downregulation of expression of critical genes, caused by dsRNA/siRNA, eventually leads to death/growth retardation of the insect and forms the basis of pest control. In this view, the efficient delivery and uptake of the dsRNA trigger is of prime importance. In contrast to the study of gene function, pest control strategies cannot depend on injection of the molecule. The deployment of pest controlling siRNA/miRNA molecules would involve oral exposure, either as transgenic plants or as sprays. Most of the nutrients from gut lumen are absorbed in the midgut tissue of the insect; therefore, this tissue is an attractive target for RNAi. After ingestion, the dsRNA enters into the gut lumen of the insect. Insect gut is divided into foregut, midgut and hindgut. While both foregut and hindgut are covered with chitin, it is only the midgut that has exposed cell surfaces. It is the site of nutrient exchange between the haemolymph and the gut contents. Therefore, midgut epithelium is an attractive target as it is the primary tissue exposed to dsRNA in the gut lumen. The stability of dsRNA molecule and the efficiency of the silencing process (discussed in section 5) is determined by the gut pH and nucleases.

A breakthrough research in RNAi-mediated pest control was published in 2007 on the western corn rootworm, *Diabrotica virgifera virgifera* (WCRW) [53], and cotton bollworm *Helicoverpa armigera* (CBW) [54]. In the former study, a candidate gene was screened based on the complete cDNA library. Out of a total of 290 dsRNAs, *Vacoular ATPase (V-ATPase)* subunit A was finally selected for the development of transgenic corn plants. The larvae reared on transformed plants caused much less damage to the roots and also showed the reduced expression of the target gene. The other study of Mao et al. [9] targeted the pesticide detoxifying gene *Cytochrome P450* (*CYP6AE14*), which provides gossypol tolerance to the insect. Transgenic plants expressing dsRNA corresponding to *CYP6AE14* levels of this transcript in insect body was decreased and the larval growth was retarded. Following these two studies, many research groups started to consider RNAi as a feasible technique which could be employed in the transgenic approaches to manage insects. As we know from the various studies conducted, the Bt (*Bacillus thuringiensis*) toxins are effective on lepidopteran and coleopteran pests but fail to work against hemipteran pests like aphids, whiteflies, phyllids, etc. [55–58].

RNAi-engineered plants can be more useful in case of these phloem-feeding hemipteran pests, which are notorious not only because of feeding damages but also because of their ability to transmit plant viruses [59]. The midgut genes of *Nilaparvata lugens* were downregulated by feeding on transgenic rice expressing dsRNA against three separate genes, but no lethal phenotype was detected in this case [60]. Pitino et al. [61] demonstrated RNAi in aphid *Myzus persicae* directed towards the receptor of activated kinase (*Rack-1*) gene by transgenic expression in *Arabidopsis thaliana*. Another important pest, the whitefly, is also now amenable to RNAi [62]. Its control was demonstrated both by feeding on artificial diet and by feeding on transgenic tobacco plants expressing dsRNA of *V-ATPase A* gene [11, 63]. RNAi experiments conducted on agricultural pests as well as on insect vectors of several human diseases are summarised in Table 2 [53–118].

Insect pests	Mode of delivery	Gene target
		Order Coleopteran
Diabrotica virgifera virgifera	Artificial diet and transgenic plant	*a*-Tubulin, vacuolar ATPase subunit A [53]
Phyllotreta striolata	Plant tissue	Arginine kinase [64]
Leptinotarsa decemlineata	Artificial diet	Vacuolar ATPase subunit A and E [53]
Diabrotica undecimpunctata howardi	Artificial diet	Vacuolar ATPase subunit A and E, *a*-tubulin [53]
Monochamus alternates	Injection	*Laccase* gene [65]
		Order Diptera
Aedes aegypti	Blood meal Artificial diet Feeding	Inverted repeat (IR) RNA derived from the premembrane protein coding region of the DENV-2 RNA genome [66] V-ATPase A [67] ATP-dependent efflux pump [68]
Anopheles gambiae	Feeding	Chitin synthase [69]
Glossina morsitans morsitans	Feeding	Midgut protein Tsetse EP; transferrin [70]
Bactrocera dorsalis	Feeding and injection	Rpl19; V-ATPase D subunit; fatty acid elongase Noa; small GTPase Rab11 [71]
		Order Hemiptera
Acyrthosiphon pisum	Injection Feeding	Calreticulin, cathepsin-L [72] C002 [73] Hunchback [74] V-ATPase [75] aquaporin [76]
Cimex lectularius	Injection	Cpr gene[77]
Diaphorina citri	Topical In planta (virus induced)	Abnormal wing disc [78] Abnormal wing disc [79]
Laodelphax striatellus	Feeding	Disembodied [80]
Rhodnius prolixus	Injection	Nitrophorins1–4 [81] *a*-Glucosidase [82] Gap gene giant [83] Phospholipase A2 [84]

Insect pests	Mode of delivery	Gene target
Sitobion avenae	Feeding In planta	Catalase [85] CbE E4 [86]
Lygus lineolaris	Injection Injection	Inhibitor of apoptosis gene (IAP) [87] Polygalacturonase (PG) [88]
Oncopeltus fasciatus	Injection	Hunchback [89]
Riptortus pedestris	Injection Injection and feeding	Circadian clock gene, mammalian-type cryptochrome; Bla [90] Gland nitrophorin 2 (*NP2*) [91]
Nilaparvata lugens	Feeding and transgenic Feeding Feeding and injection	Hexose transporter; carboxypeptidase; trypsin-like serine protease [92] ATP synthase subunit [93] Trehalose phosphate synthase [94] Cathepsin B-like protease; nicotinic acetylcholine receptors [95]
Myzus persicae	Transgenic plant	*MpC002* and *Rack-1* [96]
Bemisia tabaci	Injection Artificial diet Transgenic plant	Snap, Chickadee, CG5885, GATAd [62] Actin; ADP/ATP translocase; α-tubulin; ribosomal protein L9; V-ATPase [63] V-ATPase subunit A [11]
Bactericerca cockerelli	Injection/feeding	Actin, V-ATPase [97]
	Order Hymenoptera	
Athalia rosae	Injection	*Ar white gene*
	Order Isoptera	
Reticulitermes flavipes	Feeding	Endogenous digestive cellulase enzyme, hexamerin storage protein [98]
	Order Lepidoptera	
Ostrinia furnacalis	Spraying	LIM protein 1; myosin 3 light chain; chymotrypsin-like serine protease; chymotrypsin-like protease C1; chymortypsin-like serine protease C3; hydroxybutyrate dehydrogenase; Kazal-type serine proteinase inhibitor 1; fatty acid binding protein 1; unknown; caboxypeptidse 4 [99]
Ostrinia nubilalis	Spraying	Chitinase (*OnCht*); chitin synthase (*OnCHS2*) [100]
Epiphyas postvittana	Feeding	Carboxylesterase gene (*EposCXE1*); pheromone binding protein [101]

Insect pests	Mode of delivery	Gene target
Helicoverpa armigera	Feeding Transgenic plant Transgenic plant Feeding and transgenic plant	Acetylcholinesterase (*AChE*) [102] Cytochrome P450; gluthatione-S-transferase[9, 103] Ecdysone receptor EcR [104] HaHR3 moulting factor [105]
Hyalophora cecropia	Injection	*Haemolin* [106]
Manduca sexta	Injection	*Cadherin* [107]
Spodoptera litura	Injection	Vitellogenin receptor [108]
Spodoptera exigua	Feeding	Chitin synthase gene A [109]
Spodoptera littoralis	Injection	*β*-Actin gene [110]
Spodoptera frugiperda	Allatostatin C; allototropin 2; cytochrome	Feeding [111]
Plutella xylostella	Feeding	Rieske iron–sulphur protein (RISP) [112]
	Order Orthtoptera	
Gryllus bimaculatus	Injection Injection Injection Injection Injection	Delta; Notch [113] Insulin receptor; insulin receptor substrate; phosphatase and tensin homolog; target of rapamycin; PRS6-p70-protein kinase; forkhead box O; epidermal growth factor receptor [114] Nitric oxide synthase gene *NOS* [115] Circadian clock gene *per* [116] Sulfakinins [117]
Schistocerca americana		Eye colour gene vermilion [118]

Table 2. Different insect pests targeted by RNAi.

The choice of a suitable target gene is central to pest control strategy. The gene selection approaches can be based on choosing the gene with known function such as detoxification enzymes, cell synthesis, nutrition, metabolism and cytoskeleton structure. These types of genes can be selected as insect pest control targets. For this, expressed sequence tag (EST) library of European corn borer (*Ostrinia nubilalis*) was screened to find out that a *chitinase* gene (*OnCht*) and a *chitin synthase* gene (*OnCHS2*), which are very important in regulating the growth and development of this insect [119]. Likewise, the EST library of *Bemisia tabaci* was also used to screen out few important genes for RNAi-mediated control [63]. The cDNA library screening approach was also used. Mao et al. [9] constructed a cDNA library from RNAs expressed in the midgut of fifth-instar larvae exposed to gossypol. Several cDNA libraries of WCR (*D. virgifera virgifera*) were prepared and considered upon the underlying principle that genes encoding proteins with essential functions would be the best RNAi targets for causing lethality [8].

As an extension of the cDNA library screening approach, the next-generation sequencing (NGS) technologies have led to novel opportunities for expression profiling in organisms lacking any genome or transcriptome sequence information. It enables the direct sequencing of cDNA generated from mRNA (RNA-seq) [120, 121]. Hence, it provides the *de novo* generation of the transcriptome for a non-model organism, including various pests. Wang et al. [99] adopted Illumina's RNA-seq and digital gene expression tag profile (DGE-tag) to screen optimal RNAi targets from Asian corn borer (ACB; *Ostrinia furnacalis*). The same technique has been used for the grain aphid, *Sitobion avenae* and *Spodoptera litura* [122, 123]. It seems likely that the combination of DGE-tag with RNA-seq is a rapid, high-throughput, cost-effective and easy way to select for candidate target genes for RNAi, which may not be only limited to the midgut tissue but can also be selected from the whole insect.

The convenience of RNAi to target specific pests while not harming other species is a perfect method of pest management. However, target gene selection and efficient delivery methods are the two major cornerstones of pest management by RNAi. The candidate gene for RNAi can be tailored to be species specific or they can also have a broad spectrum. Specificity can be achieved by designing dsRNAs that target the more variable regions of genes, such as untranslated regions (UTRs). It was first demonstrated in *Drosophila* where UTR of the *gamma-tubulin* gene was targeted and even closely related species could be targeted selectively [75]. However, it can also be possible to target multiple organisms with a single gene. One such example is of *V-ATPase* gene, which is an effective target in *B. tabaci*, *D. virgifera* and *B. dorsalis* [8, 63, 124]; all of these insects belong to different orders. In this case, either a conserved region can be selected which could affect closely related species or a mixture of dsRNA fragments from different genes belonging to different species can be selected.

Delivery methods that ensure continuous supply of dsRNA/siRNA will be applicable in the fields. A more reliable and verified method would be transgenic plants as the dsRNA can be applied as bait, sprays, or supplied through irrigation systems [125, 126]. The application approach by spray could be quite practical like the spray of chemical pesticides. Gan et al. [127] have also demonstrated the control of viral infection using dsRNA spraying. Similar results were obtained with Asian corn borer, *Ostrinia furnacalis*. This study showed that larval lethality or developmental disorders can be achieved by gene-specific RNAi, and spraying can be an efficient method for continuous supply of dsRNA [99]. The coating of dsRNA molecule with liposomes is used for delivering siRNA to mammalian cells, specific tissues and some insects [128, 75]. This coating prevents the degradation of the molecule and enhances its uptake ability; spraying may also be explored for such particles. Zhang et al. [129] used the chitosan nanoparticle based RNAi technology to suppress the expression of two chitin synthase genes (*AgCHS1* and *AgCHS2*) in African malaria mosquito (*A. gambiae*) larvae. Bacterial expression or chemical synthesis allows large-scale production of dsRNA at efficient costs [75, 130, 131].

4. RNAi: Link with immunity and viral infections

The RNAi mechanisms evolved primarily as a defence mechanism against viruses and transposons [132]. Research has established that RNAi pathway also contributes to the innate immunity of the insects against the viruses having either dsRNA genome or such replicative intermediates. It was demonstrated that the *Drosophila* S2 cells utilise the endocytosis-mediated pathway involving the pattern recognition scavenger receptors for the uptake of dsRNA from the surroundings. These receptors are key players in the innate immune responses of the cell [133, 134]. Saleh et al. [135] demonstrated the strong link of dsRNA uptake pathway and the activation of the immune response in the infected cells. The normal cells used dsRNA uptake pathway to internalise viral dsRNA and subsequently showed manifestation of antiviral response in these cells. On the contrary, the mutant cells (defective genes used for dsRNA uptake) did not show activation of any antiviral response. Mutants in the core siRNA components Dicer-2, AGO-2 and R2D2 are more susceptible to viral infections [140].

Further, it was also reported that receptors such as Sr-CI and Eater, which contribute to majority of dsRNA uptake in the *Drosophila* S2 cells, were significantly down-regulated after pathogenic virus treatments, and significant changes in phagocytic activity were observed. The role of RNAi in antiviral defence has also been firmly established in mosquitoes [136]. Viruses can also affect the availability of RNAi machinery for other candidate dsRNA molecules. They can saturate the RNAi machinery and affect the efficiency of RNAi mechanism. Many viruses are known to produce viral suppressors of RNA silencing (VSRs), which bind to the key elements of the RNAi pathway rendering it unavailable. Many of the viral proteins (viz. B2 protein from Flockhouse virus, 1A proteins from *Drosophila* C virus and cricket paralysis virus) are known to interfere in the siRNA pathway of RNA-mediated silencing [137–140]. These viral proteins may affect the biogenesis of the trigger molecule by binding to important enzymes such as dicer, which generate the siRNA from long dsRNA or affect the target cleavage by binding to RISC. The viral proteins may also sequester the dsRNA signal molecule or form complexes with the replicative intermediates of the siRNA pathway.

Viruses also produce large amount of RNAs and small RNAs that accumulate in the infected cells. It has also been hypothesised that the occurrence of alternative and effective antiviral pathway may become important in controlling the viral infections and may supersede the RNAi pathway. Few of these possible pathways have been worked upon. Goic et al. [141] have reported the potential interaction of nucleic acid-based acquired immunity with the core RNAi machinery in the study of persistent infection of S2 cells by Flock House Virus (FHV). The insects also protect themselves from foreign nucleic acids by becoming refractory to RNAi. In the oriental fruit fly, *Bactrocera dorsalis*, orally administered dsRNA-targeting endogenous genes, resistance to RNAi was seen due to a blockade in the dsRNA uptake pathway. A very interesting hypothesis is presented by Swevers et al. [142] about the possible impact of persistent viral infection in the insects. In their work, the authors have analysed various factors that determine the response to exogenous dsRNA in the background of viral infection.

5. Efficiency of RNAi

Though RNAi is a conserved mechanism in eukaryotes, its efficiency is governed by various factors. The response of different insect species towards this mechanism of gene silencing is imperative for successful implementation in the study of gene function and more importantly in the pest management programs. Also, the efficacy is governed by many factors which are not intrinsic to the organism such as the delivery, dosage and choice of the candidate gene. Comprehending these factors will provide a better insight into designing the experiments for successful application of RNAi. The available reports indicate that the lower *Insecta* species such as that of *Blatella* show a much robust and persistent RNAi response, while higher *Insecta* species belonging to the orders Lepidoptera and Diptera are non-compliant [15]. The sensitivity could vary within and among the orders. For instance, many Lepidopteran insects are resistant to RNAi. Terenius et al. [143] have reviewed various factors that may be contributing to the poor responsiveness of these insects. The efficiency can vary with insect species, target gene, developmental stage of the organism, expression of RNAi machinery, method of delivery, stability of dsRNA, etc. A few factors that may be crucial in determining the efficiency of RNAi are discussed below.

5.1. The RNAi machinery

RNAi evolved in organisms as a defence mechanism against viral infections at the cellular level [144, 145]. The differences in the expression of core RNAi machinery can be a prime reason affecting the adequacy of RNAi mechanism. The systemic RNA-interference-deficient 1 (sid-1) protein forms a gated channel which is selective for dsRNA molecule. Its role is well established in the systemic spread of the RNAi signal in the model organism *Caenorhabditis elegans* [146]. The presence of *SID-1*gene orthologs in insects varies with the insect orders [52]. The dipterans lack this gene completely. The mosquito *Culex quinquefasciatus* also lacks sid-1 ortholog but shows the systemic spread of the dsRNA trigger [147]. On the one hand, honey bee (*Apis mellifera*) showed an increase in the expression of *SID-1* during the RNAi experiments, indicating its role in the uptake pathway [148]. On the other hand, in *Tribolium castaneum*, the silencing of all three orthologs of *SID-1* casted no influence on the efficiency of RNAi [149].

In *Bombyx mori*, three orthologs are present but no significant success has been found in this lepidopteran, while mosquitoes show systemic RNAi despite the absence of *sid-1* in several species [149–152]. R2D2, a cofactor of dicer-2 enzyme which cleaves long dsRNA into siRNA for loading into the RISC, is absent in *B. mori* making the insect very insensitive to RNAi. Another important enzyme RNA-dependent RNA polymerase (RdRP), which amplifies the primary siRNA signal in *C. elegans*, is entirely not reported in the insects [149]. *T. castaneum* showed a robust systemic RNAi, but a wide survey of RNAi related genes did not show any traces of RdRP [149]. However, RdRP-like activity was substituted in *Drosophila* cell lines by certain other enzymatic pathways. In many cases, the absence of certain well-known genes of the RNAi pathway is directly responsible for the poor response of the organism while in several other examples, the absence is compensated by other genes/pathways which play key roles of their counterparts.

5.2. The RNAi molecule

The exogenous dsRNA molecule is the trigger for initiating the RNAi pathway. These molecules are delivered in the form of dsRNA, siRNA or hairpin RNA. Apart from sequence specificity, other parameters are also crucial in determining the efficiency of RNAi experiments. The study on the administration of dsRNA (feeding by means of artificial diet, natural diet, droplet method, blood meal, transgenic plants, etc.) in insects has used varied length of dsRNA molecule. The nucleotide length used in these reports ranges from 134 to 1842 bp, while most of the studies used 300–500 bp as the optimal length [153]. However, silencing effects have also been observed in the case of single siRNA synthesised chemically (administration in *H. armigera*) or a cocktail of siRNA (obtained by using dicer enzyme to chop the dsRNA molecule) [154]. In the cell line experiments done on the *Drosophila* S2 cell line, 211 bp was found to be the optimum length of dsRNA that could be absorbed by the cells [135]. Not only the length but also the specificity of the RNAi molecule is a concern. It can be understood by the reports on *Drosophila* that feeding specific sequence of *V-ATPase* dsRNA caused no silencing in non-target species [75], which implies the specificity of the process. On the contrary, various other studies report non-specific silencing. Off-target effects were reported in *Rhodnius prolixus* [81] and Colorado potato beetle (*Leptinotarsa decemlineata*) [8]. Single mismatches are known to impair the RNAi effect in the mammalian cell lines [155]. Further studies will clarify whether single mismatches show similar impact in insects as well. In case of pest management programs, long dsRNAs (>200 bp) are generally used which generate many probable siRNA maximising the RNAi response [153]. The dosage of the dsRNA molecule also plays an important role in determining the efficiency of the process. Higher doses are required in case of feeding experiments as compared to injection. The silencing effect in *R. prolixus* was enhanced by multiple doses [38]. Therefore, it follows that doses and types of administration (oral or injectable) also need to be optimised according to the life stage of the organism and the target tissue.

5.3. Delivery of the molecule/uptake of silencing signal

One of the most decisive factors for inducing RNAi is the efficient delivery of the dsRNA molecule. The common methods of delivery are by microinjection, soaking, oral delivery and transgenic technique [156]. Microinjection-based delivery is the most commonly used technique in studying gene functions. It has proven to work well for *Tribolium, Drosophila* and many other lepidopteran insects. Although it works well for larger insects, success with smaller insects is limited due to the invasive nature of this technique. The survival of aphids after microinjection procedure is highly dependent on the injected volume [157].

Further, factors such as needle choice, optimal volume and place of injection are very crucial considerations and tend to vary with organisms and laboratories. Feeding-based experiments involve either *in vitro* synthesised or bacterially expressed dsRNA molecules. The success of oral delivery methods indicates the possible employment of RNAi technique for target pest control. However, the stability of the molecule will always be a concern in the gut lumen. Artificial diet mixed with dsRNA could not induce RNAi in *Drosophila* spp. Ingested dsRNA against a gut-specific *aminopeptidase N* gene also failed to develop RNAi response in *Spodoptera litura* [43]. Therefore, it can be suggested that oral delivery is not equally suitable for all species. Another convenient method of delivery is soaking. Nevertheless, this method is more applicable for cell line experiments rather than whole insects.

After the delivery of the molecules, the next step is the uptake of the molecules by insects. Huvenne and Smagghe [52] have elaborately reviewed the basic mechanisms involved in the uptake of dsRNA in the insects. The spreading of the RNAi signal, i.e., systemic RNAi, is an important determinant of the efficiency of RNAi. In cases of functional genetics, cell autonomous RNAi has been successfully employed to study the function of genes; however, for implementation in the pest control programs, non-cell autonomous RNAi is important. The systemic spread of the silencing signal is absent in the most studied model insect *Drosophila*. In contrast, the most studied insect *Tribolium* shows a powerful systemic silencing effect [149].

5.4. Potency of the silencing signal

The manifestation of the RNAi effect also depends on the stability and persistence of the dsRNA molecule. In *Acyrthosiphon pisum*, the silencing effect on the aquaporin gene began to reduce after five days [157]. The early stability of dsRNA molecule may be disrupted by the non-specific nucleases as reported in many of the lepidopteran insects [143]. These are extracellular enzymes different from dicer and digest the trigger molecule, thereby preventing the RNAi cascade. In certain cases, the activity of dsRNA degrading enzymes have been studied and their levels were measured in different stages, which was found related to the developmental stage. The dsRNase activity is also found in the digestive juices of *Bombyx mori*, saliva of *Linus lineolaris* and in haemolymph of *Manduca sexta* [87, 158, 159]. The existence/stability/mode of action of these enzymes are not sufficiently studied and future research in this direction needs to be carried out to comprehend the stability of dsRNA molecule in the *in vivo* studies. The choice of gene can also decrease the strength of the silencing signal. Ideally, the protein whose function is to be silenced should have a short half-life, whilst the mRNA turnover number should be high. The stability of protein explained the weak RNAi response in both *D. melanogaster* and *T. casteneum* [160]. However, such studies have not been conducted for the majority of the genes and therefore it can be concluded that expression of RNAi is limited by many uncovered phenomena.

6. Conclusions

The advent of RNA interference has been a crucial phase of the modern day science. The wide array of applications in the entomological research has led to many momentous findings. The functionality of many genes has been understood by this technique. Its implication in functional genomics is not only restricted to the study of a given set of genes but is also used to unveil the interaction of different genes in a particular metabolic pathway. The rapid pace of RNAi-based research suggests that it would soon facilitate better understanding of evolution, circadian rhythms, behavioural pattern, reproductive biology and interaction between host and parasites/pathogens. However, successful manifestation of RNAi is dependent on several factors. The insect species might lack the basic RNAi machinery [161] or may rapidly degrade alien dsRNA. Such factors could be intrinsic to the concerned tissue or gene. The gene might have high transcription rate and could evade the effect of RNAi or the target mRNA may be too transient.

As happens with every phenomenon, this mechanism can also undergo selection pressure. Viruliferous insects that also have RNAi suppressors would be able to thrive on RNAi-protected crops. Furthermore, single nucleotide polymorphisms (SNPs) that result in lower effectiveness of the RNAi could potentially be selected for and lead to the evolution of resistance [153]. Genetic variations among insect species are already a challenge for RNAi. Therefore, parallel research must be carried out to develop strategies, which would minimise the resistance development and selective pressures.

RNAi has proved its utility as a futuristic tool of insect pest management. However, there are several issues that need to be addressed before the implementation of this technology in fields. The knowledge gaps underlying large-scale implications of pesticidal RNAi-based crops on the environment should be identified and bridged. The off-target gene silencing is a serious concern where unintended organisms are adversely affected [162]. The non-target effects can be categorised as off-target gene silencing, silencing the target gene in non-target organisms, immune stimulation and saturation of the RNAi machinery [163]. A balanced approach should be taken with maximum effects on the target pests with minimal effects on non-target organisms.

Acknowledgements

SKU is thankful to the Department of Science and Technology, India, for DST-INSPIRE faculty fellowship and Panjab University for facility.

Author details

Nidhi Thakur[1,2], Jaspreet Kaur Mundey[3] and Santosh Kumar Upadhyay[3*]

*Address all correspondence to: skupadhyay@pu.ac.in

1 Plant Molecular Biology Lab, CSIR-National Botanical Research Institute, Lucknow, India

2 Academy of Scientific and Innovative Research, Anusandhan Bhawan, New Delhi, India

3 Department of Botany, Panjab University, Chandigarh, India

References

[1] Fire A, Xu S, Montgomery MK, Kostas SA, Driver SE, Mello CC. Potent and specific genetic interference by double-stranded RNA in Caenorhabditis elegans. *Nature* 1998:391, 806–811. DOI:10.1038/35888.

[2] Meister G, Tuschl T. Mechanisms of gene silencing by double-stranded RNA. *Nature* 2004:431(7006), 343–349. DOI:10.1038/nature02873.

[3] Kennerdell JR, Carthew RW. Use of dsRNA-mediated genetic interference to demonstrate that frizzled and frizzled 2 act in the wingless pathway. *Cell* 1998:95(7), 1017–1026. DOI: http://dx.doi.org/10.1016/S0092-8674(00)81725-0.

[4] Angaji SA, Hedayati SS, Poor RH, Madani S, Poor SS, Panahi S. Application of RNA interference in treating human diseases. *Journal of Genetics* 2010:89(4), 527–537.

[5] Ambesajir A, Kaushik A, Kaushik J, Petros S. RNA interference: A futuristic tool and its therapeutic applications. *Saudi Journal of Biological Sciences* 2012:19, 395–403. DOI: 10.1016/j.sjbs.2012.08.001.

[6] Younis A, Siddique MI, Kim C, Lim K. RNA interference (RNAi) induced gene silencing: A promising approach of hi-tech plant breeding. *International Journal of Biological Science* 2014:10(10), 1150–1158. DOI: 10.7150/ijbs.10452.

[7] Gu L, Knipple DC. Recent advances in RNA interference research in insects: Implications for future insect pest management strategies. *Crop Protection* 2013:45, 36–40. DOI:10.1016/j.cropro.2012.10.004.

[8] Baum JA, Bogaert T, Clinton W, Heck GR, Feldmann P, Ilagan O et al. Control of coleopteran insect pests through RNA interference. *Nature Biotechnology* 2007:25(11), 1322–1326. DOI: 10.1038/nbt1359.

[9] Mao YB, Cai WJ, Wang JW, Hong GJ, Tao XY, Wang LJ, Huang YP, Chen XY. Silencing a cotton bollworm P450 monooxygenase gene by plant-mediated RNAi impairs larval tolerance of gossypol. *Nature Biotechnology* 2007:25(11), 1307–1313. DOI: 10.1038/nbt1352.

[10] Chen J, Zhang D, Yao Q, Zhang J, Dong X, Tian H et al. Feeding-based RNA interference of a trehalose phosphate synthase gene in the brown planthopper, *Nilaparvata lugens*. *Insect Molecular Biology* 2010:19(6), 777–786. DOI:10.1111/j.1365-2583.2010.01038.x.

[11] Thakur N, Upadhyay SK, Verma PC, Chandrashekar K, Tuli R, Singh PK. Enhanced whitefly resistance in transgenic tobacco plants expressing double stranded RNA of v-ATPase a gene. *PLoS One* 2014:9(3), e87235. DOI: 10.1371/journal.pone.0087235.

[12] Saini RK, Yadav GS, Kumari B. Novel approaches in pest and pesticide management in agro-ecosystem. http://hau.ernet.in/coa/pdf/ento4789.pdf

[13] Sanahuja G, Banakar R, Twyman RM, Capell T, Christou P. *Bacillus thuringiensis*: A century of research, development and commercial applications. *Journal of Plant Biotechnology* 2011:9, 283–300. DOI: 10.1111/j.1467-7652.2011.00595.x.

[14] Bergé JB, Ricroch AE. Emergence of minor pests becoming major pests in GE cotton in China: What are the reasons? What are the alternatives practices to this change of status? *GM Crops* 2010:1, 214–219. DOI: 10.4161/gmcr.1.4.13421.

[15] Bellés X. Beyond drosophila: RNAi in vivo and functional genomics in insects. *Annual Review of Entomology* 2010:55, 111–128. DOI: 10.1146/annurev-ento-112408-085301.

[16] Bucher G, Scholten J, Klingler M. Parental RNAi in *Tribolium* (Coleoptera). *Current Biology* 2002:12, R85–R86. DOI: http://dx.doi.org/10.1016/S0960-9822(02)00666-8.

[17] Liu PZ, Kaufman TC. Hunchback is required for suppression of abdominal identity, and for proper germband growth and segmentation in the intermediate germband insect Oncopeltus fasciatus. *Development* 2004a:131, 1515–1527. DOI: 10.1242/dev.01046.

[18] Liu PZ, Kaufman TC. Kruppel is a gap gene in the intermediate germband insect Oncopeltus fasciatus and is required for development of both blastoderm and germband-derived segments. *Development* 2004b:131, 4567–4579. DOI: 10.1242/dev.01311.

[19] Ronco M, Uda T, Mito T, Minelli A, Noji S, Klingler M. Antenna and all gnathal appendages are similarly transformed by homothorax knock-down in the cricket *Gryllusbimaculatus. Developmental Biology* 2008:313, 80–92. DOI:10.1016/j.ydbio.2007.09.059.

[20] Mito T, Inoue Y, Kimura S, Miyawaki K, Niwa N, Shinmyo Y et al. Involvement of *hedgehog, wingless*, and *dpp* in the initiation of proximodistal axis formation during the regeneration of insect legs, a verification of the modified boundary model. *Mechanisms of Development* 2002:114, 27–35. DOI:10.1016/S0925-4773(02)00052-7.

[21] Lynch JA, Desplan C. A method for parental RNA interference in the wasp Nasonia vitripennis. *Nature Protocols* 2006:1, 486–494. DOI:10.1038/nprot.2006.70.

[22] Khila A, Grbic M. Gene silencing in the spider mite Tetranychus urticae: dsRNA and siRNA parental silencing of the Distal-less gene. *Development Genes and Evolution* 2007:217, 241–251.

[23] Grossmann D, Scholten J, Prpic NM. Separable functions of wingless in distal and ventral patterning of the *Tribolium* leg. *Development Genes and Evolution* 2009:219, 469–479. DOI: 10.1007/s00427-009-0310-z.

[24] Brent AE, Yucel G, Small S, Desplan C. Permissive and instructive anterior patterning rely on mRNA localization in the wasp embryo. *Science* 2007:315, 1841–1843. DOI: 10.1126/science.1137528.

[25] Hughes CL, Kaufman TC. RNAi analysis of deformed, proboscipedia and sex combs reduced in the milkweed bug oncopeltus fasciatus: Novel roles for Hox genes in the hemipteran head. *Development* 2000:127, 3683–3694.

[26] Tomoyasu Y, Denell RE. Larval RNAi in *Tribolium* (Coleoptera) for analyzing adult development. *Development Genes and Evolution* 2004:214, 575–578. DOI: 10.1007/s00427-004-0434-0.

[27] Tomoyasu Y, Wheeler SR, Denell RE. *Ultrabithorax* is required for membranous wing identity in the beetle *Tribolium castaneum*. *Nature* 2005:433, 643–647. DOI:10.1038/nature03272.

[28] Arakane Y, Muthukrishnan S, Beeman RW, Kanost MR, Kramer KJ. Laccase 2 is the phenoloxidase gene required for beetle cuticle tanning. *Proceedings of the National Academy of Sciences of the United States of America* 2005:102, 11337–11342. DOI: 10.1073/pnas.0504982102.

[29] Ohnishi A, Hashimoto K, Imai K, Matsumoto S. Functional characterization of the *Bombyx mori* fatty acid transport protein (*Bm*FATP) within the silkmoth pheromone gland. *The Journal of Biological Chemistry* 2009:284, 5128–5136. DOI: 10.1074/jbc.M806072200.

[30] Dong Y, Friedrich M. Nymphal RNAi: Systemic RNAi mediated gene knockdown in juvenile grasshopper. *BMC Biotechnology* 2005:5, 25. DOI: 10.1186/1472-6750-5-25.

[31] Dong Y, Friedrich M. Enforcing biphasic eye development in a directly developing insect by transient knockdown of single eye selector genes. *Journal of Experimental Zoology Part B: Molecular and Developmental Evolution* 2010:314, 104–114. DOI: 10.1002/jez.b.21313.

[32] Martin D, Maestro O, Cruz J, Mane-Padros D, Belles X. RNAi studies reveal a conserved role for RXR in molting in the cockroach *Blattella germanica*. *Journal of Insect Physiology* 2006:52, 410–416. DOI:10.1016/j.jinsphys.2005.12.002.

[33] Nakamura T, Mito T, Tanaka Y, Bando T, Ohuchi H, Noji S. Involvement of canonical Wnt/Wingless signalling in the determination of the positional values within the leg segment of the cricket *Gryllus bimaculatus*. *Development, Growth & Differentiation* 2007:49, 79–88. DOI: 10.1111/j.1440-169X.2007.00915.x.

[34] Moriyama Y, Sakamoto T, Karpova SG, Matsumoto A, Noji S, Tomioka K. RNA interference of the clock gene period disrupts circadian rhythms in the cricket Gryllus bimaculatus. *Journal of Biological Rhythms* 2008:23, 308–318. DOI: 10.1177/0748730408320486.

[35] Hamada A, Miyawaki K, Honda-sumi E, Tomioka K, Mito T, Ohuchi H et al. Loss-offunction analyses of the fragile X-related and dopamine receptor genes by RNA interference in the cricket Gryllus bimaculatus. *Developmental Dynamics* 2009:238, 2025–2033. DOI: 10.1002/dvdy.22029.

[36] Nakamura T, Mito T, Bando T, Ohuchi H, Noji S. Dissecting insect leg regeneration through RNA interference. *Cellular and Molecular Life Sciences* 2008:65, 64–72. DOI: 10.1016/j.mod.2011.07.001.

[37] Mito T, Inoue Y, Kimura S, Miyawaki K, Niwa N, Shinmyo Y et al. Involvement of *hedgehog*, *wingless*, and *dpp* in the initiation of proximodistal axis formation during

the regeneration of insect legs, a verification of the modified boundary model. *Mechanisms of Development* 2002:114, 27–35. DOI:10.1016/S0925-4773(02)00052-7.

[38] Araujo RN, Santos A, Pinto FS, Gontijo NF, Lehane MJ, Pereira MH. RNA interference of the salivary gland Nitrophorin 2 in the triatomine bug Rhodnius prolixus (Hemiptera: Reduviidae) by dsRNA ingestion or injection. *Insect Biochemistry and Molecular Biology* 2006:36, 683–693. DOI:10.1016/j.ibmb.2006.05.012.

[39] Boisson B, Jacques JC, Choumet V, Martin E, Xu J, Vernick K, et al. Gene silencing in mosquito salivary glands by RNAi. *FEBS Letters* 2006:580, 1988–1992. DOI: http://dx.doi.org/10.1016/j.febslet.2006.02.069.

[40] Belgacem YH, Martin JR. Hmgcr in the corpus allatum controls sexual dimorphism of locomotor activity and body size via the insulin pathway in Drosophila. *PLoS One* 2007:2, e187. DOI: 10.1371/journal.pone.0000187.

[41] Lee CM, Su MT, Lee HJ. Pigment dispersing factor: An output regulator of the circadian clock in the German cockroach. *Journal of Biological Rhythms* 2009:24, 35–43. DOI: 10.1177/0748730408327909.

[42] Lycett GJ, McLaughlin LA, Ranson H, Hemingway J, Kafatos FC, Loukeris TG et al. Anopheles gambiae P450 reductase is highly expressed in oenocytes and in vivo knockdown increases permethrin susceptibility. *Insect Molecular Biology* 2006:15, 321–27. DOI: 10.1111/j.1365-2583.2006.00647.x.

[43] Sivakumar S, Rajagopal R, Venkatesh GR, Srivastava A, Bhatnagar RK. Knockdown of aminopeptidase-N from Helicoverpa armigera larvae and in transfected Sf21 cells by RNA interference reveals its functional interaction with Bacillus thuringiensis insecticidal protein Cry1Ac. *Journal Biological Chemistry* 2007:282, 7312–7319. DOI: 10.1074/jbc.M607442200.

[44] Ohnishi A, Hull JJ, Matsumoto S. Targeted disruption of genes in the Bombyx mori sex pheromone biosynthetic pathway. *Proceedings of National Academy of Science of the United States of America* 2006:103, 4398–4403. DOI: 10.1073/pnas.0511270103.

[45] Turner CT, Davy MW, MacDiarmid RM, Plummer KM, Birch NP, Newcomb RD. 2006. RNA interference in the light brown apple moth, Epiphyas postvittana (Walker) induced by double-stranded RNA feeding. *Insect Molecular Biology* 2006:15, 383–391. DOI: 10.1111/j.1365-2583.2006.00656.x.

[46] Paldi N, Glick E, Oliva M, Zilberberg Y, Aubin L, Pettis J et al. Effective gene silencing in a microsporidian parasite associated with honeybee (Apis mellifera) colony declines. *Applied and Environmental Microbiology* 2010:76, 5960–5964. DOI:10.1128/AEM.01067-10.

[47] Garbian Y, Maori E, Kalev H, Shafir S, Sela I. Bidirectional transfer of RNAi between honey bee and Varroa destructor: Varroa gene silencing reduces Varroa population. *PLoS Pathogens* 2012:8, e1003035. DOI: 10.1371/journal.ppat.1003035.

[48] Goto A, Blandin S, Royet J, Reichhart JM, Levashina EA. Silencing of Toll pathway components by direct injection of double-stranded RNA into Drosophila adult flies. *Nucleic Acids Research* 2003:31, 6619–6623. DOI: 10.1093/nar/gkg852.

[49] Blandin S, Moita LF, Kocher T, Wilm M, Kafatos FC, Levashina EA. Reverse genetics in the mosquito Anopheles gambiae: Targeted disruption of the defensin gene. *EMBO Reports* 2002:3, 852–856. DOI: 10.1093/embo-reports/kvf180.

[50] Osta MA, Christophides GK, Kafatos FC. Effects of mosquito genes on Plasmodium development. *Science* 2004:303, 2030–2032. DOI:10.1126/science.1091789.

[51] Eleftherianos I, Gokcen F, Felfoldi G, Millichap PJ, Trenczek TE, ffrench-Constant RH et al. The immunoglobulin family protein hemolin mediates cellular immune responses to bacteria in the insect Manduca sexta. *Cell Microbiology* 2007:9, 1137–1147. DOI: 10.1111/j.1462-5822.2006.00855.x.

[52] Huvenne H, Smagghe, G. Mechanisms of dsRNA uptake in insects and potential of RNAi for pest control: A review. *Journal of Insect Physiology* 2010:56, 227–235. DOI: 10.1016/j.jinsphys.2009.10.004.

[53] Baum JA, Bogaert T, Clinton W, Heck GR, Feldmann P, Ilagan O et al. Control of coleopteran insect pests through RNA interference. *Nature Biotechnology* 2007:25, 1322–1326. DOI:10.1038/nbt1359.

[54] Mao YB, Cai WJ, Wang JW, Hong GJ, Tao XY, Wang LJ et al. Silencing a cotton bollworm P450 monooxygenase gene by plant-mediated RNAi impairs larval tolerance of gossypol. *Nature Biotechnology* 2007:25(11), 1307–1313. DOI: 10.1038/nbt1352.

[55] Li J, Chen Q, Lin Y, Jiang T, Wu G, Hua H. RNA interference in Nilaparvata lugens (Homoptera: Delphacidae) based on dsRNA ingestion. *Pest Management Science* 2011:67, 852–859. DOI: 10.1002/ps.2124.

[56] Elaine BA, Miguel SS, Christopher RM. Mechanisms of hopperburn: An overview of insect taxonomy, behavior, and physiology. *Annual Review of Entomology* 2005:50, 125–151. DOI: 10.1146/annurev.ento.49.061802.123310.

[57] Liu S, Ding Z, Zhang C, Yang B, Liu Z. Gene knockdown by intro-thoracic injection of double-stranded RNA in the brown planthopper, Nilaparvata lugens. *Insect Biochemistry and Molecular Biology* 2010:40, 666–671. DOI:10.1016/j.ibmb.2010.06.007.

[58] Gatehouse JA, Price DRG. Protection of crops against insect pests using RNA interference. *Insect Biotechnology* 2011:2, 145–168. DOI: 10.1007/978-90-481-9641-8_8.

[59] Navas-Castillo J, Fiallo-Olivé E, Sánchez-Campos S. Emerging virus diseases transmitted by whiteflies. *Annual Review of Phytopathology* 2011:49, 219–248. DOI: 10.1146/annurev-phyto-072910-095235.

[60] Zha W, Peng X, Chen R, Du B, Zhu L, He G. Knockdown of midgut genes by dsRNA-transgenic plant-mediated RNA interference in the hemipteran insect Nilaparvata lugens. *PLoS One* 2011:6, e20504. DOI: 10.1371/journal.pone.0020504.

[61] Pitino M, Coleman AD, Maffei ME, Ridout CJ, Hogenhout SA. Silencing of aphid genes by dsRNA feeding from plants. *PLoS One* 2011:6, e25709. DOI: 10.1371/journal.pone.0025709.

[62] Ghanim M, Kontsedalov S, Czosnek H. Tissue-specific gene silencing by RNA interference in the whitefly Bemisia tabaci (Gennadius). *Insect Biochemistry and Molecular Biology* 2007:37, 732–738. DOI:10.1016/j.ibmb.2007.04.006.

[63] Upadhyay SK, Chandrashekar K, Thakur N, Verma PC, Borgio JF, Singh PK et al. RNA interference for the control of whiteflies (Bemisia tabaci) by oral route. *Journal of Biosciences* 2011:36, 153–161. DOI: 10.1007/s12038-011-9009-1.

[64] Zhao YY, Yang G, Wang-Pruski G, You MS. Phyllotreta striolata Coleoptera: Chrysomelidae): Arginine kinase cloning and RNAi-based pest control. *European Journal of Entomology* 2008:105, 815–822. DOI: 10.14411/eje.2008.108.

[65] Niu BL, Shen WF, Liu Y, Weng HB, He LH, Mu JJ et al. Cloning and RNAi-mediated functional characterization of MaLac2 of the pine sawyer, Monochamus alternatus. *Insect Molecular Biology* 2008:17, 303–312. DOI: 10.1111/j.1365-2583.2008.00803.x.

[66] Franz AW, Sanchez-Vargas I, Adelman ZN, Blair CD, Beaty BJ, James AA et al. Engineering RNA interference-based resistance to dengue virus type 2 in genetically modified Aedes aegypti. *Proceedings of the National Academy of Sciences of the United States of America* 2006:103(11), 4198–4203. DOI: 10.1073/pnas.0600479103.

[67] Coy MR, Sanscrainte ND, Chalaire KC, Inberg A, Maayan I, Glick E et al. Gene silencing in adult Aedes aegypti mosquitoes through oral delivery of double-stranded RNA. *Journal of Applied Entomology* 2012:136(10), 741–748. DOI: 10.1111/j.1439-0418.2012.01713.x.

[68] Figueira-Mansur J, Ferreira-Pereira A, Mansur JF, Franco TA, Alvarenga ESL, Sorgine MHF et al. Silencing of P-glycoprotein increases mortality in temephos-treated Aedes aegypti larvae. *Insect Molecular Biology* 2013:22(6), 648–658. DOI: 10.1111/imb.12052.

[69] Zhang X, Zhang J, Zhu KY. Chitosan/double-stranded RNA nanoparticle-mediated RNA interference to silence chitin synthase genes through larval feeding in the African malaria mosquito (Anopheles gambiae). *Insect Molecular Biology* 2010:19(5), 683–693. DOI: 10.1111/j.1365-2583.2010.01029.x.

[70] Walshe DP, Lehane SM, Lehane MJ, Haines LR. Prolonged gene knockdown in the tsetse fly Glossina by feeding double stranded RNA. *Insect Molecular Biology* 2009:(1), 11–19. DOI: 10.1371/journal.pone.0017788.

[71] Li X, Zhang M, Zhang H. RNA interference of four genes in adult Bactrocera dorsalis by feeding their dsRNAs. *PLoS One* 2011:6(3), e17788. DOI: 10.1371/journal.pone.0017788.

[72] Jaubert-Possamai S, Le Trionnaire G, Bonhomme J, Christophides GK, Rispe C, Tagu D. Gene knockdown by RNAi in the pea aphid Acyrthosiphon pisum. *BMC Biotechnology* 2007:7, 63. DOI:10.1186/1472-6750-7-63.

[73] Mutti NS, Park Y, Reese JC, Reeck GR. RNAi knockdown of a salivary transcript leading to lethality in the pea aphid, Acyrthosiphon pisum. *Journal of Insect Science* 2006:6, 1–7. DOI: 10.1673/031.006.3801.

[74] Mao J, Zeng F. Feeding-based RNA interference of a gap gene is lethal to the pea aphid, Acyrthosiphon pisum. *Plos One* 2012:7, e48718. DOI: 10.1371/journal.pone.0048718.

[75] Whyard S, Singh AD, Wong S. Ingested double-stranded RNAs can act as species-specific insecticides. *Insect Biochemistry and Molecular Biology* 2009:39, 824–832. DOI: 10.1016/j.ibmb.2009.09.007.

[76] Shakesby A, Wallace I, Isaacs H, Pritchard J, Roberts D, Douglas A. A water-specific aquaporin involved in aphid osmoregulation. *Insect Biochemistry and Molecular Biology* 2009:39, 1–10. DOI: 10.1016/j.ibmb.2008.08.008.

[77] Zhu F, Sams S, Moural T, Haynes KF, Potter MF, Palli SR. RNA interference of NADPH-cytochrome P450 reductase results in reduced insecticide resistance in the bed bug, Cimex lectularius. *PLos One* 2012:7, e31037. DOI: 10.1371/journal.pone.0031037.

[78] El-Shesheny I, Hajeri S, El-Hawary I, Gowda S, Killiny N. Silencing abnormal wing disc gene of the Asian citrus psyllid, Diaphorina citri disrupts adult wing development and increases nymph mortality. *PLos One* 2013:8, e65392. DOI: 10.1371/journal.pone.0065392.

[79] Hajeri S, Killiny N, El-Mohtar C, Dawson WO, Gowda S. Citrus tristeza virus-based RNAi in citrus plants induces gene silencing in Diaphorina citri, a phloem-sap sucking insect vector of citrus greening disease (Huanglongbing). *Journal of Biotechnology* 2014:176, 42–49. DOI: 10.1016/j.jbiotec.2014.02.010.

[80] Wan P-J, Jia S, Li N, Fan J-M, Li G-Q. RNA interference depletion of the halloween gene disembodied implies its potential application for management of planthopper Sogatella furcifera and Laodelphax striatellus. *PLos One* 2014:9, e86675. DOI: 10.1371/journal.pone.0086675.

[81] Araujo RN, Soares AC, Paim RM, Gontijo NF, Gontijo AF, Lehane MJ et al. The role of salivary nitrophorins in the ingestion of blood by the triatomine bug Rhodnius prolixus (Reduviidae: Triatominae). *Insect Biochemistry and Molecular Biology* 2009:39, 83–89. DOI: 10.1016/j.ibmb.2008.10.002.

[82] Mury FB, da Silva JR, Ferreira LS, dos Santos Ferreira B, de Souza-Filho GA, de Souza-Neto JA et al. Alpha-glucosidase promotes hemozoin formation in a blood-suck-

ing bug: An evolutionary history. *PLoS One* 2009:4, e6966. DOI: 10.1371/journal.pone.0006966.

[83] Paim RM, Araujo RN, Lehane MJ, Gontijo NF, Pereira MH. Longterm effects and parental RNAi in the blood feeder Rhodnius prolixus (Hemiptera; Reduviidae). *Insect Biochemistry and Molecular Biology* 2013:43, 1015–1020. DOI: 10.1016/j.ibmb.2013.08.008.

[84] Defferrari M, Lee D, Fernandes C, Orchard I, Carlini C. A phospholipase A2 gene is linked to Jack bean urease toxicity in the Chagas' disease vector Rhodnius prolixus. *Biochimica et Biophysica Acta* 2014:1840, 396–405. DOI: 10.1016/j.bbagen.2013.09.016.

[85] Deng F, Zhao Z. Influence of catalase gene silencing on the survivability of Sitobion avenae. *Archives of Insect Biochemistry and Physiology* 2014:86, 46–57. DOI: 10.1002/arch.21161.

[86] Xu L, Duan X, Lv Y, Zhang X, Nie Z, Xie C, Ni Z, Liang R. Silencing of an aphid carboxylesterase gene by use of plant-mediated RNAi impairs Sitobion avenae tolerance of Phoxim insecticides. *Transgenic Research* 2014:23, 389–396. DOI: 10.1007/s11248-013-9765-9.

[87] Walker WB, Allen ML. Expression and RNA interference of salivary polygalacturonase genes in the tarnished plant bug, Lygus lineolaris. *Journal of Insect Science* 2010:10, 173. DOI: 10.1673/031.010.14133.

[88] Walker WB, Allen ML. RNA interference-mediated knockdown of IAP in Lygus lineolaris induces mortality in adult and preadult life stages. *Entomologia Experimentalis et Applicata* 2011:138, 83–92. DOI: 10.1111/j.1570-7458.2010.01078.x.

[89] Liu PZ, Kaufman TC. Hunchback is required for suppression of abdominal identity, and for proper germband growth and segmentation in the intermediate germ band insect Oncopeltus fasciatus. *Development* 2004:131, 1515–1527. DOI: 10.1242/dev.01046.

[90] Ikeno T, Numata H, Goto SG. Circadian clock genes period and cycle regulate photoperiodic diapause in the bean bug Riptortus pedestris males. *Journal of Insect Physiology* 2011a:57, 935–938. DOI: 10.1016/j.jinsphys.2011.04.006.

[91] Araujo RN, Santos A, Pinto FS, Gontijo NF, Lehane MJ, Pereira MH. RNA interference of the salivary gland nitrophorin 2 in the triatomine bug Rhodnius prolixus (Hemiptera: Reduviidae) by dsRNA ingestion or injection. *Insect Biochemistry and Molecular Biology* 2006:36, 683–693. DOI:10.1016/j.ibmb.2006.05.012.

[92] Zha W, Peng X, Chen R, Du B, Zhu L, He G. Knockdown of midgut genes by dsRNA-transgenic plant-mediated RNA interference in the hemipteran insect Nilaparvata lugens. *PLoS One* 2011:6(5), e20504. DOI: 10.1371/journal.pone.0020504.

[93] Li J, Chen Q, Lin Y, Jiang T, Wu G, Hua H. RNA interference in Nilaparvata lugens (Homoptera: Delphacidae) based on dsRNA ingestion. *Pest Management Science* 2011:67(7), 852–859. DOI: 10.1002/ps.2124.

[94] Chen J, Zhang D, Yao Q, Zhang J, Dong X, Tian H et al. Feeding-based RNA interference of a trehalose phosphate synthase gene in the brown planthopper, Nilaparvata lugens. *Insect Molecular Biology* 2010:19(6), 777–786. DOI: 10.1111/j.1365-2583.2010.01038.x.

[95] Zhang Y, Wang X, Yang B, Hu Y, Huang L, Bass C et al. Reduction in mRNA and protein expression of a nicotinic acetylcholine receptor $\alpha 8$ subunit is associated with resistance to imidacloprid in the brown planthopper, Nilaparvata lugens. *Journal of Neurochemistry*. 2015. DOI: 10.1111/jnc.13281.

[96] Pitino M, Coleman AD, Maffei ME, Ridout CJ, Hogenhout SA. Silencing of aphid genes by dsRNA feeding from plants. *PLoS One* 2011:6, e25709. DOI: 10.1371/journal.pone.0025709.

[97] Wuriyanghan H, Rosa C, Falk BW. Oral delivery of doublestranded RNAs and siRNAs induces RNAi effects in the potato/tomato psyllid, Bactericerca cockerelli. *PLoS One* 2011:6, e27736. DOI: 10.1371/journal.pone.0027736.

[98] Zhou XG, Wheeler MM, Oi FM, Scharf ME. RNA interference in the termite Reticulitermes flavipes through ingestion of double-stranded RNA. *Insect Biochemistry and Molecular Biology* 2008:38, 805–815. DOI: 10.1016/j.ibmb.2008.05.005.

[99] Wang YB, Zhang H, Li HC and Miao XX. Second generation sequencing supply an effectiveway to screen RNAi targets in large scale for potential application in pest insect control. *PLoS One* 2011:6(4), e18644. DOI: 10.1371/journal.pone.0018644.

[100] Khajuria C, Buschman LL, Chen MS, Muthukrishnan S, Zhu KY. A gut-specific chitinase gene essential for regulation of chitin content of peritrophic matrix and growth of *Ostrinia nubilalis* larvae. *Insect Biochemistry and Molecular Biology* 2010:40, 621–629. DOI: 10.1016/j.ibmb.2010.06.003.

[101] Turner CT, Davy MW, Macdiarmid RM, Plummer KM, Birch NP, Newcomb RD. RNA interference in the light brown apple moth, *Epiphyas postvittana* (Walker) induced by double-stranded RNA feeding. *Insect Molecular Biology* 2006:15, 383–391. DOI: 10.1111/j.1365-2583.2006.00656.x.

[102] Kumar M, Gupta GP, Rajam MV. Silencing of acetylcholinesterase gene of Helicoverpa armigera by siRNA affects larval growth and its life cycle. *Journal of Insect Physiology* 2009:55, 273–278. DOI: 10.1016/j.jinsphys.2008.12.005.

[103] Mao YB, Tao XY, Xue XY, Wang LJ, Chen XY. Cotton plants expressing *CYP6AE14* double-stranded RNA show enhanced resistance to bollworms. *Transgenic Research* 2011:20, 665–673. DOI: 10.1007/s11248-010-9450-1.

[104] He HJ, Wang Q, Zheng WW, Wang JX, Song QS, Zhao XF. Function of nuclear transport factor 2 and Ran in the 20E signal transduction pathway in the cotton bollworm, Helicoverpa armigera. *BMC Cell Biology* 2010:11, 1. DOI:10.1186/1471-2121-11-1.

[105] Xiong Y, Zeng H, Zhang Y, Xu D, Qiu D. Silencing the HaHR3 gene by transgenic plant-mediated RNAi to disrupt Helicoverpa armigera development. *International Journal of Biological Sciences* 2013:9(4), 370–381. DOI: 10.7150/ijbs.5929.

[106] Bettencourt R, Terenius O, Faye I. *Hemolin* gene silencing by ds-RNA injected into Cecropia pupae is lethal to next generation embryos. *Insect Molecular Biology* 2002:11, 267–271. DOI: 10.1046/j.1365-2583.2002.00334.x.

[107] Porta H, Jimenez G, Cordoba E, Leon P, Soberon M, Bravo A. Tobacco plants expressing the Cry1AbMod toxin suppress tolerance to Cry1Ab toxin of Manduca sexta cadherin-silenced larvae. *Insect Biochemistry and Molecular Biology* 2011:41, 513–519. DOI: 10.1016/j.ibmb.2011.04.013.

[108] Shu YH, Wang JW, Lu K, Zhou JL, Zhou Q, Zhang GR. The first vitellogenin receptor from a Lepidopteran insect: Molecular characterization, expression patterns and RNA interference analysis. *Insect Molecular Biology* 2011:20, 61–73. DOI: 10.1111/j.1365-2583.2010.01054.x.

[109] Tian H, Peng H, Yao Q, Chen H, Xie Q, Tang B et al. Developmental control of a lepidopteran pest *Spodoptera exigua* by ingestion of bacteria expressing dsRNA of a non-midgut gene. *PLoS One* 2009:4(7), e6225. DOI: 10.1371/journal.pone.0006225.

[110] Gvakharia BO, Bebas P, Cymborowski B, Giebultowicz JM. Disruption of sperm release from insect testes by cytochalasin and beta-actin mRNA mediated interference. *Cellular and Molecular Life Sciences* 2003:60, 1744–1751. DOI: 10.1007/s00018-003-3139-z.

[111] Griebler M, Westerlund SA, Hoffmann KH, Meyering-Vos M. RNA interference with the allatoregulating neuropeptide genes from the fall armyworm *Spodoptera frugiperda* and its effects on the JH titer in the hemolymph. *Journal of Insect Physiology* 2008:54, 997–1007. DOI: 10.1016/j.jinsphys.2008.04.019.

[112] Gong LA, Yang XQ, Zhang BL, Zhong GH, Hu MY. Silencing of Rieske iron-sulfur protein using chemically synthesised siRNA as a potential biopesticide against *Plutella xylostella*. *Pest Management Science* 2011:67, 514–520. DOI: 10.1002/ps.2086.

[113] Mito T, Nakamura T, Bando T, Ohuchi H, Noji S. The advent of RNA interference in entomology. *Entomological Science* 2011:14, 1–8. DOI: 10.1111/j.1479-8298.2010.00408.x.

[114] Dabour N, Bando T, Nakamura T, Miyawaki K, Mito T, Ohuchi H, Noji S. Cricket body size is altered by systemic RNAi against insulin signaling components and epidermal growth factor receptor. *Development Growth & Differentiation* 2011:53, 857–869. DOI: 10.1111/j.1440-169X.2011.01291.x.

[115] Takahashi T, Hamada A, Miyawaki K, Matsumoto Y, Mito T, Noji S et al. Systemic RNA interference for the study of learning and memory in an insect. *Journal of Neuroscience Methods* 2009:179, 9–15. DOI:10.1016/j.jneumeth.2009.01.002.

[116] Moriyama Y, Sakamoto T, Karpova SG, Matsumoto A, Noji S, Tomioka K. RNA interference of the clock gene period disrupts circadian rhythms in the cricket Gryllus bimaculatus. *Journal of Biological Rhythms* 2008:23, 308–318. DOI: 10.1177/0748730408320486.

[117] Meyering-Vos M, Muller A. RNA interference suggests sulfakinins as satiety effectors in the cricket *Gryllus bimaculatus*. *Journal of Insect Physiology* 2007:53, 840–848. DOI:10.1016/j.jinsphys.2007.04.003.

[118] Dong Y, Friedrich M. Nymphal RNAi: Systemic RNAi mediated gene knockdown in juvenile grasshopper. *BMC Biotechnology* 2005:5, 25. DOI:10.1186/1472-6750-5-25.

[119] Khajuria C, Buschman LL, Chen MS, Muthukrishnan S, Zhu KY. A gut-specific chitinase gene essential for regulation of chitin content of peritrophic matrix and growth of Ostrinia nubilalis larvae. *Insect Biochemistry and Molecular Biology* 2010:40, 621–629. DOI: 10.1016/j.ibmb.2010.06.003.

[120] Wang Z, Gerstein M, Snyder M. RNA-Seq: A revolutionary tool for transcriptomics. *Nature Reviews Genetics* 2009:10, 57–63. DOI:10.1038/nrg2484.

[121] Haas BJ, Zody MC. Advancing RNA-Seq analysis. *Nature Biotechnology* 2010:28, 421–423. DOI: 10.1038/nbt0510-421.

[122] Zhang M, Zhou Y, Jones HD, Gao Q, Wang D, Ma Y, et al. Identifying potential RNAi targets in grain aphid (*Sitobion aveane* F.) based on transcriptome profiling of its alimentary canal after feeding on wheat plants. *BMC Genomics* 2013:14, 560. DOI: 10.1186/1471-2164-14-560.

[123] Li H, Jiang W, Zhang Z, Xing Y, Li F. Transcriptome analysis and screening for potential target genes for RNAi-mediated pest control of the beet armyworm, *Spodoptera exigua*. *PLoS One*. 2013:8(6), e65931. DOI:10.1371/journal.pone.0065931.

[124] Li X, Zhang M, Zhang H. RNA interference of four genes in adult Bactrocera dorsalis by feeding their dsRNAs. *PLoS One* 2011:6, e17788. DOI:10.1371/journal.pone.0017788.

[125] Hunter W, Ellis J, Vanengelsdorp D, Hayes J, Westervelt D, Glick E et al. Large-scale field application of RNAi technology reducing Israeli acute paralysis virus disease in honey bees (Apis mellifera, Hymenoptera: Apidae). *PLoS Pathogens* 2010:6, e1001160. DOI: 10.1371/journal.ppat.1001160.

[126] Hunter WB, Glick E, Paldi N, Bextine BR. Advances in RNA interference: dsRNA treatment in trees and grapevines for insect pest population suppression. *Southwestern Entomologist* 2012:37, 85–87. DOI: http://dx.doi.org/10.3958/059.037.0110.

[127] Gan D, Zhang J, Jiang H, Jiang T, Zhu S, Cheng B. Bacterially expressed dsRNA protects maize against SCMV infection. *Plant Cell Reports* 2010:29, 1261–1268. DOI: 10.1007/s00299-010-0911-z.

[128] Kurreck J. RNA interference: From basic research to therapeutic applications. *Angewandte Chemie (International Edition in English)* 2009:48, 1378–1398. DOI: 10.1002/anie.200802092.

[129] Zhang X, Zhang J, Zhu KY. Chitosan/double-stranded RNA nanoparticle-mediated RNA interference to silence chitin synthase genes through larval feeding in the African malaria mosquito (Anopheles gambiae). *Insect Molecular Biology* 2010:19(5), 683–693. DOI: 10.1111/j.1365-2583.2010.01029.x.

[130] Gong LA, Yang XQ, Zhang BL, Zhong GH, Hu MY. Silencing of Rieske iron-sulfur protein using chemically synthesised siRNA as a potential biopesticide against *Plutella xylostella*. *Pest Management Science* 2011:67, 514–520. DOI: 10.1002/ps.2086.

[131] Zhu F, Xu JJ, Palli R, Ferguson J, Palli SR. Ingested RNA interference for managing the populations of the Colorado potato beetle, *Leptinotarsa decemlineata*. *Pest Management Science* 2011:67, 175–182. DOI: 10.1002/ps.2048.

[132] Obbard DJ, Gordon KH, Buck AH, Jiggins FM. The evolution of RNAi as a defence against viruses and transposable elements. *Philosophical Transactions of the Royal Society B: Biological Sciences* 2009:364(1513), 99–115. DOI: 10.1098/rstb.2008.0168.

[133] Saleh MC, Tassetto M, van Rij RP, Goic B, Gausson V, Berry B, Jacquier C, Antoniewski C, Andino R. Antiviral immunity in Drosophila requires systemic RNA interference spread. *Nature* 2009:458, 346–351. DOI: 10.1038/nature07712.

[134] Ulvila J, Parikka M, Kleino A, Sormunen R, Ezekowitz RA, Kocks C, Ramet M. Double-stranded RNA is internalized by scavenger receptor-mediated endocytosis in Drosophila S2 cells. *Journal of Biological Chemistry* 2006:281, 14370–14375. DOI: 10.1074/jbc.M513868200.

[135] Saleh MC, van Rij RP, Hekele A, Gillis A, Foley E, O'Farrell PH et al. The endocytic pathway mediates cell entry of dsRNA to induce RNAi silencing. *Nature Cell Biology* 2006:8, 793–802. DOI: 10.1038/ncbl439.

[136] Campbell CL, Keene KM, Brackney DE, Olson KE, Blair CD, Wilusz J et al. Aedes aegypti uses RNA interference in defense against Sindbis virus infection. *BMC Microbiology* 2008:8(1), 47. DOI: 10.1186/1471-2180-8-47.

[137] Aliyari R, Wu Q, Li WH, Wang XH, Li F, Green LD, et al. Mechanism of induction and suppression of antiviral immunity directed by virus-derived small RNA sin Drosophila. *Cell Host & Microbe* 2008:4, 387–397. DOI:10.1016/j.chom.2008.09.001.

[138] Li H, Li WX, Ding SW. Induction and suppression of RNA silencing by an animal virus. *Science* 2002:296, 1319–1321. DOI:10.1126/science.1070948.

[139] Nayak A, Berry B, Tassetto M, Kunitomi M, Acevedo A, Deng C, et al. Cricket paralysis virus antagonizes Argonaute2 to modulate antiviral defensein Drosophila. *Nature Structural and Molecular Biology* 2010:17, 547–554. DOI:10.1038/nsmb.1810.

[140] Wang XH, Aliyari R, Li WX, Li HW, Kim K, Carthew R, et al. RNA interference directs innate immunity against viruses in adult Drosophila. *Science* 2006:312, 452–454. DOI:10.1126/science.1125694.

[141] Goic B, Vodovar N, Mondotte JA, Monot C, Frangeul L, Blanc H, et al. RNA-mediated interference and reverse transcription control the persistence of RNA viruses in the insect model Drosophila. *Nature Immunology* 2013:14, 396–403. DOI:10.1038/ni.2542.

[142] Swevers L, Broeck JV, Smagghe G. The possible impact of persistent virus infection on the function of the RNAi machinery in insects: A hypothesis. *Frontiers in Physiology* 2013:4, 319. DOI: 10.3389/fphys.2013.00319.

[143] Terenius O, Papanicolaou A, Garbutt JS, Eleftherianos I, Huvenne H, Kanginakudru S, et al. RNA interference in Lepidoptera: An overview of successful and unsuccessful studies and implications for experimental design. *Journal of Insect Physiology* 2011:57, 231–245. DOI:10.1016/j.jinsphys.2010.11.006.

[144] Blair CD. Mosquito RNAi is the major innate immune pathway controlling arbovirus infection and transmission. *Future Microbiology* 2011:6, 267–277. DOI: 10.2217/fmb.11.11.

[145] Schnettler E, Sterken MG, Leung JY, Metz SW, Geertsema C, Goldbach RW et al. Noncoding flavivirus RNA displays RNA interference suppressor activity in insect and mammalian cells. *Journal of Virology* 2012:86, 13486–13500. DOI: 10.1128/JVI.01104-12.

[146] Winston WM, Molodowitch C, Hunter CP. Systemic RNAi in C. elegans requires the putative transmembrane protein SID-1. *Science* 2002:295, 2456–2459. DOI:10.1126/science.1068836.

[147] Barnard AC, Nijhof AM, Fick W, Stutzer C, Maritz-Olivier C. RNAi in arthropods: Insight into the machinery and applications for understanding the pathogen-vector interface. *Genes* 2012:3(4), 702–741. DOI:10.3390/genes3040702.

[148] Aronstein K, Pankiw T, Saldivar E. SID-1 is implicated in systemic gene silencing in the honey bee. *Journal of Apicultural Research* 2006:45, 20–24. DOI:10.3896/IBRA.1.45.1.05.

[149] Tomoyasu Y, Miller SC, Tomita S, Schoppmeier M, Grossmann D, Bucher G. Exploring systemic RNA interference in insects: A genome-wide survey for RNAi genes in Tribolium. *Genome Biology* 2008:9(1), R10. DOI: 10.1186/gb-2008-9-1-r10.

[150] Boisson B, Jacques JC, Choumet V, Martin E, Xu JN, Vernick K et al. Gene silencing in mosquito salivary glands by RNAi. *FEBS Letters* 2006:580, 1988–1992. DOI: http://dx.doi.org/10.1016/j.febslet.2006.02.069.

[151] Volz J, Muller HM, Zdanowicz A, Kafatos FC, Osta MA. A genetic module regulates the melanization response of Anopheles to Plasmodium. *Cellular Microbiology* 2006:8, 1392–1405. DOI: 10.1111/j.1462-5822.2006.00718.x.

[152] Zhu JS, Chen L, Raikhel AS. Posttranscriptional control of the competence factor beta FTZ-F1 by juvenile hormone in the mosquito Aedes aegypti. *Proceedings of the National Academy of Sciences of the United States of America* 2003:100, 13338–13343. DOI: 10.1073/pnas.2234416100.

[153] Scott JG, Michel K, Bartholomay LC, Siegfried BD, Hunter WB, Smagghe G et al. Towards the elements of successful insect RNAi. *Journal of Insect Physiology* 2013:59(12), 1212–1221. DOI: 10.1016/j.jinsphys.2013.08.014.

[154] Kumar M, Gupta GP, Rajam MV. Silencing of acetylcholinesterase gene of Helicoverpa armigera by siRNA affects larval growth and its life cycle. *Journal of Insect Physiology* 2009:55, 273–278. DOI: 10.1016/j.jinsphys.2008.12.005.

[155] Wu H, Ma H, Ye C, Ramirez D, Chen S, Montoya J et al. Improved siRNA/shRNA functionality by mismatched duplex. *PLoS One* 2011:6(12), e28580. DOI: 10.1371/journal.pone.0028580.

[156] Yu N, Christiaens O, Liu J, Niu J, Cappelle K, Caccia S et al. Delivery of dsRNA for RNAi in insects: An overview and future directions. *Insect Science* 2013:20(1), 4–14. DOI: 10.1111/j.1744-7917.2012.01534.x.

[157] Shakesby AJ, Wallace IS, Isaacs HV, Pritchard J, Roberts DM, Douglas AE. A water-specific aquaporin involved in aphid osmoregulation. *Insect Biochemistry and Molecular Biology* 2009:39, 1–10. DOI: 10.1016/j.ibmb.2008.08.008.

[158] Arimatsu Y, Kotani E, Sugimura Y, Furusawa T. Molecular characterization of a cDNA encoding extracellular dsRNase and its expression in the silkworm, *Bombyx mori. Insect Biochemistry and Molecular Biology* 2007:37, 176–183. DOI:10.1016/j.ibmb.2006.11.004.

[159] Garbutt JS, Belles X, Richards EH, Reynolds SE. Persistence of double stranded RNA in insect hemolymph as a potential determiner of RNA interference success: Evidence from Manduca sexta and Blattella germanica. *Journal of Insect Physiology* 2013:59, 171–178. DOI: 10.1016/j.jinsphys.2012.05.013.

[160] Rinkevich FD, Scott JG. Limitations of RNAi of a6 nicotinic acetylcholine receptor subunits for assessing the in vivo sensitivity to spinosad. *Insect Science* 2013:20, 101–108. DOI: 10.1111/j.1744-7917.2012.01523.x.

[161] Upadhyay SK, Dixit S, Sharma S, Singh H, Kumar J, Verma PC, Chandrashekar K. siRNA machinery in whitefly (*Bemisia tabaci*). Plos ONE 2013: 8(12), e83692. DOI: 10.1371/journal.pone.0083692.

[162] Lundgren JG, Duan JJ. RNAi-based insecticidal crops: Potential effects on non-target5 species. Bioscience 2013:63(8), 657–665. DOI: http://dx.doi.org/10.1525/bio.2013.63.8.8.

[163] Jackson AL, Linsley PS. Noise amidst the silence: Off-target effects of siRNAs? Trends in Genetics 2004:20(11), 521–524. DOI: http://dx.doi.org/10.1016/j.tig.2004.08.006.

Chapter 18

Management of Insect Pest by RNAi — A New Tool for Crop Protection

Thais Barros Rodrigues and Antonio Figueira

Additional information is available at the end of the chapter

http://dx.doi.org/10.5772/61807

Abstract

The fast-growing human population requires the development of new agricultural technologies to meet consumers′ demand, while minimizing environmental impacts. Insect pests are one of the main causes for losses in agriculture production, and current control technologies based on pesticide application or the use of transgenic crops expressing *Bacillus thuringiensis* toxin proteins are facing efficacy challenges. Novel approaches to control pests are urgently necessary. RNA interference (RNAi) is a gene silencing mechanism triggered by providing double-stranded RNA (dsRNA), that when ingested into insects can lead to death or affect the viability of the target pest. Transgenic plants expressing dsRNA version of insect specific target genes are the new generation of resistant plants. However, the RNAi mechanism is not conserved among insect orders, and its elucidation is the key to develop commercial RNAi crops. In this chapter, we review the core RNAi pathway in insects and the dsRNA uptake, amplification, and spread of systemic silencing signals in some key insect species. We also highlight some of the experimental steps before developing an insect pest-resistant "RNAi plant". Lastly, we review some of the most recent development studies to control agricultural insect pests by RNAi transgenic plants.

Keywords: Biotechnology, dsRNA, Entomology, Gene silencing, Insect control, RNA interference

1. Introduction

Agriculture has to continually adapt to rising environmental concerns in conjunction with meeting the increasing consumers′ demand. The fast-growing human population creates the need for the sustainable intensification of agriculture throughout the world which can be acomplished by adopting mechanization and new technologies to close yield gaps while minimizing environmental impacts. In the past few decades, insect pest control has been mainly conducted by the application of chemical pesticides because of the low cost and efficacy; but their indiscriminate use has caused escalating problems with the evolution of insect resistance to the pesticides together with secondary pest outbreaks. The development of new biotechnological approaches, with the introduction of transgenic crops expressing *Bacillus thuringiensis* (Bt) Cry toxin proteins, also known as insect-resistant transgenic Bt-plants, decreased pesticide utilization in certain key crops, such as cotton and maize, and brought economical and environmental benefits [1-3]. But once again, insect resistance has arisen, now against the Bt toxins, and outbreaks of nontarget pests have emerged [1, 4], which makes necessary the development of novel approaches to control selected agriculture pests.

RNA interference (RNAi) is a gene silencing mechanism at the cellular level triggered by double-stranded RNA (dsRNA) and is likely to be the new approach underlying the next generation of insect-resistant transgenic plants. In some studies, successful delivery of dsRNA molecules to insects by ingestion resulted in the expected essential gene target silencing [5, 6], which led to death or affected the viability of the target insect, resulting in control of the pest.

In general, long dsRNAs are processed by species-specific RNase-III-like enzymes, resulting in smaller double-stranded molecules. These shorter RNAs are loaded into RNA complexes as a guide for finding target mRNAs that are either cleaved or blocked for translation in posttranscriptional silencing, or inducing histone modifications when involved in transcriptional silencing response [7, 8]. However, the RNAi systemic spreading mechanism is not conserved across organisms, and its elucidation is an essential step in developing an efficient method to control agricultural pests by RNAi technology.

In this chapter, we review how the RNAi mechanism occurs in insects, highlighting the core RNAi pathway and components, and new developments regarding dsRNA uptake, amplification, and the spread of systemic silencing signals in some key insect species. We also discuss the critical experimental steps before developing an "RNAi plant" protected against a specific insect pest, with consideration to application. Lastly, we review some of the most recent published studies to control agriculturally important insect pests based on RNAi transgenic plants.

2. RNAi mechanism

RNAi is an important and natural antiviral defense mechanism, protecting organisms from RNA viruses, or even avoiding the random integration of transposons [9]. Over time, with the discovery of some aspects of the mechanism, RNAi has become a widely used tool to knock down and analyze the function of genes. Most of the RNAi pathways have dsRNA as the precursor triggering molecule that vary in length and origin [7, 8]. In addition, the RNAi pathways differ not only in the RNA precursor molecule, but also in genes, enzymes, and effector complexes involved throughout the process. However, some key steps are conserved. Briefly, RNA duplexes are processed into short RNA duplexes, which are then used to guide the recognition of their target, either to cleave a complementary mRNA, or to repress their target translation at a posttranscriptional silencing level, or to modify the chromatin structure at the transcriptional level [7, 8].

The RNA precursor molecules from the RNAi pathways, all of which are already identified in insects, are small RNAs, categorized into three classes [8, 10]: the first two classes are small interfering RNAs (siRNAs; 20–25 nucleotides) and microRNAs (miRNAs; 21–24 nucleotides) [7] (Figure 1). Both miRNAs and siRNAs share a common RNase-III processing enzyme, Dicer, and closely related effector complexes and both can regulate gene expression at the posttranscriptional level [8, 10, 11]. Conversely, the third class of small RNAs, the PIWI-interacting RNAs (piRNAs; 24–30 nucleotides), are generated independent of the Dicer activity [12]. piRNAs have been reported to play an essential role in germ-line development, stem cell renewal, transposon silencing, and epigenetic regulation [13-16]. These piRNAs originate from a diversity of sequences, including repetitive DNA and transposons, and they seem to act both at the posttranscriptional and chromatin levels [10]. The mechanism that generates and amplifies piRNAs is not well-understood, but involves slicer activities (Argonaute proteins associated with cleaving activity) [8, 10, 17]. Considered a specialized subclass of piRNAs, **r**epeat-**a**ssociated **si**RNAs (rasiRNAs; 25-29 nucleotides) were identified in the *Drosophila* genome [18], and suggested by Meister and Tuschl [7] to be involved in guiding chromatin modification in this insect species (Figure 1).

The most recognized RNAi pathways are the siRNA and miRNA; despite being triggered by different molecules, both precursors are long double-stranded RNAs (dsRNAs). Naturally in a cell, long dsRNAs can derive from RNA virus replication, from the transcription of convergent cellular genes or mobile genetic elements, or from self-annealing cellular transcripts [8]. In the siRNA pathway, these long dsRNA are processed by Dicer into siRNA duplexes. By contrast, in the miRNA pathway, miRNAs are generated from endogenous transcripts (primary miRNAs; pri-miRNAs) that form stem–loop structures [19, 20]. In the nucleus, these hairpin regions are recognized and cleaved into precursor mirRNAs (pre-miRNAs) by Drosha, another RNase-III-family enzyme, and the pre-miRNAs are transported to the cytoplasm through the nuclear export receptor Exportin-5 (Expo-5) [19, 20]. Subsequently, the pre-miRNA undergoes another endonucleolytic cleavage, now catalyzed by Dicer, generating an miRNA duplex [19, 20] (Figure 1).

The siRNA and miRNAs duplex containing ribonucleoprotein particles (RNPs) are subsequently rearranged into effector complexes. Although it is difficult to assign distinct functional labels, an siRNA-containing effector complex is referred to as an "RNA-induced silencing complex" (RISC), and an miRNA-containing effector complex is referred to as an miRNP [7]. In these complexes, the regulation is at a posttranscriptional level and every RISC or miRNP contains a member of the Argonaute (Ago) protein family [7]. For the regulation at the transcriptional level as guided by rasiRNAs, a specialized nuclear Argonaute-containing complex, known as the RNA-Induced Transcriptional Silencing complex (RITS) mediates gene silencing [10]. In general, one strand of the short-RNA duplex (the guide strand) is loaded onto an Argonaute protein at the core of the effector complexes. During loading, the nonguide strand is cleaved by an Argonaute protein and ejected. The Argonaute protein then uses the guide RNA to associate with target RNAs that contain a perfectly complementary sequence

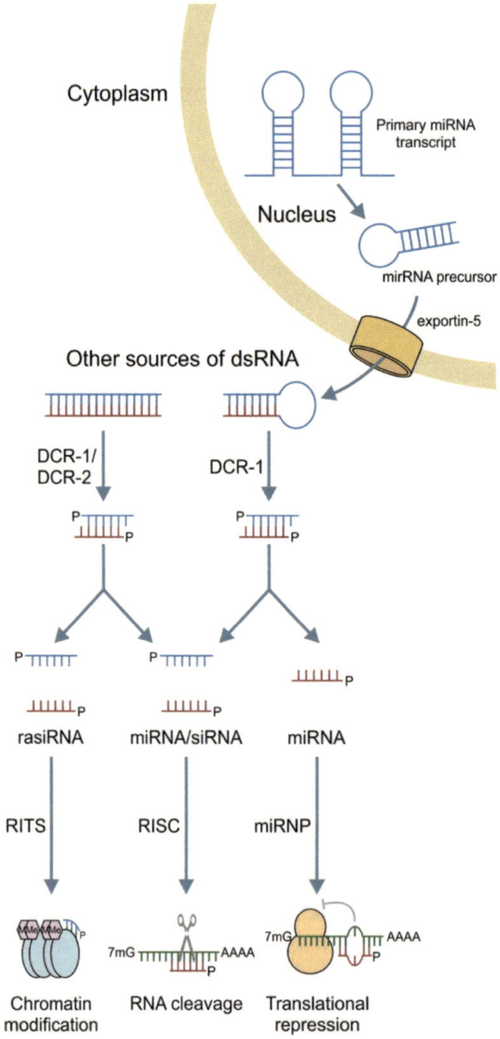

Figure 1. RNA-mediated gene silencing pathways. In the nucleus, primary miRNA transcripts (pri-miRNAs) are processed to mirRNA precursors (pre-miRNA) by the RNase-III-like enzyme Drosha. The pre-miRNA is exported through the export receptor Exportin-5 (Exp-5) to the cytoplasm, and then processed by Dicer to microRNA (miRNA). These miRNAs are unwound and assembled into miRNP (miRNA containing effector complex of RiboNucleo Protein particles) or RISC (RNA Induced Silencing Complex), triggering silencing responses by translational repression of target mRNAs or mRNA-target degradation, respectively. In the cytoplasm, long dsRNA are processed to siRNA (small interfering RNA) by the RNase-III-like enzyme Dicer. The short dsRNAs are unwound and assembled into RISC or RITS (RNA-Induced Transcriptional Silencing) complexes. The siRNA guides the RNA cleavage by the RISC complex, while rasiRNA (repeat-associated short interfering RNA) guides the condensation of heterochromatin by the RITS complex. 7mG: 7-methyl guanine; AAAA: poly-adenosine tail; Me: methyl group; P: 5'- phosphate. (Adapted from [7])

and then catalyzes the slicing of these targets, either to be cleaved by RISC, to be blocked for translation in miRNP or by inducing histone modifications in RITS [7] (Figure 1). The mechanism of miRNA-guided translational regulation is not as well-understood in the case of target-

RNA cleavage, and to make things more complicated, miRNAs can act as siRNAs, and siRNAs can act as miRNAs [7].

Dicer is one of the enzymes involved in RNAi mechanism that is encoded by a variable number of genes and presents distinct specificity among organisms [21]. For instance, mammals and *Caenorhabditis elegans,* the best characterized animal for RNAi, have each a single Dicer responsible for functions in both siRNA and miRNA pathways [12], while *Drosophila melanogaster* has two paralogues: Dicer-1 (Dcr-1) that preferentially processes miRNA precursors, and Dicer-2 (Dcr-2) required to process long dsRNA into siRNAs [22]. However, in *Tribolium castaneum,* a model organism among insects for systemic silencing by RNAi, Dcr-2 showed an important role at the RNAi pathway, whereas Dcr-1 is suggested to have an involvement in wing development, most likely through the miRNA pathway [23].

Another gene family involved in RNAi pathways is the Argonaute proteins (Ago). Ago is a central protein component of silencing complexes (RISC, RITS, miRNP) that acts in mediating target recognition and silencing [24]. Argonaute proteins contain two domains: a PAZ domain involved in dsRNA binding, and a PIWI-domain responsible for RNase activity [23]. In *Drosophila,* Ago-1 is involved in the miRNA pathway; Ago-2 in the siRNA pathway; while Piwi, Aubergine (Aub), and Ago-3 are associated in transcriptional silencing [13, 25-27]. In *Tribolium,* a single class of Argonaute was identified (Tc-Ago-1) in the miRNA pathway, while two classes of Ago-2 paralogues (Tc-Ago-2a and Tc-Ago-2b) were found in the siRNA pathway, probably deriving from gene duplication in the beetle lineage [23]. This duplicated Tc-Ago-2 might lead to higher amounts of Ago-2 protein, potentially with the enhancement of the RNAi response [23]. In the silkmoth *Bombyx mori,* a Lepidoptera species in which the RNAi response is considered much less robust [28, 29], *AGO* genes from all three main RNAi pathways were identified (*BmAGO-1* – miRNA; *BmAGO-2* – siRNA; *BmAGO-3* – piRNA), which were shown to be involved in the RNAi response in Bm5 cells [30]. Taken together, these findings, and other reviews [29], support the idea of a function overlap of the three main RNAi pathways in *B. mori* [29].

2.1. Systemic RNAi

Systemic RNAi is described as a silencing signal transmitted widely throughout a treated organism [5, 31]. The knowledge about the systemic RNAi mechanism in insects is important as it may affect the approaches adopted to develop "RNAi-mediated pest control" because the systemic mechanism is not conserved among those organisms. Systemic RNAi has two important steps to be considered: the uptake of dsRNA by the cells and the systemic spreading of the signals. Some of the main genes involved in systemic RNAi are presented below and discussed for the model organisms.

2.1.1. dsRNA uptake

In insects, two types of dsRNA uptake mechanisms have been identified [32]. The first one involves a multi-transmembrane domain protein, Systemic Interference Defective (Sid). In *C. elegans,* Sid-1 is essential and sufficient to mediate uptake and systemic spread of RNAi signal in both somatic and germ-line cells [33, 34]; conversely, in insects, Sid-1-like (Sil) proteins appear to be variable across orders [32]. For instance, Diptera do not present *SIL* genes, while *Tribolium* and *B. mori* presented three *SIL* homologues [23, 35]. However, these *Tribolium* genes share more identity with another *C. elegans* gene, *TAG-130,* not required for systemic RNAi in *C. elegans* compared to that with *SID-1* [23]. The second dsRNA uptake mechanism involves endocytosis, specific for dsRNAs acquired from the environment, known as environmental RNAi [5, 31]. First discovered in *Drosophila* S2 cells and later in *C. elegans,* this uptake of dsRNA by endocytosis appears to be evolutionary-conserved [36-38]. However, we should be cautious to conclude that all organisms have a dsRNA uptake mechanism based on endocytosis. For instance, Ulvila and colleagues [38] working with *Drosophila* S2 cells, which are hemocyte-like, described high rates of endocytosis as compared to the majority of other cell types in this species [39].

Other important proteins for systemic RNAi were identified in *C. elegans* but are specific only to germ-line cells, such as Rsd-2, Rsd-3, and Rsd-6 [40]. The Rsd-2 protein contains no particular known motifs but interacts with Rsd-6 that has a Tudor domain, suggesting that these two proteins act together [40]. The *RSD-3* gene encodes a protein that contains an epsin amino-terminal homology (ENTH) domain, found in proteins involved in vesicle trafficking, suggesting the involvement of endocytosis in systemic RNAi [40]. In *Tribolium,* a homologue for *RSD-3* (*Tc-RSD3*) has been found, but in *Drosophila,* which does not exhibit a systemic silencing response, a homologous Rsd-3 protein (Epsin-like) was identified [23]. So, the presence of Rsd-3 does not seems to determine whether or not systemic RNAi occurs in insects, and it is possible that the expression level and/or tissue specificity of this gene may affect the degree of RNAi efficiency and the dsRNA uptake from the environment [23].

2.1.2. RNAi systemic spreading: amplification and maintenance of dsRNA

Once the dsRNA overcomes all the uptake barriers, the silencing signal should be transported from treated cell to other cells, and spread to other tissues. Further, dsRNA should be constantly produced, e.g., either by the amplification of dsRNA by an RNA-dependent RNA polymerase (RdRP), and/or constantly acquired for the maintenance of the silencing responses.

In *C. elegans,* primary siRNAs processed by Dicer are used as a template for an RdRP activity to produce secondary dsRNAs [41]. The RdRP activity is key for the RNAi signal amplification. However, so far in insects, no RdRP-related protein has been found [21, 23], suggesting that strong RNAi response in insects does not rely on amplification of the trigger dsRNA, and it must be based on a different mechanism yet to be identified. Alternatively, constant supply of dsRNA may be provided by RNAi-plants to provide continuous effects.

The presence of the main genes involved in systemic RNAi and amplification in *Drosophila* and *Tribolium* fail to explain the respective absence and presence of systemic RNAi [23]. Nevertheless, the several differences in the number of these core component genes found between species suggests an interesting avenue for further investigation [23]. For instance, Ago protein that have already been shown to determine RNAi efficiency [42], was found to be duplicated in the *Tribolium* genome, while *Drosophila* carries only a copy of *AGO-2* gene, suggesting a relationship between number of *AGO* copies and RNAi response [23].

Another component that might affect RNAi efficiency in different insects are the proteins containing the dsRNA-binding motif (dsRBM), which help small molecules to properly load inside of the silencing complexes [23]. These proteins act together with Dicer, and seem to be responsible for determining Dicer specificity in *Drosophila* [23]. In the *T. castaneum* genome, two *R2D2-like* genes (a particular dsRBM) were found (*TcR2D2* and *TcC3PO*), which might help *Tribolium* to be hypersensitive to dsRNA molecule uptake by the cells [23]. However, in the *Anthonomus grandis* transcriptome, only an *R2D2* contig was identified [21]. The presence of an additional R2D2-like protein in *Tribolium* might also allow a longer-lasting RNAi effect, once dsRBM proteins are known to bind to dsRNAs, and might be involved in the maintenance of dsRNA in cells [23].

3. Factors affecting the silencing effect and RNAi efficiency as an insect control method

The RNAi approach to control insect pests had been considered for many years, but application of this technology was just realized after it was shown that ingestion of dsRNA would trigger RNAi. The concept of RNAi-plant mediated pest control was demonstrated in 2007 by the development of transgenic plants producing dsRNAs against specific insect genes, with the consequent effect on the target species [43, 44]. The main prerequisites to generate successful RNAi insect-resistant transgenic plants are: (i) identification of a specific gene with an essential function in the insect that can cause developmental deformities and/or larval lethality when knocked down or knocked out; and (ii) dsRNA delivery by oral ingestion that must be uptaken by the insect cells, and spread systemically.

The insect must uptake the dsRNA version of a target gene region by feeding. To silence the target gene, this specific dsRNA must be taken up from the gut lumen into the gut cells as what is considered as "environmental RNAi." If the target gene is expressed in a tissue distinct from the digestive system, the silencing signal should successfully spread via cells and tissues as a systemic RNAi. Both environmental and systemic RNAi are considered noncell-autonomous RNAi, which means that the interfering effect takes places in tissues/cells different from the location of application or production of the dsRNA. Conversely, in the cell-autonomous RNAi, the silencing process is limited to the cell in which the dsRNA is introduced [5]. However, the mechanism of ingested dsRNA uptake and systemic spreading of the silencing signal in the insect have yet to be fully characterized and understood.

Some factors can affect the efficiency of the dsRNA uptake and systemic silencing spread in different insects. Here, we highlight important points that must be considered in developing an RNAi approach against insect pests.

3.1. Target gene

The choice of the target gene should be carefully considered. Each gene requires particular effort to be silenced. Terenius and colleagues [28] reviewed more than 150 RNAi experimental results from RNAi of lepidopterans involving 130 genes, from which only 38% were silenced at a satisfactory level, while 48% failed to be silenced, and 14% were silenced at insufficient levels. Among the target genes, those involved in immunity were more effectively silenced, and, in contrast, genes expressed in epidermal tissues seem to be most difficult. Differences for RNAi sensitivity among genes in the same tissue was described in [28].

3.2. dsRNA design

The design of the dsRNA determines the one particular target gene to be silenced, but off-target effects can occur if siRNAs have some sequence similarity with unintended genes. Tobacco plants expressing *Helicoverpa armigera* ecdysone receptor (*EcR*) dsRNA improved resistance to another insect, *Spodoptera frugiperda*, due to the high identity shared between the nucleotide sequence of *HaEcR* and *SeEcR* genes [45]. Although this result implies that an RNAi-plant can control two or even more lepidopteran pests, this can also affect nontarget insects, becoming a biosafety issue.

3.3. dsRNA length

The length of the dsRNA fragments plays an essential role in the effectiveness of molecular uptake in insects, which is directly involved in the success of the target gene silencing. In most of the RNAi experiments, the insects are fed with long dsRNAs [5]. Some experiments showed that long dsRNAs are more efficiently uptaken than siRNAs [37, 46]. This may be due to the fact that a long dsRNA, with 100% match of the target mRNA, after processing into siRNA will provide a greater diversity of siRNAs available to cause specific suppression of target gene and increase the desired effect, and, additionally, reduce the likelihood of developing resistance [47]. In contrast, other studies reported suppression of genes in different insects via incorporation of siRNA in diet instead of dsRNA [48, 49].

3.4. dsRNA concentration

Optimal concentration of dsRNA delivered to the insect is required to induce sufficient gene target silencing. It is noteworthy to mention that exceeding the optimal dsRNA concentration may not result in more silencing [50, 51]. However, higher concentration of dsRNA decreased the duration of dsRNA exposure to reach 50% mortality of *Diabrotica virgifera virgifera* [46], suggesting an inverse relationship between dsRNA concentration and duration of exposure. In cricket (*Gryllus bimaculatus*), the highest concentrations of dsRNA yielded more efficient gene knockdown [52]. The amount of dsRNA sufficient to significantly reduce mRNA levels of *PER* and *CLK* genes were one and two μM, respectively. These concentrations reduced the expression level of the targets, but a higher concentration (20 μM) for the *CYC* gene was required, suggesting that the sensitivity to dsRNAs also depends specifically on the gene [52].

3.5. Controls

Empty vector, empty cassette, buffer only, irrelevant or nonspecific control (such as dsGFP – Green Fluorescent Protein gene region), or any other kind of negative control are essential to discriminate specific gene silencing from the simple induction of siRNA processing machinery by exposure to a dsRNA. Mainly, a negative control should demonstrate the specificity of the dsRNA designed for a target, not interfering in specific target expression, and even unspecific effects. Also, any control should have similar size and concentration of the used dsRNA [53].

3.6. Molecular silencing confirmation

An efficient molecular confirmation of the RNAi silencing should be conducted, which includes target RNA expression, and analyses of protein amount and/or enzyme activity. In RNA analysis, additional care should be taken for expression analysis. The method of choice for RNA expression analysis is the quantitative amplification of reversed transcripts or RT-qPCR, considered a very sensitive and accurate method. To provide precision in RT-qPCR, some essential care is required, such as the choice of appropriate stable reference genes and primer pair design with sufficient amplification efficiency. The reference genes should exhibit stable expression among experimental conditions, providing reliable estimate of gene expression results [54]. Additionally, primers should be designed flanking the region used to design the dsRNA to ensure that the initial cleavage of the mRNA could be detected, thus avoiding false-positives [55]. Conventional care of RT–qPCR reactions defined by the Minimum Information for Publication of Quantitative Real-Time PCR Experiments (MIQE) guidelines must be strictly followed [56].

3.7. Protein stability and phenotype analysis

Proteins can exhibit a long half-life and interfere with the phenotypic changes. However, phenotype changes are not totally related to small decrease of protein levels; haplo-sufficient genes produce proteins capable of performing the biological processes normally, even at half of the protein levels [53]. Phenotype changes could be more difficult to be observed in RNAi responses if the protein product of the target gene has a long half-life. For example, the reduction of *Da6* (nicotinic acetylcholine receptor subunit) expression in both *D. melanogaster* and *T. castaneum* exhibited weak phenotype responses [57], which may be explained based on the long stability of the nicotinic acetylcholine receptors (nAChRs) [58]. Nevertheless, for most of the genes, mRNA turnover and protein half-life are unknown and this lack of information presents one of the principal challenges for the RNAi experiments [39].

3.8. Insect issues, life stage, nucleases, and gut pH

Some insect characteristics should also be considered before starting an RNAi experiment including the developmental stage of insects. Although handling advanced developmental stages of insects is more efficient, silencing effects are more prominent in earlier stages. For instance, in second instar larvae of *Rhodnius prolixus*, the gene *nitropin 2* was knocked down for 42%, but no silencing was observed in the fourth instar individuals, even though both larval stages were treated with the same concentration of dsRNA [59]. In *Spodoptera frugiperda*, fifth instar larvae presented higher gene silencing as compared to adult moths [60].

Another consideration that can affect the RNAi silencing efficiency is the presence of insect nucleases and gut pH. For instance, feeding assays with *Lygus lineolaris* showed no mortality effects because the saliva of *L. lineolaris* contains dsRNA-degrading activity. Thus, dsRNA ingested did not result in siRNA fragments, rather were completely digested to monomers [61]. Also, dsRNA degradation is reduced during molting period and further reduced by starvation in some insects [62]. The stability of the dsRNA in the midgut could be affected not only by enzymatic but also by chemical hydrolysis [63]. In both cases, gut pH is an important factor; particularly, it is quite variable among insect orders, with variation even among gut regions [64]. For example, in general, lepidopterans exhibit a strong alkaline gut (up to pH 10.5 in some species), which provides a highly hostile environment for dsRNA [64]; therefore, this order is particularly recalcitrant to gene silencing by RNAi.

4. Overview on the use of RNAi to control insects by transgenic plants

Most of the current transgenic crops with specific control against insect pests are based on *Bacillus thuringiensis* (Bt) toxins, which act in gut epithelial cell membrane in susceptible insects. Bt toxins are highly specific against certain orders of insects, where the most successful use was achieved against Lepidoptera and Coleoptera. However, continuous exposure of those insects to Bt crops evolved field-resistance, affecting the efficiency in controlling those pests [4, 65]. Also, there are limitations of Bt transgenics to manage some other important agricultural pests, such as the sap-sucking insects (Hemiptera). This encouraged the development of new strategies to help in controlling agricultural pests.

In 2007, two studies demonstrated the concept of plants expressing dsRNAs derived from hairpin vectors that directed dsRNAs to target gene regions of economically important agricultural pests: the cotton bollworm (*Helicoverpa armigera*; Lepidoptera; [44]) and the Western corn rootworm (WCR; *Diabrotica virgifera virgifera*; Coleoptera; [43]). After the demonstration of plants resistant to insects, the application of RNAi by transgenic plants became a potential new approach to control important agricultural pests, which led to the flourishing of a new field of research. So far, searches on the publication database "Web of Science" from Thomson Reuters (August 2015), identified 543 published studies based on the combination of the topics "RNAi," "plant" and "insect," and only one quarter was published before 2008.

To implement RNAi in agricultural pest control, the target insect should uptake the dsRNA autonomously, e.g., from transgenic plants expressing dsRNA. This feeding should be continuous, since insects lack an amplification mechanism based on RdRP, such as *C. elegans*. Many of the main agricultural pest species have already been targeted by RNAi technology using various genes and delivery methods [66]. However, three orders have been the major focus of the development of transgenic plants expressing target gene regions for RNAi: Coleoptera, Hemiptera, and Lepidoptera. Here, we list some of the most recently published RNAi transgenic plants studies performed against those insect orders (Table 1).

Specie	Order	Crop	Target Gene	Remarks	Reference
Diabrotica v. virgifera	Coleoptera	*Zea mays*	*vATPase*	Mortality	[67]
Leptinotarsa decemlineata	Coleoptera	*Solanum tuberosum*	*β-actin, Shrub*	Mortality	[68]
Helicoverpa armigera *Spodoptera exigua*	Lepidoptera	*Nicotiana tabacum*	Nuclear receptor complex of 20-hydroxyecdysone (*HaEcR*)	Molting defect and larval lethality	[45]
Helicoverpa armigera	Lepidoptera	*Nicotiana tabacum*	Molt-regulating transcription factor gene (*HR3*)	Developmental deformities and larval lethality	[70]
Helicoverpa armigera	Lepidoptera	*Arabidopsis thaliana*	*HaAK*	Developmental Deformities and larval lethality	[71]
Myzus persicae	Hemiptera	*Arabidopsis thaliana and Nicotiana benthamiana*	*MpC001, Rack1*	Progeny reduced	[72]
Myzus persicae	Hemiptera	*Arabidopsis thaliana*	*serine protease*	Progeny reduced	[73]
Myzus persicae	Hemiptera	*Nicotiana tabacum*	*hunchback(hb)*	Inhibited reproduction	[74]
Bemisia tabaci	Hemiptera	*Nicotiana rustica*	*vATPase*	Mortality	[75]

Table 1. Overview of the recently published studies on the use of plant-RNAi against different insect pests

4.1. Coleoptera

The coleopterans are likely to be the first target to be controlled by the new generation of transgenics, the "RNAi-plants." *Diabrotica virgifera virgifera* (Western corn rootworm, WCR) is one of the most important agricultural pests, and this species, along with other coleopterans, requires little effort to have genes silenced by RNAi, independent of the delivery method and gene target. The significant breakthrough was demonstrated when WCR presented significant larval stunting and mortality, causing less injury to maize roots that express a hairpin version of *V-ATPase A* [43]. Since then, many studies have been conducted using various target genes, while not focusing only on pest control, but also to characterize the mechanism of action of the RNAi [46]. A recent study with WCR demonstrated that long dsRNAs of *Dv V-ATPase C* expressed in maize provides highly efficient root protection, but the siRNA population generated in the transgenic plant does not lead to lethal RNAi responses when consumed by the insect [67].

Studies have also been performed in other species, such as the important potato pest *Leptinotarsa decemlineata* (Colorado potato beetle, CPB). So far, this is the first study to compare efficacy at controlling pest insects by dsRNAs expressed either in the chloroplast or in the cytoplasm. Transgenic potato plants expressing hairpin versions of *β-actin* and *Shrub* genes (both insectidal dsRNAs) in the chloroplasts (transplastomic plants) conferred the most potent insecticidal activity (insects died after 5 days), while the conventional expression from nuclear transgenics did not affect the beetles [68].

An explanation for this result is that since choroplasts do not have cellular RNAi machinery [69], the dsRNAs produced inside these organelles are not cleaved by a plant Dicer and the beetles ingest almost entirely long dsRNA. In contrast, beetles fed on nuclear-transformed plants consumed mostly siRNAs; previous dsRNA-feeding studies already indicated that ingested long dsRNAs were much more effective than ingested siRNAs. It should be highlighted that all the other studies have been based on an efficient cytoplasm-derived dsRNA in various crops, indicating that possibly potato plants process long dsRNA more effective than the plants from those other studies (Table 1 [69]).

4.2. Lepidoptera

Plants producing *Bt* proteins were the first generation of transgenic plants to control insects, and most of the lepidopterans were successfully managed by Bt crops for years. However, the durability of Bt technology appears to be unsure. The number of pest species that evolved Bt resistance in the field, reducing transgenic efficacy, increased from one in 2005 to five in 2010 [4]. Among those five species, four are lepidopterans [4]. The lepidopterans could be the first and main targets for RNAi crops if they were not as recalcitrant to gene silencing, without any definite explanation for the limited and unstable RNAi responses [28, 29]. For instance, the concentration of dsRNA necessary to knock down a specific gene by feeding *Diatraea saccharalis* (Lepidoptera) neonate larvae is much higher than the one required for the same larval stage of *D. v. virgifera* (Coleoptera).

The first successful RNAi plant protected against a lepidopteran (*Helicoverpa armigera*) was demonstrated by silencing the *CYP6AE14* gene, necessary for detoxifying gossypol from cotton (*Gossypum hirsutum*) [44]. Studies have been conducted to explore alternative target genes to control and understand the RNAi mechanism in lepiopterans. Larval lethality and molting defects were detected in *H. armigera* fed with transgenic tobacco plants expressing dsRNA targeted to the nuclear ecdysone receptor complex (*HaEcR*), absolutely required for insect development [45]. The transgenic tobacco expressing dsRNA of *HaEcR* had an improved resistance to another lepidopteran pest, *Spodoptera exigua*. This cross-species effect might indicate a risk to affect nontarget insects, highlighting the importance of biosafety studies that should be carefully conducted [45].

The expression of dsRNA in both *Escherichia coli* and transgenic tobacco plants to silence a molt-regulating transcription factor gene (*HR3*) of *H. armigera* resulted in developmental deformity and larval lethality [70]. Transgenic *Arabidopsis thaliana* plants expressing dsRNA targeted to *arginine kinase* (*AK*) of *H. armigera* (*HaAK*) led to a 55% mortality rate in first instar larvae, while retarding growth in surviving larvae [71]. However, no lethal phenotypes were observed for the third instar larvae, although transcript levels of *HaAK* were distinctly suppressed [71].

4.3. Hemiptera

Hemipterans are characterized as piercing/sucking insects, representing major agricultural pests that inflict direct damages by sucking sap, or indirectly by acting as a vector of several viruses and bacterial infections. Since hemipterans feed through sucking the phloem, only systemic chemical insecticides are effective against these insects, resulting in high residual toxicity. The problem is further aggravated as no Bt toxin has been identified as exhibiting adequate insecticidal effects against hemipterans. Transgenic crops based on RNAi offer a large potential to control hemipteran, requiring expression of target gene dsRNAs on the phloem. One first report was published in 2011 about developing transgenic *Nicotiana benthamiana* and *A. thaliana* expressing dsRNA targeting genes expressed in *Myzus persicae* gut (*RACK1*) and salivary glands (*MpC002*) [72]. A reduction of the expression level of the target genes and a decrease in *M. persicae* fecundity were observed, but no lethal effects [72].

The same phenotype was observed when *M. persicae* fed on *A. thaliana* expressing dsRNA of a serine protease gene (*MySP*), with no lethal effects, but reduced fecundity [73]. Once again, reduced reproduction, but no lethal phenotype was observed when *M. persicae* was fed on tobacco plants expressing dsRNA targeting the *hunchback* gene [74]. A possible explanation for not achieving the expected phenotypes (mortality) after target gene depletion is that the dsRNA level produced by RNAi transgenic plants could not be sufficient for an efficient uptake of dsRNA or siRNA by sap-sucking insects [74]. However, more recently, mortality rates were observed in *Bemisia tabaci* fed in tobacco plants expressing dsRNA of *v-ATPaseA* [75]. This result provides a proof-of-concept that plants expressing dsRNA, at an efficient level and targeting crucial genes, could resist the attack of Hemipteran pests [75].

5. Conclusion and future perspectives

Since the concept of a transgenic plant expressing dsRNA targeted to a specific essential gene in the insect that affects its viability was first demonstrated in 2007, the technology has been extended to a large number of insect species from various orders. Elucidating the various mechanisms and components of the RNA interference pathway has progressed, but many aspects remain to be clarified. Many differences in components and mechanisms among insect orders and between insects and other organisms still need to be worked out. Some of these differences (e.g., genes involved, gene number, and level of expression) may explain variation in recalcitrance among insect species and need to be further investigated. Of particular interest are the mechanisms of dsRNA uptake, signal amplification, and systemic spread in the major pest species. Additional insect- or order-specific characteristics, such as gut pH, presence of dsRNA-degrading activity in digestive system, among others that could be associated with differences in recalcitrance to RNAi need to be dissected and clarified.

Due to the variety of RNAi response to RNAi in insects, no single protocol is suitable for all species. Issues related to the choice of effective target genes, including determining the size of optimal dsRNA length and ideal gene region. Assuming that the method of choice to deliver dsRNA is transgenic plants, a major question still to be addressed is the impact of plant dsRNA processing in the effective RNAi-induced silencing. There is still a need for investigation in this area. The choice of a suitable inducible promoter for expressing the dsRNA construct is another point barely explored.

Based on the recent publications reviewed in this chapter, the progress in developing "RNAi-plants" to control important insect pests widely demonstrated the potential of this technology to complement or replace Bt crops, providing resistance against a broad variety of insect pests. However, to be applied on a commercial level, several issues related to the RNAi mechanism and biosafety still need to be addressed. As a new technology, risk assessments and government regulations still have to be developed. However, RNAi transgenic crops are expected to have wider acceptance and reduced biosafety requirements for RNAi traits, in comparison to a protein incorporated into a plant, such as a Bt transgenic [39]. Thus, RNAi-mediated pest control will open a new paradigm in insect pest management.

Author details

Thais Barros Rodrigues* and Antonio Figueira

*Address all correspondence to: thaisbarros.bio@gmail.com

Centro de Energia Nuclear na Agricultura (CENA), Universidade de São Paulo, Piracicaba, SP, Brazil

References

[1] Bravo A, Soberon M. How to cope with insect resistance to Bt toxins? *Trends Biotechnol.* 2008;26:573-9. DOI: 10.1016/j.tibtech.2008.06.005

[2] Kos M, van Loon JJA, Dicke M, Vet LEM. Transgenic plants as vital components of integrated pest management. *Trends Biotechnol.* 2009;27:621-7. DOI: 10.1016/j.tibtech.2009.08.002

[3] Wu K-M, Lu Y-H, Feng H-Q, Jiang Y-Y, Zhao J-Z. Suppression of cotton bollworm in multiple crops in China in areas with Bt toxin-containing cotton. *Science.* 2008;321:1676-8. DOI: 10.1126/science.1160550

[4] Tabashnik BE, Brevault T, Carriere Y. Insect resistance to Bt crops: lessons from the first billion acres. *Natur Biotechnol.* 2013;31:510-21. DOI: 10.1038/nbt.2597

[5] Huvenne H, Smagghe G. Mechanisms of dsRNA uptake in insects and potential of RNAi for pest control: A review. *J Insect Physiol*. 2010;56:227-35. DOI: 10.1016/j.jinsphys.2009.10.004

[6] Whyard S, Singh AD, Wong S. Ingested double-stranded RNAs can act as species-specific insecticides. *Insect Biochem Mol Biol*. 2009;39:824-32. DOI: 10.1016/j.ibmb.2009.09.007

[7] Meister G, Tuschl T. Mechanisms of gene silencing by double-stranded RNA. *Nature*. 2004;431:343-9. DOI: 10.1038/nature02873

[8] Jinek M, Doudna JA. A three-dimensional view of the molecular machinery of RNA interference. *Nature*. 2009;457:405-12. DOI: 10.1038/nature07755

[9] Obbard DJ, Gordon KHJ, Buck AH, Jiggins FM. The evolution of RNAi as a defence against viruses and transposable elements. *Philo Trans Royal Soc B-Biologic Sci*. 2009;364:99-115. DOI: 10.1098/rstb.2008.0168

[10] Moazed D. Small RNAs in transcriptional gene silencing and genome defence. *Nature*. 2009;457:413-20. DOI: 10.1038/nature07756

[11] Choudhuri S. Small Noncoding RNAs: Biogenesis, Function, and Emerging Significance in Toxicology. *J Biochem Mol Toxicol*. 2010;24:195-216. DOI: 10.1002/jbt.20325

[12] Ghildiyal M, Zamore PD. Small silencing RNAs: an expanding universe. *Natur Rev Genet*. 2009;10:94-108. DOI: 10.1038/nrg2504

[13] O'Donnell KA, Boekel JD. Mighty piwis defend the germline against genome intruders. *Cell*. 2007;129:37-44. DOI: 10.1016/j.cell.2007.03.028

[14] Castaneda J, Genzor P, Bortvin A. piRNAs, transposon silencing, and germline genome integrity. *Mutat Res – Fund Mol Mech Mutagen*. 2011;714:95-104. DOI: 10.1016/j.mrfmmm.2011.05.002

[15] Shpiz S, Olovnikov I, Sergeeva A, Lavrov S, Abramov Y, Savitsky M, et al. Mechanism of the piRNA-mediated silencing of *Drosophila* telomeric retrotransposons. *Nucleic Acids Res*. 2011;39:8703-11. DOI: 10.1093/nar/gkr552

[16] Pillai RS, Chuma S. piRNAs and their involvement in male germline development in mice. *Dev Growth Different*. 2012;54:78-92. DOI: 10.1111/j.1440-169X.2011.01320.x

[17] Aravin AA, Hannon GJ, Brennecke J. The Piwi-piRNA pathway provides an adaptive defense in the transposon arms race. *Science*. 2007;318:761-4. DOI: 10.1126/science.1146484

[18] Saito K, Nishida KM, Mori T, Kawamura Y, Miyoshi K, Nagami T, et al. Specific association of Piwi with rasiRNAs derived from retrotransposon and heterochromatic regions in the *Drosophila* genome. *Genes Dev*. 2006;20:2214-22. DOI: 10.1101/gad.1454806

[19] Pasquinelli AE, Hunter S, Bracht J. MicroRNAs: a developing story. Current Opinion in Genetics & Development. 2005;15:200-5. DOI: 10.1016/j.gde.2005.01.002

[20] Hammond SM. Dicing and slicing – The core machinery of the RNA interference pathway. *Febs Lett*. 2005;579:5822-9. DOI: 10.1016/j.febslet.2005.08.079

[21] Firmino AAP, de Assis Fonseca FC, Pepino de Macedo LL, Coelho RR, Antonino de Souza JD, Jr., Togawa RC, et al. Transcriptome Analysis in Cotton Boll Weevil (*Anthonomus grandis*) and RNA Interference in Insect Pests. *Plos One*. 2013;8: e85079. DOI: 10.1371/journal.pone.0085079

[22] Lee YS, Nakahara K, Pham JW, Kim K, He ZY, Sontheimer EJ, et al. Distinct roles for *Drosophila* Dicer-1 and Dicer-2 in the siRNA/miRNA silencing pathways. *Cell*. 2004;117:69-81. DOI: 10.1016/s0092-8674(04)00261-2

[23] Tomoyasu Y, Miller SC, Tomita S, Schoppmeier M, Grossmann D, Bucher G. Exploring systemic RNA interference in insects: a genome-wide survey for RNAi genes in *Tribolium*. *Genome Biol*. 2008;9. DOI:10.1186/gb-2008-9-1-r10

[24] Peters L, Meister G. Argonaute proteins: Mediators of RNA silencing. *Mol Cell*. 2007;26:611-23. DOI: 10.1016/j.molcel.2007.05.001

[25] Pal-Bhadra M, Leibovitch BA, Gandhi SG, Rao M, Bhadra U, Birchler JA, et al. Heterochromatic silencing and HP1 localization in *Drosophila* are dependent on the RNAi machinery. *Science*. 2004;303:669-72. DOI: 10.1126/science.1092653

[26] Brennecke J, Aravin AA, Stark A, Dus M, Kellis M, Sachidanandam R, et al. Discrete small RNA-generating loci as master regulators of transposon activity in *Drosophila*. *Cell*. 2007;128:1089-103. DOI: 10.1016/j.cell.2007.01.043

[27] Lin H. piRNAs in the germ line. *Science*. 2007;316:397. DOI: 10.1126/science.1137543

[28] Terenius O, Papanicolaou A, Garbutt JS, Eleftherianos I, Huvenne H, Kanginakudru S, et al. RNA interference in Lepidoptera: An overview of successful and unsuccessful studies and implications for experimental design. *J Insect Physiol*. 2011;57:231-45. DOI: 10.1016/j.jinsphys.2010.11.006

[29] Kolliopoulou A, Swevers L. Recent progress in RNAi research in Lepidoptera: intracellular machinery, antiviral immune response and prospects for insect pest control. *Curr Opin Insect Sci*. 2014;6:28–34. DOI: http://dx.doi.org/10.1016/j.cois.2014.09.019

[30] Kolliopoulou A, Swevers L. Functional analysis of the RNAi response in ovary-derived silkmoth Bm5 cells. *Insect Biochem Mol Biol*. 2013;43:654-63. DOI: 10.1016/j.ibmb.2013.05.001

[31] Whangbo JS, Hunter CP. Environmental RNA interference. *Trends Genet*. 2008;24:297-305. DOI: 10.1016/j.tig.2008.03.007

[32] Gu L, Knipple DC. Recent advances in RNA interference research in insects: Implications for future insect pest management strategies. *Crop Protect*. 2013;45:36-40. DOI: 10.1016/j.cropro.2012.10.004

[33] Winston WM, Molodowitch C, Hunter CP. Systemic RNAi in *C. elegans* requires the putative transmembrane protein SID-1. *Science*. 2002;295:2456-9. DOI: 10.1126/science.1068836

[34] Feinberg EH, Hunter CP. Transport of dsRNA into cells by the transmembrane protein SID-1. *Science*. 2003;301:1545-7. DOI: 10.1126/science.1087117

[35] Kobayashi I, Tsukioka H, Komoto N, Uchino K, Sezutsu H, Tamura T, et al. SID-1 protein of *Caenorhabditis elegans* mediates uptake of dsRNA into *Bombyx* cells. *Insect Biochem Mol Biol*. 2012;42:148-54. DOI: 10.1016/j.ibmb.2011.11.007

[36] Jose AM, Hunter CP. Transport of sequence-specific RNA interference information between cells. *Annu Rev Genet*. 2007;41:305-30. DOI: 10.1146/annurev.genet.41.110306.130216

[37] Saleh M-C, van Rij RP, Hekele A, Gillis A, Foley E, O'Farrell PH, et al. The endocytic pathway mediates cell entry of dsRNA to induce RNAi silencing. *Natur Cell Biol*. 2006;8:793-U19. DOI: 10.1038/ncb1439

[38] Ulvila J, Parikka M, Kleino A, Sormunen R, Ezekowitz RA, Kocks C, et al. Double-stranded RNA is internalized by scavenger receptor-mediated endocytosis in *Drosophila* S2 cells. *J Biologic Chem*. 2006;281:14370-5. DOI: 10.1074/jbc.M513868200

[39] Scott JG, Michel K, Bartholomay LC, Siegfried BD, Hunter WB, Smagghe G, et al. Towards the elements of successful insect RNAi. *J Insect Physiol*. 2013;59:1212-21. DOI: 10.1016/j.jinsphys.2013.08.014

[40] Tijsterman M, May RC, Simmer F, Okihara KL, Plasterk RHA. Genes required for systemic RNA interference in *Caenorhabditis elegans*. *Curr Biol*. 2004;14:111-6. DOI: 10.1016/j.cub.2003.12.029

[41] Sijen T, Fleenor J, Simmer F, Thijssen KL, Parrish S, Timmons L, et al. On the role of RNA amplification in dsRNA-triggered gene silencing. *Cell*. 2001;107:465-76. DOI: 10.1016/s0092-8674(01)00576-1

[42] Yigit E, Batista PJ, Bei Y, Pang KM, Chen C-CG, Tolia NH, et al. Analysis of the *C. elegans* argonaute family reveals that distinct argonautes act sequentially during RNAi. *Cell*. 2006;127:747-57. DOI: 10.1016/j.cell.2006.09.033

[43] Baum JA, Bogaert T, Clinton W, Heck GR, Feldmann P, Ilagan O, et al. Control of coleopteran insect pests through RNA interference. *Natur Biotechnol*. 2007;25:1322-6. DOI: 10.1038/nbt1359

[44] Mao Y-B, Cai W-J, Wang J-W, Hong G-J, Tao X-Y, Wang L-J, et al. Silencing a cotton bollworm P450 monooxygenase gene by plant-mediated RNAi impairs larval tolerance of gossypol. *Natur Biotechnol*. 2007;25:1307-13. DOI: 10.1038/nbt1352

[45] Zhu J-Q, Liu S, Ma Y, Zhang J-Q, Qi H-S, Wei Z-J, et al. Improvement of pest resistance in transgenic tobacco plants expressing dsRNA of an insect-associated gene EcR. *Plos One*. 2012;7: e38572. DOI: 10.1371/journal.pone.0038572

[46] Bolognesi R, Ramaseshadri P, Anderson J, Bachman P, Clinton W, Flannagan R, et al. Characterizing the mechanism of action of double-stranded RNA activity against Western corn rootworm (*Diabrotica virgifera virgifer*a LeConte). *Plos One*. 2012;7: e47534. DOI: 10.1371/journal.pone.0047534

[47] Auer C, Frederick R. Crop improvement using small RNAs: applications and predictive ecological risk assessments. *Trends Biotechnol*. 2009;27:644-51. DOI: 10.1016/j.tibtech.2009.08.005

[48] Kumar M, Gupta GP, Rajam MV. Silencing of acetylcholinesterase gene of *Helicoverpa armigera* by siRNA affects larval growth and its life cycle. *J Insect Physiol*. 2009;55:273-8. DOI: 10.1016/j.jinsphys.2008.12.005

[49] Upadhyay SK, Chandrashekar K, Thakur N, Verma PC, Borgio JF, Singh PK, et al. RNA interference for the control of whiteflies (*Bemisia tabaci*) by oral route. *J Biosci*. 2011;36:153-61. DOI: 10.1007/s12038-011-9009-1

[50] Meyering-Vos M, Mueller A. RNA interference suggests sulfakinins as satiety effectors in the cricket *Gryllus bimaculatus*. *J Insect Physiol*. 2007;53:840-8. DOI: 10.1016/j.jinsphys.2007.04.003

[51] Shakesby AJ, Wallace IS, Isaacs HV, Pritchard J, Roberts DM, Douglas AE. A water-specific aquaporin involved in aphid osmoregulation. *Insect Biochem Mol Biol*. 2009;39:1-10. DOI: 10.1016/j.ibmb.2008.08.008

[52] Uryu O, Kamae Y, Tomioka K, Yoshii T. Long-term effect of systemic RNA interference on circadian clock genes in hemimetabolous insects. *J Insect Physiol*. 2013;59:494-9. DOI: 10.1016/j.jinsphys.2013.02.009

[53] Pereira TC. *Introdução à Técnica de Interferência por RNA – RNAi*. 1st ed. Ribeirão Preto: Sociedade Brasileira de Genética; 2013. 170p.

[54] Rodrigues TB, Khajuria C, Wang HC, Matz N, Cardoso DC, Valicente FH, et al. Validation of reference housekeeping genes for gene expression studies in Western corn rootworm (*Diabrotica virgifera virgifera*). *Plos One*. 2014;9: e0124187. DOI: doi:10.1371/journal.pone.0124187

[55] Holmes K, Williams CM, Chapman EA, Cross MJ. Detection of siRNA induced mRNA silencing by RT-qPCR: considerations for experimental design. *BMC Res Notes*. 2010;3. DOI: 1756-0500/3/53

[56] Bustin SA, Benes V, Garson JA, Hellemans J, Huggett J, Kubista M, et al. The MIQE guidelines: Minimum information for publication of quantitative real-time PCR experiments. *Clin Chem*. 2009;55:611-22. DOI: 10.1373/clinchem.2008.112797

[57] Rinkevich FD, Scott JG. Limitations of RNAi of a6 nicotinic acetylcholine receptor subunits for assessing the in vivo sensitivity to spinosad. *Insect Sci*. 2013;20:101-8. DOI: 10.1111/j.1744-7917.2012.01523.x

[58] Lomazzo E, Hussmann GP, Wolfe BB, Yasuda RP, Perry DC, Kellar KJ. Effects of chronic nicotine on heteromeric neuronal nicotinic receptors in rat primary cultured neurons. *J Neurochem*. 2011;119:153-64. DOI: 10.1111/j.1471-4159.2011.07408.x

[59] Araujo RN, Santos A, Pinto FS, Gontijo NF, Lehane MJ, Pereira MH. RNA interference of the salivary gland nitrophorin 2 in the triatomine bug *Rhodnius prolixus* (Hemiptera : Reduviidae) by dsRNA ingestion or injection. *Insect Biochem Mol Biol*. 2006;36:683-93. DOI: 10.1016/j.ibmb.2006.05.012

[60] Griebler M, Westerlund SA, Hoffmann KH, Meyering-Vos M. RNA interference with the allatoregulating neuropeptide genes from the fall armyworm *Spodoptera frugiperda* and its effects on the JH titer in the hemolymph. *J Insect Physiol*. 2008;54:997-1007. DOI: 10.1016/j.jinsphys.2008.04.019

[61] Allen ML, Walker WB. Saliva of Lygus lineolaris digests double stranded ribonucleic acids. *J Insect Physiol*. 2012;58:391-6. DOI: 10.1016/j.jinsphys.2011.12.014

[62] Rodriguez-Cabrera L, Trujillo-Bacallao D, Borras-Hidalgo O, Wright DJ, Ayra-Pardo C. RNAi-mediated knockdown of a *Spodoptera frugiperda* trypsin-like serine-protease gene reduces susceptibility to a *Bacillus thuringiensis* Cry1Ca1 protoxin. *Environ Microbiol*. 2010;12:2894-903. DOI: 10.1111/j.1462-2920.2010.02259.x

[63] Price DRG, Gatehouse JA. RNAi-mediated crop protection against insects. *Trends Biotechnol*. 2008;26:393-400. DOI: 10.1016/j.tibtech.2008.04.004

[64] Katoch R, Sethi A, Thakur N, Murdock LL. RNAi for insect control: Current perspective and future challenges. *Appl Biochem Biotechnol*. 2013;171:847-73. DOI: 10.1007/s12010-013-0399-4

[65] Gordon KHJ, Waterhouse PM. RNAi for insect-proof plants. *Natur Biotechnol*. 2007;25:1231-2. DOI: 10.1038/nbt1107-1231

[66] Zhang H, Li H-C, Miao X-X. Feasibility, limitation and possible solutions of RNAi-based technology for insect pest control. *Insect Sci*. 2013;20:15-30. DOI: 10.1111/j.1744-7917.2012.01513.x

[67] Li H, Khajuria C, Rangasamy M, Gandra P, Fitter M, Geng C, et al. Long dsRNA but not siRNA initiates RNAi in western corn rootworm larvae and adults. *J Appl Entomol*. 2015;139:432-45. DOI: 10.1111/jen.12224

[68] Zhang J, Khan SA, Hasse C, Ruf S, Heckel DG, Bock R. Full crop protection from an insect pest by expression of long double-stranded RNAs in plastids. *Science*. 2015;347:991-4. DOI: 10.1126/science.1261680

[69] Whyard S. Insecticidal RNA, the long and short of it. *Science*. 2015;347:950-1. DOI: 10.1126/science.aaa7722

[70] Xiong Y, Zeng H, Zhang Y, Xu D, Qiu D. Silencing the HaHR3 Gene by transgenic plant-mediated RNAi to disrupt *Helicoverpa armigera* development. *Int J Biologic Sci*. 2013;9:370-81. DOI: 10.7150/ijbs.5929

[71] Liu F, Wang X, Zhao Y, Li Y, Liu Y, Sun J. Silencing the HaAK gene by transgenic plant-mediated RNAi impairs larval growth of *Helicoverpa armigera*. *Int J Biologic Sci*. 2015;11:67-74. DOI: 10.7150/ijbs.10468

[72] Pitino M, Coleman AD, Maffei ME, Ridout CJ, Hogenhout SA. Silencing of aphid genes by dsRNA feeding from plants. *Plos One*. 2011;6:e25709. DOI: 10.1371/journal.pone.0025709

[73] Bhatia V, Bhattacharya R, Uniyal PL, Singh R, Niranjan RS. Host generated siRNAs attenuate expression of serine protease gene in *Myzus persicae*. *Plos One*. 2012;7: e46343. DOI: 10.1371/journal.pone.0046343

[74] Mao J, Zeng F. Plant-mediated RNAi of a gap gene-enhanced tobacco tolerance against the *Myzus persicae*. *Transg Res*. 2014;23:145-52. DOI: 10.1007/s11248-013-9739-y

[75] Thakur N, Upadhyay SK, Verma PC, Chandrashekar K, Tuli R, Singh PK. Enhanced whitefly resistance in transgenic tobacco plants expressing double stranded RNA of v-ATPase A gene. *Plos One*. 2014;9: e87235. DOI: 1756-0500/3/53

Chapter 19

RNA Interference – Natural Gene-Based Technology for Highly Specific Pest Control (HiSPeC)

Eduardo C. de Andrade and Wayne B. Hunter

Additional information is available at the end of the chapter

http://dx.doi.org/10.5772/61612

Abstract

RNAi technologies are more environmentally friendly, as the technology provides greater specificity in pest targeting, while reducing the potential negative effects on ecosystems and leaving beneficial insects and other organisms unharmed in crop ecosystems. Consequently, the increase in native fauna improves the efficacy of biological control agents against pests and pathogens. A growing understanding of the ubiquitous nature of RNAi, along with evidence for efficient, non-transgenic, topical applications has already begun to garner support among organic and industry producers. Designing solutions to agricultural problems based upon the same mechanisms used in nature provides newer, safer solutions to pests and pathogens for all agricultural industries.

Keywords: Future, Crops, Organic, Non-transgenic, RNAi

1. Introduction

A phenomenon initially reported in plants [1] called the attention of the scientific community, leading to the discovery of a sophisticated mechanism of gene regulation and protection against invasive nucleic acids [2–4]. Furthermore, the mechanism described in plants, referred to as post-transcriptional gene silencing (PTGS), or virus-induced gene silencing (VIGS), had been described in the 1990s [5] and was often referred to as pathogen-derived resistance [6].

RNAi is a natural process of gene regulation and antiviral defense system of eukaryotic cells. RNAi is a mechanism that functions as a "gene silencer" by targeting specific RNA sequences. RNAi results in degradation, and in some situations, translation inhibition, resulting in a reduction or complete elimination of the expression of a targeted RNA [7]. RNAi is also linked to suppressing gene expression at transcriptional level by directing epigenetic alterations on chromatin [8].

The basic RNAi process consists of the trigger molecule, a long endogenous or exogenous double-strand RNA (dsRNA) molecule that is expressed in, or introduced into, the cell, which is processed by Dicer, a ribonuclease III (RNase III) enzyme into small RNA duplexes of 21–23 nucleotides in length. These duplexes are separated with one strand (the guide strand), producing a protein complex known as the RNA-induced silencing complex (RISC). The RISC complex uses the specific sequence of the guide strand to determine potential target messenger RNAs (mRNA). Once bound to the mRNA, the guide strand directs a RISC-bound endonuclease [called "slicer", an Argonaute (AGO) protein] to cleave the mRNA which has homology to the guide strand [9]. Thus, the RISC complex can target the messenger RNA (mRNA), an invasive virus RNA, or a transposable element transcript (Please note that RNAi cannot eliminate transposons itself, but its transcripts.) [10]. These components appear to be cosmopolitan in their distribution across the RNAi spectrum of the eukaryotic phyla. This implies that a common ancestor had a functional RNAi pathway [11], estimated to have occurred over a billion years or more ago [12].

The generation of virus-resistant transgenic plants, by expressing fragments of viral genomes, was the first demonstration of the beneficial use of the RNAi [13,14]. However, with the demonstration that ingestion of dsRNAs can robustly silence genes in *Caenorhabditis elegans* [7], RNAi became not only an important tool in genetic studies to identify gene function but also opened a new field of application in plant protection against insects, arthropods, and pathogens.

In this chapter, we outlined some aspects on the development of RNAi-based strategies to control insects, presenting some considerations and research steps that are important to be addressed.

2. RNAi-based products for agricultural management of insect pest

Advances in genomics and initiatives to sequence genomes of agriculturally important organisms created big breakthroughs within the entomology fields of study, including taxonomy, insect physiology, toxicology, immunology, pest management, and microbe–host interactions. This new paradigm affected how research could be conducted, to make discoveries and increase the speed by which these could be accomplished. With these breakthroughs, entomologists, pathologists, and biologists are rapidly advancing toward better, safer, and more specific pest and pathogen management. Development of gene-based methods was dependent upon having the knowledge to understand how the cells in a living organism respond to the threats from viral pathogens, how they regulate their own gene expression, and how they maintain these natural complex systems throughout their lives.

The initial genomes which were sequenced and annotated to elucidate these very complicated interactions from: the nematode – *C. elegans*, the fruit fly – *Drosophila melanogaster*, the red flour beetle – *Tribolium castaneum*, the silkworm – *Bombyx mori*, the pea aphid – *Acyrthosiphon pisum*, the honey bee – *Apis mellifera*, to bumble bee – *Bombus terrestris* and including a few more examples from the world of agriculture [15]. Current genome initiatives, like the i5K

Arthropod initiative [15] and the Beijing Institute of Genomics, BGI, China, plan to sequence thousands of arthropod and plant genomes. The enormous amount of new information produced will also increase the understanding of the genetic basis of the mechanisms nature uses to solve problems at the cellular and organismal levels.

The number of arthropod species which have had successful RNAi reports continues to increase, and this trend will carry agriculture into the future, covering five Classes, in four Subphyla of the Arthropoda phylum, which includes eight insect orders and over 30 insect species [16–17].

3. Pitfalls and solutions – Relevant considerations for development of RNAi in insects

Though the use of RNAi strategies to control a desired insect pest seems to be very straightforward; however, some issues should be taken into considerations: (1) for oral treatments the dsRNA must survive ingestion, then be absorbed by the epithelial cells, and depending upon the target translocated through the hemolymph to reach other tissues. In insects, the dsRNA is mainly introduced through feeding, but dermal application has already been reported to possibly bypass gut issues [18–21]; (2) once inside the body, the dsRNA must enter into the cell to activate the RNAi mechanism. In insects, cell uptake of dsRNA varies widely between species, because there are different mechanisms of systemic absorption and translocation of dsRNAs within and between cells, respectively, leading to differences in response and influencing the efficiency in silencing the target gene [17,22]; (3) once the RNAi mechanisms are triggered in a group of cells, it has been demonstrated that a systemic spread of silencing may also occur, so that other tissues / cells are also affected, which may increase the RNA effect. Successful studies have shown that dsRNA can circulate in the hemolymph, and cause a suppression of genes in tissues distant from initial entry sites in the insect gut, affecting cuticle formation, the nervous system, or ovaries[23–26]. However, in insects results can be highly variable and research efforts continue to elucidate the effects of systemic signaling.

In theory, any cellular mRNA can be inactivated in a precise and controlled manner. With this in mind, the use of the RNAi mechanism to manage an insect pest relies on the capacity to design the dsRNA. The sequence of the dsRNA provides specificity and the researcher must determine the active concentration needed to obtain the desired RNAi outcome; thus, proper design and evaluation of the dsRNA becomes critical.

Identification of vitally important (i.e., with high mortality) target genes of a particular insect is a crucial step toward development of RNAi-based control strategy. Thanks to world science development and increasing efforts of the research community, the identification of an essential target can be achieved by an extended literature search and analyses of available DNA/RNA sequence databases [27]. Once identified, "candidate" target sequences are used to design potent "RNAi causing structures". Then, the dsRNAs must be experimentally validated for functionality, specificity, and stability, toward the specific RNAi target of interest. Furthermore, the development of an efficient delivery system for "RNAi causing structures" is another key step. There are several methods available that include, but are not limited to: microinjection [28], soaking (for mosquito larvae, and nematodes) [29,30], and feeding (chewing and piercing-sucking insects) [17,17,27,31,32].

One approach to identify potential target genes which will function under field conditions is to perform bioassays that closely mimic the conditions in the field, for example, using a bioassay that mimics the feeding of a hemipteran insect acquiring the dsRNA during the natural feeding process performed on the crop plant. One problem with delivering dsRNA through feeding is that, depending on the bioassay, it may be difficult to measure the dose of dsRNA ingested, from the dose absorbed by the gut cells and the target cells [33].

Oral delivery of dsRNA through feeding can be performed by using artificial diet, detached plant parts (leaves, buds, roots), or intact plants [17,24,34,35]. Delivering dsRNA through the diet provides an easy procedure to screen large numbers of dsRNAs in insect larvae and adults [23,24,34,37]. In addition, it allows addressing different issues, such as effective length of dsRNA, determine regions of the gene to be target which may provide better suppression, and to determine the effective lethal concentration (LC50) [23,38].

Although oral feeding provides a more natural screening system, it is important to take into consideration that for some insect species from across all taxonomic orders, they may not provide an effective RNAi response when conducting oral feeding bioassays regardless of the dosage of dsRNA, as the dsRNA may not enter, or be detected in the insect's body [22]. In contrast, in these same insects when dsRNA was injected directly into the insect's body, a potent RNAi response was observed [23,39,40]. Indeed, lack of positive results using feeding bioassays does not necessarily indicate that the insect is insensitive to RNAi, but in a majority of the situations, insects have nucleases in the saliva, in the midgut, or even in the hemolymph that degrades dsRNA before it can be absorbed by the cells [40–42].

Wynant et al. [40] discussed the interactions of enzymes and RNAi-causing dsRNAs in the alimentary tract and hemolymph of insects and other arthropods using oral delivery. The elucidation of the roles of microbes and host enzymes on RNAi efficacy across arthropod species continues to be a challenging field of research [43].

Where information about absorption of dsRNA or presence of nucleases is not available for a particular insect species, the use of reporter dsRNAs molecules are useful to clarify possible issues. It is essential that the dsRNAs sequence should not match with any insect's transcript sequence. The dsRNA "movement" can be monitored (detected), or quantified in the insect's body by RT-qPCR, showing that the insect has acquired the potent, fully functional, systemically spreading dsRNA during feeding (plant, diet, drop of water, etc.) (Figure 1).

When conducting a RT-PCR detection of reporter dsRNA after insect feeding, it is important to sample a tissue other than the gut such as the hemolymph, fat body, or ovary. Careful collection of tissues which are not in direct contact with the gut provides evidence that the dsRNA was truly absorbed by the cells, and you are not just detecting dsRNA just in the digestive tract.

With small insects, as the Asian Citrus Psyllid (ACP) *Diaphorina citri* (whitefly or aphids), collection of material can be difficult without bringing in gut tissues, so another option is to

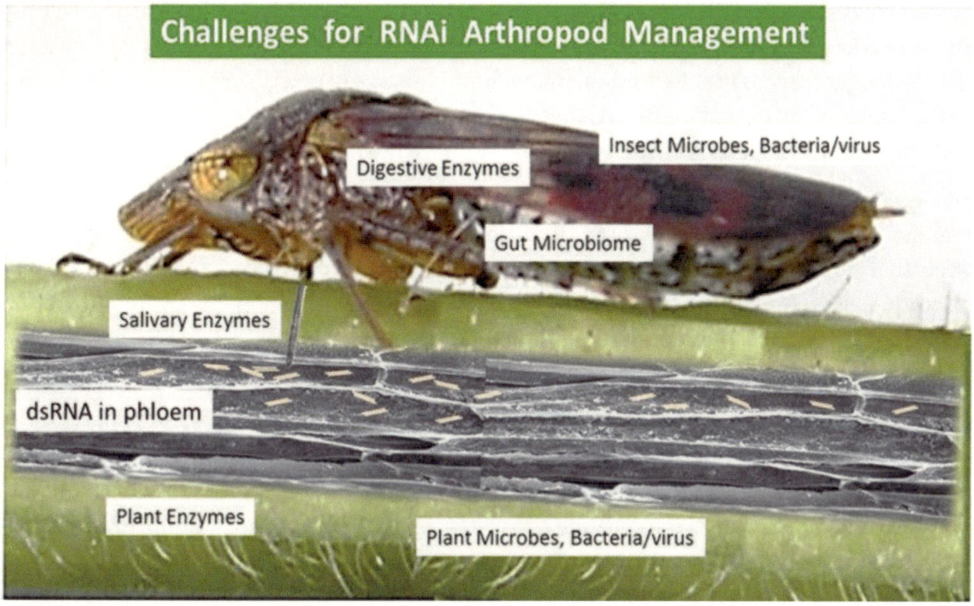

Figure 1. Topically applied RNA, provides long dsRNAs for insect ingestion. If absorbed into the plant, then long dsRNA persists in plant vascular tissues, xylem, and phloem, for several weeks due to lower metabolic activity, fewer enzymes, and microbes. Once the dsRNA enters a plant or insect cell, the RNAi mechanism is triggered, and the dsRNA processed [Image: Hunter, W.B., USDA-ARS, 2015].

let the insects feed on the source of the dsRNA (plant, diet, etc.) for a period of 24–48 h, then transfer them to an untreated food source. After feeding for 36 h, or more, the insect should excrete any food residue from the treated food source, which contains dsRNA. After this period, proceed with sample collection for dsRNA detection.

The reporter dsRNA is designed so that the sequence does not match with any known mRNA transcript in your insect. This is to avoid off target of other transcripts in the insect. Some commonly used dsRNAs which are used as negative controls in RNAi experiments are: green fluorescent protein (GFP), β-glucuronidase (GUS), and enhanced yellow fluorescent protein (EYFP) [44].

When designing RNAi experiments, important questions arise regarding the design of dsRNA, including: the length of the molecule and the region targeted within the mRNA. The minimal required length to achieve an RNAi effect will vary depending on insect species [45]. For example, in *Tribolium castaneum*, analysis showed that the dsRNA length had a strong influence on the efficacy of the RNAi response, with longer dsRNA proven to be more effective on curtailing gene expression [46]. In *T. castaneum* dsRNA, it was observed that length was crucial for cellular uptake; a minimum of 70 nucleotides were necessary to achieve the desired interference. However, other studies in the potato/tomato psyllid, *Bactericera cockerelli* [47], the pea aphid *Acyrthosiphon pisum* [48], and the lepidopteran *Manduca sexta* [49] have reported gene suppression using shorter dsRNAs, between 21 and 27 nucleotides in length. These molecules are called small interfering RNAs (siRNA). Overall, the majority of studies demonstrate success with dsRNA ranging from 140 to 520 nucleotides in length. Interestingly, Huvenne and Smagghe [31] reported success using a dsRNA 1,842 nucleotides in length. dsRNAs longer than 200 nucleotides provide the advantage of resulting in many siRNAs, post-cleavage against the targeted mRNA, thus maximizing the RNAi response and preventing the development of individuals with "resistance" due to the natural genetic variation.

There is no consensus on the mRNA region that the dsRNA should match to (e.g., 5′ or 3′). For example, in the pea aphid, *A. pisum,* no difference in mortality was observed in groups of insects that received dsRNA matching the 5′ or 3′ end of the *hunchback* (hb) gene [27]. In the mosquito, *Aedes aegypti* greater RNAi effects were achieved when insect larvae ingested dsRNA targeting the 3′ end versus 5′ end of an apoptosis gene, *AaeIAP1* [18]. These different results highlight the need to screen several dsRNA molecules across the entire mRNA [50].

In the context of field applications of RNAi for insect management, dsRNAs can be designed to be highly specific to both the target gene and the insect species. If desired, the RNAs can be designed to have a broader spectrum to affect several pest species. For example, RNAi strategies can be designed to remove one aphid species from a cropping system, or be designed to remove multiple aphid species from that same ecosystem [24,38].

4. Bioassays for dsRNA screening

For RNAi research attempting the development of a viable pest management product. It is of utmost importance to identify the best delivery mechanisms (i.e., topical sprays, baits, or transgenic plants) as early as possible; this will expedite the entire process and can cut years off of the development and commercialization timeline.

The example outlined below highlights RNAi bioassays directed toward two citrus insect pests, each one with different feeding behaviors: piercing-sucking plant-feeding (the Asian citrus psyllid *Diaphorina citri,* Hemiptera) and a chewing beetle pest (the weevil *Diaprepes abbreviatus,* Coleoptera). In both situations, the bioassays were designed to evaluate the efficacy of oral ingestion of dsRNAs under "natural feeding conditions" which mimic conditions the insects will encounter in the field.

4.1. Bioassays for piercing-sucking insects

The artificial feeding bioassay is being widely used for studies on insect nutrition, pathogen acquisition, toxicity, and RNAi (Figure 2A) [51–53].

It is notable that liquid feeding bioassays (dsRNAs mixed in a liquid diet or a sucrose solution) frequently result in high mortality levels in the controls, and increased degradation of dsRNA in the solution due to bacterial or fungal contaminations [42,57]. In addition, these bioassays require significantly high dsRNA concentrations to achieve insect mortality. Concentrations up to 1μg/μL [58–60] cannot be reproduced inside plant vascular tissues.

Hemipteran pests in citrus (psyllids, leafhoppers, aphids, whiteflies) have piercing-sucking mouthparts that are inserted into the plant vascular system to feed. The development of an

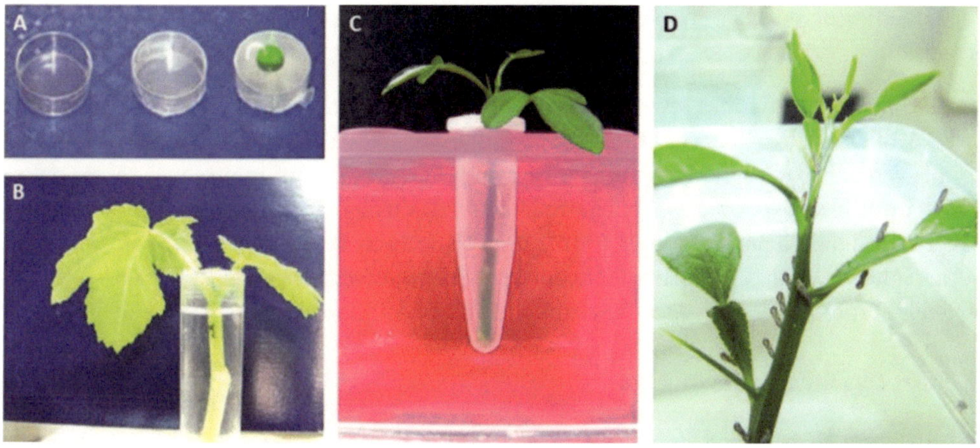

Figure 2. RNAi feeding assays used at the USDA lab, ARS, Ft. Pierce, FL (2007-2014), to successfully screen dsRNA constructs rapidly and under controlled conditions: (A) sucrose solutions within artificial membranes (5 ng dsRNA/μL) [54], (B) rooted okra plant cuttings, (C) citrus flush (5 ng to 100 ng dsRNA/ 0.25 g plant tissue). Plant cuttings absorb dsRNA directly providing systemic movement of dsRNA, (D) insects are given a feeding access period to ingest the dsRNA across 10 days to observe mortality (Hunter and Andrade, USDA-ARS 2015) [54–56].

RNAi control strategy against these insects relies on effective delivery of the dsRNA through the vascular tissues.

Demonstration of the first dsRNA delivery into full-sized citrus trees and grapevines, without a delivery vector, expression vector, or transformation event was performed in 2008 [56]. These results showed that two hemipteran insects, the xylem-feeding leafhopper (*H. vitripennis*), and the phloem-feeding Asian citrus psyllid (*D. citri*), tested positive for ingested dsRNA after feeding from host plants treated with dsRNA as either a foliar spray or root drench. These results along with other studies that demonstrated successful RNAi through oral ingestion in insects [24,34,36,61,62] support the potential for exogenously delivered RNAi control strategies.

Use of cut plant feeding bioassays for hemipteran pests enables the screening of a large number of dsRNAs molecules at a reduced cost of materials and time. The bioassay, can use leaf disks, whole leaf, new growth leaves and stem, or rooted cuttings, to absorb and deliver dsRNAs. In citrus, the "flush", which are new growth foliar shoots, are collected from potted citrus seedlings grown in a glasshouse (USDA-ARS, Fort Pierce, FL). The leaves and stem material are about 7–8 cm long. The plant material is washed in 0.2% bleach water, for 10 min. Then the base of each stem is cut at a 45 degree angle while submerged in filtered water. The material is then placed into a 1.5 mL tube containing 0.5 mL water (Figure 2B and C). The dsRNA solution, 300 μL, is added to the water, the tube top is wrapped with plastic or Parafilm™ and placed under artificial lighting to stimulate absorption of dsRNA solution. The next day the tube is filled with water using a 26 gauge syringe needle and syringed filtered (0.45 μ). The treated cuttings are then placed into a cage and adult insects provided feeding access for 10 days (Figure 2D). The plant material can remain viable for up to 40 days on average. While most bioassays may terminate after eight to 10 days of observations for mortality, having a longer feeding access time enables observations on insect oviposition, egg viability, or nymph development.

Each dsRNA molecules has an optimal concentration. So each dsRNA molecule is evaluated across a range of total concentrations (i.e., 5, 20, 50, 100 nanograms/ tissue). The bioassay permits screening for synergistic effects of multiple dsRNAs and to screen a single dsRNA against multiple insect species. For example, the assay using citrus flush permits screening of dsRNAs designed against psyllids for off target effects in the citrus aphid (*Toxoptera citricidus*) and glassy-winged sharpshooter leafhopper (*Homalodisca vitripennis* (Germar), two closely related hemipterans, which also use citrus trees as a host plant.

4.2. Bioassays for chewing insects

For insects which are foliage feeders, the delivery of dsRNA can be achieved as a foliar topical spray. In this scenario, the dsRNAs are evaluated similarly as topical insecticides. The dsRNA solution is sprayed on leaves, and then fed to the insects. An example of the effectiveness of this approach was reported by Bolognesi [45] working with the coleopteran *Diabrotica virgifera*, in which dsRNA administered through feeding, silenced genes in tissues far from the gut epithelium.

Similar results were obtained while developing an RNAi strategy against the Diaprepes root weevil (DRW), *Diaprepes abbreviatus* L., (Curculionidae: Coleoptera) (Andrade and Hunter). The adults feed and oviposition on mature citrus leaves. Topically applied dsRNA was sprayed on a bouquet of citrus leaves for delivery to DRW adults (Figure 3A). RNA's have been shown to move through the plant xylem and phloem [6].

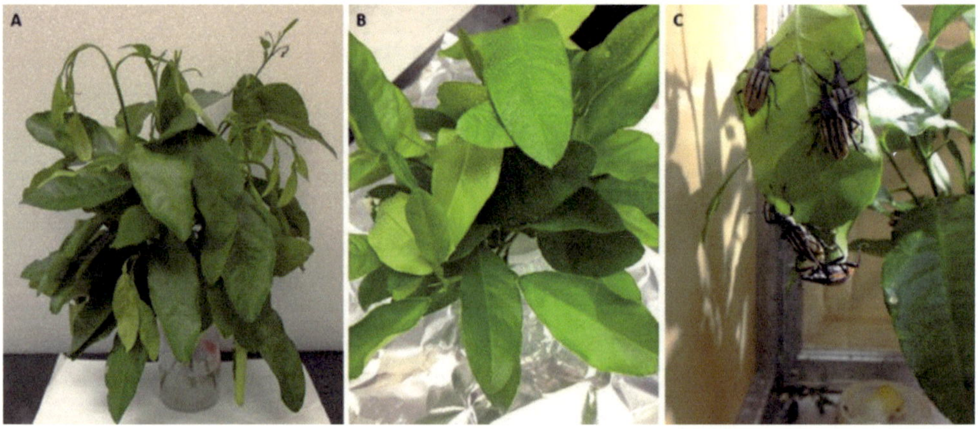

Figure 3. Citrus *"leaf bouquet"* feeding bioassay for *Diaprepes* root weevil. **(A)** Fresh stems with leaves are washed in 0.2% bleach water, rinsed with Nanopure™ filtered water, then the stems are freshly cut while submerged in water. The leaf bouquets are placed in water-filled containers and placed under artificial lighting for 24 h prior to use. **(B)** Topical foliar treatment: the dsRNA is mixed with water and applied using a low-volume aerosol sprayer. **(C)** After the leaves dry, the "bouquets" are caged with adult insects.

A test spray using only water established the volume needed to provide full coverage of leaf bouquets without excessive run off (Figure 3B). After the leaves have dried, they are caged with adult insects (Figure 3C). Freshly treated citrus leaf bouquets replaced previous bouquets every five to seven days for a 5-week period. The total amount of dsRNA to be sprayed over the leaf bouquet was determined by evaluating a range of concentrations in a pretest experiment for efficacy. The effects from RNAi in insects usually start to appear within 4 to 5 days post-ingestion, which suggests there may be a dose response [63]. Since foliage feeding insects tend to eat a lot of leaf material each day, a low-dose spray may be able to deliver a significant amount of dsRNA.

5. Final considerations on RNAi applied to agriculture

Efficient delivery and increased stability of dsRNA need to be developed if non-transgenic, topically delivered, RNAi strategies are to be established. Increased stability and superior delivery into some insects can be achieved using nanoparticle-mediated RNAi [63–65], traditional crop improvement strategies, in which plants express hairpin dsRNAs, will continue to be a mainstay of agricultural approaches [63,65,66].

Transgenic plants have successfully used RNAi strategies to produce crops with improved virus resistance, increased nutrition and fiber content [67]; biotechnology companies are trying to move towards a faster, more natural process of topically applied RNAi. dsRNA molecules are part of naturally occurring processes in all living organisms. They exist in our foods, and our bodies [66]. The short persistence time of dsRNA in the environment is demonstrated by the fact that analyses of soils and plant debris, treated with dsRNA have consistently shown rapid breakdown of dsRNAs within 2–3 days [68], also means less concerns about unintended contamination of water supplies, soils, or adverse air quality effects. Furthermore, since all living things have evolved to break down dsRNA and use the nucleic acids as cellular nutrients, this technology will be safer than conventional chemistries for those who apply RNAi products, or eat the produce [66–69].

RNAi technologies have greater specificity in pest targeting, which reduces negative impacts on crop ecosystems by leaving more insects and other organisms unharmed in the field. The increased fauna consequently improves the efficacy of pollination, and biological control agents that help suppress a broad range of pests. The increased understanding of the ubiquitous nature of RNAi, along with evidence of efficient topical application, has already begun to garner support for this technology among members of the organic grower's communities, which desperately need a truly natural, innovative breakthrough, to manage many of the pests and pathogens which plague the organic industries.

5.1. Cost-effective methods for the mass production and formulation of dsRNA

Cost-efficient methods for mass production of vast amounts of dsRNA are being developed, and include bacterial, plant, and synthetic production [65]. While small amounts of dsRNA can be easily produced in the laboratory for research purposes, commercially available kits are not a viable, cost-effective method for the production of large quantities of dsRNA [65]. The costs associated with the commercialization and implementation of RNAi products are decreasing rapidly. The costs of dsRNA production have dropped from $500,000 USD for 40 g in 2008 to less than $4,000 USD for 40 g today. *For example, see* [70]. As interests in commercialization of RNAi-based products increase, better production systems will be developed to meet the predicted demands of these growing markets [17,65,71]. One of the most cost-effective methods for production is in bacteria, since for most countries bacteria-produced dsRNA would provide an affordable production system which could advance RNAi as, "*The* novel biological insecticide of the future!" Most agricultural companies interested in the future of RNAi are working on developing their own technologies that will further reduce production costs predicted to be near $4 USD per one gram by the end of 2015. *For example, see* [72].

5.2. Other applications

Future applications of RNAi and other gene-based targeting biotechnologies will add value to existing beneficial insects (pollinators, predators, parasitoids). A real-world example is a study conducted over several years in which an RNAi product designed to reduce Israeli acute paralysis virus replication was fed to honey bees. The treated bees had significantly greater survival and produced significantly more honey [73]. RNAi strategies have also reduced honey bee parasites, like *Varroa* mites [74,75], and internal microsporidian parasites [76] without deleterious effects to the bees. The highly specific nature of RNAi approaches can be exploited to reduce pests with no harmful effects on non-target species. The use of RNAi in combination with beneficial pollinators and natural enemies has the potential to raise the level of all pest management efforts [17].

Biotechnology has demonstrated the safe production of plants which are more nutritious, less toxic, more resistant to drought, and more efficient for biofuel production [66, 67]. RNAi has already been successfully used to produce crops which are virus- and drought-resistant [66]. However, plants expressing dsRNAs while stable and safe take years to develop and millions of dollars to commercialize [65]. Development of topically applied RNAi, which is a non-transgenic approach improves crop traits and provides a major step forward for environmentally sound crop management [66, 67].

6. Conclusions

As more insects and mites develop chemical resistance to one or more insecticides, now estimated to be over 500 species with resistance to one or more products [77], it is imperative that new types of pest control are developed. The public would like the world to be filled with environmentally friendly technologies, safe for human and animal consumption, technologies which are safe for use around animals and beneficial insects, safe for each type of ecosystem, forest, field, crop, or backyard, a technology that will not endanger water or food quality, a more natural solution, with a natural approach toward problem-solving. So enters RNA interference!

RNA interference, or gene silencing, is a way to reduce specific mRNAs so that a particular protein is either not made or it is reduced. The RNAi mechanism is a natural one which occurs in the cells of humans, animals, insects, and plants, and appears to have evolved as a primary defense system against virus replication [78]. Andrew Fire and Craig Mello, won the Nobel Prize in 2006 [79] for explaining how the RNAi mechanism is triggered, when a cell encounters double-stranded RNA, and how this could be used to benefit humanity. Humanity's greatest discoveries have come from observing the natural world; while RNAi will not solve every problem, it certainly can help improve plant health, reduce insect pests and pathogens [17, 66, 67, 80]. Some of the benefits from developing RNAi as topically applied products are: 1) The rapid degradation of the molecules ensures low environmental risks. All cells have the capacity to degrade dsRNA, and the salvage pathways to recycle these bases and nucleosides to form new nucleotides. Thus, cells constantly breaking down DNA and RNA into recycled nucleotides [81]. 2) Topical RNAi applications do not insert genes, so do not produce proteins. RNAi reduces the expression of the targeted proteins, a modulation effect of the natural system. 3) RNAi can be designed and tested faster (in about 2–3 years) than producing transgenic crops, which can take 10 to 20 years and cost hundreds of millions of dollars [65]. 4) Finally, RNAi strategies as topical sprays would, for the first time, be able to remove one or two closely related insect species, while leaving all the other insects unharmed [38]. The ability to design RNAi as highly specific pest control will finally provide relief to biological control agents and beneficial insects [17, 44, 73], significantly improving integrated pest management programs.

The advantages and promises from RNAi technology sound amazing. However, serious efforts in outreach and education are needed to better inform the different stake holders including the general public, and agricultural industry, leaders as well as decision makers in the regulatory and political communities to help expedite the release and adoption of RNAi products and technology.

7. Disclaimer

Mention of trade names or commercial products herein is solely for the purpose of providing specific information and does not imply recommendation or endorsement, to the exclusion of other similar products or services by the U.S. Department of Agriculture. USDA is an equal opportunity provider and employer.

Acknowledgements

We thank Dr. Xiomara Sinisterra-Hunter, AgTec, LLC, Plant Biotechnology Consultant, Port St. Lucie, FL, for critical reviews of the manuscript, and Maria Gonzalez, Biological science technician, USDA, Fort Pierce, FL, for technical assistance.

Author details

Eduardo C. de Andrade[1] and Wayne B. Hunter[2]

*Address all correspondence to: eduardo.andrade@embrapa.br

1 Embrapa Cassava and Fruits, Rua Embrapa, s/n, Cruz das Almas,BA, Brasil

2 USDA, ARS, U.S. Horticultural Research Laboratory, Fort Pierce, FL, USA

References

[1] Napoli C, Lemieux C, Jorgensen, R. Introduction of a chimeric chalcone synthase gene into petunia results in reversible co-suppression of homologous genes in trans. Plant Cell 1990;2:279–89. DOI: http://dx.doi.org/10.1105/tpc.2.4.279.

[2] Voinnet O, Pinto YM, Baulcombe DC. Suppression of gene silencing: a general strategy used by diverse DNA and RNA viruses of plants. Proc Nat Acad Sci USA 1999;96:14147–52. DOI: 10.1073/pnas.96.24.14147.

[3] Voinnet O. Induction and suppression of RNA silencing: insights from viral infections. Nat Rev Genetics 2005;6:206–20. DOI: 10.1038/nrg1555.

[4] Sidahmed AM, Wilkie B. Endogenous antiviral mechanisms of RNA interference: a comparative biology perspective. Method Molecul Biol 2010;623:3–19. DOI: 10.1007/978-1-60761-588-0_1.

[5] Baulcombe DC. RNA as a target and an initiator of post-transcriptional gene silencing in trangenic plants. Plant Molecul Biol 1996;32:79–88. DOI 10.1007/BF00039378.

[6] Molnar A, Melnyk C, Baulcombe DC. Silencing signals in plants: a long journey for small RNAs. Genome Biol 2011;12:215. DOI 10.1186/gb-2010-11-12-219.

[7] Fire A, Xu S, Montgomery MK, Kostas SA, Driver SE, Mello CC. Potent and specific genetic interference by double-stranded RNA in *Caenorhabditis elegans*. Nature 1998;391:806–11. DOI: 10.1038/35888.

[8] Castel SE, Martienssen RA. RNA interference in the nucleus: roles for small RNAs in transcription, epigenetics and beyond. Nat Rev Genetics 2013;14:100–12. DOI: 10.1038/nrg3355.

[9] Tomari Y, Zamore PD. Perspective: machines for RNAi Genes Develop 2005;19:517–29. DOI: 10.1101/gad.1284105.

[10] Buchon N, Vaury C. RNAi: a defensive RNA-silencing against viruses and transposable elements. Heredity 2006;96:195–202. DOI:10.1038/sj.hdy.6800789.

[11] Cerutti H, Casas-Mollano, J.A. On the origin and functions of RNA-mediated silencing: from protists to man. Current Genetics 2006;50:81–99. DOI: 10.1007/s00294-006-0078-x.

[12] Roger AJ, Hug LA. The origin and diversification of eukaryotes: problems with molecular phylogenetics and molecular clock estimation. Philosoph Transac Royal Soc B 2006;361:1039–1054. DOI: 10.1098/rstb.2006.1845.

[13] Hamilton AJ, Baulcombe DC. A species of small antisense RNA in posttranscriptional gene silencing in plants. Science 1999;286:950–952. DOI: 10.1126/science.286.5441.950.

[14] Bonfim K, Faria JC, Nogueira EO, Mendes EA, Aragão FJL. RNAi-mediated resistance to bean golden mosaic virus in genetically engineered common bean (*Phaseolus vugaris*). Molecul Plant-Microbe Interact 2007;20:717–26. DOI: http://dx.doi.org/10.1094/MPMI-20-6-0717.

[15] i5K Consortium. The i5K initiative: advancing arthropod genomics for knowledge, human health, agriculture, and the environment. J Heredity 2013;104:595–600. DOI: 10.1093/jhered/est050.

[16] Zhang H, Li H, Miao X. Feasibility, limitation and possible solutions of RNAi-based technology for insect pest control. Insect Sci 2013:20:15–30. DOI 10.1111/j.1744-7917.2012.01513.x.

[17] Zotti M, Smagghe G. RNAi technology for insect management and protection of beneficial insects from diseases: lessons, challenges and risk assessments. Neotropic Entomol 2015;44. DOI 10.1007/s13744-015-0291-8.

[18] Pridgeon JW, Zhao L, Becnel JJ, Strickman DA, Clark GG, Linthicum KJ. Topically applied *AaeIAP1* double-stranded RNA kills female adults of *Aedes aegypti*. J Med Entomol 2008;45:414–20. DOI:http://dx.doi.org/10.1093/jmedent/45.3.414.

[19] Wang Y, Zhang H, Li H, Miao X. Second-generation sequencing supply an effective way to screen RNAi targets in large scale for potential application in pest insect control. PLoS One 2011;6:e18644. DOI: 10.1371/journal.pone.0018644.

[20] El-Shesheny I, Hajeri S, El-Hawary I, Gowda S, Killiny N. Silencing abnormal wing disc gene of the Asian citrus psyllid, *Diaphorina citri* disrupts adult wing development and increases nymph mortality. PLoS One 2013;8:e65392. DOI:10.1371/journal.pone.0065392.

[21] Killiny N, Hajeri S, Tiwari S, Gowda S, Stelinski LL. Double-stranded RNA uptake through topical application, mediates silencing of five *CYP4* genes and suppresses insecticide resistance in *Diaphorina citri*. PLoS One 2014;9:e110536. DOI:10.1371/journal.pone.0110536.

[22] Terenius O, Papanicolaou A, Garbutt JS, Eleftherianos I, Huvenne H, et al. RNA interference in Lepidoptera: an overview of successful and unsuccessful studies and

implications for experimental design. J Insect Physiol 2011;57:231–245. DOI: 10.1016/j.jinsphys.2010.11.006.

[23] Araujo RN, Santos A, Pinto FS, Gontijo NF, Lehane MJ, Pereira MH. RNA interference of the salivary gland nitrophorin 2 in the triatomine bug *Rhodnius prolixus* (Hemiptera: Reduviidae) by dsRNA ingestion or injection. Insect Biochem Molecul Biol 2006;36:683–93. ISSN 0965-1748; 0965-1748. DOI:10.1016/j.ibmb.2006.05.012

[24] Whyard S, Singh AD, Wong S. Ingested double-stranded RNAs can act as species-specific insecticides. Insect Biochem Molecul Biol 2009;39:824–32. DOI: 10.1016/j.ibmb.2009.09.007.

[25] Paim RM, Pereira MH, Di Ponzio R, Rodrigues JO, Guarneri AA, Gontijo NF, Araujo RN. Validation of reference genes for expression analysis in the salivary gland and the intestine of *Rhodnius prolixus* (Hemiptera, Reduviidae) under different experimental conditions by quantitative real-time PCR. BMC Res Notes 2012;5:128. DOI: 10.1186/1756-0500-5-128.

[26] Paim RM, Pereira MH, Araujo RN, Gontijo NF, Guarneri AA. The interaction between *Trypanosoma rangeli* and the nitrophorins in the salivary glands of the triatomine *Rhodnius prolixus* (Hemiptera; Reduviidae). Insect Biochem Molecul Biol 2013;43:229–36. DOI:10.1016/j.ibmb.2012.12.011.

[27] Mao J, Zeng F. Feeding-based RNA interference of a gap gene is lethal to the pea aphid, *Acyrthosiphon pisum*. PLoS One 2012;7:e48718. DOI:10.1371/journal.pone.0048718.

[28] Liu S, Ding Z, Zhang C, Yang B, Liu, Z. Gene knockdown by introthoracic injection of double-stranded RNA in the brown planthopper, *Nilaparvata lugens*. Insect Biochem Molecul Biol 2010;40:666–71. DOI: 10.1016/j.ibmb.2010.06.007.

[29] Singh AD, Wong S, Ryan CP, Whyard S. Oral delivery of double-stranded RNA in larvae of the yellow fever mosquito, *Aedes aegypti*: implications for pest mosquito control. J Insect Sci 2013;13:69. Available from: http://www.insectscience.org/13.69.

[30] Dutta TK, Banakar P, Rao U. The status of RNAi-based transgenic research in plant nematology. Front Microbiol 2015;5:1–7. DOI: 10.3389/fmicb.2014.00760.

[31] Huvenne H, Smagghe G. Mechanisms of dsRNA uptake in insects and potential of RNAi for pest control: a review. J Insect Physiol 2010;56:227–35. DOI:10.1016/j.jinsphys.2009.10.004.

[32] Pitino M, Coleman AD, Maffei ME, Ridout CJ, Hogenhout SA. Silencing of aphid genes by dsRNA feeding from plants. PLoS ONE 2011;6:e25709. DOI: 10.1371/journal.pone.0025709.

[33] Li H, Guan R, Guo H, Miao X. New insights into an RNAi approach for plant defence against piercing-sucking and stem-borer insect pests. Plant Cell Environ 2015:38:1–9. DOI: 10.1111/pce.12546.

[34] Baum JA, Roberts, J.K. Chapter Five- progress towards RNAi-mediated insect pest management. Adv Insect Physiol 2014;47:249–95. DOI: 10.1016/B978-0-12-800197-4.00005-1.

[35] Zhu F, Xu JJ, Palli R, Ferguson J, Palli S.R. Ingested RNA: interference for managing the populations of the Colorado potato beetle, *Leptinotarsa decemlineata*. Pest Manage Sci 2011;67:175–82. DOI: 10.1002/ps.2048.

[36] Turner CT, Davy MW, MacDiarmid RM, Plummer KM, Birch NP, Newcomb RD. RNA interference in the light brown apple moth, *Epiphyas postvittana* (Walker) induced by double-stranded RNA feeding. Insect Molecul Biol 2006;15:383–91. DOI: 10.1111/j.1365-2583.2006.00656.x

[37] Aronstein K, Oppert B, Lorenzen MD. RNAi in Agriculturally-Important Arthropods, RNA Processing, Prof. Paula Grabowski (Ed.), 2011, ISBN: 978-953-307-557-0, InTech, [Available from: http://www.intechopen.com/books/rna-processing/rnai-in-agriculturally-important-arthropods. Accessed 2015/08/25.

[38] Bachman PM, Bolognesi R, Moar WJ, Mueller GM, Paradise MS, et al. Characterization of the spectrum of insecticidal activity of a double-stranded RNA with targeted activity against western corn rootworm (*Diabrotica virgifera virgifera* LeConte). Transgenic Res 2013;22:1207–22. DOI: 10.1007/s11248-013-9716-5.

[39] Wynant N, Verlinden H, Breugelmans B, Simonet G, Vanden Broeck J. Tissue-dependence and sensitivity of the systemic RNA interference response in the desert locust, *Schistocerca gregaria*. Insect Biochem Molecul Biol 2012;42:911–7. DOI:10.1016/j.ibmb.2012.09.004.

[40] Wynant N, Santos D, Verdonck R, Spit J, Van Wielendaele P, Vanden Broeck, J. Identification, functional characterization and phylogenetic analysis of double stranded RNA degrading enzymes present in the gut of the desert locust, *Schistocerca gregaria*. Insect Biochem Molecul Biol 2014;46:1–8.DOI: http://dx.DOI.org/10.1016/j.ibmb.2013.12.008.

[41] Garbutt JS, Bellés X, Richards EH, Reynolds SE. Persistence of double-stranded RNA in insect hemolymph as a potential determiner of RNA interference success: evidence from *Manduca sexta* and *Blattella germanica*. J. Insect Physiology 2012. DOI: http://dx.doi.org/10.1016/j.jinsphys.2012.05.013.

[42] Christiaens O, Swevers L, Smagghe G. DsRNA degradation in the pea aphid (*Acyrthosiphon pisum*) associated with lack of response in RNAi feeding and injection assay. Peptides 2014;53:307–14. DOI: 10.1016/j.peptides.2013.12.014.

[43] Sharma P, Sharma S, Maurya RK, De TD, Thomas T, Lata S, Singh N, Pandey KC, Valecha N, Dixti R. Salivary glands harbor more diverse microbial communities than gut in *Anopheles culicificacies*. Parasites Vectors 2014;7:235. DOI: 10.1186/1756-3305-7-235.

[44] Scott JG, Michel K, Bartholomay LC, Siegfried BD, Hunter WB, Smagghe G, Zhu KY, Douglas AE. Towards the elements of successful insect RNAi. J Insect Physiol 2013;59:1212–21. http://dx.doi.org/10.1016/j.jinsphys.2013.08.014.

[45] Bolognesi R, Ramaseshadri P, Anderson J, Bachman P, Clinton W, Flannagan R, Ilagan O, Lawrence C, Levine S, Moar W, et al. Characterizing the mechanism of action of double-stranded RNA activity against western corn rootworm (*Diabrotica virgifera virgifera* LeConte). PLoS One 2012;7: e47534. DOI:10.1371/journal.pone.0047534.

[46] Miller SC, Miyata K, Brown SJ, Tomoyasu Y. Dissecting systemic RNA interference in the red flour beetle *Tribolium castaneum*: parameters affecting the efficiency of RNAi. PLoS One 2012;7:e47431. DOI:10.1371/journal.pone.0047431.

[47] Wuriyanghan H, Rosa C, Falk BW. Oral delivery of double-stranded RNAs and siRNAs induces RNAi effects in the potato/tomato psyllid, *Bactericerca cockerelli*. PLoS One 2011;6:e27736. DOI: 10.1371/journal.pone.0027736.

[48] Mutti NS, Park Y, Reese JC, Reeck GR. RNAi knockdown of a salivary transcript leading to lethality in the pea aphid, *Acyrthosiphon pisum*. J Insect Sci 2006;6:1–7. DOI: 10.1673/031.006.3801.

[49] Kumar P, Pandit SS, Baldwin I.T. Tobacco rattle virus vector: a rapid and transient means of silencing *Manduca sexta* genes by plant mediated RNA interference. PLoS One 2012;7:e31347. DOI:10.1371/journal.pone.0031347.

[50] Noh MY, Beeman RW, Arakane Y. RNAi-based functional genomics in *Tribolium castaneum* and possible applications for controlling insect pests. Entomol Res 2012;42:1–10. DOI: 10.1111/j.1748-5967.2011.00437.x.

[51] Hamilton MA. Further experiments on the artificial feeding of *Myzus persicae* (Sulz.) Annal Appl Biol 1935;32:243–58. DOI:10.1111/j.1744-7348.1935.tb07160.x.

[52] Li J, Wang W-P, Wang M-Q, Ma W-H, Hua H-X. Advances in the use of the RNA interference technique in Hemiptera. Insect Sci 2013;20:31–9. DOI 10.1111/j. 1744-7917.2012.01550.x.

[53] Christiaens O, Smagghe G. The challenge of RNAi-mediated control of hemipterans. Curr Opin Insect Sci 2014;6:15–21. DOI: http://dx.doi.org/10.1016/j.cois.2014.09.012.

[54] Hall DG, Shatters RG, Carpenter JE, Shapiro JP. Research toward an artificial diet for adult Asian Citrus Psyllid. Annal Entomol Soc Am 2010;03: 611–17. DOI:http://dx.doi.org/10.1603/AN10004.

[55] Hall DG, Richardson ML, Ammar E-D, Halbert SE. Asian citrus psyllid, *Diaphorina citri*, vector of citrus huanglongbing disease. Entomol Experiment Applic 2012;146:207–23. DOI: 10.1111/eea.12025.

[56] Hunter WB, Glick E, Paldi N, Bextine BR. Advances in RNA interference: dsRNA treatment in trees and grapevines for insect pest suppression. Southwest Entomol 2012;37:85–7. DOI: http://dx.doi.org/10.3958/059.037.0110.

[57] Upadhyay SK, Chandrashekar K, Thakur N, Verma PC, Borgio JF, Singh PK, Tuli R. RNA interference for the control of whiteflies (*Bemisia tabaci*) by oral route. J Biosci 2011;36:153–61. DOI:10.1007/s12038-011-9009-1.

[58] Borgio JF. RNAi mediated gene knockdown in sucking and chewing insect pests. J Biopesticides 2010;3:386–93. Available from: http://www.jbiopest.com/users/lw8/efiles/francis_borgio.pdf.

[59] Katoch R, Sethi A, Thakur N, Murdock LL. RNAi for insect control: current perspective and future challenges. Appl Biochem Biotechnol 2013;171:847–73. DOI:10.1007/s12010-013-0399-4.

[60] Tomizawa M, Noda H. High mortality caused by high dose of dsRNA in the green rice leafhopper *Nephotettix cincticeps* (Hemiptera: Cicadellidae). Appl Entomol Zoo 2013;48:553–59. DOI:10.1007/s13355-013-0211-5.

[61] Zhou X, Wheeler MM, Oi FM, Scharf ME. RNA interference in the termite *Reticulitermes flavipes* through ingestion of double-stranded RNA. Insect Biochem Molecul Biol 2008;38:805–15. DOI:10.1016/j.ibmb.2008.05.005.

[62] Zha W, Peng X, Chen R, Du B, Zhu L, He, G. Knockdown of midgut genes by dsRNA-transgenic plant-mediated RNA interference in the Hemipteran insect *Nilaparvata lugens*. PLoS One 2011;6(5):e20504. DOI:10.1371/journal.pone.0020504.

[63] Yu N, Christiaens O, Lui J, Niu J, Cappelle K, Caccia S, Huvenne H, Smagghe G. Delivery of dsRNA for RNAi in insects: an overview and future directions. Insect Sci 2013;20:4–40. Doi 10.1111/j.1744-7917.2012.01534.x.

[64] Zhang X, Zhang J, Zhu KY. Chitosan/double-stranded RNA nanoparticle-mediated RNA interference to silence chitin synthase genes through larval feeding in the African malaria mosquito (*Anopheles gambiae*). Insect Molecul Biol 2010;19:683–93. DOI: 10.1111/j.1365-2583.2010.01029.x

[65] Palli SR. RNA interference in Colorado potato beetle: steps toward development of dsRNA as a commercial insecticide. Curr Opin Insect Sci 2014;3. DOI: 10.1016/j.cois.2014.09.011.

[66] Petrick JS, Brower-Toland B, Jackson A, Kier LD. Safety assessment of food and feed from biotechnology-derived crops employing RNA-mediated gene regulation to achieve desired traits: a scientific review. Regul Toxicol Pharmacol 2013;66:167–76. DOI: http://dx.doi.org/10.1016/j.yrtph.2013.03.008.

[67] Koch A, Kogel K-H. New wind in the sails: improving the agronomic value of crop plants through RNAi-mediated gene silencing. Plant Biotechnol J 2014;12:821–31. DOI:10.1111/pbi.12226.

[68] Dubelman S, Fischer J, Zapata F, Huizinga K, Jiang CJ, et al. Environmental fate of double-stranded RNA in agricultural soils. PLoS ONE 2014;9. DOI:10.1371/journal.pone.0093155.

[69] Ivashuta SI, Petrick JS, Heisel SE, Zhang Y, Guo L, Reyholds TL, Rice JF, Allen E, Roberts JK. Endogenous small RNAs in grain: Semi-quantification and sequence homology to human and animal genes. Food Chem Toxicol 2009;47:353–60. DOI: 10.1016/j.fct.2008.11.025.

[70] AgroRNA, South Korea, [Internet]. Available from: http://www.agrorna.com/. Accessed: 2015/08/25.

[71] Nguyen TA, Fruehauf JH. *transkingdom* RNA interference (*tk*RNAi): a novel method to induce therapeutic gene silencing. T-Cell Protocols. Method Molecul Biol 2009;514:27–34. Available from: http://link.springer.com/protocol/10.1007%2F978-1-60327-527-9_3.

[72] APSE, LLC, [Internet]. Available from: http://www.apsellc.com/. Accessed: 2015/08/25.

[73] Hunter W, Ellis J, VanEngelsdorp D, Hayes J, Westervelt D, Glick E, Paldi N. Large-scale field application of RNAi technology reducing Israeli acute paralysis virus disease in honey bees (*Apis mellifera,* Hymenoptera: Apidae). PLoS Pathogens 2010;6:e1001160. DOI:10.1371/journal.ppat.1001160.

[74] Campbell EM, Budge GE, Bowman AS. Gene-knockdown in the honey bee mite *Varroa destructor* by a non-invasive approach: studies on a glutathione S-transferase. Parasites Vectors 2010;3:73. DOI:10.1186/1756-3305-3-73.

[75] Garbian Y, Maori E, Kalev H, Shafir S, Sela I. Bidirectional transfer of RNAi between honey bee and *Varroa destructor*: *Varroa* gene silencing reduces *Varroa* population. PLoS Pathogens 2012;8(12):e1003035. DOI: 10.1371/journal.ppat.1003035.

[76] Paldi N, Glick E, Oliva M, Zilberberg Y, Aubin L, Pettis JS, Chen YP, Evans JD. 2010. Effective gene silencing of a microsporidian parasite associated with honey bee (*Apis mellifera*) colony declines. Appl Environ Microbiol 2010;76:5960–4. DOI:10.1128/AEM.01067-10.

[77] Elzen GW, Hardee DD. United States Department of Agriculture–Agricultural Research Service, Research on managing insect resistance to insecticides. Pest Management Sci 2003;59:770–6.

[78] Blair CD, Olson KE. The role of RNA interference (RNAi) in Arbovirus-vector interactions. Viruses 2015;7:820–43. DOI: 10.3390/v7020820.

[79] The Nobel Prize in Physiology or Medicine 2006. Andrew Z. Fire and Craig C. Mello "For their discovery of RNA interference - gene silencing by double-stranded RNA". Available from: http://www.nobelprize.org/nobel_prizes/medicine/laureates/2006/. [Accessed: 2015-08-25].

[80] Whyard S. Insecticidal RNA, the long and short of it. Science 2015;347:950–91. DOI: 10.1126/science.aaa7722.

[81] Lane AN, Fan TW-M. Survey and summary. Regulation of mammalian nucleotide metabolism and biosynthesis. Nucleic Acids Res 2015;43:1–20. DOI: 10.1093/nar/gkv047.

Chapter 20

RNA Interference – A Powerful Functional Analysis Tool for Studying Tick Biology and its Control

Remil Linggatong Galay, Rika Umemiya-Shirafuji, Masami Mochizuki, Kozo Fujisaki and Tetsuya Tanaka

Additional information is available at the end of the chapter

http://dx.doi.org/10.5772/61577

Abstract

Ticks (Acari: Ixodida) are blood-sucking arthropods globally recognized as vectors of numerous diseases. They are primarily responsible for the transmission of various pathogens, including viruses, rickettsiae, and blood parasites of animals. Ticks are second to mosquitoes in terms of disease transmission to humans. The continuous emergence of tick-borne diseases and acaricide resistance of ticks necessitates the development of new and more effective control agents and strategies; therefore, understanding of different aspects of tick biology and their interaction with pathogens is very crucial in developing effective control strategies. RNA interference (RNAi) has been widely used in the area of tick research as a versatile reverse genetic tool to elucidate the functions of various tick proteins. During the past decade, numerous studies on ticks utilized RNAi to evaluate potentially key tick proteins involved in blood feeding, reproduction, evasion of host immune response, interaction with pathogens, and pathogen transmission that may be targeted for tick and pathogen control. This chapter reviewed the application of RNAi in tick research over the past decade, focusing on the impact of this technique in the advancement of knowledge on tick and pathogen biology.

Keywords: Acari, ticks, Ixodidae, RNA interference, tick-borne diseases

1. Introduction

Ticks belong to the class of Arachnida together with spiders, scorpions, and mites. To date, there are about 900 species of ticks, majority of which are hard ticks belonging to the Ixodidae family, as well as about 200 species are soft ticks belonging to the Argasidae family, and a single species belonging to the Nuttalliellidae family [1]. Most of the ticks of medical and veterinary importance are hard ticks. Through their blood-feeding behavior, ticks can directly affect their host by causing anemia, irritation, and allergic reactions particularly in heavy infestation. The saliva of some tick species may also contain neurotoxic substances that may cause the condition termed "tick paralysis" [2]. Additionally, the transmission of pathogens including viruses, bacteria, and parasitic protozoa also occurs during blood feeding [1]. Ticks are considered second to mosquitoes in terms of their impact on public health, but they are the most important vectors of different pathogens in both domestic and wild animals [3]. Tick infestation and tick-borne diseases (TBDs) continue to have great economic impact on livestock production, particularly on cattle and small ruminants, in several continents [2]. The annual loss in cattle production worldwide due to ticks and TBDs has been estimated to be worth billions of USD [4].

The complete dependence of ticks to host blood for the completion of their life cycle and generation of offspring is the reason for their notoriety as vectors of several diseases. Depending on the species, a tick may utilize one to three hosts during their life cycle. Most of the pathogens they transmit can be carried on throughout their life cycle through transstadial (from one stage to the next) transmission and to the next generation through transovarial (from adults to eggs) transmission [5]. A single tick may carry multiple pathogens [6], thereby having the potential of infecting a host with a cocktail of pathogens. Most tick-borne infections are zoonotic in nature, and more of these are being recognized in recent years [1, 7]. Among the TBDs that are well-known in the veterinary and medical field are anaplasmosis, borreliosis, rickettsiosis, ehrlichiosis, babesiosis, theileriosis, and tick-borne encephalitis.

The significant impact of ticks and TBDs underscores the importance of tick control. For several decades, the application of chemical acaricides has been the primary tick control method, and acaricides were used extensively in livestock production. However, the continuous emergence of resistant tick strains makes most chemical acaricides ineffective [8]. Moreover, the increasing concerns for animal product and environmental contamination set limitations for this control method. To search for new and more effective means of controlling ticks and TBDs, researchers have actively expanded the understanding on tick biology.

RNA interference (RNAi) is a reverse genetic approach for manipulation of genes that commonly utilizes double-stranded RNA (dsRNA) to induce post-transcriptional gene-specific silencing [9]. RNAi has been extensively employed in many studies on tick biology and pathogen interaction since the first report of RNAi application in the hard tick *Amblyomma americanum* [10]. In fact, it is evident that a number of laboratories in different countries working on tick research are routinely performing RNAi, as shown by an increasing number of recent publications utilizing this technique. Typically, functional studies using RNAi involve gene knockdown with subsequent infestation and evaluation of phenotypes, such as blood feeding and reproduction success (Figure 1). Indeed, RNAi has been particularly useful in searching for tick proteins that can be targeted for control of tick development and TBDs [11].

This chapter aims to show the extent of RNAi application in tick research, emphasizing the progress of advanced knowledge on tick biology and tick-pathogen interaction. We first discussed so far known RNAi mechanisms and the current RNAi inducing methods in ticks; then, briefly described the studies on tick physiology, immunity, and pathogen interaction that employed RNAi, highlighting the prospects of applications of RNAi in tick research.

http://dx.doi.org/10.5772/61577

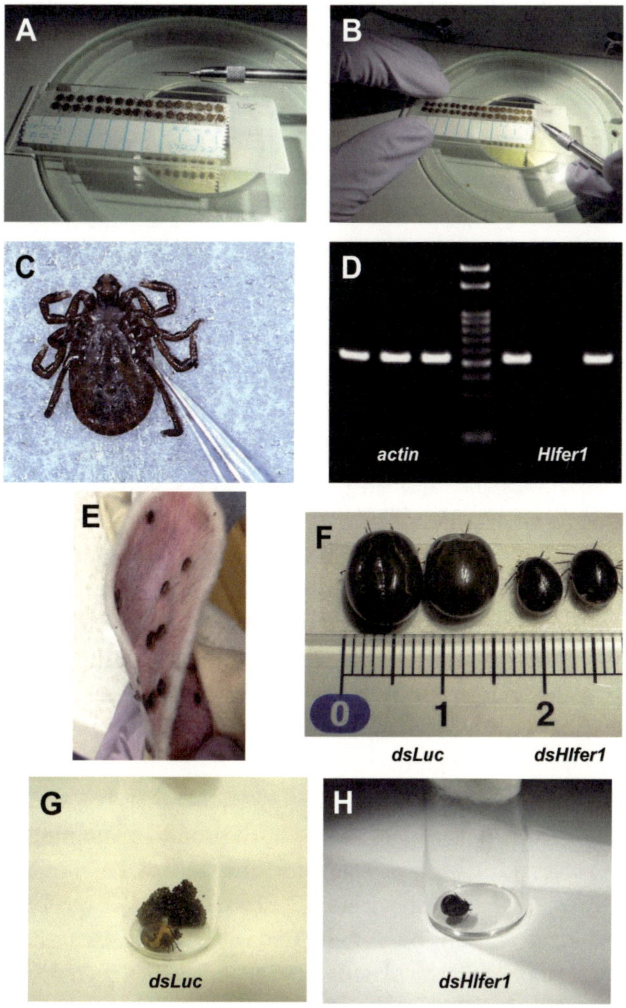

Figure 1. A typical RNAi experiment in the hard tick *Haemaphysalis longicornis*. The double-stranded RNA (dsRNA) is introduced to adult ticks by microinjection. Unfed adult ticks, placed on a double adhesive tape attached on a glass slide (A), are injected with dsRNA using a pointed microcapillary glass attached to a microinjector (B) through the membrane of the fourth coxa under a stereomicroscope (C). Successful silencing, as shown by the absence of a band for the target gene, such as *Hlfer1*, is confirmed around 4 d post-injection through RT-PCR after adjusting the cDNA level using an internal control, such as actin (D). Ticks were infested on a host and allowed to feed to repletion (E) and after dropping, parameters such as engorged body weight (F), survival, egg laying (G, H), and hatch were compared.

2. RNAi pathway in ticks

The mechanism of RNAi has been well studied in the nematode *Caenorhabditis elegans* and the fruit fly *Drosophila melanogaster* [9, 12]. RNAi begins with the uptake of dsRNA by the cell, followed by its cleavage to produce small interfering RNAs (siRNAs). Cleavage of dsRNA is accomplished by an RNAse III enzyme called Dicer. The siRNAs are then incorporated into RNA-induced silencing complex (RISC), which then drives the degradation or translational inhibition of the target mRNA that results to gene silencing. This silencing signal may spread among the cells and different tissues, leading to systemic gene silencing in the whole organism [13]. The mechanism of RNAi in ticks has not been fully elucidated, but the study of Kurscheid et al. [14] revealed that several components of RNAi machinery in other invertebrates are also present in the ticks, and they proposed a putative tick RNAi pathway. Here, we briefly describe the available knowledge on key components of RNAi machinery in ticks, in comparison of other invertebrates.

2.1. dsRNA uptake

There are two recognized dsRNA uptake mechanisms in invertebrates: a transmembrane channel-mediated uptake through systemic RNA interference defective (SID) transmembrane proteins described in *C. elegans*, and an endocytosis-mediated uptake described in most arthropods [15, 16]. Several SIDs identified in *C. elegans* have been shown to be involved in the spread of RNAi [17]. SID-1, SID-3, and SID-5, which have wide tissue distribution, are involved in the systemic spread of RNAi [18–20], whereas SID-2, localized mainly in the gut, is involved primarily in the intestinal uptake of ingested dsRNA [21]. The multi-domain SID-1 along the plasma membrane facilitates the traffic of dsRNA into and out of the cells. Homologs of SID-1 are present in some arthropods and vertebrates [18]. Both SID-3, a conserved tyrosine kinase, and SID-5 have intracytoplasmic localization, the latter being associated with late endosomes [19, 20]. SID-2 has luminal localization in the intestinal cells, and it was also found in the lower levels of excretory duct cells [21]. In addition to SIDs, endocytosis has also been also implicated as a dsRNA uptake mechanism in *C. elegans* through a protein containing an epsin N-terminal homology (ENTH) domain [22]. In *D. melanogaster*, dsRNA uptake in cells is facilitated mainly by scavenger receptor-mediated endocytosis [23]. Two scavenger receptors, Eater and Sr-CI, have been identified to be responsible for the majority of dsRNA uptake. These scavenger receptors are mainly expressed in the plasmatocytes and have a primary role in the phagocytosis of bacterial pathogens [24, 25].

SID homologues have not been identified in ticks. However, a homologue of ENTH, Epn-I, has been identified in the hard ticks *Rhiphicephalus* (*Boophilus*) *microplus* and *Ixodes scapularis* [14]. A class B scavenger receptor identified in *Haemaphysalis longicornis* (HlSRB) has been demonstrated to mediate systemic RNAi in this tick [26, 27]. Combined injection of dsRNA against *HlSRB* and other target genes, *Vitellogenin*-1 (*HlVg-1*) and *Vitellogenin Receptor* (*HlVgR*) effectively silenced these genes. However, silencing *HlSRB* prior to injection of dsRNA against *HlVg-1* and *HlVgR* inhibited the silencing of the latter two genes, suggesting that the uptake of the injected dsRNA is dependent on HlSRB in ticks. Similar to *D. melanogaster* scavenger receptors, HlSRB is also involved in the phagocytosis of bacteria [28], but it is expressed not only in the hemocytes but also in the other organs such as midguts, salivary glands, and ovary [26]. The presence of ENTH homologue and scavenger receptor indicates that the uptake of dsRNA in ticks is through endocytosis. Additionally, the presence of scavenger receptor in different tick tissues strongly implies its involvement in systemic RNAi, particularly after dsRNA injection. Introduction of dsRNA into the hemocoel of ticks directly exposes the different tick organs to dsRNA, and the scavenger receptor in these organs most likely mediates the entry of dsRNA into the cells.

2.2. dsRNA processing and RISC assembly

The recommended length of dsRNA to effectively induce silencing of the target gene in non-mammalian systems is more than 200 bp [15]. A study in *R. (B.) microplus* showed, however, that short dsRNAs between 100 and 200 bp were also effective in inducing silencing of *Ubiquitin-63E* homologue, with minimal off-target effects, but short hairpin dsRNAs were not able to induce silencing effects [29]. After cellular uptake, dsRNAs are cleaved into 21–25 nt siRNAs by an RNAse III enzyme called Dicer. In contrast to *C. elegans* and mammals that have only one Dicer, *D. melanogaster* and mosquitoes have two Dicers [15]. Dicer-2 is the one involved in the generation of siRNA, whereas Dicer-1 acts on stem loop RNA precursors to generate micro RNA (miRNA). Both, however, are required for siRNA-induced gene silencing due to their distinct roles in siRISC assembly [30]. Only a single putative Dicer has been identified so far in the hard tick *I. scapularis*, which is more similar to mammalian Dicer-1 [14].

The RNAi inhibition of a target mRNA is accomplished by RISC formed by siRNAs and Argonaute (AGO) proteins. AGO proteins are highly conserved between species, encoded by multiple genes in most organisms. All AGO proteins are characterized by two domains: the PAZ domain and the PIWI domain [31]. Upon ATP activation, AGO mediates RISC recognition of mRNA target that are homologous to siRNAs, subsequently leading to the cleavage of the mRNA target [9]. In most insects, including *D. melanogaster* and mosquitoes, five AGO genes have been identified [15, 31]. In ticks, a homologue of AGO-1 has been identified in *I. scapularis* and *R. (B.) microplus*, and a homologue of AGO-2 has been identified in *I. scapularis* [14]. However, the functions of these tick AGOs remains to be confirmed.

2.3. Amplification of RNAi signal

The ability to spread throughout the whole organism, inducing total systemic silencing of the target gene in spite of introducing only a relatively small amount of dsRNA, is an important aspect of RNAi observed in plants and invertebrates. This systemic RNAi-induced gene silencing in both plants and *C. elegans* involves RNA-directed RNA polymerase (RdRP) that amplifies the RNAi signal [9]. RdRP function in RNAi has not been found in arthropods, but a putative homologue of RdRP EGO-1 protein of *C. elegans* has been identified in the hard tick *I. scapularis*, and a partial sequence was also identified from *R. (B.) microplus* [14].

3. Methods of introducing dsRNA in ticks

3.1. Injection

Direct injection is the most widely used technique for introducing dsRNA for in vivo gene silencing, not only in ticks but also in insects [11, 32]. Through this method, dsRNA is usually introduced directly into the hemocoel of ticks allowing the dsRNA to circulate within the hemolymph. In most reports, a high concentration of at least 1 μg dsRNA per tick has been shown to be effective in inducing gene silencing [33], but in some reports, lower concentration has been found to be similarly effective [34–36]. Injection has been accomplished using a 33–36-gauge needle attached to a Hamilton syringe particularly in large tick species, such as *Amblyomma americanum*[37], *Dermacentor variabilis*, and *D. marginatus* [38], while microinjection using a microcapillary drawn to a fine point needle and inserted to a micromanipulator has been commonly employed in smaller tick species, including *Ixodes* [39], and *Haemaphysalis* [26] ticks. Different injection sites include the lower right quadrant of the ventral surface of the exoskeleton [40], the groove between the basis capituli and the scutum [37], the ventral torso of the idiosoma, away from the anal opening [39], and the coxal membrane in the fourth coxae [26, 41]. In some reports, dsRNA was injected through the spiracle [29, 42, 43] and anal pore; the latter inducing midgut-specific silencing of the target gene [44]. Injection of dsRNA has been commonly performed in unfed adult ticks, subsequently allowed to recover for at least 24 h before infestation or use in succeeding experiments. Exceptionally, dsRNA has been also injected in engorged *R. (B.) microplus* [42, 45-47], *A. americanum, I. scapularis*, and *D. variabilis* adults [43], which produced significant effects on the eggs and larvae, and microinjection has also been accomplished in *I. scapularis* [48-52] and engorged *O. moubata* nymphs [53].

3.2. Soaking

Soaking in dsRNA has been previously employed to study RNAi in the cell lines of *D. melanogaster* [23, 54]. In tick research, this method has been applied to induce in vitro RNAi not only in cell cultures [55-57], but also in some organs including whole salivary glands [36, 58-60] and midguts [61]. Soaking live *Varroa destructor* [62] and *Dermanyssus gallinae* [63] mites, as well as *Aedes aegypti* larvae [64] in a solution of dsRNA has been already demonstrated in producing effective silencing of the target genes in these organisms. However, soaking whole ticks in a solution of dsRNA has not been commonly performed. Soaking *Haemaphysalis longicornis* nymphs in a solution of dsRNA for 24 h resulted to significant transcript reduction of the target gene, although the effect on the phenotype was not observed in all the nymphs [65]. In our laboratory, we have attempted to soak *H. longicornis* larvae, nymphs, and adults in a dsRNA solution overnight, which resulted to a significant decrease in the mRNA level of a targeted gene (Galay et al., unpublished results). Soaking offers a simpler and less invasive method of introducing dsRNA without injuring the ticks and is applicable to immature tick stages. Furthermore, it does not require injection equipment; therefore, it is less laborious.

3.3. Electroporation

Electroporation is a technique that employs electric impulses to promote DNA uptake of cells and has been primarily used with in vitro cell transfection [66]. In tick research, this technique has been first applied to facilitate the introduction of dsRNA in *I. scapularis* eggs and nymphs [67]. After electroporation, fluorescein-labeled dsRNA was visualized all over the nymph's body and eggs, indicating the successful entry of dsRNA. In a more recent report, the wax coating of the eggs was first removed using heptane and hypochlorite prior to electroporation

[68]. Using heptane alone did not significantly decrease the hatching rate. Thus, heptane may be more helpful in evaluating the effect of a particular dsRNA to egg hatching. This technique also offers a less invasive method of dsRNA introduction that can be applied to immature tick stages and eggs.

3.4. Feeding

Feeding dsRNA in insects has been achieved in different species using diets mixed with dsRNA, liposome-embedded or lipophilic siRNAs, and bacteria and transgenic plants that can synthesize dsRNA [32, 69]. Although in vitro feeding assays have been shown to be useful in studying different tick molecules and tick-pathogen interaction [70], its application in RNAi study in ticks has been limited. A study on the Lyme disease vector *I. scapularis* employed capillary feeding of dsRNA to nymphs to suppress anticomplement gene *isac* [71]. In another study, adult *R.* (*B.*) *microplus* ticks were capillary fed with *ubiquitin* dsRNA mixed in whole blood or *Bm86* dsRNA mixed in bovine serum [72]. In both cases, ticks were pre-fed in an animal host before capillary feeding was performed. While this method may be advantageous over injection due to very minimal injury, drawbacks may arise from the uncertainty whether an individual tick will ingest the amount of dsRNA that will effectively induce silencing, and the possibility of variation in the amount of dsRNA ingested by the ticks within a treatment group. Furthermore, capillary feeding is difficult to perform and may not be applicable in ticks with short hypostome.

4. RNAi and study of tick physiology

4.1. Genes related to salivary functions

The saliva is an important arsenal of ticks containing hundreds of pharmacologically potent substances that facilitate attachment to their hosts and blood-sucking [73]. Different salivary proteins have redundant functions in counteracting the hemostatic [74], inflammatory, and immune mechanisms [75] of the host. Aside from its function in tick feeding, the salivary glands are also involved in osmoregulation and transmission of pathogens [76].

Many studies on characterization of salivary proteins in the recent years employed RNAi (Table 1). In fact, the first report on the application of RNAi in tick research described a tick inhibitor of inflammatory mediator, a salivary histamine-binding protein, wherein researchers induced in vitro RNAi by soaking salivary glands in dsRNA [10, 58]. Soluble N-ethylmaleimide-sensitive factor attachment receptors (SNARE) complex proteins, which mediate exocytosis in secretory pathways of the salivary glands, have been characterized in *Amblyomma* ticks. These include N-ethylmaleimide-sensitive fusion (NSF) protein, Synaptosomal Associated Protein of 25 kDa (SNAP-25) [77], Ykt6 [65], and vesicle transport through interaction with t-SNAREs (Vti) [78]. Silencing various genes such as Salp14, Salp9pac [39], Neuronal isoform munc18-1 (nSec1) [59], and synaptobrevin [36] affected the secretion of anticoagulant or the anticoagulant activity of salivary gland extracts, indicating that these genes are important in tick anti-hemostatic mechanism.

Longistatin [79] and acidic chitinases [80] have been found to be important in the formation of blood pool and tick cement cone, respectively. The attachment site of *longistatin*-silenced *H. longicornis* ticks did not show pathological changes, such as hemorrhagic lesions corresponding to the blood pool, while the attachment site of ticks simultaneously silenced acidic chitinases exhibited blood leakage and these ticks can be easily removed. Various protease inhibitors that have roles in anti-hemostatic, anti-inflammatory, and immunomodulatory mechanism have been also characterized using RNAi, including a cystatin, sialostatine L [81], a Kunitz type protease inhibitor, rhipilin [82], and serine protease inhibitors (serpin) [83, 84].

Other salivary proteins with immunomodulatory function, such as the anti-complement protein, isac [71], and two proteins that can inhibit neutrophil function, ISL 929 and 1373 [85], have also been knockdowned in *I. scapularis*. Silencing of *isac* in nymphs, induced by capillary feeding of dsRNA, not only reduced blood feeding, but also decreased the load of the spirochete *Borrelia burgdorferi* in the tick. Meanwhile, the saliva of ticks devoid of ISL 929 and 1373 had reduced ability in inhibiting host integrin. An osmoregulatory protein aquaporin, characterized in *I. ricinus* through RNAi, showed that suppression of this protein impaired the concentration of blood meal due to failure in removing water [86].

4.2. Genes related to digestion and midgut function

The midgut of ticks houses various kinds of enzymes that act on a large amount of ingested host blood, which contains great quantities of hemoglobin [151]. Functional studies on these enzymes and other midgut proteins using RNAi have expanded the understanding of tick digestive physiology (Table 1). Silencing hemoglobinolytic enzymes, such as leucine aminopeptidase [91, 92], longipain [95], and cathepsin L [96, 97] had negative impact on tick feeding. Moreover, the longipain of *H. longicornis* was found to have a protective role in *Babesia* infection through its babesiacidal activity [95]. Other proteins important in tick digestion that have been characterized using RNAi are thrombin inhibitors that prevent blood coagulation and serine proteinase, which induce erythrocyte degradation. Silencing of thrombin inhibitor hemalin from *H. longicornis* [93] and boophilin from *R.* (*B.*) *microplus* [47] prolonged the blood feeding period and decreased the oviposition of these ticks, respectively. Silencing serine protease reduced the weight of ticks after blood feeding due to impaired erythrocyte degradation [94].

4.3. Genes related to reproductive function

Ticks are known for their high fecundity, laying hundreds of eggs per batch in the case of soft ticks and up to thousands in the case of hard ticks. A series of physiological events takes place in female ticks during and after blood feeding that initiate ovarian maturation and subsequent oviposition. Vitellogenesis, the synthesis and oocyte deposition of the yolk protein precursor (vitellogenin), is a key process for ovarian development and oocyte maturation induced by blood meal in ticks [152]. Three genes encoding vitellogenin have been identified and characterized in *H. longicornis* [102].

Target gene	Tick species	RNAi Effect	Refs
Salivary proteins			
Histamine-binding protein (HBP)	*Amblyomma americanum*	Altered feeding pattern and longer feeding period; decreased histamine-binding activity in the salivary glands	[10, 58]
Salp14/ Salp9pac	*Ixodes scapularis*	Impaired feeding, decreased post-blood meal weight, decreased anticoagulant activity of salivary gland extract	[39]
Neuronal isoform munc18-1 (nSec1)	*A. americanum*	Decreased post-blood meal weight and prolonged feeding time, decreased anticoagulant secretion of salivary gland	[59]
Synaptobrevin	*A. americanum*	Inhibited secretion of anticoagulant stimulated by PGE	[36]
Cystatin	*A. americanum*	Decreased post-blood meal weight, mortality during feeding, low feeding success rate	[61]
Anticomplement protein (Isac)	*I. scapularis*	Decreased post-blood meal weight, decreased *Borrelia burgdorferi* infection	[71]
Sialostatin L (cystatin)	*I. scapularis*	Failure to feed on the host, decreased post-blood meal weight and failed oviposition	[77]
Aquaporin	*I. ricinus*	Decreased post-blood meal weight, decreased volume of ingested blood	[78]
HlYkt6 (SNARE)	*Haemaphysalis longicornis*	Decreased post-blood meal weight, high mortality, supressed salivary secretion and anticoagulant activity	[65]
ISL 929 and 1373	*I. scapularis*	Supressed PMN inhibitory activity of saliva from knockdowned ticks	[79]
Rhipilin (Kunitz type protease inhibitor)	*Rhipicephalus haemaphysaloides*	Prolonged attachment time, decreased post-blood meal weight	[80]
Longistatin	*H. longicornis*	Mortality after attachment, failure to engorge, poor blood pool formation	[81]
Serine protease inhibitor (serpin)	*A. americanum*	No effect on tick attachment, feeding and oviposition	[82]
	R. haemaphysaloides	Decreased attachment rate and engorgement weight	[83]
Reprolysin	*Rhipicephalus* (*Boophilus*) *microplus*	Decreased egg weight and egg conversion ratio	[84]
N-ethylmaleimide sensitive fusion protein (NSF)	*A. maculatum*	Inhibition of engorgement, failure of oviposition	[85]

Target gene	Tick species	RNAi Effect	Refs
Synaptosomal Associated Protein of 25 kDa (SNAP-25)	*A. maculatum*	Decreased post-blood meal weight, decreased egg weight, failure in hatching	[85]
Vti (SNARE)	*A. americanum, A. maculatum*	Decreased post-blood meal weight and survival, failed oviposition	[86]
Glutaminyl cyclase (QC)	*A. maculatum, I. scapularis*	Decreased post-blood meal weight, egg weight and hatch	[87]
AV422	*A. americanum*	Decreased post-blood meal weight	[88]
Acidic chitinase (Ach)	*A. americanum*	Leakage of blood from the mouthparts in late feeding phase, loose attachment in the host's skin	[89]
Digestive activity			
Longepsin	*H. longicornis*	No effects reported	[90]
Leucine aminopeptidase	*H. longicornis*	Extended pre-oviposition period, decreased egg weight and egg conversion ratio, morphological abnormalities in the oocytes	[91, 92]
Hemalin (thrombin inhibitor)	*H. longicornis*	Longer blood feeding period, failure to engorge, decreased inhibitory activity of fibrinogen clot formation in the midgut	[93]
Boophilin (thrombin inhibitor)	*R. (B.) microplus*	Decreased oviposition	[47]
Serine proteinase	*H. longicornis*	Suppressed erythrocyte degradation; decreased post-blood meal weight	[94]
Longipain	*H. longicornis*	Impaired blood feeding, decreased post-blood meal weight, increased *B. gibsoni* infection level and transovarial transmission	[95]
Cathepsin L	*I. ricinus*	Decreased weight gain	[96]
	H. longicornis	Decreased post-blood meal weight	[97]
Astacin	*R. (B.) microplus*	Decreased egg weight and egg conversion ratio	[84]
Tick reproduction			
Follistatin-related protein (FRP)	*H. longicornis*	Decreased egg conversion ratio	[98]
Vitellogenin receptor (VgR)	*Dermacentor variabilis*	Failure of Vg uptake by oocytes; failed oviposition	[34]
	H. longicornis	Suppressed oocyte maturation and failed oviposition, failure of *B. gibsoni* transovarial transmission	[99]

Target gene	Tick species	RNAi Effect	Refs
	A. hebraeum	Suppressed oocyte maturation, long pre-oviposition period,	[100]
Voraxin	*A. americanum*	Failure to engorge and lay eggs in females fed with males injected with a combination of subolesin and voraxin dsRNA	[101]
Vitellogenin (Vg)	*H. longicornis*	Decreased post-blood meal weight, abnormal oocytes, decreased egg conversion ratio	[102]
GATA factor	*H. longicornis*	Disrupted egg development	[103]
S6 kinase	*H. longicornis*	Disrupted egg development	[103]
Target of rapamycin (TOR)	*H. longicornis*	Decreased post-blood meal weight, mortality after engorgement, Failure of oocytes to mature and failure to lay eggs	[104]
Structural and metabolic function			
Glutamine:fructose-6-phosphate aminotransferase (HlGFAT)	*H. longicornis*	Decreased post-blood meal weight and survival	[105]
β-Actin	*I. scapularis*	Decreased post-blood meal weight and oviposition	[106]
Na^+K^+ATPase	*I. scapularis*	Decreased post-blood meal weight and oviposition	[106]
Valosin-containing protein (HlVCP)	*H. longicornis*	Decreased post-blood meal weight	[107]
Cyclophilins (Immunophilin)	*H. longicornis*	Lower post-blood meal weight, low survival after blood feeding and failure to lay eggs after silencing cyclophilin A	[108]
Ribosomal protein P0	*H. longicornis*	Decreased post-blood meal weight, low engorgement rate, and high mortality	[109]
Protein disulphide isomerases (PDI)	*H. longicornis*	Mortality after engorgement, leakage of blood from the midgut, little egg output	[110]
Organic anion transporter polypeptide (OATP)	*A. americanum*	Decreased post-blood meal weight, oviposition and egg conversion ratio	[37]
Ferritins (FER)	*I. ricinus*	Decreased post-blood meal weight, oviposition and hatch	[111]
	H. longicornis	Decreased post-blood meal weight, survival, oviposition and hatch	[112, 113]
Iron regulatory protein (IRP1)	*I. ricinus*	Decreased post-blood meal weight and hatching of eggs	[111]

Target gene	Tick species	RNAi Effect	Refs
Elongation factor 1-α	*R. annulatus, R. (B.) microplus*	High post-blood meal mortality, decreased post-blood meal weight and failure of oviposition	[45]
Lysine-ketoglutarate reductase/saccharopine dehydrogenase (LKR/SDH)	*H. longicornis*	Longer blood feeding period, decreased post-blood meal weight, longer pre-oviposition period, decreased oviposition and hatch after SDH silencing; higher volume of hemolymph after LKR silencing	[114]
Ubiquitin	*R. (B.) microplus*	Shorter post-blood meal survival, decreased or absence of egg output, impaired embryogenesis	[14, 29, 45, 72];
	R. annulatus	High mortality	[45]
Glycogen synthase kinase-3 (GSK-3)	*R. (B.) microplus*	Decreased oviposition and hatching	[115]
CD147 receptor	*A. americanum*	Inhibited feeding, low post-blood meal weight tender cuticle	[116]
Insulin-like growth factor binding protein-related proteins	*A. americanum*	Decreased post-blood meal weight	[117]
Putative 5.8S, ITS2 and 28S rRNA	*A. americanum*	High mortality and very low post-blood meal weight	[118]
Putative 2B7 60S ribosomal protein L13e	*A. americanum*	High mortality and very low post-blood meal weight	[118]
Putative interphase cytoplasm foci protein 45	*A. americanum*	High mortality and very low post-blood meal weight	[118]
Putative threonyl-tRNA synthetase	*A. americanum*	High mortality and very low post-blood meal weight	[118]
Putative 60S ribosomal protein L13a	*A. americanum*	100% mortality	[118]
Putative mitochondrial 12S rRNA	*A. americanum*	High mortality and very low post-blood meal weight	[118]
Chymotrypsin inhibitor (HlChI)	*H. longicornis*	Mortality after attachment, retarded blood feeding and longer feeding period, decreased post-blood meal weight, decreased egg weight and egg conversion ratio	[119]
Scavenger receptor	*H. longicornis*	Decreased post-blood meal weight, mortality after engorgement, decreased oviposition and hatch; inhibited bacterial phagocytosis of granulocytes	[26, 28]

Target gene	**Tick species**	**RNAi Effect**	**Refs**
4E-BP (eIF4E-binding protein)	*H. longicornis*	Decreased lipid accumulation in the midgut and fat bodies after long starvation period	[120]
Protein kinase B (AKT)	*H. longicornis*	Inhibition of engorgement and growth of organs during blood feeding; decreased expression of *longepsin*, *HlMIF* and *HlVgs*	[121]
	R. (B.) microplus	Decreased cell glycogen content and viability, and altered cell membrane permeability	[57]
Spook (Spo)	*Ornithodoros moubata*	Arrested development and molting	[53]
Shade (Shd)	*O. moubata*	Abnormal ecdysis and delayed molting	[53]
Cystatin (RHCyst)	*R. haemaphysaloides*	Decreased attachment and hatching rate	[122]
Tropomyosin	*H. longicornis*	Longer feeding time, decreased engorgement rate and post-blood meal weight, high mortality after blood feeding, failed oviposition	[123]
Protective antigens			
Subolesin (4D8)	*I. scapularis*	Decreased post-blood meal weight, oviposition and survival; failure of embryogenesis; silencing in eggs and larvae when dsRNA injected to engorged females	[43, 124]
	A. americanum	Decreased post-blood meal weight, oviposition and survival	[43, 101, 124]
	D. marginatus	Decreased post-blood meal weight, oviposition and survival	[124]
	D. variabilis	Decreased post-blood meal weight, oviposition and survival; decreased fertility; silencing in eggs and larvae when dsRNA injected to engorged females	[43, 124]
	R. sanguineus	Decreased post-blood meal weight, oviposition and survival; more dramatic effect when simultaneously silenced with Rs86	[124, 125]
	R. (B.) microplus	High mortality, decreased post-blood meal weight, oviposition and hatch in dsRNA-injected adults and progeny of dsRNA-injected adults	[42, 45, 46]
	R. annulatus,	Decreased post-blood meal weight	[45, 126]
	O. erraticus	Decreased egg output	[127]
	O. moubata	Decreased egg output	[127]

Target gene	Tick species	RNAi Effect	Refs
Midgut protein Rs86	*R. sanguineus*	Decreased post-blood meal weight and oviposition	[125]
Midgut protein Hl86	*H. longicornis*	Decreased post-blood meal weight	[128]
Midgut protein Bm86	*R. (B.) microplus*	Decreased number of engorging ticks, lower post-blood meal body weight and survival after feeding in *B. bovis*-infected host, decreased egg weight	[129]
Midgut protein Ree86	*R. evertsi evertsi*	No significant effect	[130]
Midgut protein ReeATAQ	*R. evertsi evertsi*	No significant effect	[130]
Longicin	*H. longicornis*	Decreased post-blood meal weight, increased *B. gibsoni* infection in the midgut and ovary, and transmission in the eggs	[131]
α2-macroglobulin proteins	*I. ricinus*	Decreased phagocytic action of hemocytes	[132, 133]
Macrophage migration inhibitory factor	*A. americanum*	No effect on phenotypes	[134]
Janus kinase (JAK)–signaling transducer activator of transcription (STAT) pathway	*I. scapularis*	Increased *A. phagocytophilum* infection level	[135]
Dual oxidase (Duox)	*I. scapularis*	Decreased level of *B. burgdorferi*	[136]
Peroxidase ISCW017368	*I. scapularis*	Decreased level of *B. burgdorferi*	[136]
Glutathione S-transferase	*R. (B.) microplus*	Decreased tick attachment and post-blood meal weight	[45]
	R.sanguineus	Increased susceptibility to permethrin	[137]
Selenoprotein W	*R. (B.) microplus*	Decreased tick attachment and post-blood meal weight	[45]
Selenoprotein K	*A. maculatum*	Decreased oviposition	[138]
Selenoprotein M	*A. maculatum*	Decreased oviposition	[138, 139]
Thioredoxin reductase	*A. maculatum*	Decreased native microbial load in midguts and salivary glands	[139]
Rmcystatin3 (cysteine protease inhibitor)	*R. (B.) microplus*	Increased resistance to bacteria	[140]
Pathogen acquisition/ transmission			
Subolesin	*D. variabilis*	Inhibited *Anaplasma marginale* infection in salivary glands	[141, 142]

Target gene	Tick species	RNAi Effect	Refs
	R. (B.) microplus	Decreased *A. marginale* infection level in salivary glands and tick cells	[143]
Salp15	*I. scapularis*	Decreased *Borrelia burgdorferi* transmission to the host	[52]
Salp14	*I. scapularis*	No effect on acquisition of *A. phagocytophilum* and *B. burgdorferi* in nymphs	[49]
Salp16	*I. scapularis*	Reduced *A. phagocytophilum* acquisition	[48]
Salp25D	*I. scapularis*	Decreased acquisition of *B. burgdorferi* after knockdown in salivary glands	[44]
Varisin	*D. variabilis*	Decreased *A. marginale* infection level	[144]
Immunophilin	*R. (B.) microplus*	Decreased hatch, decreased larval survival, increased *B. bovis* infection in larval progeny	[41]
Kunitz-type serine protease inhibitor (Spi)	*R. (B.) microplus*	Inhibition of engorgement, decreased egg weight	[41]
Glutathione S-transferase	*D. variabilis*	Inhibited *A. marginale* infection	[142]
H^+ transporting lysosomal vacuolar proton pump (vATPase)	*D. variabilis*	Inhibited *A. marginale* infection in the midgut after acquisition feeding	[142]
Selenoprotein M	*D. variabilis*	Inhibited *A. marginale* infection and multiplication in salivary glands	[142]
Putative von Willebrand factor (94Will)	*R. (B.) microplus*	Decreased *A. marginale* infection level in salivary glands	[143]
Flagelliform silk protein (100Silk)	*R. (B.) microplus*	Decreased *A. marginale* infection level in salivary glands and tick cells	[143]
Putative metallothionein (93 Meth)	*R. (B.) microplus*	Increased *A. marginale* infection level in tick cells	[143]
Tick salivary lectin pathway inhibitor (TSLPI)	*I. scapularis*	Decreased load of *B. burgdorferi* and transmission to host	[145]
Kunitz-type serine protease inhibitor (DvKPI)	*D. variabilis*	Increased rickettsial infection in the midgut	[146]
Kunitz-type protease inhibitor 5 (KTPI)	*R. annulatus, R. (B.) microplus*	Decreased post-blood meal weight	[126]
Histamine release factor	*I. scapularis*	Decreased post-blood meal weight, decreased *B. burgdorferi* transmission	[147]
TROSPA	*R. annulatus, R. (B.) microplus*	Decreased *B. bigemina* infection level; Decreased post-blood meal weight in *R. microplus*	[126]

Target gene	Tick species	RNAi Effect	Refs
Serum amyloid A	*R. annulatus, R. (B.) microplus*	Decreased *B. bigemina* infection level	[126]
Ricinusin	*R. annulatus, R. (B.) microplus*	Decreased post-blood meal weight in *R. annulatus*	[126]
Calreticulin	*R. annulatus, R. (B.) microplus*	Decreased *B. bigemina* infection level in *R. microplus*; decreased post-blood meal weight in *R. annulatus*	[126]
Chitin deacetylase-like protein (IsCDA)	*I. scapularis*	No significant effect on *B. burgdorferi* acquisition or transmission	[50]
Antifreeze glycoprotein	*I. scapularis*	Decreased survival and mobility of ticks in extremely cold temperature; decreased *A. phagocytophilum* infection level	[148]
x-linked inhibitor of apoptosis protein (E3 ubiquitin ligase, XIAP)	*I. scapularis*	Increased *A. phagocytophilum* infection	[149]
Cytochrome c oxidase subunit III	*R. (B.) microplus*	Failure in transmission of *A. marginale*	[150]

Table 1. Genes functionally characterized through RNAi in different tick species.

Silencing these genes through RNAi greatly reduced the reproductive capacity of female ticks, which showed immature and light-colored oocytes. The uptake of vitellogenin in the oocytes is facilitated by vitellogenin receptor, which has been characterized in *D. variabilis* [34], *H.longicornis* [99], and *A. hebraeum* [100]. Aside from the negative impact in oviposition consistently induced by RNAi in all these studies, silencing of *H. longicornis* vitellogenin receptor also reportedly inhibited the transovarial transmission of *Babesia gibsoni*. Three factors involved in the initiation of vitellogenesis, the GATA factor, S6 kinase [103], and target of rapamycin (TOR) pathway [104], have been also characterized in *H. longicornis* ticks using RNAi. The significance of other proteins to reproduction, such as a tick homologue of the human follistatin-related protein [98] and the engorgement protein voraxin [101] from the male gonad, has been also demonstrated using RNAi.

4.4. Genes related to structural and metabolic functions

Various gene encoding proteins important in cellular structure and metabolism have been characterized using RNAi. Due to their wide distribution and systemic function, knockdown of these proteins caused detrimental effects on different tick physiological functions and some even proved to be lethal (Table 1). Among these proteins is the multifunctional ubiquitin, which has been first targeted based on a homologous gene of *D. melanogaster* in a study investigating the components of tick RNAi pathway [14]. Ubiquitin knockdown in *R. (B.)*

microplus shortened the post-blood meal survival of ticks and impaired egg viability and hatch. In separate studies, ubiquitin has also been the subject in examining off-target effects of RNAi [29] and the feasibility of dsRNA feeding in *R.* (*B.*) *microplus* [72]. RNAi-mediated silencing of ribosomal proteins in *A. americanum* [118], and ubiquitin, elongation factor-1 alpha and several other proteins in *R.* (*B.*) *microplus* and *R. annulatus* [45] has been employed to screen potential antigens for tick control.

In the hard tick *H. longicornis,* individual knockdown of glutamine:fructose-6-phosphate aminotransferase [105], cyclophilin A [108], the ribosomal protein P0 [109], protein disulphide isomerases [110], and tropomyosin [123] resulted to decreased survival of ticks after engorgement. Two proteins with apparent roles in withstanding long starvation period, lysine-ketoglutarate reductase/saccharopine dehydrogenase (LKR/SDH) [114] and 4E-BP [120], have also been characterized in *H. longicornis*. LKR/SDH mRNA expression is higher in starved ticks than in unfed ticks and knockdown of LKR resulted to high volume of hemolymph after blood feeding, suggesting its role in osmoregulation. Meanwhile, 4E-BP knockdown led to decreased lipid storage in the midguts and fat bodies of ticks during longer starvation period. An interesting report on the application of RNAi in studying tick neurobiology targetedβ-actin and Na^{+}-K^{+}-ATPase of *I. scapularis* using fluorescently labeled dsRNAs to monitor the uptake in tick synganglia [106].

The significance of proteins involved in iron metabolism to tick feeding and reproduction has been also demonstrated using RNAi in two hard tick species, *I. ricinus* [111] and *H. longicornis* [112]. Silencing two types of the iron storage protein ferritin greatly reduced the ticks' capacity to engorge and produce eggs, also affecting post-blood meal survival due to occurrence of iron-mediated oxidative stress [113]. An iron regulatory protein responsible for translation of iron binding proteins was characterized in *I. scapularis,* with its knockdown greatly reducing egg hatchability [111]. Two enzymes, spook and shade, were characterized in the soft tick *O. moubata* and were shown to be important in ecdysteroidogenesis through RNAi [53]. Silencing spook protein in nymphs caused arrested development and molting, whereas silencing shade delayed molting and led to abnormal ecdysis.

5. RNAi studies on tick protective antigens and immunity

The immune system of ticks has a vital role of protecting them from harmful substances in the blood, including components of their host's immune system, and from various pathogens that they acquire in their blood feeding activity. Tick protective antigens, therefore, gain wide interest due to their potential as target for tick control. The highly conserved tick protective antigen subolesin, previously known as 4D8, was first identified from *I. scapularis* through cDNA expression library immunization (ELI) [153], after which, it has been also identified in other hard tick species, and using RNAi, was found to be important in the success of blood feeding and reproduction [124]. An ortholog of subolesin has also been characterized in two soft tick species and RNAi demonstrated that subolesin is also important in the reproduction of soft ticks [127]. The function of subolesin is unclear, but a report showed that subolesin knockdown affected the expression of several genes involved in multiple cellular pathways, suggesting a role in gene expression by interacting with regulatory proteins [154]. Aside from being reported as a promising anti-tick vaccine antigen candidate in many studies, it has been also proposed that subolesin may be targeted in ticks that subsequently will be released for sterile acarine technique (SAT) [38].

The membrane-bound glycoprotein Bm86 expressed mainly in the midgut of *R.* (*B.*) *microplus* [155] is the first, and until recently, the only tick antigen that is commercially available as an anti-tick vaccine in some countries. The exact function of Bm86, however, remains unclear yet. RNAi has been employed to knockdown *Bm86* and its homologues in other tick species, including *R. sanguineus*, *H. longicornis*, and *R. evertsi evertsi*, which in most cases affected the blood feeding and reproduction of adult ticks, except in *R. evertsi evertsi* wherein knockdown of two homologues did not yield significant effects [130]. A study in *R.* (*B.*) *microplus* also showed that knockdown of *Bm86* decreased the blood feeding capacity and survival of ticks after feeding on a *B. bovis*-infected host, suggesting that Bm86 may have a critical role in the fitness of ticks after feeding from an acutely *B. bovis*-infected host [129].

The function of some components of immunity, such as α2-macroglobulin proteins [132, 133], antimicrobial peptides [131], Janus kinase (JAK)-signaling transducer activator of transcription (STAT) pathway [135], dityrosine network [136], and cysteine protease inhibitor in the hemocytes [140] have been analyzed using RNAi. The α2-macroglobulin proteins of *I. ricinus*, related to vertebrate complement system, were shown to be involved in the phagocytic activity of hemocytes against Gram-negative bacteria [132, 133]. In contrast, a cysteine protease Rmcystatin3 identified in *R.* (*B.*) *microplus* was implicated as a negative modulator of tick immune response after its silencing greatly reduced the number of bacterial load in the ticks [140]. The role of a defensin from *H. longicornis*, longicin, in ticks' immune defense against *Babesia* parasites was demonstrated through RNAi, as exhibited by a higher load of *B. gibsoni* in the midgut and ovary of *longicin*-silenced ticks after infestation in an infected host [131]. Meanwhile, JAK-STAT pathway was shown to be important in *Anaplasma phagocytophilum* infection in ticks after its knockdown increased the infection in the salivary glands of nymphs that fed on infected mice [135]. A dual oxidase and a peroxidase, ISCW017368, which together forms a dityrosine network, were separately silenced in *I. scapularis*, both resulting to reduced *Borrelia burgdorferi* persistence in ticks [136].

The obligatory blood feeding lifestyle of ticks exposes them to high levels of pro-oxidants that may trigger oxidative stress. Antioxidant enzymes function to protect them from the harmful effects of oxidative stress. Furthermore, these antioxidant enzymes provide detoxification mechanisms to counteract toxins that they encounter in the environment, such as chemical acaricides. RNAi has been very useful in evaluating the function of these antioxidants. Silencing a selenoprotein in *R.* (*B.*) *microplus* reduced the engorged body weight and egg output [45]. In contrast, a study on *A. maculatum* showed that silencing two selenoproteins did not alter blood feeding, although the egg output was reduced. Interestingly, the total antioxidant capacities of the saliva from knockdowned ticks were higher, indicating that other antioxidant enzymes may have compensated for the absence of selenoproteins [138]. In another study, silencing thioredoxin reductase, another selenoprotein, in *A. maculatum* did not have a negative impact on blood feeding and reproduction. Likewise, variations in transcriptional expression of some antioxidant enzymes were also observed, suggesting compensatory mechanism in the absence of thioredoxin reductase [139]. However, the more interesting finding in that study was the decreased microbiota population following thioredoxin reductase knockdown, possibly because of disturbed redox homeostasis balance. Meanwhile, silencing a glutathione S-transferase (GST) gene affected the attachment of ticks and reduced the post-blood meal bodyweight of *R.* (*B.*) *microplus* [45]. It also made *R. sanguineus* ticks more susceptible to permethrin, although no significant effects on tick attachment, feeding and reproductive capacity were observed [137].

6. Understanding tick-pathogen interaction through RNAi

RNAi has undoubtedly paved a way to better understand the different aspects of ticks' association with various pathogens. Numerous tick proteins with different functions have been found to be involved in the acquisition, establishment, and transmission of pathogens. Several proteins have been studied through RNAi to determine their importance in the development cycle of different pathogens. The knockdown of subolesin [142, 156], GST, vATPase, and selenoprotein M [142] in *D. variabilis*, and putative von Willebrand factor, flagelliform silk protein and subolesin in *R.* (*B.*) *microplus* [143] decreased the infection level of *A. marginale* in these hard ticks, implying that these proteins are significant in the establishment of infection of this rickettsia.

RNAi also demonstrated that the Lyme disease agent *B. burgdorferi* can utilize several proteins of *I. scapularis* to facilitate its transmission to the host. These include salivary proteins such as tick histamine release factor [147], Salp15 [52], and the lectin complement pathway inhibitor (TSLPI) [145]; the latter two provide protection for *B. burgdorferi* against components of the host immune system. Salivary proteins Salp14 [49], Salp16 [48], and Salp25D [44] have been examined for their function in acquiring *A. phagocytophilum* or *B. burgdorferi* through RNAi. Knockdown of Salp14 did not affect the acquisition of either rickettsiae, whereas the knockdown of Salp16 and Salp25D decreased the infection level of *A. phagocytophilum* and *B. burgdorferi* in the tick, respectively.

An interesting study on *I. scapularis* showed that *A. phagocytophilum* promotes cold tolerance through an antifreeze glycoprotein [148]. In the absence of this antifreeze glycoprotein, the survival rate of ticks after exposure to extremely cold temperature and the infection level of *A. phagocytophilum* following exposure was reduced. Tick defensins, varisin from *D. variabilis* [144], and ricinusin from *Rhipicephalus* ticks [126] have been silenced to examine their functions in pathogen establishment; the former reduced *A. marginale* infection level, while the latter did not have an effect on *B. bigemina* infection.

Several reports also demonstrated the interaction of *Babesia* parasites and tick proteins through RNAi. Knockdown of the immunophilin gene in *R.* (*B.*) *microplus* had negative impact on the reproductive performance of the tick and also increased the infection rate of *B. bovis* in larval progeny [41], while knockdown of TROSPA, serum amyloid A, and calreticulin reduced the infection level of *B. bigemina* in *Rhipicephalus* ticks [126]. Silencing a Kunitz-type serine protease inhibitor from *D. variabilis* increased the rickettsial infection in the midgut [146], whereas in *R. (B.) microplus*, silencing a Kunitz-type serine protease inhibitor, Spi, tended to increase the infection rate of *B. bovis* in larval progeny [41], but silencing of another Kunitz-type protease inhibitor 5 (KTPI) did not have any effect on *Babesia* infection [126].

7. Future directions in tick research and application in tick control

Indeed, great progress in understanding tick biology has been already accomplished in the past. However, many aspects of tick physiology and host-tick-pathogen interaction need to be unraveled yet. Moreover, several optimizations can still be done to improve RNAi in tick research. While being the most widely used method of introducing dsRNA, the injection method (particularly microinjection) that requires elaborate equipment may not be accessible to all laboratories. Moreover, injection is mostly applicable to adult and sometimes nymphal stages, and may be injurious to the ticks, especially when performed by an inexperienced researcher. The soaking method is simpler, less invasive, and less laborious. Electroporation has been recently shown to be effective in introducing dsRNA in eggs [66] and may be useful in studying the function of genes that are involved in embryogenesis and physiology of immature tick stages.

RNAi may also prove to be a promising tick control method and not just a research tool. In pest insect management, the possibility of using RNAi as a novel tool of pest control is already being explored by feeding liposome-coated dsRNA or dsRNA expressed in transgenic plants or bacteria [32]. RNAi targeting several genes have been accomplished by feeding plants expressing dsRNA in several species of economically important crop pests [16]. Feeding dsRNA to ticks is still an underdeveloped approach, which has been yet accomplished only by artificial feeding. Coating dsRNAs with liposomes or nanocarriers may increase dsRNA stability that may make it feasible for administration to the host. Genes that are highly conserved across different tick species, and are of importance in tick survival are good candidate targets. These include proteins with structural and metabolic functions, such as ubiquitin, tropomyosin, and ferritin. However, the specificity of dsRNA to the tick gene should be highly considered. Additional consideration would be the establishment of a minimum effective dose, since the synthesis of dsRNA is costly.

Additionally, RNAi has been proposed as an alternative method for the sterile insect technique in blood-sucking mosquitoes that will produce sterile males by feeding dsRNA in mosquito larvae [64]. Quite similarly, the application of RNAi for tick control was also proposed in a single report on *D. variabilis*, wherein the highly conserved subolesin was targeted leading to reproductive incapacity [38]. In conclusion, the authors suggested that RNAi may be used to massively produce sterile ticks (SAT) that may be released in the field. Releasing subolesin-silenced ticks may also aid in the control of *A. marginale*, since it has been reported that subolesin knockdown reduced the infection level of this pathogen [141–143]. Introducing dsRNA to eggs through electroporation described above may be a more convenient way of producing knockdowned ticks.

http://dx.doi.org/10.5772/61577

8. Summary

In this chapter, we have reviewed the application of RNAi in tick research and described the significant contribution of RNAi in advancing our knowledge on tick biology and tick-pathogen interaction. RNAi has revolutionized the advancement of our understanding of various aspects of tick blood feeding and digestion, reproduction, metabolism, and immunity. As a functional analysis tool, RNAi has become very handy in elucidating the functions of different proteins from more than 10 hard tick species and a few soft tick species. It has been particularly helpful in screening potential target antigens for anti-tick and tick-borne pathogen vaccine development [157]. Several methods of introducing dsRNA in ticks have been employed but injection has remained to be the most widely used technique. The number of published research on ticks that involves the application of RNAi has been continuously increasing through the years, and it is expected to continue doing so. A great majority of the published reports focused on hard ticks, but due to some physiological differences, more research using RNAi on soft ticks should be conducted. Finally, with numerous potential target genes already identified, the application of RNAi as a tick control method should be investigated in the future, starting with optimization of dsRNA delivery method for practical use.

Acknowledgements

This work was supported by the Japan Society for the Promotion of Science (JSPS) KAKENHI Grant Numbers 22580335, 25292173, and 26660229. We also thank our colleague, Melbourne R. Talactac, at the Laboratory of Infectious Diseases, Joint Faculty of Veterinary Medicine, Kagoshima University, for his assistance in writing this chapter.

Author details

Remil Linggatong Galay[1,2], Rika Umemiya-Shirafuji[3], Masami Mochizuki[1], Kozo Fujisaki[4] and Tetsuya Tanaka[2*]

*Address all correspondence to: tetsuya@ms.kagoshima-u.ac.jp

1 Department of Veterinary Paraclinical Sciences, College of Veterinary Medicine, University of the Philippines Los Baños, Los Baños, Philippines

2 Laboratory of Infectious Diseases, Joint Faculty of Veterinary Medicine, Kagoshima University, Kagoshima, Japan

3 National Research Center for Protozoan Diseases, Obihiro University of Agriculture and Veterinary Medicine, Inada-cho, Obihiro, Hokkaido, Japan

4 National Agricultural and Food Research Organization, Tsukuba, Ibaraki, Japan

References

[1] Dantas-Torres F, Chomel B, Otranto D. Ticks and tick-borne diseases: A One Health perspective. Trends Parasitol. 2012;28:437-46. doi:10.1016/j.pt.2012.07.003.

[2] Jonjegan F, Uilenberg G. The global importance of ticks. Parasitology 2004;129:S3-S14.

[3] de la Fuente J. The fossil record and the origin of ticks (Acari: Parasitiformes: Ixodida). Exp Appl Acarol. 2003;29:437-46.

[4] Estrada-Peña A, Salman M. Current limitations in the control and spread of ticks that affect livestock: A review. Agriculture. 2013;3:221-35. doi:10.3390/agriculture3020221.

[5] Estrada-Peña A, de la Fuente J. The ecology of ticks and epidemiology of tick-borne viral diseases. Antiviral Res. 2014;108:104-28. doi:10.1016/j.antiviral.2014.05.016.

[6] Kim E, Bauer C, Grevelding CG, Quack T. Improved PCR/nested PCR approaches with increased sensitivity and specificity for the detection of pathogens in hard ticks. Ticks Tick Borne Dis. 2013;4:409-16. doi:10.1016/j.ttbdis.2013.04.004.

[7] Baneth G. Tick-borne infections of animals and humans: A common ground. Int J Parasitol. 2014;44:591-6. doi:10.1016/j.ijpara.2014.03.011.

[8] Guerrero FD, Lovis L, Martins JR. Acaricide resistance mechanisms in *Rhipicephalus (Boophilus) microplus*. Rev Bras Parasitol Vet. 2012;21:1-6. doi:10.1590/S1984-29612012000100002.

[9] Hannon GJ. RNA interference. Nature. 2002;418:244-51. doi:10.1038/418244a.

[10] Aljamali MN, Sauer JR, Essenberg RC. RNA interference: Applicability in tick research. Exp App Acarol. 2002;28:89-96.

[11] de la Fuente J, Kocan KM, Almazan C, Blouin EF. RNA interference for the study and genetic manipulation of ticks. Trends Parasitol. 2007;23:427-33. doi:10.1016/j.pt.2007.07.002.

[12] Mello CC, Conte Jr. D. Revealing the world of RNA interference. Nature. 2004;431:338-42. doi:10.1038/nature02872.

[13] Whangbo JS, Hunter CP. Environmental RNA interference. Trends Genetics. 2008;24:297-305. doi:10.1016/j.tig.2008.03.007.

[14] Kurscheid S, Lew-Tabor AE, Valle MR, Bruyeres AG, Doogan VJ, Munderloh UG, et al. Evidence of a tick RNAi pathway by comparative genomics and reverse genetics screen of targets with known loss-of-function phenotypes in *Drosophila*. BMC Mol Biol. 2009;10:26. doi:10.1186/1471-2199-10-26.

[15] Barnard AC, Nijhof AM, Fick W, Stutzer C, Maritz-Olivier C. RNAi in arthropods: Insight into machinery and applications for understanding the pathogen-vector interface. Genes. 2012;3:704-41. doi:10.3390/genes3040702.

[16] Aronstein K, Oppert B, Lorenzen MD. RNAi in agriculturally-important arthropods. In: Grabowski P, editor. RNA Processing: InTech; 2011. p. 157-80. doi:10.5772/19768.

[17] Rocheleau CE. RNA interference: Systemic RNAi SIDes with endosomes. Curr Biol. 2012;22:R873-R5. doi:10.1016/j.cub.2012.08.039.

[18] Hunter CP, Winston WM, Molodowitch C, Feinberg EH, Shih J, Sutherlin M, et al. Systemic RNAi in *Caenorhabditis elegans*. Cold Spring Harb Symp Quant Biol. 2006;71:95-100. doi:10.1101/sqb.2006.71.060.

[19] Jose AM, Smith JJ, Hunter CP. Export of RNA silencing from *C. elegans* tissues does not require the RNA channel SID-1. Proc Natl Acad Sci USA. 2009;106:2283-8. doi: 10.1073/pnas.0809760106.

[20] Hinas A, Wright AJ, Hunter CP. SID-5 is an endosome-associated protein required for efficient systemic RNAi in *C. elegans*. Curr Biol. 2012;22:1938-43. doi:10.1016/j.cub. 2012.08.020.

[21] Winston WM, Sutherlin M, Wright AJ, Feinberg EH, Hunter CP. *Caenorhbaditis elegans* SID-2 is required for environmental RNA interference. Proc Natl Acad Sci USA. 2007;104:10565-70. doi:10.1073/pnas.0611282104.

[22] Tijsterman M, May RC, Simmer F, Okihara KL, Plasterk RHA. Genes required for systemic RNA interference in *Caenorhabditis elegans*. Curr Biol. 2004;14:111-6. doi: 10.1016/j.cub.2003.12.029.

[23] Ulvila J, Parikka M, Kleino A, Sormunen R, Ezekowitz RA, Kocks C, et al. Double-stranded RNA is internalized by scavenger receptor-mediated endocytosis in *Drosophila* S2 cells. J Biol Chem. 2006;281:14370-5. doi:10.1074/jbc.M513868200.

[24] Ramet M, Pearson A, Manfruelli P, Li X, Koziel H, Gobel V, et al. *Drosophila* scavenger receptor CI is a pattern recognition receptor for bacteria. Immunity. 2001;15:1027-38. doi:10.1016/S1074-7613(01)00249-7.

[25] Kocks C, Cho JH, Nehme N, Ulvila J, Pearson A, Meister M, et al. Eater, a transmembrane protein mediating phagocytosis of bacterial pathogens in Drosophila. Cell. 2005;123:335-46. doi:10.1016/j.cell.2005.08.034.

[26] Aung KM, Boldbaatar D, Liao M, Umemiya-Shirafuji R, Nakao S, Matsuoka T, et al. Identification and characterization of class B scavenger receptor CD36 from the hard tick, *Haemaphysalis longicornis*. Parasitol Res. 2011;108:272-85. doi:10.1007/ s00436-010-2053-1.

[27] Aung KM, Boldbaatar D, Umemiya-Shirafuji R, Liao M, Xuan X, Suzuki H, et al. Scavenger receptor mediates systemic RNA interference in ticks. PLoS ONE. 2011;6:e28407. doi:10.1371/journal.pone.0028407.

[28] Aung KM, Boldbaatar D, Umemiya-Shirafuji R, Liao M, Tsuji N, Xuan X, et al. HlSRB, a Class B Scavenger Receptor, is Key to the Granulocyte-Mediated Microbial Phagocytosis in Ticks. PloS ONE. 2012;7:e33504. doi:10.1371/journal.pone.0033504.

[29] Lew-Tabor AE, Kurscheid S, Barrero R, Gondro C, Moolhuijzen PM, Valle MR, et al. Gene expression evidence for off-target effects caused by RNA interference-mediated gene silencing of *Ubiquitin-63E* in the cattle tick *Rhipicephalus microplus*. Int J Parasitol. 2011;41:1001-14. doi: 10.1016/j.ijpara.2011.05.003.

[30] Lee YS, Nakahara K, Pham JW, Kim K, He Z, Sontheimer EJ, et al. Distinct roles for *Drosophila* Dicer-1 and Dicer-2 in the siRNA/miRNA silencing pathways. Cell. 2004;117:69-81. doi:10.1016/S0092-8674(04)00261-2.

[31] Hock J, Meister G. The Argonaute protein family. Genome Biology. 2008;9:210. doi: 10.1186/gb-2008-9-2-210.

[32] Xue X, Mao Y, Tao X, Huang Y, Chen X. New approaches to agricultural insect pest control based on RNA interference. In: Zayed A, Kent CF, editors. Advances in insect physiology. 42: Elsevier; 2012. p. 73-117. doi:10.1016/B978-0-12-387680-5.00003-3.

[33] Karim S, Adamson SW. RNA interference in ticks: A functional genomics took for the study of physiology. In: Zayed A, Kent CF, editors. Advances in insect physiology. 42: Elsevier; 2012. p. 120-54. doi:10.1016/B978-0-12-387680-5.00004-5.

[34] Mitchell III RD, Ross E, Osgood C, Sonenshine DE, Donohue KV, Khalil SM, et al. Molecular characterization, tissue-specific expression and RNAi knockdown of the first vitellogenin receptor from a tick. Insect Biochem Mol Biol. 2007;37:375-88. doi: 10.1016/j.ibmb.2007.01.005.

[35] Decrem Y, Beaufays J, Blasioli V, Lahaye K, Brossard M, Vanhamme L, et al. A family of putative metalloproteases in the salivary glands of the tick *Ixodes ricinus*. FEBS J. 2008;275:1485-99. doi:10.1111/j.1742-4658.2008.06308.x.

[36] Karim S, Ramakrishnan VG, Tucker JS, Essenberg RC, Sauer JR. *Amblyomma americanum* salivary glands: Double-stranded RNA-mediated gene silencing of synaptobrevin homologue and inhibition of PGE_2 stimulated protein secretion. Insect Biochem Mol Biol. 2004;34:407-13. doi:10.1016/j.ibmb.2004.01.005.

[37] Mulenga A, Khumthong R, Chalaire KC, Strey O, Teel P. Molecular and biological characterization of the *Amblyomma americanum* organic anion transporter polypeptide. J Exp Biol. 2008;211:3401-8. doi:10.1242/jeb.022376.

[38] de la Fuente J, Almazan C, Naranjo V, Blouin EF, Meyer JM, Kocan KM. Autocidal control of ticks by silencing of a single gene by RNA interference. Biochem Biophys Res Comm. 2006;344:332-28. doi:10.1016/j.bbrc.2006.03.109.

[39] Narasimhan S, Montgometry RR, DePonte K, Tschudi C, Marcantonio N, Anderson JF, et al. Disruption of *Ixodes scapularis* anticoagulation by using RNA interference. Proc Natl Acad Sci USA. 2004;101:1141-6. doi:10.1073/pnas.0307669100.

[40] Kocan KM, Blouin EF, de la Fuente J. RNA interference in ticks. J Vis Exp. 2011;20:2472. doi:10.3791/2474.

[41] Bastos RG, Ueti MW, Guerrero FD, Knowles DP, Scoles GA. Silencing of a putative immunophilin gene in the cattle tick *Rhipicephalus* (*Boophilus*) *microplus* increases the infection rate of *Babesia bovis* in larval progeny. Parasit Vectors. 2009;2:57. doi: 10.1186/1756-3305-2-57.

[42] Nijhof AM, Taoufik A, de la Fuente J, Kocan KM, de Vries E, Jonjegan F. Gene silencing of the tick protective antigens, *Bm86*, *Bm91* and *subolesin* in the one-host tick *Boophilus microplus* by RNA interference. Int J Parasitol. 2007;2007:653-62. doi:10.1016/j.ijpara.2006.11.005.

[43] Kocan KM, Manzano-Roman R, de la Fuente J. Transovarial silencing of the subolesin gene in three-host ixodid tick species after injection of replete females with subolesin dsRNA. Parasitol Res. 2007;100:1411-5. doi:10.1007/s00436-007-0483-1.

[44] Narasimhan S, Sukumaran B, Bozdogan U, Thomas V, Liang X, DePonte K, et al. A tick antioxidant facilitates the lyme disease agent's successful migration from the mammalian host to the arthropod vector. Cell Host Microbe. 2007;2:7-18. doi:10.1016/j.chom.2007.06.001.

[45] Almazan C, Lagunes R, Villar M, Canales M, Rosario-Cruz R, Jonjegan F, et al. Identification and characterization of *Rhipicephalus* (*Boophilus*) *microplus* candidate protective antigens for the control of cattle tick infestations. Parasitol Res. 2010;106:471-9. doi:10.1007/s00436-009-1689-1.

[46] Merino O, Almazan C, Canales M, Villar M, Moreno-Cid JA, Estrada Pena A, et al. Control of *Rhipicephalus* (*Boophilus*) *microplus* infestations by the combination of subolesin vaccination and tick autocidal control after subolesin gene knockdown in ticks fed on cattle. Vaccine. 2011;29:2248-54. doi:10.1016/j.vaccine.2011.01.050.

[47] Soares TS, Watanabe RMO, Tanaka-Azevedo AM, Torquato RJS, Lu S, Figueiredo AC, et al. Expression and functional characterization of boophilin, a thrombin inhibitor from *Rhipicephalus* (*Boophilus*) *microplus* midgut. Vet Parasitol. 2012;187:521-8. doi: 10.1016/j.vetpar.2012.01.027.

[48] Sukumaran B, Narasimhan S, Anderson JF, DePonte K, Marcantonio N, Krishnan MN, et al. An *Ixodes scapularis* protein required for survival of *Anaplasma phagocytophilum* in tick salivary glands. J Exp Med. 2006;203:1507-17. doi:10.1084/jem.20060208.

[49] Pedra JOF, Narasimhan S, DePonte K, Marcantonio N, Kantor FS, Fikrig E. Disruption of the salivary protein 14 in *Ixodes scapularis* nymphts and impact on pathogen acquisition. Am J Trop Med Hyg. 2006;75:677-82.

[50] Kariu T, Smith A, Yang X, Pal U. A chitin deacetylase-like protein is a predominant constituent of tick perotrophic membrane that influences the persistence of Lyme disease pathogens within the vector. PLoS ONE. 2013;8:e78376. doi:10.1371/journal.pone.0078376.

[51] Pal U, Li X, Wang T, Montgometry RR, Ramamoothi N, Desilva AM, et al. TROSPA, an *Ixodes scapularis* receptor *Borrelia burgdorferi*. Cell. 2004;119:457-68. doi:10.1016/j.cell.2004.10.027.

[52] Ramamoorthi N, Narasimhan S, Pal U, Bao F, Yang XF, Fish D, et al. The Lyme disease agent exploits a tick protein to infect the mammalian host. Nature. 2005;436:573-7. doi:10.1038/nature03812.

[53] Ogihara MH, Hikiba J, Suzuki Y, Taylor D, Kataoka H. Ovarian ecdysteroidogenesis in both immature and mature stages of an Acari, *Ornithodoros moubata*. PLoS ONE. 2015;10:e0124953. doi:10.1371/journal.pone.0124953.

[54] Clemens JC, Worby CA, Simonson-Leff N, Muda M, Maehama T, Hemmings BA, et al. Use of double-stranded RNA interference in *Drosophila* cell lines to dissect signal transduction pathways. Proc Natl Acad Sci USA. 2000;97:6499-503. doi:10.1073/pnas.110149597.

[55] Blouin EF, Manzano-Roman R, De la Fuente J, Kocan KM. Defining the role of subolesin in tick cell culture by use of RNA interference. Ann NY Acad Sci. 2008;1149:41-4. doi:10.1196/annals.1428.058.

[56] Barry G, Alberdi P, Schnettler E, Weisheit S, Kohl A, Fazakerley JK, et al. Gene silencing in tick cell lines using small interfering or long double-stranded RNA. Exp App Acarol. 2013;59:319-38. doi:10.1007/s10493-012-9598-x.

[57] de Abreu LA, Calixto C, Waltero CF, Noce BPD, Githaka NW, Seixas A, et al. The conserved role of the AKT/GSK3 axis in cell survival and glycogen metabolism in *Rhipicephalus* (*Boophilus*) *microplus* embryo tick cell line BME26. Biochim Biophys Acta. 2013;1830:2574-82. doi:10.1016/j.bbagen.2012.12.016.

[58] Aljamali MN, Bior AD, Sauer JR, Essenberg RC. RNA interference in ticks: A study using histamine binding protein dsRNA in the female tick *Amblyomma americanum*. Insect Mol Biol. 2003;12:299-305. doi:10.1046/j.1365-2583.2003.00416.x.

[59] Karim S, Ramakrishnan VG, Tucker JS, Essenberg RC, Sauer JR. *Amblyomma americanum* salivary gland homolog of nSec1 is essential for saliva protein secretion. Biochem Biophys Res Comm. 2004;324:1256-63. doi:10.1016/j.bbrc.2004.09.189.

[60] Ramakrishnan VG, Aljamali MN, Sauer JR, Essenberg RC. Application of RNA interference in tick salivary gland research. J Biomol Tech. 2005;16:297-305.

[61] Karim S, Miller NJ, Valenzuela J, Sauer JR, Mather TN. RNAi-mediated gene silencing to assess the role of synaptobrevin and cystatin in tick blood feeding. Biochem Biophys Res Commun. 2005;334:1336-42. doi:10.1016/j.bbrc.2005.07.036.

[62] Campbell EM, Budge GE, Bowman AS. Gene-knockdown in the honey bee mite *Varroa destructor* by a non-invasive approach: Studies on a glutathione S-transferase. Parasit Vectors. 2012;3:73. doi:10.1186/1756-3305-3-73.

[63] Kamau LM, Wright HW, Nisbet AJ, Bowman AS. Development of an RNA-interference procedure for gene knockdown in the poultry red mite, *Dermanyssus gallinae*: Studies on histamine releasing factor and Cathepsin-D. Afr J Biothechnol. 2013;12:1350-6. doi:10.5897/AJB12.2693.

[64] Whyard S, Erdelyan CNG, Partridge AL, Singh AD, Beebe NW, Capina R. Silencing the buzz: A new approach to population suppression of mosquitoes by feeding larvae double-stranded RNAs. Parasit Vectors. 2015;8:96. doi:10.1186/s13071-015-0716-6.

[65] Gong H, Umemiya R, Zhou J, Liao M, Zhang H, Jia H, et al. Blocking the secretion of saliva by silencing the *HlYkt6* gene in the tick *Haemaphysalis longicornis*. Insect Biochem Mol Biol. 2009;39:372-81. doi:10.1016/j.ibmb.2009.03.002.

[66] Neumann E, Schaeffer-Ridder M, Wang Y, Hofschneider PH. Gene transfer into mouse lyoma cells by electroporation in high electric fields. EMBO J. 1982;1:841-5.

[67] Karim S, Troiano E, Mather TN. Functional genomics tool: Gene silencing in *Ixodes scapularis* eggs and nymphs by electroporated dsRNA. BMC Biotech. 2010;10:1. doi: 10.1186/1472-6750-10-1.

[68] Ruiz N, de Abreu LA, Parizi LF, Kim TK, Mulenga A, Braz GRC, et al. Non-invasive delivery of dsRNA into de-waxed tick eggs by electroporation. PLoS ONE. 2015. doi: 10.1371/journal.pone.0130008.

[69] Yu N, Christiaens O, Liu J, Niu J, Cappelle K, Caccia S, et al. Delivery of dsRNA for RNAi in insects: An overview and future directions. Insect Sci. 2013;20:4-14. doi: 10.1111/j.1744-7917.2012.01534.x.

[70] Krober T, Guerin PM. *In vitro* feeding assays for hard ticks. Trends Parasitol. 2007;23:445-9. doi:10.1016/j.pt.2007.07.010.

[71] Soares CAG, Lima CMR, Dolan MC, Piesman J, Beard CB, Zeidner NS. Capillary feeding of specific dsRNA induces silencing of the *isac* gene in nymphal *Ixodes scapularis* ticks. Insect Mol Biol. 2005;14:443-52. doi:10.1111/j.1365-2583.2005.00575.x.

[72] Lew-Tabor AE, Bruyeres AG, Zhang B, Valle MR. *Rhipicephalus* (*Boophilus*) *microplus* tick in vitro feeding methods for functional (dsRNA) and vaccine candidate (antibody) screening. Ticks Tick Borne Dis. 2014;5:500-10. doi:10.1016/j.ttbdis.2014.03.005.

[73] Francischetti I, Sa-Nunes A, Mans B, Santos I, Ribeiro J. The role of saliva in tick feeding. Front Biosci. 2010;14:2051-88.

[74] Chmelar J, Calvo E, Pedra J, Francischetti I, Kotsyfakis M. Tick salivary secretion as a source of antihemostatics. J Proteomics. 2012;75:3842-54. doi:10.1016/j.jprot.2012.04.026.

[75] Kazimirova M, Stibraniova I. Tick salivary compounds: Their role in modulation of host defences and pathogen transmission. Front Cell Infect Microbiol. 2013;3:43. doi: 10.3389/fcimb.2013.00043.

[76] Kaufman WR. Ticks: Physiological aspects with implications for pathogen transmission. Ticks Tick Borne Dis. 2010;1:11-22. doi:10.1016/j.ttbdis.2009.12.001.

[77] Browning R, Karim S. RNA interference mediated depletion of NSF and SNAP-25 results in the inhibition of blood feeding of the Gulf-Coast tick, *Amblyomma maculatum*. Insect Mol Biol. 2013;22:245-57. doi:10.1111/imb.12017.

[78] Villareal AM, Adamson SW, Browning RE, Budachetri K, Sajid MS, Karim S. Molecular characterization and functional significance of the Vti family of SNARE proteins in tick salivary glands. Insect Biochem Mol Biol. 2013;2013:483-93. doi:10.1016/j.ibmb.2013.03.003.

[79] Anisuzzaman, Islam MK, Alim MA, Miyoshi T, Hatta T, Yamaji K, et al. Longistatin, a plasminogen activator, is key to the availability of bloodmeals for ixodid ticks. PloS Pathog. 2011;7:e1001312. doi:10.1371/journal.ppat.1001312.

[80] Kim TK, Curran J, Mulenga A. Dual silencing of long and short *Amblyomma americanum* acidic chitinase forms weakens the tick cement cone stability. J Exp Biol. 2014;217:3493-503. doi:10.1242/jeb.107979.

[81] Kotsyfakis M, Karim S, Andersen JF, Mather TN, Ribeiro JMC. Selective cysteine protease inhibition contributes to blood-feeding success of the tick *Ixodes scapularis*. J Biol Chem. 2007;282:29256-63. doi:10.1074/jbc.M703143200.

[82] Gao X, Shi L, Zhou Y, Zhang H, Zhou J. Characterization of the anticoagulant protein Rhipilin-1 from the *Rhipicephalus haemaphysaloides* tick. J Insect Physiol. 2011;57:339-43. doi:10.1016/j.jinsphys.2010.12.001.

[83] Chalaire KC, Kim TK, Garcia-Rodriguez H, Mulenga A. *Amblyomma americanum* (L.) (Acari: Ixodidae) tick salivary gland serine protease inhibitor (serpin) 6 is secreted into tick saliva during feeding. J Exp Biol. 2011;214:665-73. doi:10.1242/jeb.052076.

[84] Yu Y, Y.J. C, Zhou Y, Zhang H, Zhou J. Isolation and characterization of two novel serpins from the *Rhipicephalus haemaphysaloides*. Ticks Tick Borne Dis. 2013;4:297-303. doi:10.1016/j.ttbdis.2013.02.001.

[85] Guo X, Booth CJ, Paley MA, Wang X, DePonte K, Fikrig E, et al. Inhibition of neutrophil function by two tick salivary proteins. Infect Immun. 2009;77:2320-9. doi:10.1128/IAI.01507-08.

[86] Campbell EM, Burdin M, Hoppler S, Bowman AS. Role of an aquaporin in the sheep tick *Ixodes ricinus*: Assessment as a potential control target. Int J Parasitol. 2010;40:15-23. doi:10.1016/j.ijpara.2009.06.010.

[87] Barnard AC, Nijhof AM, Gaspar ARM, Neitz AWH, Jonjegan F, Maritz-Olivier C. Expression profiling, gene silencing and transcriptional networking of metzincin metal-

loproteases in the cattle, *Rhipicephalus* (*Boophilus*) *microplus*. Vet Parasitol. 2012;186:403-14. doi:10.1016/j.vetpar.2011.11.026.

[88] Adamson SW, Browning RE, Chao CC, Bateman Jr. RC, Ching WM, Karim S. Molecular characterization of tick salivary gland glutaminyl cyclase. Insect Biochem Mol Biol. 2013;43:781-93. doi:10.1016/j.ibmb.2013.05.011.

[89] Mulenga A, Kim TK, Ibelli AMG. Deorphanization and target validation of cross-tick species conserved novel *Amblyomma americanum* tick saliva protein. Int J Parasitol. 2013;43:439-51. doi:10.1016/j.ijpara.2012.12.012.

[90] Boldbaatar D, Sikasunge CS, Battsetseg B, Xuan X, Fujisaki K. Molecular cloning and functional characterization of an aspartic protease from the hard tick *Haemaphysalis longicornis*. Insect Biochem Mol Biol. 2006;36:25-36. doi:10.1016/j.ibmb.2005.10.003.

[91] Hatta T, Umemiya R, Liao M, Gong H, Harnnoi T, Tanaka M, et al. RNA interference of cytosolic leucine aminopeptidase reduces fecundity in the hard tick, *Haemaphysalis longicornis*. Parasitol Res. 2007;100:847-54. doi:10.1007/s00436-006-0336-3.

[92] Hatta T, Tsuji N, Miyoshi T, Islam MK, Alim MA, Yamaji K, et al. Leucine aminopeptidase, HlLAP, from the ixodid tick *Haemaphysalis longicornis*, plays vital roles in the development of oocytes. Parasitol Int. 2010;59:286-9. doi:10.1016/j.parint.2010.03.001.

[93] Liao M, Zhou J, Gong H, Boldbaatar D, Shirafuji R, Battur B, et al. Hemalin, a thrombin inhibitor isolated from a midgut cDNA library from the hard tick *Haemaphysalis longicornis*. J Insect Physiol. 2009;55:165-74. doi:10.1016/j.jinsphys.2008.11.004.

[94] Miyoshi T, Tsuji N, Islam MK, Alim MA, Hatta T, Huang X, et al. A set of serine protease paralogs are required for blood-digestion in the ixodid tick *Haemaphysalis longicornis*. Parasitol Int. 2008;57:499-505. doi:10.1016/j.parint.2008.08.003.

[95] Tsuji N, Miyoshi T, Battsetseg B, Matsuo T, Xuan X, Fujisaki K. A Cysteine Protease Is Critical for *Babesia* spp. Transmission in *Haemaphysalis* Ticks. PLoS Pathog. 2008;4(5):e1000062.

[96] Franta Z, Sojka D, Frantova H, Dvorak J, Horn M, Srba J, et al. *Ir*CL1—the haemoglobinolytic cathepsin L of the hard tick, *Ixodes ricinus*. Int J Parasitol. 2011;41:1253-62. doi:10.1016/j.ijpara.2011.06.006.

[97] Yamaji K, Miyoshi T, Hatta T, Matsubayashi M, Alim MA, Anisuzzaman, et al. HlCPL-A, a cathepsin L-like cysteine protease from the ixodid tick *Haemaphysalis longicornis*, modulated midgut proteolytic enzymes and their inhibitors during blood meal digestion. Infect Genet Evol. 2013;16:206-11. doi:10.1016/j.meegid.2013.01.018.

[98] Zhou J, Liao M, Hatta T, Tanaka M, Xuan X, Fujisaki K. Identification of a follistatin-related protein from the tick *Haemaphysalis longicornis* and its effect on tick oviposition. Gene. 2006;372:191-8. doi:10.1016/j.gene.2005.12.020.

[99] Boldbaatar D, Battsetseg B, Matsuo T, Hatta T, Umemiya-Shirafuji R, Xuan X, et al. Tick vitellogenin receptor reveals critical role in oocyte development and transovarial transmission of *Babesia* parasite. Biochem Cell Biol. 2008;86:331-44.

[100] Smith AD, Kaufman WR. Molecular characterization of the vitellogenin receptor from the tick, *Amblyomma hebraeum* (Acari: Ixodidae). Insect Biochem Mol Biol. 2013;43:1133-41. doi:10.1016/j.ibmb.2013.10.002.

[101] Smith A, Guo X, de la Fuente J, Naranjo V, Kocan KM, Kaufman WR. The impact of RNA interference of the subolesin and voraxin genes in the male *Amblyomma hebraeum* (Acari: Ixodidae) on female engorgement and oviposition. Exp App Acarol. 2009;47:71-86. doi:10.1007/s10493-008-9195-1.

[102] Boldbaatar D, Umemiya-Shirafuji R, Liao M, Tanaka T, Xuan X, Fujisaki K. Multiple vitellogenins from the *Haemaphysalis longicornis* tick are crucial for ovarian development. J Insect Physiol. 2010;56:1587-98. doi:10.1016/j.jinsphys.2010.05.019.

[103] Boldbaatar D, Battur B, Umemiya-Shirafuji R, Liao M, Tanaka T, Fujisaki K. GATA transcription, translation and regulation in *Haemaphysalis longicornis* tick: Analysis of the cDNA and an essential role for vitellogenesis. Insect Biochem Mol Biol. 2010;40:49-57. doi:10.1016/j.ibmb.2009.12.009.

[104] Umemiya-Shirafuji R, Boldbaatar D, Liao M, Battur B, Rahman MS, Kuboki T, et al. Target of rapamycin (TOR) controls vitellogenesis via activation of the S6 kinase in the fat body of the tick, *Haemaphysalis longicornis*. Int J Parasitol. 2012;42:991-8. doi: 10.1016/j.ijpara.2012.08.002.

[105] Huang X, Tsuji N, Miyoshi T, Motobu M, Islam MK, Alim MA, et al. Characterization of glutamine:fructose-6-phosphate aminotransferase from the ixodid tick, *Haemaphysalis longicornis*, and its critical role in host blood feeding. Int J Parasitol. 2007;37:383-92. doi:10.1016/j.ijpara.2006.11.012.

[106] Karim S, Kenny B, Troiano E, Mather TN. RNAi-mediated gene silencing in tick synganglia: A proof of concept study. BMC Biotech. 2008;8:30. doi: 10.1186/1472-6750-8-30.

[107] Boldbaatar D, Battsetseg B, Hatta T, Miyoshi T, Tsuji N, Xuan X, et al. Valosin-containing protein from the hard tick *Haemaphysalis longicornis*: Effects of dsRNA-mediated HlVCP gene silencing. Biochem Cell Biol. 2007;85:384-94.

[108] Boldbaatar D, R.M. K, Battur B, Umemiya R, Liao M, Tanaka T, et al. Identification of two forms of cyclophilin from the hard tick *Haemaphysalis longicornis*. Process Biochemistry. 2008;43:615-25.

[109] Gong H, Liao M, Zhou J, Hatta T, Huang P, Zhang G, et al. Gene silencing of ribosomal protein P0 is lethal to the tick *Haemaphysalis longicornis*. Vet Parasitol. 2008;151:268-78. doi:10.1016/j.vetpar.2007.11.015.

[110] Liao M, Boldbaatar D, Gong H, Huang P, Umemiya R, Harnnoi T, et al. Functional analysis of protein disulfide isomerases in blood feeding, viability and oocyte devel-

opment in *Haemaphysalis longicornis* ticks. Insect Biochem Mol Biol. 2008;38:285-95. doi:10.1016/j.ibmb.2007.11.006.

[111] Hajdusek O, Sojka D, Kopacek P, Buresova V, Franta Z, Sauman I, et al. Knockdown of proteins involved in iron metabolism limits tick reproduction and development. Proc Natl Acad Sci U S A 2009;106:1033-8. doi:10.1073/pnas.0807961106.

[112] Galay RL, Aung KM, Umemiya-Shirafuji R, Maeda H, Matsuo T, Kawaguchi H, et al. Multiple ferritins are vital to successful blood feeding and reproduction of the hard tick *Haemaphysalis longicornis*. J Exp Biol. 2013;216:1905-15. doi:10.1242/jeb.081240.

[113] Galay RL, Umemiya-Shirafuji R, Bacolod ET, Maeda H, Kusakisako K, Koyama J, et al. Two kinds of ferritin protect ixodid ticks from iron overload and consequent oxidative stress. PLoS ONE. 2014;9:e90661. doi:10.1371/journal.pone.0090661.

[114] Battur B, Boldbaatar D, Umemiya-Shirafuji R, Liao M, Battsetseg B, Taylor D, et al. LKR/SDH plays important roles throughout the tick life cycle including a long starvation period. PLoS ONE. 2009;4:e7136. doi:10.1371/journal.pone.0007136.

[115] Fabres A, De Andrade CP, Guizzo M, Sorgine MH, Paiva-Silva GO, Masuda A, et al. Effect of GSK-3 activity, enzymatic inhibition and gene silencing y RNAi on tick oviposition and egg hatching. Parasitology. 2010;137:1537-46. doi:10.1017/S0031182010000284.

[116] Mulenga A, Khumthong R. Disrupting the *Amblyomma americanum* (L.) CD147 receptor homolog prevents ticks from feeding to repletion and blocks spontaneous detachment of ticks from their host. Insect Biochem Mol Biol. 2010;40:524-42. doi:10.1016/j.ibmb.2010.04.012.

[117] Mulenga A, Khumthong R. Silencing of three *Amblyomma americanum* (L.) insulin-like growth factor binding protein-related proteins prevents ticks from feeding to repletion. J Exp Biol. 2010;213:1153-61. doi:10.1242/jeb.035204.

[118] de la Fuente J, Manzano-Roman R, Naranjo V, Kocan KM, Zivkovic Z, Blouin EF, et al. Identification of protective antigens by RNA interference for control of the lone star tick, *Amblyomma americanum*. Vaccine. 2010;28:1786-95. doi:10.1016/j.vaccine.2009.12.007.

[119] Alim MA, Islam MK, Anisuzzaman, Miyoshi T, Hatta T, Yamaji K, et al. A hemocyte-derived Kunitz-BPTI-type chymotrypsin inhibitor, HlChl, from the ixodid tick *Haemaphysalis longicornis*, plays regulatory functions in tick blood-feeding processes. Insect Biochem Mol Biol. 2012;42:925-34. doi:10.1016/j.ibmb.2012.09.005.

[120] Kume A, Boldbaatar D, Takazawa Y, Umemiya-Shirafuji R, Tanaka T, Fujisaki K. RNAi of the translation inhibition gene *4E-BP* identified from the hard tick, *Haemaphysalis longicornis*, affects lipid storage during the off-host starvation period of ticks. Parasitol Res. 2012;111:889-96. doi:10.1007/s00436-012-2915-9.

[121] Umemiya-Shirafuji R, Tanaka T, Boldbaatar D, Tanaka T, Fujisaki K. Akt is an essential player in regulating cell/organ growth at the adult stage in the hard tick *Haema-*

physalis longicornis. Insect Biochem Mol Biol. 2012;42:164-73. doi:10.1016/j.ibmb.2011.12.001.

[122] Wang Y, Zhou Y, Gong H, Cao J, Zhang H, Li X, et al. Functional characterization of a cystatin from the tick *Rhipicephalus haemaphysaloides*. Parasit Vectors. 2015;8:140. doi:10.1186/s13071-015-0725-5.

[123] Tian M, Tian Z, Luo J, Xie J, Yin H, Zeng Q, et al. Idenfification of the tropomyosin (Hl-Tm) *Haemaphysalis longicornis*. Vet Parasitol. 2015;207:318-23. doi:10.1016/j.vetpar.2014.10.007.

[124] de la Fuente J, Almazan C, Blas-Machado U, Naranjo V, Mangold AJ, Blouin EF, et al. The tick protective antigen, 4D8, is a conserved protein involved in modulation of tick blood ingestion and reproduction. Vaccine. 2006;24:4082-95. doi:10.1016/j.vaccine.2006.02.046.

[125] de la Fuente J, Almazan C, Naranjo V, Blouin EF, Kocan KM. Synergistic effect of silencing the expression of tick protective antigens 4D8 and Rs86 in *Rhipicephalus sanguineus* by RNA interference. Parasitol Res. 2006;99:108-13. doi:10.1007/s00436-006-0132-0.

[126] Antunes S, Galindo RC, Almazan C, Rudenko N, Golovchenko M, Grubhoffer L, et al. Functional genomics studies of *Rhipicephalus* (*Boophilus*) *annulatus* ticks in response to infection with the cattle protozoan parasite, *Babesia bigemina*. Int J Parasitol. 2012;42:187-95. doi:10.1016/j.ijpara.2011.12.003.

[127] Manzano-Roman R, Diaz-Martin V, Oleaga A, Siles-Lucas M, Perez-Sanchez R. Subolesin/akirin orthologs from *Ornithodoros* spp. soft ticks: Cloning, RNAi gene silencing and protective effect of the recombinant proteins. Vet Parasitol. 2012;185:248-59. doi:10.1016/j.vetpar.2011.10.032.

[128] Liao M, Zhou J, Hatta T, Umemiya R, Miyoshi T, Tsuji N, et al. Molecular characterization of *Rhipicephalus* (*Boophilus*) *microplus Bm86* homologue from *Haemaphysalis longicornis* ticks. Vet Parasitol. 2007;146:148-57. doi:10.1016/j.vetpar.2007.01.015.

[129] Bastos RG, Ueti MW, Knowles DP, Scoles GA. The *Rhipicephalus* (*Boophilus*) *microplus Bm86* gene plays a critical role in the fitness of ticks fed on cattle during acute *Babesia bovis* infection. Parasit Vectors. 2010;3:111. doi:10.1186/1756-3305-3-111.

[130] Nijhof AM, Balk JA, Postigo M, Rhebergen AM, Taoufik A, Jonjegan F. Bm86 homologues and novel ATAQ proteins with multiple epidermal growth factor (EGF)-like domains from hard and soft ticks. Int J Parasitol. 2010;40:1587-97. doi:10.1016/j.ijpara.2010.06.003.

[131] Tsuji N, Battsetseg B, Boldbaatar D, Miyoshi T, Xuan X, Oliver Jr. JH, et al. Babesial vector tick defensin against *Babesia* sp. parasites. Infect Immun. 2007;75:3633-40. doi:10.1128/IAI.00256-07.

[132] Buresova V, Hajdusek O, Franta Z, Loosova G, Grunclova L, Levashina EA, et al. Functional genomics of tick thioester-containing proteins reveal the ancient origin of the complement system. J Innate Immun. 2011;3:623-30. doi:10.1159/000328851.

[133] Buresova V, Hajdusek O, Franta Z, Sojka D, Kopacek P. IrAM-An alpha2-macroglobulin from the hard tick *Ixodes ricinus*: Characterization and function in phagocytosis of a potential pathogen *Chryseobacterium indologenes*. Dev Comp Immunol. 2009;33:489-98. doi:10.1016/j.dci.2008.09.011.

[134] Bowen CJ, Jaworski DC, Wasala NB, Coons LB. Macrophage migration inhibitory factor expression and protein localization in *Amblyomma americanum* (Ixodidae). Exp Appl Acarol. 2010;50:343-52. doi:10.1007/s10493-009-9324-5.

[135] Liu L, Dai J, Zhao YO, Narasimhan S, Yang Y, Zhang L, et al. *Ixodes scapularis* JAK-STAT pathway regulates tick antimicrobial peptides, thereby controlling the agent of human granulocytic anaplasmosis. J Infect Dis. 2012;206:1233-41. doi:10.1093/infdis/jis484.

[136] Yang X, Smith AA, Williams MS, Pal U. A dityrosine network mediated by dual oxidase and peroxidase influences the persistence of Lyme disease pathogens within the vector. J Biol Chem. 2014;289:12813-22. doi:10.1074/jbc.M113.538272.

[137] Duscher GG, Galindo RC, Tichy A, Hummel K, Kocan KM, de la Fuente J. Glutathione S-transferase affects permethrin detoxification in the brown dog tick, *Rhipicephalus sanguineus*. Ticks Tick Borne Dis. 2014;5:225-33. doi:10.1016/j.ttbdis.2013.11.006.

[138] Adamson S, Browning R, Singh P, Nobles S, Villareal A, Karim S. Transcriptional activation of antioxidants may compensate for selenoprotein deficiencies in *Amblyomma maculatum* (Acari: Ixodidae) injected with *selK*- or *selM*-dsRNA. Insect Mol Biol. 2014;23:497-510. doi:10.1111/imb.12098.

[139] Budachetri K, Karim S. An insight into the functional role of thioredoxin reductase, a selenoprotein, in maintaining normal native microbiota in the Gulf Coast tick (*Amblyomma maculatum*). Insect Mol Biol. 2015. doi:10.1111/imb.12184.

[140] Liu S, Soares TS, Vaz Jr. Id, Lovato DV, Aparecida ST. Rmcystatin3, a cysteine protease inhibitor from *Rhipicephalus microplus* hemocytes involved in immune response. Biochimie. 2014;106:17-23. doi:10.1016/j.biochi.2014.07.012.

[141] de la Fuente J, Ayoubi P, Blouin EF, Almazan C, Naranjo V, Kocan KM. Anaplasmosis: Focusing on host-vector-pathogen interactions for vaccine development. Ann NY Acad Sci. 2006;1078:416-23. doi:10.1196/annals.1374.081.

[142] Kocan KM, Zivkovic Z, Blouin EF, Naranjo V, Almazan C, Mitra R, et al. Silencing of genes involved in *Anaplasma marginale*-tick interactions affects the pathogen developmental cycle in *Dermacentor variabilis*. BMC Dev Biol. 2009;9:42. doi:10.1186/1471-213X-9-42.

[143] Zivkovic Z, Esteves E, Almazan C, Daffre S, Nijhof AM, Kocan KM, et al. DIfferential expression of genes in salivary glands of male *Rhipicephalus* (*Boophilus*) *microplus* in

response to infection with *Anaplasma marginale*. BMC Genomics. 2010;11:186. doi: 10.1186/1471-2164-11-186.

[144] Kocan KM, de la Fuente J, Manzano-Roman R, Naranjo V, Hynes WL, Sonenshine DE. Silencing expression of the defensin, varisin, in male *Dermacentor variabilis* by RNA interference results in reduced *Anaplasma marginale* infections. Exp App Acarol. 2008;46:17-28. doi:10.1007/s10493-008-9159-5.

[145] Schuijt TJ, Coumou J, Narasimhan S, Dai J, DePonte K, Wouters D, et al. A tick mannose-binding lectin inhibitor interferes with the vertebrate complement cascade to enhance transmission of the lyme disease agent. Cell Host Microbe. 2011;10:136-46. doi:10.1016/j.chom.2011.06.010.

[146] Ceraul SM, Chung A, Sears KT, Popov VL, Beier-Sexton M, Rahman MS, et al. A kunitz protease inhibitor from *Dermacentor variabilis,* a vector for spotted fever group Rickettsiae, limits *Rickettsia montanensis* infection. Infect Immun. 2011;79:321-9. doi: 10.1128/IAI.00362-10.

[147] Dai J, Narasimhan S, Zhang L, Liu L, Wang P, Fikrig E. Tick histamine release factor is critical for *Ixodes scapularis* engorgement and transmission of the Lyme diseases agent. PloS Pathog. 2010;6:e1001205. doi:10.1371/journal.ppat.1001205.

[148] Neelakanta G, Sultana H, Fish D, Anderson JF, Fikrig E. *Anaplasma phagocytophilum* induces *Ixodees scapularis* ticks to express an antifreeze glycoprotein gene that enhances their survival in the cold. J Clin Invest. 2010;120:3179-90. doi:10.1172/JCI42868.

[149] Severo MS, Choy A, Stephen sKD, Sakhon OS, Chen G, Chung DD, et al. The E3 ubiquitin ligase XIAP restricts *Anaplasma phagocytophilum* colonization of *Ixodes scapularis* tick. J Infect Dis. 2013;208:1830-40. doi:10.1093/infdis/jit380.

[150] Bifano TD, Ueti MW, Esteves E, Reif KE, Braz GRC, Scoles GA, et al. Knockdown of the *Rhipicephalus microplus* cytochrome c oxidase subunit III gene is associated with a failure of *Anaplasma marginale* transmission. PLoS ONE. 2014;9:e98614. doi:10.1371/journal.pone.0098614.

[151] Sojka D, Franta Z, Horn M, Caffrey C, Mares M, Kopacek P. New insights into the machinery of blood digestion by ticks. Trends Parasitol. 2013;29:276-85. doi:10.1016/j.pt.2013.04.002.

[152] Friesen KJ, Kaufman WR. Quantification of vitellogenesis and its control by 20-hydroxyecdysone in the ixodid tick, *Amblyomma hebraeum*. J Insect Physiol. 2002;48:773-82. doi:10.1016/S0022-1910(02)00107-5.

[153] Almazan C, Kocan KM, Bergman DK, Garcia-Garcia JC, Blouin EF, de la Fuente J. Identification of protective antigens for the control of *Ixodes scapularis* infestations using cDNA expression library immunization. Vaccine. 2003;21:1492-501. doi:10.1016/S0264-410X(02)00683-7.

[154] de la Fuente J, Maritz-Olivier C, Naranjo V, Ayoubi P, Nijhof AM, Almazan C, et al. Evidence of the role of tick subolesin in gene expression. BMC Genomics. 2008;9:372. doi:10.1186/1471-2164-9-372.

[155] Willadsen P, Riding GA, McKenna RV, Kemp DH, Tellam RL, Nielsen JN, et al. Immunologic control of a parasitic arthropod. Identification of a protective antigen from *Boophilus microplus*. J Immunol. 1989;143:1346-51.

[156] de la Fuente J, Blouin EF, Manzano-Roman R, Naranjo V, Almazan C, de la Lastra JMP, et al. Functional genomic studies of tick cells in response to infection with the cattle pathogen, Anaplasma marginale. Genomics. 2007;90:712-22. doi:10.1016/j.ygeno.2007.08.009.

[157] de la Fuente J, Merino O. Vaccinomics, the new road to tick vaccines. Vaccine. 2013;31:5923-9. doi:10.1016/j.vaccine.2013.10.049.